PITUITARY DISORDERS

Comprehensive Management

PITUITARY DISORDERS

Comprehensive Management

Ali F. Krisht, M.D.

Assistant Professor
Department of Neurosurgery
Director of Neuroendocrine Clinic
University of Arkansas for Medical Sciences
Little Rock, Arkansas

George T. Tindall, M.D.

Professor
Department of Neurosurgery
Emory University School of Medicine
Atlanta, Georgia

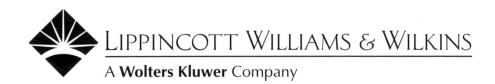

LIPPINCOTT WILLIAMS & WILKINS
A **Wolters Kluwer** Company

Editor: Charles W. Mitchell
Managing Editor: Grace E. Miller
Marketing Manager: Pete Darcy
Project Editor: Karen Ruppert

Copyright © 1999 Lippincott Williams & Wilkins

351 West Camden Street
Baltimore, Maryland 21201–2436 USA

The publisher is not responsible (as a matter of product liability, negligence or otherwise) for any injury resulting from any material contained herein. This publication contains information relating to general principles of medical care which should not be construed as specific instructions for individual patients. Manufacturers' product information and package inserts should be reviewed for current information, including contraindications, dosages and precautions.

Printed in the United States of America

First Edition

Library of Congress Cataloging-in-Publication Data

Pituitary disorders : comprehensive management / [edited by] Ali F.
   Krisht, George T. Tindall. — 1st ed.
      p.   cm.
   Includes bibliographical references and index.
   ISBN 0-683-30143-8
   1. Pituitary gland—Tumors.   I. Krisht, Ali F.   II. Tindall,
George T., 1928—
   [DNLM: 1. Pituitary Neoplasms—diagnosis.   2. Pituitary Neoplasms—
therapy.   3. Pituitary Gland—physiopathology.   WK 585 P6932   1999]
RC280.P5P575   1999
616.99'247—dc21
DNLM/DLC
for Library of Congress   98-3826
                                                           CIP

The publishers have made every effort to trace the copyright holders for borrowed material. If they have inadvertently overlooked any, they will be pleased to make the necessary arrangements at the first opportunity.

To purchase additional copies of this book, call our customer service department at **(800) 638–0672** or fax orders to **(800) 447–8438.** For other book services, including chapter reprints and large quantity sales, ask for the Special Sales department.

Canadian customers should call **(800) 665–1148,** or fax **(800) 665–0103.** For all other calls originating outside of the United States, please call **(410) 528–4223** or fax us at **(410) 528–8550.**

99 00 01 02 03
1 2 3 4 5 6 7 8 9 10

To my parents who opened the way,
To my teachers who guided my way,
To my family, Nashwa, Geenah, and Liana,
whose love filled my way.

Ali F. Krisht

In the last 100 years, the role of the pituitary gland evolved from being considered a small and poorly understood anatomic entity to being described as "The Master Gland of the Body." The last three decades witnessed an explosion in our knowledge of the pituitary gland and its disorders. This led to the development of medical treatments with dramatic responses, best exemplified by the efficacy of dopamine agonists in melting even the giant and invasive prolactinomas. The evolution of our understanding of the pituitary gland and its disorders was escorted, hand in hand, by advances in radiologic studies and refinements in surgical techniques. The results are favorable clinical outcomes in the majority of patients with pituitary adenomas and an increased number of patients who are cured of their tumors.

Pituitary Disorders: Comprehensive Management is an in-depth review and an update of our present knowledge of the pituitary gland and its disorders. It serves as a comprehensive reference and a clinical guide for medical students, internists, endocrinologists, gynecologists, pediatricians, neurologists, ophthalmologists, neuroradiologists, and neurosurgeons. The editors are greatly indebted to the contribution of such well-known pituitary experts as presented in this text.

ACKNOWLEDGMENTS

We are grateful and indebted to all the contributors who provided their valuable time to the making of this book.

We are especially indebted to Mrs. Ronalda Williams, who spent countless hours organizing, revising, contacting, and editing, from the book's conception to its completion.

Special thanks to Grace Miller, Managing Editor, and Karen Ruppert, Project Editor, from Lippincott Williams & Wilkins for their help and guidance.

CONTRIBUTORS

Ossama Al-Mefty, M.D.
Professor and Chairman
Department of Neurosurgery
University of Arkansas for Medical Sciences
Little Rock, Arkansas

Joseph M. Alexander, Ph.D.
Assistant Professor of Medicine
Harvard Medical School
Assistant in Biochemistry Medicine
Massachusetts General Hospital
Boston, Massachusetts

Cargill H. Alleyne Jr, M.D.
Resident in Neurosurgery
Department of Neurosurgery
Emory University School of Medicine
Atlanta, Georgia

Thomas E. Andreoli, M.D.
Professor and Chairman
Department of Internal Medicine
University of Arkansas for Medical Sciences
Little Rock, Arkansas

Edgardo J.C. Angtuaco, M.D.
Professor
Head Section of Neuroradiology
University of Arkansas for Medical Sciences
Little Rock, Arkansas

Baha M. Arafah, M.D.
Associate Professor of Medicine
Division of Clinical and Molecular Endocrinology
Case Western Reserve University
University Hospitals of Cleveland
Cleveland, Ohio

Marc S. Arginteanu, M.D.
Resident
Department of Neurosurgery
Mount Sinai Medical Center
New York, New York

Kenan I. Arnautović, M.D.
Clinical Research Fellow
Department of Neurosurgery
University of Arkansas for Medical Sciences
Little Rock, Arkansas

Lewis S. Blevins Jr, M.D.
Associate Professor of Medicine
Departments of Internal Medicine and Neurosurgery
Division of Endocrinology and Diabetes
Vanderbilt University School of Medicine
Nashville, Tennessee

Frederick A. Boop, M.D.
Associate Professor of Neurosurgery and Anatomy
University of Arkansas for Medical Sciences
Chief, Pediatric Neurosurgery
Arkansas Children's Hospital
Little Rock, Arkansas

Michael Buchfelder, M.D.
Neurosurgery Clinic
The University Erlagen
Nurnberg, Germany

C. Michael Cawley, M.D.
Assistant Professor
Department of Neurosurgery
Emory University School of Medicine
Atlanta, Georgia

Rita M. Chidiac, M.D.

Fellow, Division of Clinical and Molecular
Endocrinology
Case Western Reserve University
University Hospitals of Cleveland
Cleveland, Ohio

William T. Couldwell, M.D., Ph.D.

Professor and Chairman
Department of Neurological Surgery
New York Medical College
Valhalla, New York

Rudolf Fahlbusch, M.D.

Neurosurgery Clinic
The University Erlagen
Nurnberg, Germany

John C. Flickinger, M.D.

Professor of Radiation Oncology
University of Pittsburgh Medical Center
Pittsburgh, Pennsylvania

Roger H. Frankel, M.D.

Resident, Department of Neurosurgery
Emory University School of Medicine
Atlanta, Georgia

Ghaleb A. Ghani, M.B., B.Ch.

Associate Professor of Anesthesiology
Emory University School of Medicine
Atlanta, Georgia

Kathryn E. Graham, M.D.

Assistant Professor of Medicine
Oregon Health Sciences University
Portland, Oregon

Michael J. Harrison, M.D.

Assistant Professor
Department of Neurosurgery
University of Arkansas for Medical Sciences
Little Rock, Arkansas

Mary Louise Hlavin, M.D.

Assistant Professor of Neurological Surgery
Case Western Reserve University
University Hospitals of Cleveland
Cleveland, Ohio

Jurgen Honegger, M.D.

Neurosurgery Clinic
The University Erlagen
Nurnberg, Germany

Muhammad Husain, M.D.

Associate Professor of Pathology
John L. McClellan Memorial Veteran's Hospital
Little Rock, Arkansas

Scott Isaacs, M.D.

Fellow, Department of Internal Medicine
Emory University School of Medicine
Atlanta, Georgia

Sivakumar Jaikumar, M.D.

Resident, Department of Neurosurgery
University of Arkansas for Medical Sciences
Little Rock, Arkansas

Hae-Dong Jho, M.D., Ph.D.

Professor of Neurological Surgery
Director of Minimally Invasive Innovative
Microneurosurgery
University of Pittsburgh School of Medicine
Pittsburgh, Pennsylvania

Larry Katznelson, M.D.

Instructor in Medicine
Harvard Medical School
Assistant in Medicine
Neuroendocrine Unit
Boston, Massachusetts

Anne Klibanski, M.D.

Associate Professor of Medicine
Harvard Medical School
Chief, Neuroendocrine Unit
Massachusetts General Hospital
Boston, Massachusetts

Douglas Kondziolka, M.D., M.Sc., F.R.C.S.(C), F.A.C.S.
Associate Professor of Neurological Surgery and Radiation Oncology
University of Pittsburgh
Pittsburgh, Pennsylvania

Ali F. Krisht, M.D.
Assistant Professor of Neurosurgery
Director of Neuroendocrine Clinic
University of Arkansas for Medical Sciences
Little Rock, Arkansas

Edward R. Laws Jr, M.D.
Professor of Neurosurgery and Medicine
University of Virginia Health Sciences Center
Charlottesville, Virginia

L. Dade Lunsford, M.D.
Lars Leksell Professor and Chairman
Department of Neurological Surgery
University of Pittsburgh School of Medicine
Presbyterian University Hospital
Pittsburgh, Pennsylvania

Ian E. McCutcheon, M.D., F.R.C.S.(C)
Assistant Professor
Department of Neurosurgery
University of Texas
M.D. Anderson Cancer Center
Houston, Texas

Nancy J. Newman, M.D.
Associate Professor of Ophthalmology and Neurology
Emory University School of Medicine
Atlanta, Georgia

Panos Nomikos, M.D.
Neurosurgery Clinic
The University Erlagen
Nurnberg, Germany

Edward H. Oldfield, M.D.
Chief, Department of Neurosurgery
Surgical Neurology Branch
National Institutes of Health
Bethesda, Maryland

Nelson M. Oyesiku, M.D.
Assistant Professor
Department of Neurosurgery
Emory University School of Medicine
Atlanta, Georgia

T. Glenn Pait, M.D.
Assistant Professor
Department of Neurosurgery
University of Arkansas for Medical Sciences
Little Rock, Arkansas

Catherine Pihoker, M.D.
Assistant Professor
Department of Pediatrics
University of Washington
Seattle, Washington

Kalmon D. Post, M.D.
Professor and Chairman
Department of Neurosurgery
Mount Sinai Medical Center
New York, New York

W. Brian Reeves, M.D.
Associate Professor of Internal Medicine
University of Arkansas for Medical Sciences
Little Rock, Arkansas

Albert L. Rhoton Jr, M.D.
R.D. Keene Family Professor and Chairman
Department of Neurological Surgery
University of Florida College of Medicine
Gainesville, Florida

Mary H. Samuels, M.D.
Associate Professor of Medicine
Division of Endocrinology
Diabetes and Clinical Nutrition
Oregon Health Sciences University
Portland, Oregon

Warren R. Selman, M.D.
Professor and Vice Chairman
Department of Neurological Surgery
Case Western Reserve University
University Hospitals of Cleveland
Cleveland, Ohio

David Shore, M.D.
Fellow, Department of Internal Medicine
Emory University School of Medicine
Atlanta, Georgia

Charles Teo, M.D.
Vice-Chief, Pediatric Neurosurgery
Arkansas Children's Hospital
Little Rock, Arkansas

Kamal Thapar, M.D., Ph.D.
Division of Neurosurgery
St. Michael's Hospital
University of Toronto
Toronto, Ontario, Canada

George T. Tindall, M.D.
Professor of Neurosurgery
Department of Neurosurgery
Emory University School of Medicine
Atlanta, Georgia

Ugur Türe, M.D.
Assistant Professor
Department of Neurosurgery
Marmara University School of Medicine
Istanbul, Turkey

Mary Lee Vance, M.D.
Professor of Medicine and Neurosurgery
Department of Internal Medicine
University of Virginia Medical Center
Charlottesville, Virginia

Michael Vaphiades, M.D.
Assistant Professor
Department of Ophthalmology and Neurology
University of Arkansas for Medical Sciences
Little Rock, Arkansas

Jonathon Weinstein, M.D.
Fellow, Department of Internal Medicine
Emory University School of Medicine
Atlanta, Georgia

Martin H. Weiss, M.D.
Professor and Chairman
Department of Neurological Surgery
University of Southern California
Los Angeles, California

CONTENTS

SECTION I. Historical Perspectives

SECTION II. Evolution and Phylogeny

SECTION III. Basic Considerations

Anatomy

Pathophysiology

Pathology

Radiology

Clinical Aspects

SECTION IV. Management of Pituitary Tumors

SECTION V. Surgery of Pituitary Lesions

SECTION VI. Radiation Therapy of Pituitary Tumors

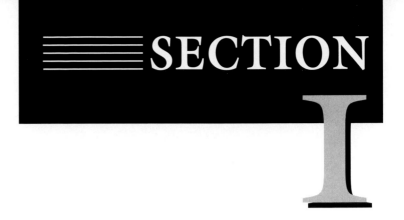

SECTION

I

Historical Perspectives

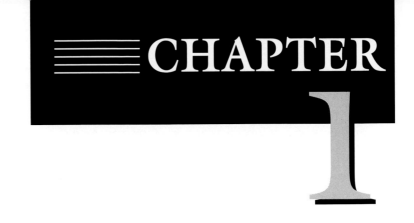

CHAPTER 1

The Pituitary: Historical Notes

T. Glenn Pait and Kenan I. Arnautović

PRIMITIVE UNDERSTANDING OF THE PITUITA

It is no wonder that early anatomists and physicians did not appreciate the small, well-hidden pituitary. Harvey Cushing (1869–1939) said it best in a Lister Memorial Lecture delivered at the Royal College of Surgeons of England on July 9, 1930:

> *Nature saw fit to enclose the central nervous system in a bony case lined by a tough, protecting membrane, and within this case she concealed a tiny organ which lies enveloped by an additional bony capsule and membrane like the nugget in the innermost of a series of Chinese boxes (1).*

He further noted that no other single structure in the body is so well protected and well hidden (1).

Hippocrates (460–370 BC) associated the brain with intelligence, thoughts, and dreams. He also believed the brain to be a cooling gland, which carried out its task by secreting phlegm or *pituita* (2). This concept is historically preserved in our anatomic term the *pituitary body.*

Galen (130–200 AD), the founder of experimental physiology, wrote that "nature" had established a special space for the gland hypophysis. He believed that the entire encephalon and the cranium lie above the gland and that the bone of the plate is located below. Thus, an animal could die many times before an injury from an external object could penetrate these parts. Galen considered the infundibulum to be a common, hollow, steeply sloping canal or space joining the encephalon to the gland hypophysis. He stated that the upper rim of the infundibulum is a perfect circle that continually narrows as it grows into the gland. Furthermore, the gland is a flattened sphere with a cavity and is succeeded by a bone that ends in the plate. Galen thought that the sella turcica of the sphenoid bone was pierced by foramina, through which blood vessels carried thick residues of pituita (3). The *pneuma*, or spirit, is brought into the body through the lungs, flows into the vascular canals, and is transformed into the Vital Spirit. The Vital Spirit passes into the brain, where the "rete mirabile" changes it into Animal Spirit (3, 4). Galen described the rete mirabile as the "most wonderful of bodies," which encircles the gland hypophysis and covers the whole base of the brain. It is not a simple structure but resembles several superimposed fishermen's nets. The waste from the production of Animal Spirit emerges from the nasopharynx as *pituita*, or nasal mucus. This concept of the function of the pituitary gland was accepted as truth for some 1500 years.

3

THEORIES FROM THE RENAISSANCE

Conrad Schreiber of Wittenberg (1614–1680) and Richard Lower of Oxford (1631–1691) eventually disproved a communication between the ventricles of the brain to the nasopharynx. They postulated that substances pass from the brain through the infundibulum to the pituitary, where they were distilled back into the blood (4). Theirs is a most remarkable early hypothesis of neurosecretory substances.

Andreas Vesalius (1514–1564) named the pituitary the "glandula pituitam cerebri excipiens" (4, 5). He continued to accept the ancient doctrine that pituita was secreted through the nose. Galen believed that phlegm was filtered through the cribriform plate of the ethmoid. Vesalius, however, disagreed because of the anatomic relationships of the pituitary. He substituted a more likely pathway, through the palatine canal and the superior orbital fissure into the sphenopalatine fossa and finally out the nose (6). Vesalius first illustrated the pituitary in 1538: "rete mirabile, in quo vitalis spiritus ad animalem preparatur" (1) (Fig. 1.1). In 1541, Walter Ryff of Strasburg stole the diagram of Vesalius and transposed it, line for line, onto the drawn surface of a human body (Fig. 1.2). This action greatly annoyed Vesalius, causing him to change his illustration in his *Fabrica*, which was published in 1543. He removed the rete from his arterial plate and gave a separate rendering of the structure. He also included a drawing to show the process of pituitary distillation (2) (Figs. 1.3 and 1.4).

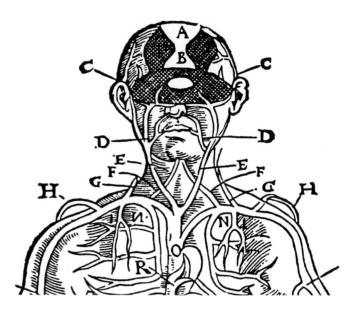

Figure 1.2. Ryff's adaptation (1541) of Vesalius' pituitary. *A*, blood vessels in both anterior cavities of the brain; *B*, wonderful network.

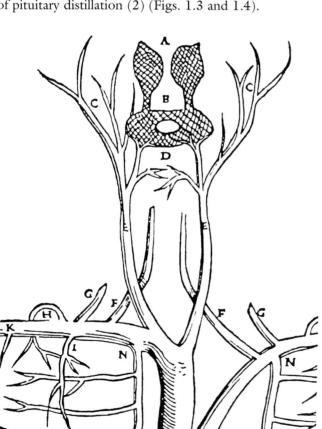

Figure 1.1. Vesalius' first illustration of the pituitary, 1538: *A*, blood vessels in both anterior cavities of the brain; *B*, wonderful network.

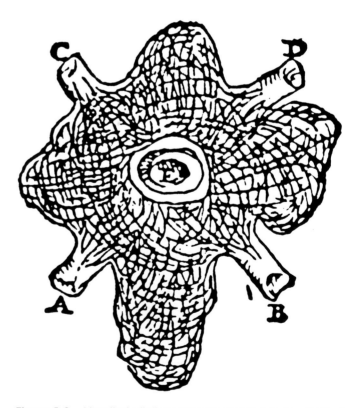

Figure 1.3. Vesalius' pituitary changes in his *Fabrica*, 1543. *A* and *B*, the arteries entering the skull and then breaking up into the remarkable plexus; *C* and *D*, the branches into which the shoots of the plexus are reunited and that correspond exactly in size to the arteries indicated in A and B; *E*, the gland receiving the pituita from the brain.

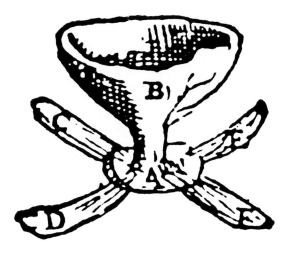

Figure 1.4. Vesalius' representation of the infundibulum demonstrating the process of pituitary distillation. The pelvis or cup (cyathus) set upright by which the brain distills into the gland underlying it. *A*, the gland into which the pituita is distilled; *B*, the pelvis along which it is led; *C, D, E*, and *F*, the passages provided for the easier exit of the pituita.

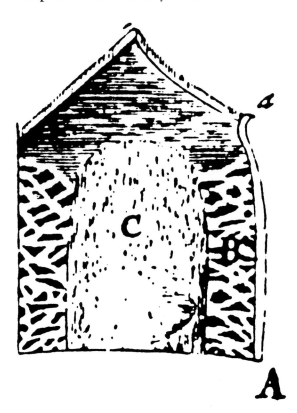

Figure 1.5. Lower and Willis' diagram of the pituitary (1664). *A*, arteria canalis directus; *B*, vasorum plexus restiformis; *C*, glandula pituitaria.

Richard Lower (1631–1691), an associate and friend of Sir Thomas Willis (1621–1675), confirmed Schneider's view that the pituitary was not a cavity filled with liquid. Willis agreed with his colleague and voiced this opinion in his writings. Harvey Cushing translated one of Willis' sentences, which perhaps credited Willis and Lower with the suggestion of pituitary hormones:

> *The ramification of the carotids into a reticulated plexus shows . . . that the blood . . . before it is let onto the cerebrum takes some part of the superfluous serum of the pituitary gland and instills another part into the various shoots to be led back toward the heart (1) (Fig. 1.5).*

Hans Simmer reported that the phrase "of the pituitary" was incorrectly translated. According to Simmer, S. Pordage translated the remaining works of Thomas Willis in 1681 and used the words "to the pituitary." Willis spoke of uptake by the pituitary and not of discharge—a receptive, not a secretory, function (7). Thomas Gibson (1647–1722), a Fellow of the Royal College of Physicians in London, wrote that the function of the pituitary was perhaps to secrete cerebrospinal fluid. This belief was also held by other noted anatomists of the 17th century, such as Raymond Vieussens (1641–1715) and Sylvius (Franciscus de le Boe) (1614–1672).

VIEWS OF THE 18TH CENTURY

Joseph Lieutaud (1703–1780), an anatomist and professor of medicine at the University of Aix-en-Provence, named the infundibulum the "tige pituitaire" (pituitary stalk), stating that "I have given the name pituitary stalk to this part because I believe that the term funnel would not be suitable for it" (4, 8, 9). He noted that the pituitary stalk was not canalized, but was a solid cylinder composed of gray substance that was covered by pia mater. Surrounding the stalk are small, longitudinal blood vessels that communicate with the pituitary gland (8, 9). This was perhaps an early description of the pituitary portal system.

Toward the end of the 18th century, the pituitary began to generate more interest. Many noted men of medicine and science wrote and speculated about the functions and possible maladies of the gland. Franz Joseph Gall (1758–1828), a noted French physician and anatomist, believed that the pituitary was a large ganglion (4, 5). In 1778, Samuel Thomas von Soemmering (1755–1830) introduced the term "hypophysis cerebri" (4). Joseph Wenzel (1768–1808) suggested that the pituitary was the cause of epilepsy (4). In his doctoral thesis of 1839, Joseph Engel proposed that the pituitary was actually a small cerebellum involved in balance and movements. He observed that alcoholic patients often had pituitary diseases (4). Carl Gustav Carus (1789–1869) proposed that the small gland was the cranial part of the nervus sympaticus (4). Ernst Burdach (1801–1876) suggested that the pituitary was the beginning of the spinal cord and that the anterior and posterior lobes were a replica of the anterior and posterior tracts of the spinal cord (4, 10).

In 1797, Matthew Baillie (1761–1823), physician to King George III, recorded in his text, *Morbid Anatomy*, that "this gland is very little liable to be affected by disease" (4, 11). He reported only one patient in which the gland was enlarged to twice the normal size (4, 11). Early accounts of blindness caused by pituitary enlargement were remarked on by Jean Louis Petit (1674–1750), Raymond Vieussens (1641–1715), and T. H. Hedlund (1791–1847) (4). Anton de Haen (1704–1776), professor of medicine at the University of Vienna, mentioned finding a pituitary tumor during a postmortem examination of a patient with a history of amenorrhea. The cause of the syndrome, however, was not established (4). In 1864, Andrea Verga described the first postmortem examination of a pituitary tumor that had destroyed the sphenoid and pressed on the optic chiasm. He called such a disease "Prosopectasia" (12).

THE FRENCH INFLUENCE

It was the great French neurologist Pierre Marie (1853–1940) who recognized a relationship between the pituitary and a type of gigantism, acromegaly. In an acromegalic patient, he found that the pituitary had been replaced by tumor tissue. He therefore felt justified in concluding that the normal function of the gland was to inhibit somatic growth and that gigantism was the result of a lack of this inhibition because of tumor destruction. His paper aroused much interest and was published in 1886 (13). Jose Dantas de Souza-Leite, a pupil of Marie from Bahia, Brazil, wrote his doctoral thesis on Marie's malady. His work contained a total of 48 cases. In 1891, Pierre Marie and de Souza-Leite combined their work and published their findings under the title *Essays on Acromegaly* (14). In their landmark paper, they described a disease characterized by hypertrophy of the hands, feet, and face, which they called "acromegaly." They did not understand the cause of the disease and stated, "we have nothing definite" (14). Although Marie's and de Souza-Leite's assumption about the role of the pituitary was exactly the opposite of the truth, they did recognize that the little gland at the skull base was indeed a regulator of growth. This historic error clearly demonstrates that even erroneous theories may be of value in bringing about interest and directing further investigations.

It was Oscar Minkowski (1858–1931) who recognized a constant relationship between acromegaly and enlargement of the pituitary (15). However, the syndrome continued to be thought of as a result of glandular insufficiency until 1894, when Augusto T. Tamburini (1848–1919) suggested that acromegaly was caused by overactivity of the gland (16).

THE MODERN ERA

Further clinical observations and necropsy findings began to provide more insight into pituitary problems, and patients with pituitary tumors but without acromegaly began to be reported. In 1900, Joseph Francois Felix Babinski (1857–1932) observed the case of an obese young woman with genital hypoplasia (17). The following year, Alfred Froehlich (1871–1953) also wrote about a pituitary tumor in a patient without acromegaly (18) (Fig. 1.6). Neither Babinski nor Froehlich considered that the patient's symptoms were the result of hypofunction of the gland. These new findings of pituitary problems added a degree of confusion to a rather already confused picture (19). It was Harvey Cushing who shed some light in the dark room of the pituitary gland at a gathering of the American Medi-

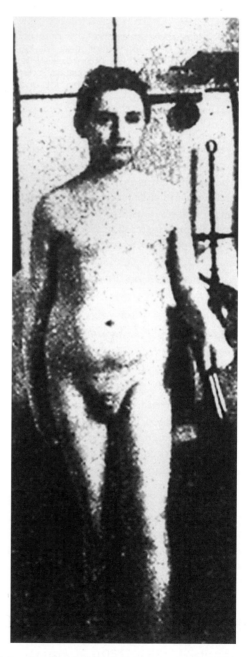

Figure 1.6. A patient of Froehlich's who had a pituitary tumor without acromegaly. (Courtesy of the Royal Society of Medicine, London.)

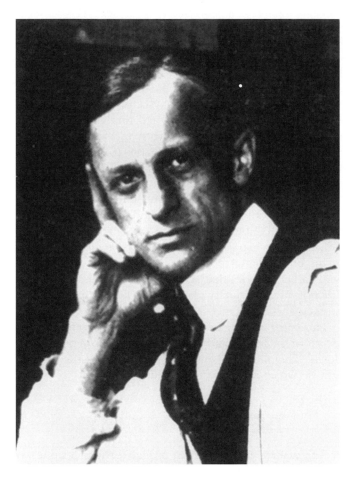

Figure 1.7. Harvey W. Cushing (1869–1939). (H.C. at his Laboratory Desk 1907.) (Adapted from Fulton JF. Harvey Cushing. Springfield, IL: Charles C Thomas, 1946:244.)

cal Association in June of 1909 (20) (Fig. 1.7). On this occasion, Cushing introduced the new terms "hypopituitarism" and "hyperpituitarism." He declared that "two conditions, one due to a pathological increased activity of the pars anterior of the hypophysis (hyperpituitarism), the other to a diminished activity of the same epithelial structure (hypopituitarism), seem capable of clinical differentiation" (20). Cushing continued his work on the pituitary and, in 1912, published his now classic monograph on the pituitary body, in which he incorporated the concepts of pituitary function at that time (21).

HISTOLOGIC CHARACTERISTICS

The understanding of the histologic characteristics of the pituitary gland progressed just as slowly as did the understanding of its physiologic aspects. In 1844, Adolph Hannover (1814–1994) recognized two types of cells in the anterior lobe of the gland (22). In 1884 and 1886, Flesh, Lothringer, and Dostoiewsky described the two types of cells as either nongranular, clear chromophobe cells or granular chromophil cells (4, 23–25). Shortly thereafter, Schoenemann divided the chromophil cells into

eosinophil, which stain with acid dyes, and basophil, which stain with basic dyes (4, 25, 26). In 1900, Carl Benda (1857–1933) discovered that pituitary tumors were composed of specific pituitary cells and thus were true adenomas of the gland itself (27). He showed that, in patients with acromegaly, the tumor stained as eosinophilic (25, 27). He was the first to strongly emphasize the need to use histologic methods to study such tumors. Thus began the era of the histopathology of the pituitary gland.

EXPERIMENTAL STUDIES

The pituitary was long regarded as a gland without a function. Two methods were developed to study its physiologic characteristics. In the first, the gland itself was introduced or an extract of the gland was injected into an organism or fed to the subject. This was the so-called "positive method," which was used to bring about a reaction comparable to normal glandular activity. In the "negative method," the gland was partially or completely removed or destroyed. Numerous experimental hypophysectomies were carried out on a variety of animals (28). Emil Goetsch (1883–1963), a colleague of Harvey Cushing, fed rats 0.05 g of acetone-dried powder of whole pituitary glands. He documented that growth and sexual development were stimulated through such a positive method of testing (29). Within a short time, however, Goetsch's claims were refuted by other investigators (30).

To study the results of the negative method of investigation, a procedure had to be developed by which the gland could be approached and manipulated in such a fashion as to ensure a clean lesion without complications, such as hemorrhage, infection, or trauma, to neighboring structures. Such complications might confuse the results. This presented a rather difficult task for early investigators. The technical challenges were obvious; hypophysectomy proved far more difficult than other surgical interventions such as adrenalectomy. A satisfactory surgical route to the pituitary gland had to be developed in an acceptable animal model. These approaches were divided into an extracranial and an intracranial pathway to the sella turcica. The extracranial approach was from below in the midline through the nasal, buccal, hyoid, and pharyngeal regions or from one side by a lateral pharyngeal and sphenopalatine route (31). The intracranial method was from above through a median opening in the cranial vault or laterally through a temporal craniotomy with elevation of the subjacent lobe. In 1881, Julius v. Michel attempted hypophysectomies on numerous cats, dogs, and rabbits through the frontal approach (31, 32). Most of the animals died of operative complications, but a few survived. Still, it was difficult to determine if all or only a part of the gland had been removed.

Sir Victor Horsley (1857–1916) was the first to publish a note about the experimental removal of the pituitary gland (33). In a paper largely dealing with the thyroid gland, he made a brief statement that he had removed the pituitary gland from two dogs with no disturbing symptoms (33).

The debate about the loss of the gland and compatibility with life continued. Perhaps the first major contribution on this subject was made by Marienesco, an associate of Marie, in an early study of acromegaly. In his article of 1892, he mentions experiments by Dastres, who approached the gland through the mouth without success (31, 34). Marienesco also approached the pituitary through the buccal route. In this route, the soft palate was divided, the sella turcica opened, and the gland destroyed with heat. Three of the animals in Marienesco's operations survived, living 3, 5, and 18 days. The investigator concluded that the loss of the pituitary was compatible with life for some weeks (31, 34). Also in 1892, Gley reported a study on the hypophysis of a rabbit. He made a trephine opening in the midcranial vault and introduced an instrument through the brain and into the sella turcica. Such a blind attempt to destroy the target had unsatisfactory results (35).

The first studies to suggest the symptoms of apituitarism were reported by Giulio Vassale (1862–1912) and Ercole Sacchi in 1892 and 1894 (36, 37). Their approach was similar to that of Mariensco with an attempt to destroy the gland with thermocautery and chromic acid. Most of the animals died of operative complications. The symptoms observed in the surviving animals included apathy, motor disturbances with irregular muscle twitching, lowering of temperature, polydipsia, anorexia, weight loss, and coma. The authors concluded that, regardless of the postoperative complications, the hypophysis was of great physiologic importance. The gland produced a secretion, and its absence was incompatible with life (36, 37). Nicolas C. Paulesco (1869–1931), a physiologist from Bucharest, in collaboration with Balacesco, a surgeon, developed an intracranial approach to the pituitary gland in dogs through a temporal route. Their method proved to be a major advancement for cranial surgery (38). They used a technique of "cerebral dislocation" to expose parts that would be otherwise inaccessible. The animals were divided into two groups, those with total and those with partial hypophysectomies. The group undergoing total hypophysectomy died within 24 hours. The group undergoing partial hypophysectomy lived for a period of time according to the amount and vitality of the remaining glandular tissue. Paulesco concluded that the pituitary was indeed essential for life, its absence being fatal (4, 38).

In 1909, Reford and Cushing reported a series of 20 cases of experimental hypophysectomies performed in the manner of Paulesco and Balacesco (39). They agreed with the premise that total loss of the pituitary in the canine was incompatible with life (39). In the following year, Cushing reported to the American Association for the Advancement of Science an extensive series of hypophysectomies carried out with his colleagues, Samuel Crowe and John Homans, at the Hunterian Surgical Laboratories at the Johns Hopkins University. Again, the results showed that apituitarism leads to death. Death was preceded by loss of appetite, loss of weight, and listlessness, which was defined as "cachexia hypophysiopriva" (40).

In 1912, G. Ascoli and T. Legnani noted atrophy of the adrenal cortex after hypophysectomy (41). In 1917, William Bell (1871–1936) reported that clamping of the pituitary stalk had the same effects as hypophysectomy, with atrophy of the uterus and ovaries (42).

In 1912, Bernhard Aschner (1883–1960) improved the technique of hypophysectomy. He used a transbuccal approach, which injured the brain only minimally. He carried out extensive studies on canines, and his animals survived for months. Radiographs were obtained to follow the cessation of growth in puppies. He also noted genital hypoplasia in his experimental population (43). Aschner disagreed with earlier theories that acromegaly was caused by hypofunction of the pituitary gland. He believed that the cause was actually hyperfunction of the gland.

Laboratory work continued, and the unraveling of the secrets of the little gland at the base of the skull progressed slowly. This all-important work, however, laid the foundation on which others would stand.

THE EFFECT OF X-RAYS

The medical milestone that provided the first noninvasive window through which to see the pituitary gland was the discovery of X-rays on November 8, 1895, by Wilhelm Conrad Roentgen (1845–1923) (44). This sensational discovery was announced to the world on January 6, 1896 (44) and was greeted with universal enthusiasm. Soon afterward, no part of the body escaped being X-rayed. Roentgen's discovery laid bare the silhouette of the skull to direct inspection. In 1899, Hermann Oppenheim (1858–1919) called attention to the fact that tumors of the hypophysis may dilate the sella turcica (45). It became evident that many patients with well-defined acromegaly had enlarged pituitary fossae. Even more shocking, many patients without signs of acromegaly also had evidence of a tumor-expanded sella. Clinicians began to take note that patients with these large fossae had an accompanying, characteristic, definable set of symptoms. The first physicians to clearly focus on these peculiar combinations of symptoms were gynecologists and ophthalmologists. Women with unaccountable amenorrhea often complained of visual disturbances and thus would be sent to an ophthalmologist for an evaluation. The eye examination often revealed pressure against the optic chiasm. It did not take long before patients with these symptoms began to be routinely subjected to roentgenographic studies. The enlarged pituitary fossa was often the reported finding. From this clinical experience, others with such problems, particularly men, were also found to have a large pituitary fossa. It became clear that comparable disturbances in the attributes of sex were present (1).

With roentgenographic studies, clinical syndromes became better defined, and solid evidence that a mass was causing mischief became available. With a mass compressing the gland and the symptoms and signs consistent with such a diagnosis, as well as supporting radiologic data, surgical intervention became an option for treatment. Surgeons now had the evidence and support to operate. And so, ways of operating on these lesions had to be devised. To this end, the earlier animal studies would be of immeasurable value.

ENTER THE SURGEON

Early surgical intervention for pituitary tumors was met with disbelief that such an undertaking could be successful. Lane, a surgeon, expressed his thoughts in 1892:

> *Where the growth lies in contact with the base of the skull, that is, springs from the inferior surface of the brain, conservation would pronounce the word inaccessible. This warning, however, is quite unheeded by the gens audax omnia perpeti; for example, by such an announcement that they think operations for removal of tumors from the bases of the brain are feasible; such daring characterized a specialist in cerebral surgery, whom the writer heard say that he believed it possible to open the skull and lift up the brain as to catch a view of the foramen magnum. The reader may ask, Did he mean this of a living subject? (46).*

Earlier surgical laboratory experience was of immense value for the transition to the human operating theaters. Surgeons began to appreciate the gross anatomy of this small ovoid structure, flattened from above downward, lying transversely along its axis, and occupying the sella turcica of the sphenoid bone in the middle of the two middle fossae. Two avenues of attack were devised to approach the hypophysis—intracranial and transsphenoidal. The intracranial approach was through the anterior or temporal fossae. The transsphenoidal approach involved temporary displacement of the nose to the right, downward, or upward or splitting of the nose medially. Other transsphenoidal avenues were the endonasal, sublabial, or pharyngeal route (47).

In 1889, Sir Victor Horsley was the first to operate on a pituitary tumor pressing on the optic chiasm. However, he waited 17 years before reporting this operative case in a paper published in 1906 (48). He used the technique of cerebral dislocation as he approached the pituitary through a frontal craniotomy: "For this purpose I raised the frontal lobe, but found that the tumor was really a cystic adenosarcoma of the pituitary gland, and was inoperable" (48). Horsley experienced a great deal of difficulty ligating veins

entering the longitudinal sinus with the frontal approach to the gland and referred to this approach as the "prehistoric way" (48). Thereafter, he advocated the temporal approach because it did not involve the same degree of venous disturbance as transfrontal exposure. According to those who observed him in the operating theater, he carried out the pituitary surgery in two stages (49–51). The first stage included the craniotomy; the second stage involved lifting the temporal lobe and viewing the pituitary.

As with neurosurgery today, special surgery needed special instruments, and good illumination is essential. Horsley used a strong headlight to inspect the operative field (50). The instruments used had long handles and slender bodies. He used slender spatulas and small rhinoscopic mirrors to inspect the skull base. In 1906, Horsley stated that he had performed 10 operations on the pituitary gland with 2 deaths (48). He advocated surgical intervention for such lesions and stated that the surgeon's duty in such cases was to relieve the mechanical pressure brought about by the tumor and to do it in such a manner as to avert blindness (48). The same obligations hold true today.

EARLY CASES

In 1893, Richard Caton (1842–1926) and Frank Thomas Paul (1851–1941) reported the case of a 34-year-old woman with acromegaly who had severe facial pain, headaches, and failing vision (52) (Fig. 1.8). Caton, a phy-

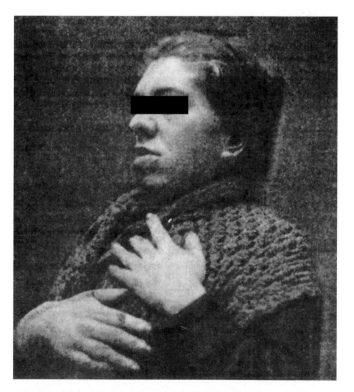

Figure 1.8. A patient with acromegaly treated by Caton and Paul. (Courtesy of Caton R, Paul FT. Notes of a case of acromegaly treated by operation. BMJ 1893;2:1421.)

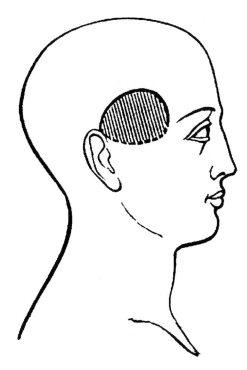

Figure 1.9. The operative site of a patient with acromegaly treated by Caton and Paul. (Courtesy of Caton R, Paul FT. Notes of a case of acromegaly treated by operation. BMJ 1893;2: 1422.)

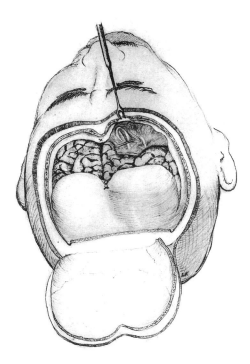

Figure 1.10. Proposed method of reading tumors of optic chiasm by Kiliani. (Courtesy of Kiliani OGT. Some remarks on tumors of the chiasm, with a proposal how to reach the same by operation. Ann Surg 1904;39.)

sician at the Royal Infirmary, requested a surgical opinion from Paul, a surgeon at the same institution. Sir Victor Horsley was also consulted and agreed to the surgical plan. After a temporal craniectomy was done, Paul did not think that the tumor could be attacked directly (Fig. 1.9). The patient's pain improved, but her vision was lost, and she died about 3 months after the surgery. During the autopsy, a large pituitary tumor the size of a tangerine was discovered. The final diagnosis was a "round-cell sarcoma," a diagnosis often made during this era (52).

As pituitary abnormalities became more recognized, other surgeons began to show interest in developing approaches for surgical exploration of the skull base. In 1903, Otto Kiliani, a New York surgeon, practiced an intracranial approach on a cadaver. He used a bifrontal osteoplastic craniotomy, opened the dura, ligated the longitudinal sinus, and elevated the frontal lobes (51, 53) (Fig. 1.10). He unsuccessfully attempted his rehearsed procedure on a patient who lapsed into a coma after an episode of pituitary apoplexy (51, 53). The patient did not survive the hemorrhage.

In January of 1900 in Berlin, Fedor Victor Krause (1857–1937) had the occasion to expose the pituitary body of a young technician, 20 years old, who became depressed after an unsatisfactory love affair and fired a bullet into his right temporal lobe (53). The young man survived the gunshot injury and developed headaches, mental status changes, and periods of unresponsiveness several weeks later. A roentgenogram showed a bullet located in

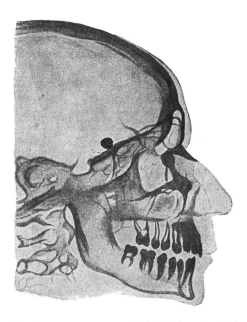

Figure 1.11. Roentgenogram with bullet located in the region of the right optic foramen. (Courtesy of Krause FV. Surgery of the Brain. Vol. 1. New York: Rebman, 1900:Table XVII, facing page 118.)

the region of the right optic foramen (Fig. 1.11). A right frontal osteoplastic flap was developed (Fig. 1.12). The approach was extradural to the sphenoid wing, and the bullet was removed without any difficulties. The patient did remarkably well and was free of symptoms at a follow-up examination in 1907. Krause was quick to recognize

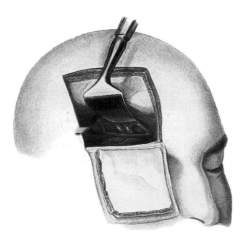

Figure 1.12. Right frontal osteoplastic flap as developed by Krause (1900).

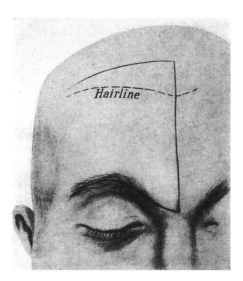

Figure 1.13. Frontal approach of Frazier demonstrating the relationship of the incision to the eyebrow and hairline. (Courtesy of Frazier CH. Lesions of the hypophysis from the viewpoint of the surgeon. Surg Gynecol Obstet 1913;17:730.)

vania Hospital in Philadelphia, reported his experience with lesions of the hypophysis in 1913 (57). He first used a frontal extradural approach but later changed to a frontal intradural operation (51, 58, 59) (Figs. 1.13–1.15). Frazier's modified procedure was similar to that of Louis Linn McArthur (1858–1934), a surgeon in Chicago who resected the supraorbital rim and a part of the orbital roof

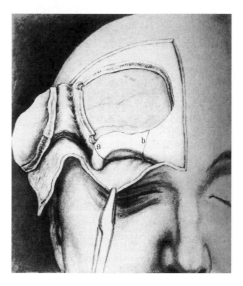

Figure 1.14. Frontal approach of Frazier demonstrating the osteoplastic flap and the supraorbital ridge. *a* and *b*, supraorbital ridge bone cuts. (Courtesy of Frazier CH. Lesions of the hypophysis from the viewpoint of the surgeon. Surg Gynecol Obstet 1913; 17:730.)

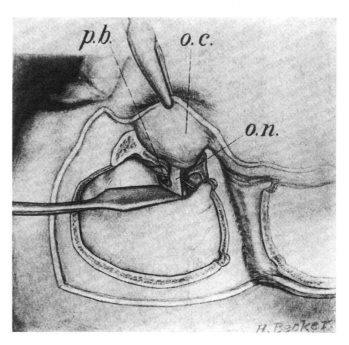

Figure 1.15. Frazier's frontal approach with elevation of the frontal lobe exposing the optic nerve (*o.n.*) and the pituitary body (*p.b.*). *o.c.*, orbital context. (Courtesy of Frazier CH. Lesions of the hypophysis from the viewpoint of the surgeon. Surg Gynecol Obstet 1913;17:731.)

the importance of this operation and the exposure of the pituitary gland that was offered: "As I had succeeded in reaching the optic foramen from in front, in order to extract the bullet, it seemed feasible to approach the pituitary body in the same way" (53). In 1904, Krause used his approach to remove a "fibrosarcoma" from the region of the sella turcica (53).

In 1904, W. Braun, a student of Krause, showed in cadavers that the extradural approach to the sella turcica could be made through the temporal route by going beneath the cavernous sinus (54). The next year, Krause performed the first intracranial, transfrontal approach for a pituitary tumor, but he did not publish the case until several years later (55). Silbermark, another European surgeon, proposed addressing the pituitary through a transSylvian avenue (56). Charles Frazier (1870–1936), of the Pennsyl-

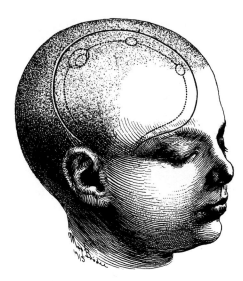

Figure 1.16. Heuer's outline of scalp and bone flap to attack the chiasmal region. (Courtesy of Heuer GJ. Surgical experiences with an intracranial approach to chiasmal lesions. Arch Surg 1920;1:370.)

(51, 60, 61). Frazier always preferred the transcranial approach to other routes to the pituitary (58).

The search continued for a better cranial route to the skull base gland. George Heuer (1882–1950), of the Johns Hopkins Hospital, introduced an intradural approach using Frazier's cutaneous incision but a much larger bone flap so that the brain might be dislocated as the frontal lobe was elevated (62) (Fig. 1.16). In Heuer's absence, Walter E. Dandy (1886–1946), another Hopkins' man, presented this modified approach to the members of the Johns Hopkins Medical Society on February 4, 1918 (63). Heurer and Dandy did this operation on 24 patients between 1914 and 1918. Dandy later became critical of Heuer's large frontoparietal bone flap. He stated that, at first glance, the problem of exposure seemed to be solved by providing adequate room through cerebral displacement during the operation (64). This exposure, however, allowed a greater amount of trauma to the brain during retraction of the frontal lobe, thereby producing significant postoperative edema (Fig. 1.17). This injury increased the operative mortality and morbidity of such procedures. Of concern in such cases was the increased chance of injury to the motor area, which was pressed against the mesial margin of the bone flap (Fig. 1.18). Another concern was the potential for increased seizure activity. Dandy also believed that the huge bone flap was more time-consuming and a frequent source of extradural hemorrhage. Dandy avoided such large bone flaps, making a small craniotomy as far anteriorly and laterally as possible. If the brain was tense, he would remove cerebrospinal fluid to obtain the needed room. This fluid was obtained through evacuation of the cisterna chiasmatis by tapping the anterior horn of the opposite ventricle or through a lumbar drain (64). Dandy stated that the "nasal route was impractical and can never be otherwise" (64).

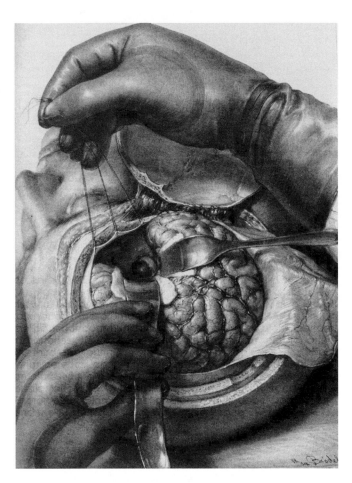

Figure 1.17. Exposure of the chiasmal region by Heuer and Dandy. (Courtesy of Heuer GJ. Surgical experiences with an intracranial approach to chiasmal lesions. Arch Surg 1920;1:374.)

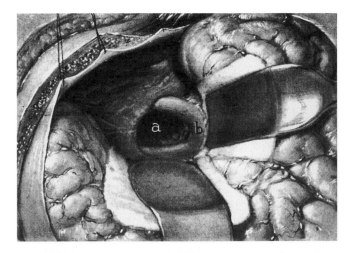

Figure 1.18. Exposure of the sella turcica by Heuer and Dandy. *a,* hypophyseal tumor; *b,* optic chiasm. (Courtesy of Heuer GJ. Surgical experiences with an intracranial approach to chiasmal lesions. Arch Surg 1920;1:375.)

THE HIGH ROAD VERSUS THE LOW ROAD

A tug-of-war arose between surgeons promoting the "high road" (cranial surgeons) and those advocating the "low road" (nasal surgeons). The attack against the low road approach centered around contamination by the nasal mucosa of the hypophyseal field. The greatest danger arose when cerebrospinal fluid was exposed to the nasal environment. The concern of the high road proponents was the fact that adequate exposure was not optimal and illumination was poor.

Arguments against the cranial procedures centered around the fact that they were too dangerous, producing postoperative edema and placing the optic chiasm in harm's way. This view was strongly expressed by David Giordano (1864–1954) (65). He had carried out cadaver studies to demonstrate the feasibility of the transnasal approach to the pituitary gland. His work consisted of resecting the anterior wall of the frontal sinuses and nose, opening the ethmoid cells and removing their walls, and opening the sphenoid (65). Other experimental procedures to reach the pituitary were carried out by Friedmann and Mass and by Koenig (45, 66). Friedmann and Mass removed the hypophysis in cats by splitting the soft palate and drilling the body of the sphenoid. Koenig did the same in adult cadavers (66). Another cadaver study came from Loewe in 1905 (21, 67). He described a superior nasal approach in which the nose was split with a long incision to one side of the median line. The maxillae were separated, the maxillary sinus walls were destroyed, the septum was taken back to the vomer, the vomer was then removed, and the sinuses were entered (21, 67).

THE NASAL APPROACH

Herman Schloffer (1868–1937) studied the various cadaver operations and surveyed the topic of pituitary surgery for a review published in 1906 (68). In Austria the following year, he performed the first transnasal operation to remove a pituitary tumor (69) (Fig. 1.19). The patient was

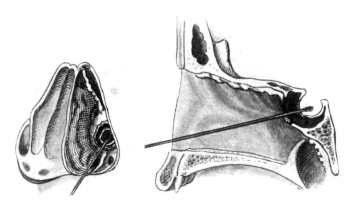

Figure 1.19. Schloffer's operation. (Courtesy of Cope VZ. Surgery of the pituitary fossa. Br J Surg 1916;4:131.)

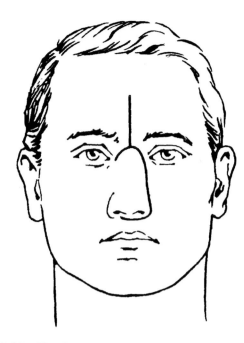

Figure 1.20. Von Eiselsperg's incision. (Courtesy of Cope VZ. Surgery of the pituitary fossa. Br J Surg 1916;4:129.)

a young man with hypopituitarism who had visual changes, headache, loss of libido, and loss of body hair. Results of an examination revealed bitemporal hemianopia and genital atrophy (69). The incision was carried around the root, left side, and base of the nose at its junction with the face. The nose was then entirely freed of its connections and turned over to the right side. The septum and turbinates were cut; hemorrhage was controlled with temporary gauze packing. The ethmoidal and sphenoidal cells were opened, leading to the anterior wall of the sella turcica. A good X-ray plate of the bony field of work was recommended to find the sella. The sphenoid sinus was cleaned with a spoon, and the thin wall of the floor of the sella was easily opened. The tumor was excised, and the cavity was closed with a tampon soaked in balsam from Peru. The 30-year-old man did well immediately after surgery. About 2 months afterward, however, his headaches returned and he subsequently died of intracranial hyperation caused by hydrocephalus, which was caused by progression of the tumor. Schloffer noted that his operation only temporarily alleviated the patient's symptoms. Regardless of the final outcome of this first transnasal operation, the procedure was received with enthusiasm. A method to approach the small gland at the skull base was now available.

Anton von Eiselsberg (1860–1939) was the next surgeon to expose a pituitary tumor through a superior nasal approach (Fig. 1.20). Many surgeons used an electric forehead lamp to provide the light so necessary for the operating field. According to Krause, the best artifical illumination apparatus of the day was manufactured by Zeiss for von Eiselsberg (45). In July of 1907, von Eiselsberg operated on a 20-year-old man with adiposogenital dystrophy. He modified Schloffer's approach to use a tuning fork incision with the nose reflected downward. This incision left a poor cosmetic appearance with an unsightly dent in the patient's head (70). The surgeon returned the patient to the operating theater for a second transnasal procedure, and again for a craniotomy to further decompress the aggressive adenomatous tumor (71). The patient died after the third operation, having survived 15 years after the initial surgical undertaking. In 1910, before the American Surgical Association, von Eiselsberg reported six cases (72). The first patient with acromegaly to be treated with surgical therapy was a patient of von Eiselsberg's on December 12, 1907 (73). The patient did not fare well and died a few days after surgery (73).

On February 14, 1908, Julius von Hochenegg (1859–1940), of Vienna, modified the von Eiselsberg technique by plugging the nasopharynx and turning down the anterior wall of the frontal sinus (74). The patient, a woman affected with acromegaly, was plagued with its unsightly changes. She improved, with visual changes for the better, resolution of her headaches, and regression of some of the acromegalic symptoms (74).

Emil Theodor Kocher (1841–1917) changed the superior transnasal approach of his colleagues into a submucous resection of the septum, therefore avoiding the nasal cavity (75). The first use of the submucous procedure was on January 9, 1909, on a patient with acromegaly. The event was indeed a complicated operation. A T-shaped incision was made above and an inverted Y-shaped incision was made below (75). The patient benefited from the surgery with improvement in her symptoms.

Harvey Cushing performed an extracranial approach to the pituitary on March 26, 1909 (76) (Fig. 1.21). He modified Schloffer's approach to reflect the frontonasal flap downward. This patient also suffered from acromegaly. Cushing's first transnasal patient had only a partial resection of the tumor but lived another 21 years, which proved that a patient could improve even with incomplete removal of the lesion (76). Cushing remarked in a letter to his father that the pituitary "seems to be an important gland and one which is surgically accessible" (77).

The superior nasal approaches were complex procedures incorporating a considerable amount of resection of the nasal sinuses. Oscar Hirsch, an otolaryngologist, proposed that the large opening in use at that time for transnasal operations was too large and not necessary for the exposure (51, 78). His endonasal operation consisted of two or three stages done with the patient under local anesthesia. His procedure involved resection of the median septum and an opening into the sphenoid through a single nostril. His suggestions were not enthusiastically received. On March 10, 1910, he performed the first inferior transnasal approach without the need to reflect the nose on a patient who would prove to harbor an adenoma (79). The operation was done in three separate stages and no definitive tumor could be found. The patient died 15 months after the third stage. An autopsy identified the elusive tumor, a large adenoma consisting of eosinophilic cells.

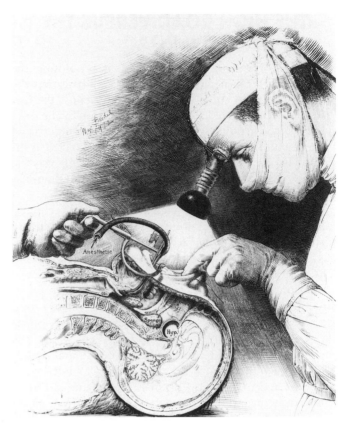

Figure 1.21. Cushing's transsphenoidal operation. (Courtesy of Br'del Archives, Department of Art as Applied to Medicine, Johns Hopkins University School of Medicine, Baltimore, MD.)

Hirsch soon modified his operation to a submucous septal approach, which could be completed in one stage, and performed his first operation using this approach on June 4, 1910 (79). The patient was a woman with a history of headaches, visual field disturbances, secondary amenorrhea, and galactorrhea (80). Hirsch used submucosal septum resection, opened the sphenoid sinus, took down the sphenoid septum, and opened the floor of the sinus and the dura. The tumor revealed itself to the young surgeon and came forth spontaneously. Hirsch was able to retain the visualization of the operative field by using a well-known tool of a rhinologist, a nasal speculum (80).

Allen B. Kanavel (1874–1938), a surgeon from Chicago, introduced another intranasal route in which a U-shaped incision was placed beneath the alae of the nose, allowing the nose to be elevated (81). Kanavel worked out his approach on cadavers and thought that infection would be less of a problem because the ethmoid cells would be opened. On July 21, 1909, Albert E. Halstead (1869–1926) and Allen Kanavel used a sublabial incision (82).

Harvey Cushing performed his first extracranial (or transsphenoidal) procedure on March 26, 1909 (21, 76) (Figs. 1.21 and 1.22). He used a modification of the Schloffer technique. The patient had acromegaly and was referred by Charles Mayo of Rochester, Minnesota. The

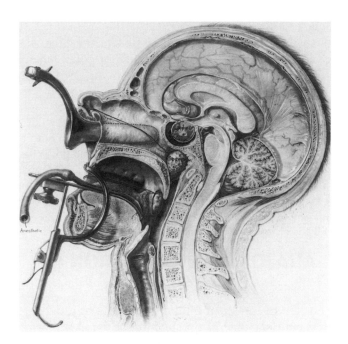

Figure 1.22. Cushing's transsphenoidal operation. (Courtesy of Br'del Archives, Department of Art as Applied to Medicine, Johns Hopkins University School of Medicine, Baltimore, MD.)

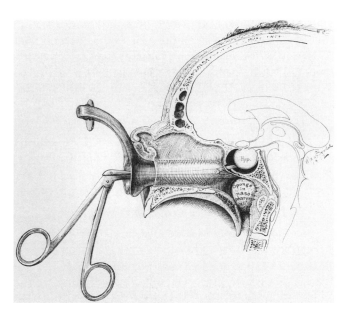

Figure 1.23. Cushing's transsphenoidal operation. (Courtesy of Br'del Archives, Department of Art as Applied to Medicine, Johns Hopkins University School of Medicine, Baltimore, MD.)

patient did well after surgery, and Cushing continued to refine the approach using many of the earlier techniques (76). On June 4, 1910, Cushing carried out the sublabial incision of Halstead (Fig. 1.23). The patient died shortly after surgery of complications from hydrocephalus (21, 83). This procedure has become known as the "Cushing procedure." Cushing made no such claims about the procedure and noted that it was a combination of the techniques of many others (21, 83).

ARGUMENT ENSUES

The interest in operative approaches for treating pituitary disorders continued and in fact was stirring a great deal of excitement among surgeons. Other techniques, such as the transpalatal and the superior and inferior extra-axial transethmoidal, were developed (32, 51, 84–89). Schools of surgery were established—the high road (intracranial) and the low road (extracranial, transnasal). The cranial proponents espoused the fact that a craniotomy was safer and provided better exposure for removing tumors with intracranial extensions. In addition, infection was less of a concern and visual recovery seemed to be better. Those in favor of the transsphenoidal operation argued that it was the safer procedure, better for cyst removal and drainage, and allowed symptoms to improve. The arguments comprised a long list and resembled a law school class with debates on both sides of the issue.

The high road surgeons began to gain momentum with their campaign. Perhaps this can be explained by the growth of neurologic surgery as a specialty. About this time, some surgeons started to devote a greater part of their clinical work to neurologic disorders. Therefore, a strong emphasis was placed on refining and developing intracranial operations. Men such as Cushing, Frazier, von Eiselsberg, and Krause, to name a few, directed their attention to the young field of neurologic surgery. V. Z. Cope remarked:

> *Whether the benefit occurring from the fronto-orbital operation will prove to be greater or more long lasting than that from the trans-sphenoidal method is yet impossible to say; but since the general intracranial pressure is more easily relieved, and growth can be removed from the more immediate neighborhood of the chiasma by the fronto-orbital method it is likely that this operation may have the advantage. Experience will prove (5).*

Cushing eventually concentrated his attention on the cranial methods to address lesions of the pituitary. In a 1939 review of Cushing's pituitary cases, W. R. Henderson perhaps gave some insight into the reason for the famous surgical pioneer to change his tack: the adoption of the transfrontal operation as the routine procedure during later years arose out of the experience that had been gained from chiasmal explorations in patients with unexplained bitemporal hemianopia (and a normal sella), many of whom were found to have removal of suprasellar tumors (for example, meningiomas or adenomas). The recovery of vision seemed to be more complete than was customarily obtained after transsphenoidal operations, and experience soon showed the importance of removing the supradiaphragmatic extrusions that are commonly present around the optic nerves. The intracranial approach was eventually used, therefore, for nearly all pituitary tumors, irrespective of whether the growth of the tumor was chiefly upward (with a small sella) or downward as well (with a large sella) (90).

REFINING THE LOW ROAD

Many surgeons were influenced by the leaders in surgery, particularly Cushing, who preferred the intracranial method to the transsphenoidal technique. A few neurosurgeons, however, continued to follow the low road to the pituitary. Norman Dott (1897–1973), a student of Cushing, improved visualization along the low road by attaching two small light bulbs to Cushing's nasal speculum (51). Dott operated on 120 patients with adenomas without mortality (51). Gerard Guiot (1912–1996) was introduced to the transsphenoidal procedure by Dott in 1956 (51). Guiot adopted the technique and revived interest in the low road to pituitary tumors (51). Jules Hardy of Montreal, a student of Guiot, brought the transsphenoidal approach back to North America. The introduction of microsurgical techniques and instrumentation greatly advanced the transsphenoidal operation (91), and improved instrumentation and better visualization with the surgical microscope brought about an increase in the number of transsphenoidal operations.

RADIATION THERAPY

Roentgen ray therapy has also played a role in the treatment of pituitary tumors. The first case of a pituitary adenoma treated with radiation therapy was in 1909 (92). This was the same year that Krause performed the first successful intracranial operation on a pituitary tumor. A. Gramegna reported the case of a patient with acromegaly who improved after irradiation (92). The patient was a young woman with severe headaches. She received two courses of radiotherapy through the mouth, and her headaches improved after each course of therapy. A. Beclere apparently treated a patient in 1909 but did not publish the case until 1922 (93). This patient was a young girl of 16 years who was plagued with visual problems, headaches, and acromegaly. The therapy was successful, and 13 years later she was doing well and menstruation had returned. She also had improved vision and regression of her symptoms of acromegaly (93). These early cases were isolated events; it was several years before clinicians began to investigate any series of treatment to determine whether such therapy was worthwhile.

The first large group of patients with pituitary lesions treated with radiation was reported by J. Heinismann and L. Czerny in 1926 (94). Also in 1926, Towne reported two cases in which the patients' symptoms, visual field defects and acuity, improved (95). Other reports soon appeared in journals (96–101). Most of the authors agreed that such therapy perhaps should be given postoperatively and considered preoperatively if the situation was not criti-

cal; there were no immediate threats to the patients. Roentgen ray therapy for pituitary tumors was not accepted. Frazier warned physicians about the limitations of irradiation as a means of preserving vision (100). After performing 2000 brain tumor operations, Cushing commented on the use of Roentgen therapy for pituitary tumors: "So far as concerns radiotherapeusis, at least in the case of the chromophobe adenomas, it is safe to say that it will come to be discarded just as radiation for exophthalmic goitre has been, so soon as neurosurgeons as a class perfect themselves in the details of the operative procedure" (102). Radiation therapy for the treatment of pituitary lesions was not without controversy.

ANATOMY AND FUNCTION OF THE GLAND

For the treatment of pituitary disorders to progress, a better understanding of the function of the gland was vitally needed. That the glandula pituitaria consisted of two parts seems to have been appreciated by Thomas Willis (103). Willis belonged to the iatrochemical school, which believed that the vital phenomena was chemical in essence (4). The Venetian anatomist Giovanni Domenico Santorini (1681–1737) recognized in 1724 that the anterior section of the pituitary was not a continuation of the infundibulum (4, 103, 104). Albrecht von Haller (1708–1777) clearly distinguished the pars anterior from the pars posterior by 1766 (103). In 1779, William Cullen (1712–1790) stated:

> This (the pituitary glandule) is compressed on both sides, simple, of uncertain structure; in the anterior part almost round, and of reddish colour; the posterior part less, cinereous, broad transversely, covered with the pia mater of the brain: it lies upon the proper impression of the sella turcica, and seems to be a kind of appendix to the brain (103).

A major advance in the physiologic significance of the pituitary was made in 1895 by George Oliver (1841–1915) and Edward Albert Schafer (1850–1935). They demonstrated that extracts of fresh, whole pituitary glands, when given intravenously to mammals under anesthesia, produced a rapid rise in blood pressure, a vasopressive action (105). This discovery was a major turning point in endocrine research. The participation of Schafer, a leading English professor of physiology, meant that the use of organ extracts was now acceptable and soon became a serious preoccupation of the physiologist (4). Researchers and clinicians directed their attention to prove that an organ extract may be a replacement or a potent drug for the cure of a specific disease. A new era of endocrine research was heralded by Schafer's address to the British Medical Association on August 2, 1895: "My definite subject—the subject of internal secretions—is one of far-reaching interest, although its full importance has only lately come to be recognised" (106).

The possibility of pituitary substitution therapy was investigated. An extensive study was conducted by Emil Goetsch (1883–1963), a coworker of Cushing, in 1916 (29). He claimed that the growth and sexual development of rats were stimulated by feeding them acetone-dried powder of whole pituitary glands (29). In 1921, Herbert McLean Evans (1882–1971) and Joseph Abraham Long proved that the anterior lobe of the hypophysis contains a growth-promoting hormone (107). Subsequently, the dedicated work of Philip E. Smith (1884–1970) and his colleague Earl T. Engle (1896–1957) showed that hypophysectomy inhibited somatic growth, as well as the development of the gonads, thyroid, and adrenal cortex (108). In 1933, Oscar Riddle identified the pituitary hormone controlling the secretion of milk as prolactin (109). This work would later play an important part in the development of a bioassay for prolactin (110).

The laboratory of Evans continued to contribute to the understanding of pituitary physiology (4, 111). In 1940, Choh Hao Li, Miriam Simpson, and Evans isolated the interstitial cell-stimulating (luteinizing) hormone (112). This remarkable team of investigators went on to discover and isolate the adrenocorticotropic, growth, and follicle-stimulating hormones in 1943, 1944, and 1949, respectively (113–115).

In 1794, Johann Peter Frank (1745–1821) distinguished diabetes insipidus from diabetes mellitus (116). It was Alfred Erich Frank, 1912, who first clearly expressed the view that polyuria in patients with diabetes insipidus was probably caused by a hypophyseal lesion (117). In 1928, Oliver Kamm succeeded in separating the posterior lobe extract of pituitrin into vasopressor and oxytocic fractions (118). The synthesis of vasopressin was achieved between 1953 and 1954 by Vincent du Vigneaud and his coworkers (119). This accomplishment has greatly contributed to the reduction of morbidity after pituitary surgery.

IMPROVEMENT THROUGH ADVANCEMENTS

Better methods of diagnosis have brought about improvements in the treatment and outcome of those suffering from pituitary disorders. The development of computed tomography and magnetic resonance imaging allowed clinicians to see the area of concern better than at any time in history (120, 121). These new radiologic methods have allowed physicians and scientists not only the ability to see the pathologic disorder but also the chance to evaluate their work. The development of special tests to measure the amounts of circulating hormones, first by bioassays and then with radioimmunoassay methods, has brought about a new era in recognition and treatment. The study of the chemical composition and structures of pituitary hormones began in the 1950s, stimulated by the work on insulin (122). The discovery of the chemical composition and structure of hormones led to the inquiry as to how these substances could act on other cell complexes. This inquiry would lead to the discovery of receptors and receptor sites (4). The keys to the doors of exciting new worlds were found, but there are more keys to be discovered and more doors to be opened. Perhaps a reader of this chapter will be the next finder of a key.

CONCLUSION

Many have contributed to the progress in understanding the treatment of the well-hidden, protected little gland at the base of the skull. Their names may not appear in this chapter, but their work is indeed a part of its history. Although this chapter is at an end, the story is far from complete.

ACKNOWLEDGMENTS

We thank Julie Yamamoto for her editorial assistance and excellent suggestions; Edwina Walls Mann, Historical Research Center, UAMS Library, for her diligence in finding that which could not be found; Jann Bell, graphic artist, for her assistance in preparing figures; and Betty Patterson for her typing talents.

REFERENCES

1. Cushing H. Papers Relating to the Pituitary Body, Hypothalamus and Parasympathetic Nervous System. Springfield, IL: Charles C. Thomas, 1932:3–5.
2. McHenry L. Garrison's History of Neurology. Springfield, IL: Charles C. Thomas, 1969:3–24.
3. May MT. Galen on the Usefulness of the Parts of the Body (de usu partium): The Ninth Book (the Encephalon, Cranial Nerves, and Cranium). Ithaca, NY: Cornell University Press, 1968: 424–461.
4. Medvei VC. A History of Endocrinology. Lancaster, MA: MTP Press, 1982:55–76, 149–211.
5. Abderhalden R. Internal Secretion. Bombay: CIBA Monographs, 1951:308–310.
6. Saunders JB deCM, O'Malley CD. The Illustrations from the Works of Andreas Vesalius of Brussels. Cleveland: World Publishing, 1950:60.
7. Simmer HH. The beginnings of endocrinology. In: Medicine in Seventeenth Century England: Symposium in Honor of C.D. O'Malley, 30 March 1 April. Berkeley: University of California Press, 1974:215–236.
8. Zuckerman S. The secretions of the brain: relation of hypothalamus to pituitary gland. Lancet 1954;1:739–743, 789–795.
9. Lietaud J. Essais Anatomiques, Contenant L'histoire Exact de Toutes les Parties qui Composent le Corps de L'homme, Avec la Maniere de Dissequer. Paris: Huart, 1742.
10. Burdach E. Beitrag zur mikroskopischen anatomie der nerven. Koenigsberg: International Medical Publishers, 1837.

11. Baillie M. The Morbid Anatomy of Some of the Most Important Parts of the Human Body. 2nd ed. London: 1797:451.
12. Verga A. Caso singolare di prosopectasia. Rendicont: 1st di Lombardia. Milano: 1864;1:111.
13. Marie P. Sur deux cas d'acromegalie: hypertrophie singuliere non congenitale des extremites superieures, inferieures et cephaliques. Rev Med 1886;6:297–333.
14. Marie P, de Souza-Leite JD. Essays on Acromegaly. London: New Sydenham Society, 1891.
15. Minkowski O. Uber einen fall von akromegalie. Berl Klin Wochenschr 1887;24:371–374.
16. Tamburini A. Contributo alla pathogenesi dell' acromegalia. Riv Sper Freniat 1894;20:559–574.
17. Babinski J. Tumeur du corps pituitaire sans acromegalie et avec arret de developement des organes genitaux. Rev Neurol 1900;8:531–533.
18. Froehlich A. Ein fall von tumor der hypophysis cerebri ohne akromegalie. Wien Klin Wochenschr 1901;15:883–906.
19. Lewis DD. Hyperplasia of the chromophile cells of the hypophysis as the cause of acromegaly, with report of a case. Bull Johns Hopkins Hosp 1905;16:157–164.
20. Cushing HW. The hypophysis cerebri. JAMA 1909;53:250–255.
21. Cushing H. The pituitary body and its disorders, clinical states produced by disorders of the hypophysis cerebri. Philadelphia: JB Lippincott, 1912.
22. Hannover A. Recherches microscopiques sur le systeme nerveux. Copenhagen: P.G. Philipsen, 1844.
23. Flesch M. Einige Beobachtungen Uber der Bau der Hypophyse des Pferdes. Magdeburg, Germany: Tagebl. d. Versamml. Deutscher Naturforscher und Aerzte, 1884:195–196.
24. Dostoiewsky A. Uber den bau der vorderlappen des hirnanhanges. Arch Mikr Anat Bonn 1885/86;26:592–598.
25. Johnson HC. Surgery of the hypophysis. In: Walker AE, ed. A History of Neurosurgery. New York: Hafner, 1967;152–177.
26. Schonemann A. Hypophysis und thyroidea. Virchows Arch Pathol Anat 1892;129:310–336.
27. Benda C. Beitrage zur normalen und pathologischen histologie der menschlichen hypophysis cerebri. Berl Klin Wochenschr 1900;37:1205–1210.
28. Jocobson D. The techniques and effects of hypophysectomy, pituitary stalk section and pituitary transplantation in experimental animals. In: Harris GW, Donovan BT, eds. The Pituitary Gland. Berkeley: University of California Press, 1966:1–21.
29. Goetsch E. The influence of pituitary feeding upon growth and sexual development. Bull Johns Hopkins Hosp 1916;27:29–50.
30. Sisson R, Broyles EN. The influence of the anterior lobe of the hypophysis upon the development of the albino rat. Bull Johns Hopkins Hosp 1921;32:22–30.
31. Crowe SJ, Cushing H, Homans J. Experimental hypophysectomy. Bull Johns Hopkins Hosp 1910;21:127–169.
32. Koenig F. Zur totalestirpation der hypophysis cerebri. Berl Klin Wochenschr 1900;37:1040.
33. Horsley V. Functional nervous disorders due to loss of thyroid gland and pituitary body. Lancet 1886;2:5.
34. Marienesco MG. De la destruction de la glande pituitaire chez le chat. C R Hebd Seances Mem Soc Biol 1892;9:509–510.
35. Gley E. Recherches sur la function de la glande thyroide. Arch Physiol Norm Pathol 1892;4:311–326.
36. Vassale G, Sacchi E. Sulla distruzione della ghiandola pituitaria. Riv Sper Freniat 1892;18:525–561.
37. Vassale G, Sacchi E. Ulteriori esperienze sulla ghiandola pituitaria. Riv Sper Freniat 1894;20:83–88.
38. Paulesco NC. L'hypophyse du cerveau. J Physiol Pathol Genet 1907;9:441–456.
39. Reford LL, Cushing H. Is the pituitary gland essential to the maintenance of life. Bull Johns Hopkins Hosp 1909;20:105–107.
40. Cushing HW. The hypophysis cerebri. JAMA 1909;53:250–255.
41. Ascoli G, Legnani T. Die folgen d. exstirpation d. hypophyse. Muenchn Med Wochenschr 1912;59:518–521.
42. Bell WB. Experimental operations on the pituitary. Q J Exp Physiol 1917;11:77–126.
43. Aschner B. Ueber die funktion der hypophyse. Fleugers Arch Ges Physiol 1912;146:1–146.
44. Castiglioni A. A History of Medicine. 2nd ed. New York: Alfred A. Knopf, 1947:1065–1074.
45. Krause F. Surgery of the Brain and the Spinal Cord. New York: Rebman, 1909:115–130.
46. Lane LC. The Surgery of the Head and Neck. San Francisco: LC Lane, 1892:296.
47. Bickham WS. Operative Surgery: Covering the Operative Technic Involved in the Operations of General and Special Surgery. Philadelphia: WB Saunders, 1924:687–703.
48. Horsley V. On operative technique of operations on the central nervous system. BMJ 1906;2:411–423.
49. Tooth GW. The treatment of tumours of the brain, and the indications of operation. In: XVIII International Congress of Medicine: Neuropathology, Part 1. London: Oxford University Press, 1913:161–257.
50. Cope VZ. The pituitary fossa, and the methods of surgical approach. Br J Surg 1916;4:107–144.
51. Landolt AM. History of pituitary surgery. In: Greenblatt SH, ed. A History of Neurosurgery: In Its Scientific and Professional Contexts. Park Ridge, IL: American Association of Neurological Surgeons, 1997:373–400.
52. Caton R, Paul FT. Notes of a case of acromegaly treated by operation. BMJ 1893;2:1421–1423.
53. Kiliani OGT. Some remarks on tumors of the chiasm, with a proposal how to reach the same by operation. Ann Surg 1904;40:35–43.
54. Braun W. For exposure of the central portion of the middle cranial fossa, gasserian ganglion and cavernous, and the hypophysis. Dtsch Zeitschr Chir 1907;87:157.
55. Krause F. Bemerkungen zur operation der hypophysengeschwulste. Dtsch Med Wochenschr 1927;53:691–694.
56. Silbermark M. Die intrakranielle exstirpation der hypophyse. Wien Klin Wochenschr 1910;23:467–468.
57. Frazier CH. Lesions of the hypophysis from the viewpoint of the surgeon. Surg Gynecol Obstet 1913;17:724–736.
58. Frazier CH. Choice of method in operations upon the pituitary body. Surg Gynecol Obstet 1919;29:9–16.
59. Frazier CH. Surgery of the pituitary lesion. Ann Surg 1928;88:1–5.
60. McArthur LL. An aseptic surgical access to the pituitary body and its neighborhood. JAMA 1912;58:2009–2011.
61. McArthur LL. Tumor of the pituitary gland: technic of operative approach. Surg Clin Chicago 1918;2:691–699.
62. Heuer GJ. Surgical experiences with an intracranial approach to chiasmal lesions. Arch Surg 1920;1:368–381.
63. Dandy WE. A new hypophysis operation. Bull Johns Hopkins Hosp 1918;29:154–155.
64. Dandy WE. The brain. In: Lewis D, ed. Practice of Surgery. Hagerstown, MD: WF Prior, 1934:556–605.
65. Giordano D. Compendio di chirurgia operatoria. Torino: Unione Tipografico-Editrice Torinese, 1897:100–104.
66. Koenig F. Zur total estirpation der hypophysis cerebri. Berl Klin Wochenschr 1900;37:1040.
67. Loewe L. Zur Chirurgie der Nase. Berlin: O. Coblentz, 1905:46.
68. Schloffer H. Zur frage der operation an der hypophyse. Beitr Klin Chir 1906;50:767–817.
69. Schloffer H. Erfolgreiche operation eines hypophysentumors auf nasalem wege. Wien Klin Wochenschr 1907;20:621–624.
70. von Eiselsberg AF, Frankl-Hochwart L. Ein neuer fall von hypophysisoperation bei degeneratio adiposo-genitalis. Wien Klin Wochenschr 1908;21:1115–1116.
71. von Eiselsberg AF. Uber den endausgang und obduktion meines ersten operierten falles von hypophysistumor. Beitr Pathol Anat 1922;71:619–626.
72. von Eiselsberg AF. My experience about operation upon the hypophysis. Trans Am Surg Assoc 1910;28:55–72.
73. von Eiselsberg F. Operations upon the hypophysis. Ann Surg 1910;52:1–14.
74. Hochenegg J. The operative cure of acromegaly by removal of a hypophysial tumor. Ann Surg 1908;48:781–784.
75. Kocher T. Ein fall von hypophysistumor mit operativer heilung. Dtsch Zeitschr Chir 1909;100:13–37.
76. Cushing H. Partial hypophysectomy for acromegaly: with remarks on the functions of the hypophysis. Ann Surg 1909;50:1002–1017.
77. Fulton JF. Harvey Cushing. Springfield, IL: Charles C. Thomas, 1946:288.

78. Hirsch O. (Meeting of the K.K. Society of Physicians in Vienna, March 26, 1909.) Wien Klin Wochenschr 1909;22:473–474.

79. Hirsch O. Endonasal method of removal of hypophyseal tumors: with report of two cases. JAMA 1910;55:772–774.

80. Hirsch O. Uber methoden der operativen behandlung von hypophysistumoren auf endonasalem wege. Arch Laryngol Rhinol 1911;24:129–177.

81. Kanavel AB. The removal of tumors of the pituitary body by an infranasal route. JAMA 1909;53:1704–1707.

82. Halstead AE. Remarks on the operative treatment of tumors of the hypophysis: with the report of two cases operated on by an oro-nasal method. Trans Am Surg Assoc 1910;28:73–93.

83. Cushing H. Surgical experiences with pituitary disorders. JAMA 1914;63:1515–1525.

84. Chiari O. Ueber eine modifikation der Schlofferschen operation von tumoren der hypophyse. Wien Klin Wochenschr 1912;25:5–6.

85. Fein J. Zur operation der hypophyse. Wien Klin Wochenschr 1910;23:108–109.

86. Krogius A. Neue methode, den nasopharyngealraum fur doe operation von basalfibromen und hypophysengeschwulsten freizulegen. Zentralbl Chir 1909;36:1420.

87. Preysing H. Beitrage zur operation der hypophyse. Verh Verein Dtsch Laryngol 1913;20:51–73.

88. Denker A. Hypophysentumoren. Int Zentralbl Laryngol Rhinol 1921;37:225.

89. Lautenschlager A. Die permaxillare hypophysenoperation. Chirurgie 1928;1:30–33.

90. Henderson WR. The pituitary adenoma: a follow-up study of the surgical results in 338 cases (Harvey Cushing's series). Br J Surg 1939;26:811–921.

91. Yasargil MG. Microsurgery: Applied to Neurosurgery. Stuttgart: Georg Thieme Verlag, 1969.

92. Gramegna A. Un cas d'acromegalie par radiotherapie. Rev Neurol 1909;17:15–17.

93. Beclere A. Technique, resultats, indications et contre-indications de la Roentgen therapie des tumeurs hypophysaires. Rev Neurol 1922;39:808–816.

94. Heinemann JI, Czerny LI. Die Rontgen therapie der hypophysentumoren. Strahlentherapie 1926;24:331–335.

95. Towne EB. Treatment of pituitary tumors: the role of the Roentgen ray and of surgery therein. Ann Surg 1930;91:29–36.

96. Dyke CG, Gross SW. The Roentgenotherapy of pituitary tumors. Bull Neurol Inst New York 1931;1:211–228.

97. Bailey P. The results of Roentgen therapy on brain tumors. Ann J Roentgenol Radiol Ther 1925;13:48–53.

98. Rand CW, Taylor RG. Irradiation in the treatment of tumors of the pituitary gland. Arch Surg 1935;30:103–150.

99. Sosman MC. The Roentgen therapy of pituitary adenomas. JAMA 1939;113:1282–1285.

100. Frazier CH. A series of pituitary pictures: commentaries on the pathologic, clinical and therapeutic aspects. Arch Neurol Psychiatry 1930;23:656–695.

101. Grant FC. The surgical treatment of pituitary adenomas. JAMA 1939;113:1279–1282.

102. Cushing H. Intracranial Tumors: Notes Upon a Series of Two Thousand Verified Cases With Surgical Mortality Percentages Pertaining Thereto. Springfield, IL: Charles C. Thomas, 1932.

103. Heller H. Remarks on the history of the neurohypophysial research. In: G. Peters, ed. Pharmacology of the Endocrine System and Related Drugs: The Neurohypophysis. Oxford: Pergamon Press, 1970:1–17.

104. Santorini GD. Observationes anatomicae. Venetis: JB Recurti, 1724:70.

105. Oliver G, Schaefer E. On the physiological actions of extracts of the pituitary body and certain other glandular organs. J Physiol (Lond) 1895;18:277–279.

106. Schafer EA. Address in physiology: on internal secretions. Lancet 1895;2:321–324.

107. Evans HM, Long JA. Characteristics effects upon growth, oestrus, and ovulation induced by the intraperitoneal administration of fresh anterior hypophyseal substance. Proc Natl Acad Sci USA 1922;8:38–39.

108. Smith PE, Engle ET. Experiential evidence regarding the role of the anterior pituitary in the development and regulation of the genital system. Am J Anat 1927;40:159–217.

109. Riddle O. The preparation, identification and assay of prolactin—a hormone of the anterior pituitary. Am J Physiol 1933;105:191–216.

110. Riddle O. Prolactin in vertebrate function and organization. J Natl Cancer Inst 1963;31:1039–1110.

111. Seyle H. The hypophysis. In: Textbook of Endocrinology. Montreal: University of Montreal, 1947:197–319.

112. Li CH, Simpson ME, Evans HM. Interstitial cell stimulating hormone: method of preparation and some physico-chemical studies. Endocrinology 1940;27:803–808.

113. Li CH, Simpson ME, Evans HM. Adrenocorticotrophic hormone. J Biol Chem 1943;149:413–424.

114. Li CH, Evans HM, Simpson ME. Isolation and properties of the anterior hypophyseal growth hormone. J Biol Chem 1945;159:353–366.

115. Li CH, Simpson ME, Evans HM. Isolation of pituitary follicle-stimulating hormone (FSH). Science 1949;109:445–446.

116. Frank JP. De Curandis Hominum Morbis Epitome. Mannheim: CF Schwann and CG Goetz, 1794:38–67.

117. Frank AE. Uber beziehungen der hypophyse zum diabetes insipidus. Berl Klin Wochenschr 1912;49:393–397.

118. Kamm O, Aldrich TB, Grote IW, Rowe LW, Bugbee EP. The active principles of the posterior lobe of the pituitary gland, I: the demonstration of the presence of two active principles, II: the separation of the two principles and their concentration in the form of potent solid preparations. J Am Chem Soc 1928;66:573–601.

119. Du Vigneaud V, Gish DT, Katsoyannis PG. A synthetic preparation possessing biological properties associated with arginin-vasopressin. J Am Chem Soc 1954;76:4751–4752.

120. New PFJ, Scott WR. Computed tomography of the brain and orbit (EMI scanning). Baltimore: Williams & Wilkins, 1975:3–7.

121. Damadian R, Goldsmith M, Minkoff L. Fonar images of the live human body. Physiol Chem Phys Med NMR 1977;9:97.

122. Ryle AP, Sanger F, Smith LF, Kitai R. The disulphide bonds of insulin. Biochem J 1955;60:541–556.

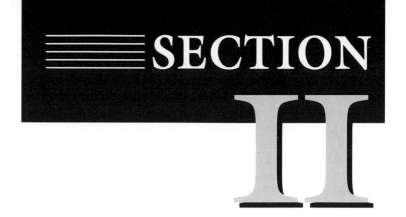

SECTION II

Evolution and Phylogeny

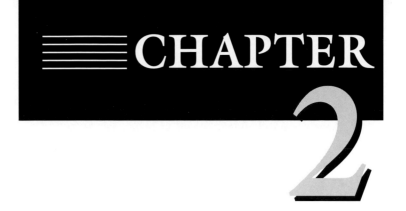

CHAPTER 2

The Pituitary Gland and Its Phylogenetic Role

Ali F. Krisht and Sivakumar Jaikumar

INTRODUCTION

Hunger and love make the world go around.

Schiller

Hunger is one of the essential drives that help with the preservation of the individual; love, on the other hand, leads to the drives that help our preservation as a species. Clearly, their presence is vital for our individual existence and for the existence of our species, which is what makes our "world go around," as Schiller indicated.

The pituitary gland has an integral role in these functions. In its intimate relationship with the brain, the pituitary gland contributes to the translation of the brain orders that drive us as individuals to the different acts that lead to the stability and homeostasis of our internal environment and thus to our preservation as individuals. It also translates the sexual drive arising from the brain into physical changes and actions that lead to our preservation as a species.

In the Galenic time, the pituitary gland was considered a secretory organ that produced a mucous substance (pituita) that was filtered into the nasal cavity (1). Sylvius and others later assumed that the pituitary gland was related to formation of cerebrospinal fluid (1). It was not until Richard Lower in 1672 that the Galenic doctrine was disproved (1).

> *For whatever serum is separated into the ventricles of the brain and tissues out of them through the infundibulum to the glandula pituitaria distills not upon the Palat but it's poured again into the blood and mixed with it.*

The clinical role of the pituitary gland came to light with Marie's paper (1888–1889), in which acromegaly was related to a pituitary tumor or pathologic disorder (1). Cushing later realized the value of the pituitary gland in the existence of the species. Realizing the presence of the gland in all vertebrates, he most elegantly expressed the role the pituitary gland must have:

Indeed, its extraordinarily well protected position, its presence in all vertebras and persistence throughout life, its remarkably disposed and abundant blood supply, would of themselves be enough to stamp the hypophysis as an organ of vital importance (1).

THE BRAIN AND THE PITUITARY GLAND

Rathke in 1838 was among the first to describe the embryologic background of the pituitary gland (2). He indicated, and this was later shown by Mihalkowics (3), that this part of the gland arises from the roof of the buccopharyngeal cavity (stomodeum), which buds off to meet and envelop the infundibular extension from the base of the brain, the part that later becomes the neurohypophysis, or the pars nervosa. The epithelial outpouching from the stomodeum develops to become the anterior lobe of the pituitary gland.

The intimate relationship of the pituitary gland with the brain is well recognized throughout the evolutionary process. The larval petromyzon (Ammocoetes) neurohypophysis developed as a thickening in the floor of the third ventricle. This was innervated by the neurosecretory cells in the preoptic region without the presence of an infundibular recess (succus infundibuli). In higher species, this developed to become the median eminence and the neural lobe. This is the case in tetrapods and lungfish. In humans, this process evolved further to form the stalk, which is just an extension of these layers leading to the formation of the posterior lobe of the pituitary gland. The extension of the stalk is accompanied by the differentiated glial brain cells, which are present in the vicinity of and around the axonal endings in the posterior lobe. With these facts, clearly the evolution of the brain is going to affect the evolution of the pituitary gland. Such evidence is seen throughout the evolutionary process. More recently, our better understanding of the physiologic nature of the gland and our ability to identify the genetic background of these processes revealed that although the pituitary gland evolved significantly, it still has substantial similarities in higher and lower vertebrates.

The growth and development of the pituitary gland is directly influenced by the events that occur at the hypothalamic level. This relationship is shown in its absence in anencephalic fetuses. Pilavdzic et al. found that anencephalic fetuses did not develop posterior lobes (neurohypophysis) (4). This was recognized as early as 17 to 18 weeks' gestation. Conversely, the growth of the anterior lobe until 17 to 18 weeks was not affected and seemed to have been programmed to run until that stage, without the influence of the hypothalamic input. When fetuses were checked later at 26 to 28 weeks' gestation, there was a reduction in cells staining for glycoprotein hormones and their α- and/or β-

subunits. After 32 weeks' gestation, the corticotrophs were reduced in number and size and the gonadotrophs were almost absent. The somatotrophs, lactotrophs, and thyrotrophs were numerous. This proves the vital role the hypothalamus has in the maintenance of the newly differentiated gonadotrophs and corticotrophs (4). Other studies comparing normal and anencephalic fetuses confirmed that the development and differentiation of the lactotrophs is not significantly hindered by the absence of the early hypothalamic inputs, at least at the structural and cellular levels (5).

THE PITUITARY IN EVOLUTION

Developmental changes and interactions of the hypothalamic–pituitary–gonadal axis undergo several evolutionary changes at the individual and species levels (6). The hypothalamic-releasing hormones comprise a subgroup of neural peptides that have a wide anatomic and phylogenetic distribution. It seems that initially they played a role in neurocrine or paracrine functions, and later in evolution they acquired the role of regulating pituitary hormone secretion. However, more recent evolutionary studies at the molecular level show a high degree of conservation of these neuropeptides not only at the structural level but also at the level of their physiologic response.

Although the pituitary hormones were shown to be less conserved in evolution compared with the hypothalamic-releasing hormones, still they revealed a high level of structural and functional similarity in different species.

Prolactin (PRL) in Evolution

In fish, PRL hormone plays a role in calcium and electrolyte metabolism. Those functions have not been recognized in higher animals, although PRL receptors are found in kidneys of higher mammals (7).

The role of PRL in breast-feeding is well established in humans. The infant's sucking of the nipple stimulates PRL secretion, which leads to stimulation of milk production through the effects of PRL on the breasts. A similar role is also seen in lower vertebrates. The crop sac of pigeons and doves (family: *Columbidae*) has a specialized epithelial cell lining, the growth and development of which is stimulated by PRL. This helps in the formation of "crop milk," which is used to feed the newly hatched squab. In addition to the crop milk feeding, a complex array of related behavioral adaptations that are relevant to the parenting role are supported by the high levels of PRL secretion in the Columbids family. These behavioral adaptations include increased food intake (hyperphagia); nesting behavior, including nest attendance; and regurgitation of food for the squabs. These behavioral adaptations, and the associated physiologic changes, bare significant similarities to the milk feeding and parenting seen in mammals.

PRL effect has also been studied at the molecular level by analyzing the avian (pigeon) PRL receptor family, which was found to be of the cytokine receptor superfamily, and by analyzing the transcription factors that are activated after PRL treatment. PRL in crop sac epithelium leads to the activation of signal transducer and activation proteins and transcription of signal transducer and activator of transcription proteins via phosphorylation of tyrosine. This same fundamental signaling step is shared with the mammalian PRL target tissues. This is a fascinating finding of the convergence of the evolution of milk feeding and behaviors related to parenting in both the Columbids and mammals (8).

The role that PRL hormone plays is far from fully defined. In lower animals, it has a developmental role that is becoming more recognized. Amphibious metamorphosis induced with exogenous thyroid hormones is retarded when PRL is given. Studies suggest that PRL plays a role in morphogenesis, tissue remodeling, gene programming, and programmed cell death or apoptosis (9).

The immunoregulatory effects of PRL and its ability to potentiate the immune system are functions that are becoming more recognized in humans. There are reports of patients with PRL-producing tumors in whom treatment of the hyperprolactinemia leads to improvement in their autoimmune disease, such as systemic lupus erythematosus. The autoimmune disease is thought to have flared up as a result of the hyperprolactinemic state (10). On the positive side, it became recognized that infants who are breast fed are more protected from infections and allergic diseases compared with infants who are not breast fed. Studies done in lower mammals showed that immunoglobulin production by the mammary glands at the end of pregnancy is influenced not only by the decrease in steroid levels but also by an increase in the serum PRL level (11).

Growth Hormone in Evolution

The growth hormone-releasing hormone (GHRH) is made up of 44 amino acids. Two forms of GHRH are found in the human hypothalamus. In rats, GHRH has 43 amino acids and a free acid terminal (12, 13). This hormone seems to be well conserved in the evolutionary process. Analysis of a carp GHRH-like peptide revealed a 44 amino acid hormone similar to the other vertebrate sequence (14).

GH and PRL are thought to belong to the same multigene family and thus to have evolved from a common ancestor. The functional aspect of this common background is related to "neuroimmunomodulation" (15). Lactogenic hormones and GHs have a role in the development of the immune system, especially in the initial signals that stimulate cells to proliferate, differentiate, and assume their functions. Their role also involves the fine tuning of the immune system to help with specific mechanisms of immune recognition that have been perfected in evolution. The role of GH and other lactogenic hormones in immune cell recognition is counterbalanced by the effects of the adrenocorticotropic–adrenal axis, which antagonizes their

immunostimulatory effects and thus enables the immune system to perform within the homeostatic limits that will help with the preservation of the organism.

Evidence exists that the pituitary GH evolution occurred as a result of an underlying slow rate superimposed by bursts of rapid evolution during which the rate increased at least 25-fold. These burst occasions are thought to be during the evolution of primates (to at least $10.8 \pm 1.3 \times 10^{-9}$ substitutions per amino acid site per year) and artiodactyl ruminants (to at least $5.6 \pm 1.3 \times 10^{-9}$ substitutions per amino acid site per year) (16, 17).

The Corticotrophs in Evolution

Corticotropin releasing factor (CRF) contains 41 amino acids. The CRF molecule stimulates the release of adrenocorticotropic hormone (ACTH), beta-endorphin, and pro-opiomelanocortin cleavage products from the pituitary. In mammals, the molecule is well conserved. Studies have shown minimum variations among different species, including rats, pigs, sheep, cows, and humans (18).

Okawara et al. showed that the fish *Catostomus commersoni* has CRF with 41 amino acids that differs from the human CRF by only two amino acids (19). This suggests 400 million years of evolution with a tightly conserved neuropeptide. Other molecules found in lower animals show a significant sequence identity with the CRF molecule as well as similarities in their functions. Urotensin I (41 amino acids) seen in suckers and carp has 51% identity with CRF (20, 21). Sauvagine (40 amino acids) in frogs has 41% identity with human CRF. Both molecules have functions related to CRF and cause release of ACTH in rats and ACTH and alpha–melanocyte-stimulating hormone in fish (22). Unlike other vertebrates, mammals have only one form of CRF.

Glucocorticoid hormones play a major role in the complex processes involved with the reaction of the neuroendocrine system to stress. Evidence indicates that the basic mechanisms and molecules involved in stress are fundamentally similar and well preserved throughout evolution in different species (23). The role of ACTH in stress and the immune response is recognized in organisms as early as the freshwater snails (*Planorbarius corneus* and *Lymnaea stagnalis*). In these animals, ACTH increased phagocytosis of *Staphylococcus aureus* and induced the release of biogenic amines. These data support the fact that the neural and endocrine systems share a common evolutionary origin (24). The role of pro-opiomelanocortin–derived peptides, including ACTH, beta-endorphin, and alpha–melanocyte-stimulating hormone, and cytokines such as IL-2, IL-6, and tumor necrosis factor–alpha in the development of the immune system was studied in higher and lower vertebrates (25). Results of these studies indicate that the above-mentioned peptides and cytokines are present in the thymus of fish, amphibians, chickens, and rats. They were also found in the apoptotic cells in the thymus of both higher and lower animals. This is additional evidence of the role of neuroendocrine cells in the development of the immune system through selection and apoptosis of thymic lymphocytes, and through slight differences in different species.

The Gonadotrophs in Evolution

Gonadotropin-releasing hormone (GnRH) is a small molecule that is made up of 10 amino acids. One would assume that because GnRH is essential for reproduction it would be highly conserved in evolution. In some species, GnRH is found in more than one molecular form. For example, in birds such as chickens, GnRH has two molecular forms. Although there were two forms of the molecule, conservation occurred in its length, in the amino acids at the ends of the molecule, and in the N- and C-terminal posttranslational modifications. An identical GnRH molecule has been found in five mammalian species, including man (26–28). Results of studies on the genetic background of this hormone suggest that the genes coding for the other forms of the GnRH are the result of a duplication that occurred before the appearance of vertebrates (29). In lower animals such as amphibians, the chicken form of the hormone (GnRH II) is concentrated outside the hypothalamus and may function as a neurotransmitter (30).

It seems that the evolution of the GnRH family involved a duplication of the gene of a neurotransmitter that was present before the vertebrates, and the new forms acquired the hormonal functions and became concentrated in hypothalamic regions such as the preoptic and infundibular regions. Although the new forms of the GnRH developed some structural changes, the hormone maintained conservation of its basic amino acid sequence.

Luteinizing hormone–releasing hormone–like material present in frog ganglia seems to function as a neurotransmitter and not as luteinizing hormone–releasing hormone. Evidence suggests that the mammalian version of this hormone is different than that found in lower species.

The Thyrotrophs in Evolution

Thyrotropin-releasing hormone is present in high concentrations in the hypothalamus and brains of amphibians and fish species. Unlike the case with the mammalian hypothalamus, in lower vertebrates these hormones do not have a hypophysiotropic hormonal function. Somatostatin, conversely, is an ancient molecule, which stayed identical in mammalian and other lower species and plays an important role in the neuronal, pancreatic, and digestive functions (31).

The most impressive role of the thyroid hormone in lower animals is seen in the complex developmental programs of the metamorphosis in frogs and toads. This process is an example of the interaction of the hypothalamus, the pituitary, and the thyroid gland. The process involves several dramatic steps, which include programmed cell death (apoptosis) and organogenesis (32).

Posterior Lobe Hormones in Evolution

Vasopressin and oxytocin molecules are made up of nine amino acids, with cysteines in the 1 and 6 positions and interconnecting S-S sulfide bridges. These sequences are fully conserved in mammals. The only exception is in the pig family, in which vasopressin has lysine for arginine. In mammals, the two hormones differ in only two positions. Evidence exists that the vasopressin/oxytocin hormones may be conserved in evolution from as early as lower invertebrates. A diuretic hormone in the insect *Locusta migratoria* (32) has the same sequence identity in five or six of nine amino acids of the vasopressin/oxytocin mammalian hormones with cysteine in the same position.

CONCLUSION

The existence of multicellular organisms hinges on coordinating systems to integrate the function of different cells to perform their function as one cohesive unit. Two of the basic regulatory systems that perform this complex and delicate task are the nervous system and the endocrine system. The nervous system uses neurotransmitters and electrical impulses to convey its commands to peripheral organs and to receive information from them. The endocrine system uses hormones to exert its influence on the target organs. These two systems intersect at the hypothalamic–pituitary junction. The hypothalamic hypophysiotropic hormones are released in the portal blood vessels of the pituitary gland and are transported to the anterior pituitary lobe, where they help regulate the secretion of its hormones. The hypothalamus also extends its neuronal projections to the posterior lobe of the pituitary gland, where the neural peptides are directly released into the circulation. This complex relationship between the nervous system and the humeral system allows the brain to keep tight control of the internal environment of the organism in response to external stimuli. After those stimuli are received, they are processed and used to help generate the appropriate responses of the hypothalamic–pituitary system and to help with the different preservation functions, including reproduction, growth and development, maintenance of the internal environment, and regulation of energy production.

Obviously, the pituitary gland has dramatic input into the evolutionary process. This role is seen at the level of the evolution of the different species as well as in the developmental changes seen in the evolution of the individual organism during its lifetime within the species. Two major evolutionary steps seen with the GH molecule suggest a major evolutionary step at the level of transition from invertebrates to vertebrates and then at the level of evolution of the mammalian species. On the other hand, because of the important role the pituitary gland has in the preservation of the species and the organism, its evolution shows significant conservation at the molecular and cellular levels. Its early role in the development of the immune system contributes to its role in evolution of multicellular organisms and the preservation of the individual organism. Its role in reproduction helps with the preservation of the species. Indeed, one can rewrite Darwin's theory of evolution as the success of the hypothalamic–pituitary system over nature, and the process of natural selection could very well be the success story of an optimal neuroendocrine system.

REFERENCES

1. Cushing H. The Pituitary Body and Its Disorders. Philadelphia: JB Lippincott, 1910:1–22.
2. Rathke H. Ueber Die Entstehung Der Glandula Pituitaria. Arch F Anat Physiol U Wissensch Med 1838;5:482–485.
3. Mihalkowics V. Wirbelsaite Und Hirnanhang. Arch F Mikr Anat 1875;XI:389–441.
4. Pilavdzic D, Kovacs K, Asa SL. Pituitary morphology in anencephalic human fetuses. Neuroendocrinology 1997;65(3):164–172.
5. Begeot M, Dubois MP, Dubois PM. Evolution of lactotrophs in normal and anencephalic human fetuses. J Clin Endocrinol Metab 1984;58(4):726–730.
6. Forest MG. Sexual maturation of the hypothalamus: pathophysiological aspects and clinical implications. Acta Neurochir (Wien) 1985;75(1–4):23–42.
7. Dunand M, Kraehenbuhl JP, Roissier BC, et al. Purification of prolactin receptors from toad kidney: comparisons with rabbit memory prolactin receptors. Am J Physiol 1998;254:C372–C382.
8. Horseman ND, Buntin JD. Regulation of pigeon crop milk secretion and parental behaviors by prolactin. Annu Rev Nutr 1995;15:213–238.
9. Tata JR. Metamorphosis: an exquisite model for hormonal regulation of post embryonic development. Biochem Soc Symp 1996;62:123–136.
10. Compan Gonzalez DA, Martinez Aguilar NE, Vargas Camano ME, et al. Hyperprolactinemia and autoimmunity. Rev Alerg Mex 1996;43(5):128–132.
11. Rosato R, Jammes H, Belair L, et al. Polymeric-Ig receptor gene expression in rabbit mammary gland during pregnancy and lactation: evolution and hormonal regulation. Mol Cell Endocrinol 1995;10(1–2):81–87.
12. Guillemin R. Hypothalamic Control of Pituitary Function: The Growth Hormone Releasing Factor. Liverpool: Liverpool University Press, 1981:1–73.
13. Spiess J, Rivier J, Vale W. Characterization of rat hypothalamic growth hormone-releasing factor. Nature 1983;303:532–535.
14. Vaughan J, Rivier J, Spiess J, et al. Purification and characterization of a GRF like immunoreactive peptide from carp hypothalamus. In: The Endocrine Society, 69th Annual Meeting, and p 50. Abstract 116.
15. Berezi I. The role of the growth and lactogenic hormone family in immune function. Neuroimmunomodulation 1994;1(4):201–216.
16. Wallis M. Variable evolutionary rates in the molecular evolution of mammalian growth hormones. J Mol Evol 1994;38(6):619–627.
17. Wallis M. The molecular evolution of vertebrate growth hormones: a pattern of near stasis interrupted by sustained bursts of rapid change. J Mol Evol 1996;43(2):93–100.
18. Jingami H, Mizuno N, Takahashi H, et al. Cloning and sequence analysis of cDNA for rat corticotropin releasing factor precursor. FEBS Lett 1985;191(1):63–66.
19. Okawara Y, Ko D, Morley SD, et al. In situ hybridization of corticotropin-releasing factor-encoding messenger RNA in the hypothalamus of the white sucker, *Catostomus commersoni*. Cell Tissue Res 1992;267(3):545–549.
20. Ishida I, Ichikawa T, Deguchi T. Cloning and sequence analysis cDNA encoding Urotensin I precursor. Proc Natl Acad Sci USA 1986;83:308–312.
21. Ling N, Esch F, Bohlen P, et al. Isolation and characterization of caprine corticotropin releasing factor. Biochem Biophys Res Commun 1984;122:1218–1224.
22. Tran TN, Fryer JN, Lederis K, et al. CRF, Urotensin I and sauvagin stimulate the release of POMC-peptides from goldfish neurointermediate lobe cells. Gen Comp Endocrinol 1990;78(3):351–360.
23. Ottaviani E, Franceschi C. The neuroimmunology of stress problem invertebrates to man. Prog Neurobiol 1996;48(4–5):421–440.
24. Ottaviani E, Cossarizza A, Ortolani C, et al. ACTH-like molecules in gastropod molluscs: a possible role in ancestral immune response and stress. Proc R Soc Lond B Biol Sci 1992;23:(247):1320–1323.
25. Ottaviani E, Franchini A, Franceschi C. Evolution of neuroendocrine thymus: studies on POMC-derived peptides, cytokines and apoptosis in lower and higher vertebrates. J Neuroimmunol 1997;72(1):67–74.
26. Matsuo H, Baba Y, Nair RMG, et al. Structure of the porcine LH and FSH releasing hormone: the proposed amino acid sequence. Biochem Biophys Res Commun 1971;43:1336–1339.
27. Burgus R, Butcher M, Amoss M, et al. Primary structure of the ovine hypothalamus luteinizing hormone-releasing factor (LRF). Proc Natl Acad Sci USA 1972;69:278–282.
28. Seeburg PH, Mason AJ, Stewart TA, et al. The mammalian GnRH and the pivotal role in production. Recent Prog Horm Res 1987;43:69–98.
29. White RB, Eisen JA, Katsen TL, et al. Second gene for gonadotropin-releasing hormone in humans. Proc Natl Acad Sci USA 1998;95(1):305–309.
30. Muske LE, King JA, Moore FL, et al. Gonadotropin-releasing hormones in microdissected brain regions of an amphibian: concentration and anatomical distribution of immunoreactive mammalian GnRH and chicken GnRH II. Regul Pept 1994;54(2–3):373–384.
31. Jackson IM. Evolutionary significance of the phylogenetic distribution of the mammalian hypothalamic releasing hormones. Fed Proc 1981;40(11):2545–2552.
32. Kanamori A, Brown DD. The analysis of complex developmental programmes: amphibian metamorphosis. Genes Cells 1996;1(5):429–435.
33. Proux JP, Miller CA, Li JP, et al. Identification of an arginine vasopressin like diuretic hormone from *Locusta Migratoria*. Biochem Biophys Res Commun 1987;149:180–186.

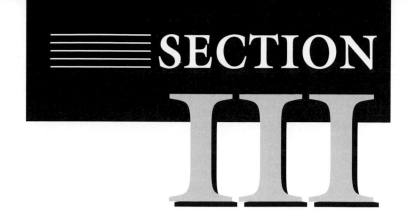

SECTION III

Basic Considerations

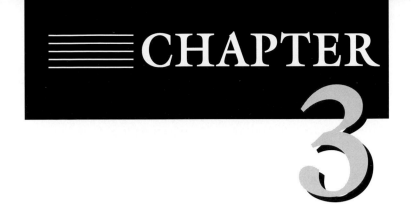

CHAPTER 3

Anatomy

Microsurgical Anatomy of the Pituitary Gland and the Sellar Region

Albert L. Rhoton, Jr.

INTRODUCTION

This chapter is divided into two sections. The first section deals with the relationships in the sellar region that are important in performing the various transcranial and subcranial approaches to pituitary tumors. The second section deals with the neural, arterial, and venous relationships in suprasellar and third ventricular regions that are important in planning surgery for tumors extending from the pituitary gland into these areas.

SELLAR REGION

Sphenoid Bone

The sphenoid bone is located in the center of the cranial base (1–4) (Figs. 3.1 and 3.2). The intimate contact of the body of the sphenoid bone with the nasal cavity below and the pituitary gland above has led to the transsphenoidal route being the operative approach of choice for most pituitary adenomas. Some part of it is also exposed in the transcranial approaches to the sellar region.

The neural relationships of the sphenoid bone are among the most complex of any bone: the olfactory tracts, gyrus rectus, and posterior part of the frontal lobe rest against the smooth upper surface of the lesser wing; the pons and mesencephalon lie posterior to the clival portion; the optic chiasm lies posterior to the chiasmatic sulcus; and cranial nerves II through VI are intimately related to the sphenoid bone. All exit the skull through the optic canal, superior orbital fissure, foramen rotundum, or foramen ovale, all foramina located in the sphenoid bone.

The sphenoid bone has many important arterial and venous relationships: the carotid arteries groove each side of the sphenoid bone and often form a serpiginous prominence in the lateral wall of the sphenoid sinus; the basilar artery rests against its posterior surface; the circle of Willis is located above its central portion; and the middle cerebral artery courses parallel to the sphenoid ridge of the lesser wing. The cavernous sinuses rest against the sphenoid bone, and intercavernous venous connections line the walls of the pituitary fossa and dorsum sellae.

In the anterior view, the sphenoid bone resembles a bat with wings outstretched (Figs. 3.1 and 3.2). It consists of a central portion, called the body; the lesser wings, which spread outward from the superolateral part of the body; the two greater wings, which spread upward from the lower part of the body; and the superior orbital fissure, which is situated between the greater and lesser wings. The vomer, the pterygoid processes, and the medial and lateral pterygoid plates are directed downward from the body. The body of the sphenoid bone is more or less cubical and con-

tains the sphenoid sinus. The superior orbital fissure, through which the oculomotor, trochlear, and abducens nerves and the ophthalmic division of the trigeminal nerve pass, is formed on its inferior and lateral margins by the greater wing and on its superior margin by the lesser wing. The inferior surface of the lesser wing forms the posterior part of the roof of each orbit, and the exposed surface of the greater wing forms a large part of the lateral wall of the orbit. The optic canals are situated above and are separated from the superomedial margin of the superior orbital fissure by the optic strut, a bridge of bone that extends from the lower margin of the base of the anterior clinoid process to the body of the sphenoid. The sphenoid ostia open from the nasal cavity into the sinus.

In the superior view, the pituitary fossa occupies the central part of the body and is bound anteriorly by the

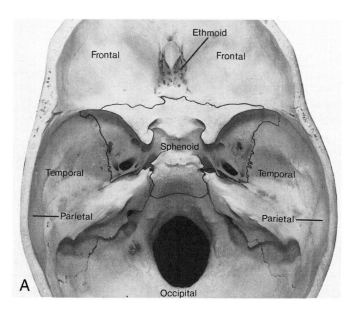

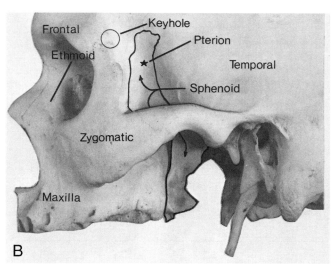

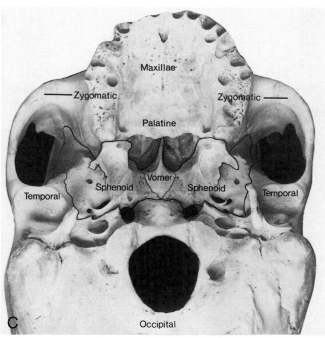

Figure 3.1. Osseous relationships of the sphenoid bone. The sphenoid bone is outlined in each view. **A.** Superior view. **B.** Lateral view. **C.** Inferior view. (Reprinted with permission from Rhoton AL Jr, Hardy DG, Chambers SM. Microsurgical anatomy and dissection of the sphenoid bone, cavernous sinus and sellar region. Surg Neurol 1979;12:63–104.)

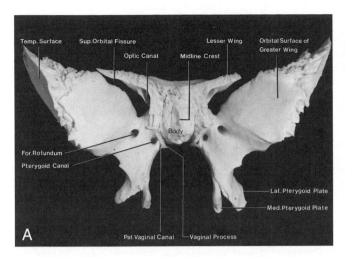

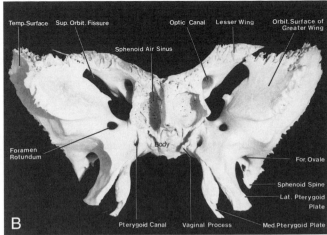

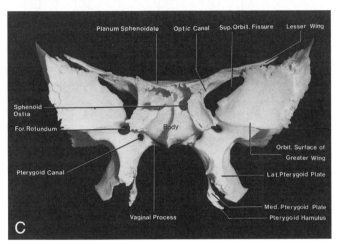

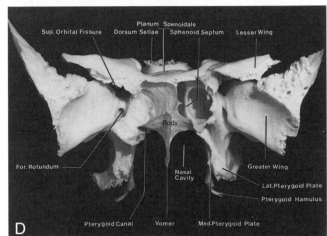

Figure 3.2. Sphenoid bone. Anterior views. **A.** Conchal-type sphenoid bone. **B.** Bone with presellar-type sphenoid sinus. **C.** Bone with sellar-type sphenoid sinus and well-defined sphenoid ostia. **D.** Bone with sellar-type sphenoid sinus with poorly defined sphenoid ostia and obliquely oriented sphenoidal septae.

Temp., temporal; *Sup.,* superior; *For.,* foramen; *Pal.,* palatal; *Lat.,* lateral; *Med.,* medial; *Orbit.,* orbital. (Reprinted with permission from Rhoton AL Jr, Hardy DG, Chambers SM. Microsurgical anatomy and dissection of the sphenoid bone, cavernous sinus and sellar region. Surg Neurol 1979;12:63–104.)

tuberculum sellae and posteriorly by the dorsum sellae (Fig. 3.1). The chiasmatic groove, a shallow depression between the optic foramina, is bound posteriorly by the tuberculum sellae and anteriorly by the planum sphenoidale. The frontal lobes and the olfactory tracts rest against the smooth upper surface of the lesser wing and the planum sphenoidale. The posterior margin of the lesser wing forms a free edge called the sphenoid ridge, which projects into the sylvian fissure to separate the frontal and temporal lobes. The anterior clinoid processes are located at the medial end of the lesser wings, the middle clinoid processes are lateral to the tuberculum sellae, and the posterior clinoid processes are situated at the superolateral margin of the dorsum sellae. The dorsum sellae is continuous with the clivus. The upper part of the clivus is formed by the sphenoid bone and the lower part by the occipital bone. The carotid sulcus extends along the lateral surface of the body of the sphenoid.

The superior aspect of each greater wing is concave upward and is filled by the tip of each temporal lobe. The foramen rotundum, through which the maxillary division of the trigeminal nerve passes, is located at the junction of the body and greater wing. The foramen ovale transmits the mandibular division of the trigeminal nerve, and the foramen spinosum transmits the middle meningeal artery. When viewed inferiorly, the vomer, a separate bone, frequently remains attached to the anterior half of the body of the sphenoid, and its most anterior portion separates the sphenoid ostia.

The pterion and the "keyhole" are two important anatomic landmarks in the region of the greater wing in the lateral view (Fig. 3.1). The pterion is located over the upper part of the greater wing. The keyhole is located just behind the junction of the temporal line and the zygomatic process of the frontal bone, several centimeters anterior to the pterion. A burr hole placed over the pterion will be located at the lateral end of the sphenoid ridge. A burr hole placed at the keyhole will expose the orbit at its lower margin and the dura over the frontal lobe at its upper margin.

Sphenoid Sinus

The sphenoid sinus is subject to considerable variation in size and shape and to variation in the degree of pneumatization (5–7) (Fig. 3.2). It is present as minute cavities at birth, but its main development takes place after puberty. In early life, it extends backward into the presellar area and subsequently expands into the area below and behind the sella turcica, reaching its full size during adolescence. As the sinus enlarges, it may partially encircle the optic canals. When the sinus is exceptionally large, it extends into the roots of the pterygoid processes or greater wing of the sphenoid bone and may even extend into the basilar part of the occipital bone. As age advances, the sinus frequently undergoes further enlargement associated with absorption of its bony walls. Occasionally, gaps exist in its bony wall, with the mucous membrane lying directly against the dura mater.

There are three types of sphenoid sinus in the adult: conchal, presellar, and sellar, depending on the extent to which the sphenoid bone is pneumatized (Fig. 3.2). In the conchal type the area below the sella is a solid block of bone without an air cavity. In the presellar type of sphenoid sinus, the air cavity does not penetrate beyond a vertical plane parallel to the anterior sellar wall. The sellar type of sphenoid sinus is the most common, and here the air cavity extends into the body of sphenoid below the sella and as far posteriorly as the clivus. In our previous study in adult cadavers, this sinus was of the presellar type in 24% and of the sellar type in 75% (8). In the conchal type, which is infrequent in the adult, the thickness of bone separating the sella from the sphenoid sinus is at least 10 mm.

The septae within the sphenoid sinus vary greatly in size, shape, thickness, location, completeness, and relation to the sellar floor (Fig. 3.3). The cavities within the sinus are seldom symmetric from side to side and are often subdivided by irregular minor septae. The septae are often located off the midline as they cross the floor of the sella. In our previous study, a single major septum separated the sinus into two large cavities in only 68% of specimens, and even in these cases the septae were often located off the midline or were deflected to one side (8). The most common type of sphenoid sinus has multiple small cavities in the large paired sinuses. The smaller cavities are separated by septae oriented in all directions. Computed tomography or magnetic resonance imaging of the sella provide the definition of the relationship of the septae to the floor of the sella needed for transsphenoidal surgery. Major septae may be found as far as 8 mm off the midline (8).

The carotid artery frequently produces a serpiginous prominence into the sinus wall below the floor and along the anterior margin of the sella (8, 9) (Figs. 3.4 and 3.5). Usually, the optic canals protrude into the superolateral portion of the sinus, and the second division of the trigeminal nerve protrudes into the inferolateral part. A diverticulum of the sinus, called "the opticocarotid recess," often

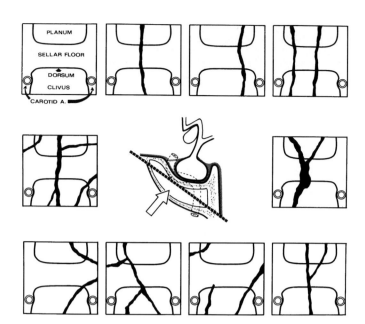

Figure 3.3. Septae in the sphenoid sinus. The *heavy broken line* on the central diagram shows the plane of the section of each specimen from which the drawings were taken, and the *large arrow* shows the direction of view. The planum is above, the dorsum and clivus are below, and the sella is in an intermediate position on each diagram. The *heavy dark lines* on the drawings show the location of the septae in the sphenoid sinus. A variety of septae separate the sinus into cavities that vary in size and shape, seldom being symmetric from side to side. A., artery. (Reprinted with permission from Renn WH, Rhoton AL Jr. Microsurgical anatomy of the sellar region. J Neurosurg 1975;43: 288–298.)

projects laterally between the optic canal and the carotid prominence.

Removing the mucosa and bone from the lateral wall of the sinus exposes the dura mater covering the medial surface of the cavernous sinus and optic canals (Figs. 3.4 and 3.5). Opening this dura exposes the carotid arteries and optic and trigeminal nerves within the sinus. The abducent nerve is located between the lateral side of the carotid artery and the medial side of the first trigeminal division. The second and third trigeminal divisions are seen in the lower margin of the opening through the lateral wall of sphenoid sinus. In half of the cases, the optic and trigeminal nerves and the carotid arteries have areas in which bone 0.5 mm or less in thickness separates them from the mucosa of the sphenoid sinus; in a few cases, the bone separating these structures from the sinus is absent (8, 9). The absence of such bony protection within the walls of the sinus may explain some of the cases of cranial nerve deficits and carotid artery injury after transsphenoidal operations (10). The bone is often thinner over the carotid arteries than over the anterior margin of the pituitary gland.

Diaphragma Sellae

The diaphragma sellae forms the roof of the sella turcica. It covers the pituitary gland, except for a small central

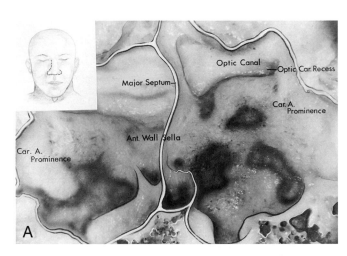

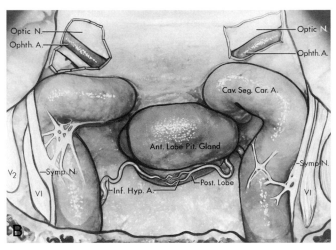

Figure 3.4. Transnasal view of the sphenoid sinus and sellar region. **A.** Orientation is as shown in the insert. Anterior view into a sphenoid sinus with the mucosa removed. The structures in the exposure include the major sphenoidal septum, anterior sellar wall (*Ant. Wall Sella*), and the bony prominences over the carotid artery (*Car. A. Prominence*) and optic canal. The optico-carotid recess (*Optic Car. Recess*) is located between the carotid artery and the optic nerve. **B.** The bone of the skull base has been removed, showing the cavernous segment of the carotid arteries (*Cav. Seg. Car. A.*), the anterior (*Ant. Lobe*) and posterior (*Post. Lobe*) lobes of the pituitary (*Pit.*) gland, and the sympathetic (*Symp. N.*) and abducent (*VI*) nerves. *N.*, nerve; *Ophth. A.*, ophthalmic artery; *Inf. Hyp. A.*, inferior hypophyseal artery; V_1 and V_2, branches of the trigeminal nerve. (Reprinted with permission from Inoue T, Rhoton AL Jr, Theele D, Barry ME. Surgical approaches to the cavernous sinus: a microsurgical study. Neurosurgery 1990;26:903–932.)

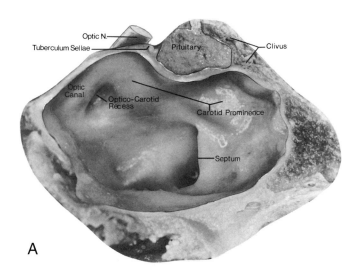

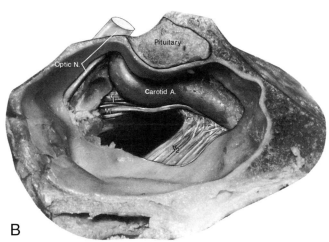

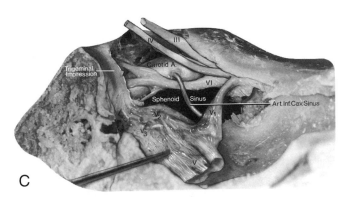

Figure 3.5. Stepwise dissection of the lateral wall of the right half of a sellar-type sphenoid sinus. **A.** The opticocarotid recess separates the carotid prominence and the optic canal. The optic nerve (*Optic N.*) is exposed proximal to the optic canal. The septum in the posterior part of the sinus is incomplete. **B.** The dura has been opened to expose the carotid artery (*Carotid A.*), the optic nerve in the optic canal, the second trigeminal division below the carotid artery, and the abducens nerve (*VI*) between the first trigeminal division (V_1) and the carotid artery. **C.** The trigeminal nerve has been reflected forward to expose the carotid artery, the trigeminal impression, the artery of the inferior cavernous sinus (*Art. Inf. Cav. Sinus*), and the abducens nerve, which splits into three bundles as it passes around the carotid artery. (Reprinted with permission from Fujii K, Chambers SM, Rhoton AL Jr. Neurovascular relationships of the sphenoid sinus: a microsurgical study. J Neurosurg 1978;50:31–39.)

Figure 3.6. Superior view of the sellar region. The ophthalmic artery arises below the optic nerve. The dorsum was removed to expose the posterior lobe of the pituitary. The meningohypophyseal trunk arises from the carotid artery and gives rise to the inferior hypophyseal, tentorial, and dorsal meningeal arteries. Cranial nerve VI (*CN VI*) receives a branch from the dorsal meningeal artery. The oculomotor nerve (*CN III*) passes through a dural ostium in the roof of the cavernous sinus. *A.*, artery. (Reprinted with permission from Harris FS, Rhoton AL Jr. Anatomy of the cavernous sinus: a microsurgical study. J Neurosurg 1976; 45:169–180.)

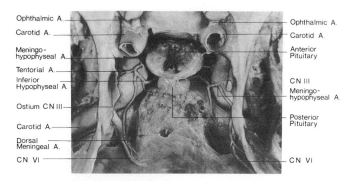

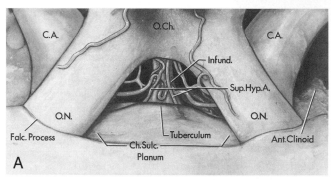

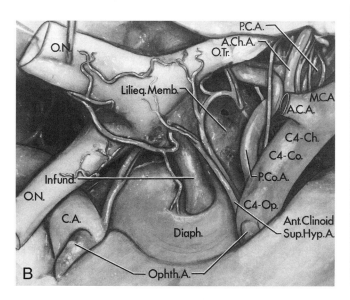

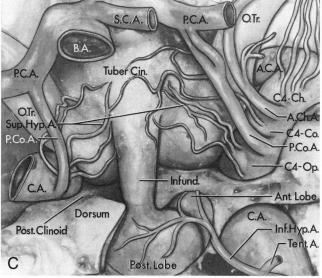

Figure 3.7. Relationships in the sellar and suprasellar areas. **A.** Anterior view. The optic nerves (*O.N.*) enter the optic canals medial to the anterior clinoid processes (*Ant. Clinoid*). The infundibulum (*Infund.*) is exposed below the optic chiasm (*O.Ch.*) and behind the planum sphenoidale, the chiasmatic sulcus (*Ch. Sulc.*), and the tuberculum sellae. The superior hypophyseal arteries (*Sup. Hyp. A.*) pass from the carotid artery (*C.A.*) to the infundibulum. The falciform process (*Falc. Process*) is a fold of dura mater that passes above the optic nerve proximal to the optic foramen. **B.** The optic nerves have been divided and elevated to show the perforating branches of the carotid arteries. The supraclinoid portion of the carotid artery is divided into three segments based on the origin of its major branches: the ophthalmic segment (*C4-Op.*) extends from the origin of the ophthalmic artery (*Ophth. A.*) to the origin of the posterior communicating artery (*P.Co.A.*), the communicating segment (*C4-Co.*) extends from the origin of the posterior communicating artery to the origin of the anterior choroidal artery (*A.Ch.A.*), and the choroidal segment (*C4-Ch.*) extends from the origin of the anterior choroidal artery to the bifurcation of the carotid artery into the anterior (*A.C.A.*) and middle (*M.C.A.*) cerebral arteries. The perforating

branches arising from the ophthalmic segment pass to the optic nerve, chiasm, infundibulum, and floor of the third ventricle. The perforating branches arising from the communicating segment pass to the optic tract (*O.Tr.*) and the floor of the third ventricle. The perforating branches arising from the choroidal segment pass upward and enter the brain through the anterior perforated substance. The diaphragma sellae (*Diaph.*) surrounds the infundibulum above the pituitary gland. Liliequist's membrane (*Lilieq. Memb.*) is situated between the infundibulum and the posterior cerebral arteries (*P.C.A.*). **C.** The right half of the dorsum and the right posterior clinoid process (*Post. Clinoid*) have been removed to expose the anterior (*Ant. Lobe*) and posterior (*Post. Lobe*) lobes of the pituitary gland. The basilar (*B.A.*), posterior cerebral, and superior cerebellar (*S.C.A.*) arteries have been elevated to expose the pituitary stalk and the floor of the third ventricle. The inferior hypophyseal (*Inf. Hyp. A.*) and the tentorial arteries (*Tent. A.*) arise from the carotid artery. *Tuber Cin.*, tuber cinereum. (Reprinted with permission from Gibo H, Lenkey C, Rhoton AL Jr. Microsurgical anatomy of the supraclinoid portion of the internal carotid artery. J Neurosurg 1981;55:560–574.)

opening in its center, which transmits the pituitary stalk (Figs. 3.6 and 3.7). The diaphragma is more rectangular than circular, tends to be convex or concave rather than flat, and is thinner around the infundibulum and somewhat thicker at the periphery. It frequently is a thin, tenuous structure that would not be an adequate barrier for protecting the suprasellar structures during transsphenoidal operation. In a prior anatomic study, Renn and Rhoton found that the diaphragma was at least as thick as one layer of dura in 38% of the cases and in these would furnish an adequate barrier during transsphenoidal hypophysectomy (8). In the remaining 62%, the diaphragma was extremely thin over some portion of the pituitary gland. It was concave when viewed from above in 54% of the specimens, convex in 4%, and flat in 42%.

The opening in its center is large compared with the size of the pituitary stalk. The diaphragmal opening is 5 mm or greater in 56%, and in these cases it would not form a barrier during transsphenoidal pituitary surgery. The opening was round in 54% of the cases and elliptical (with the short diameter of the ellipse oriented in an anteroposterior direction) in 46%. A deficiency of the diaphragma sellae is assumed to be a precondition to formation of an empty sella. An outpouching of the arachnoid protrudes through the central opening in the diaphragma into the sella turcica in about half of the patients. This outpouching represents a potential source of postoperative cerebrospinal fluid leakage (10).

Pituitary Gland

When exposed from above by opening the diaphragma, the superior surface of the posterior lobe of the pituitary gland is lighter in color than the anterior lobe. The anterior lobe wraps around the lower part of the pituitary stalk to form the pars tuberalis (11, 12) (Figs. 3.8 and 3.9). The posterior lobe is more densely adherent to the sellar wall than to the anterior lobe. The gland's width is equal to or greater than either its depth or its length in most patients. Its inferior surface usually conforms to the shape of the sellar floor, but its lateral and superior margins vary in shape because these walls are composed of soft tissue rather than bone. If there is a large opening in the diaphragma, the gland tends to be concave superiorly in the area around the stalk. The superior surface may become triangular as a result of being compressed laterally and posteriorly by the carotid arteries (Fig. 3.6). As the anterior lobe is separated from the posterior lobe, there is a tendency for the pars tuberalis to be retained with the posterior lobe. Intermediate lobe cysts are frequently encountered during separation of the anterior and posterior lobes.

Pituitary Gland and Carotid Artery

The distance separating the medial margin of the carotid artery and the lateral surface of the pituitary gland usually varies from 1 to 3 mm; however, in some cases the artery

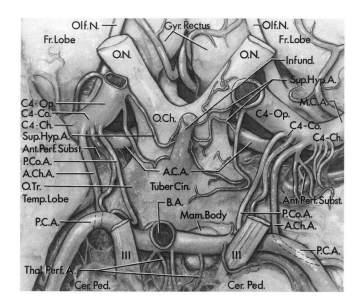

Figure 3.8. Relationships in the sellar and suprasellar areas. Inferior view. The superior hypophyseal arteries (*Sup. Hyp. A.*) pass to the infundibulum (*Infund.*) of the hypophysis. The communicating segment sends one perforating branch on each side to the optic tracts and the region around the mamillary bodies (*Mam. Body*). The choroidal segment sends its perforating branches into the anterior perforated substance (*Ant. Perf. Subst.*). The thalamoperforating arteries (*Thal. Perf. A.*) arise from the basilar artery (*B.A.*). Other structures in the exposure include the temporal (*Temp. Lobe*) and frontal (*Fr. Lobe*) lobes, gyrus rectus (*Gyr. Rectus*), and olfactory nerves (*Olf. N.*). M.C.A., middle cerebral arteries; A.C.A., anterior cerebral arteries; P.C.A., posterior cerebral arteries; Cer. Ped., cerebral peduncle; III, oculomotor nerve; A.Ch.A., anterior choroidal artery; O.Tr., optic tract; C4-Op., ophthalmic segment; C4-Co., communicating segment; C4-Ch., choroidal segment; P.Co.A., posterior communicating artery; O.N., optic nerve; O.Ch., optic chiasm. (Reprinted with permission from Gibo H, Lenkey C, Rhoton AL Jr. Microsurgical anatomy of the supraclinoid portion of the internal carotid artery. J Neurosurg 1981;55:560–574.)

will protrude through the medial wall of the cavernous sinus to indent the gland (5, 8, 13) (Fig. 3.6). Heavy arterial bleeding during transsphenoidal surgery has been reported to be caused by carotid artery injury but may also be caused by a tear in an arterial branch of the carotid artery (e.g., the inferior hypophyseal artery) or by avulsion of a small capsular branch from the carotid artery (10).

If the carotid arteries indent the lateral surfaces of the gland, the gland loses its rounded shape and conforms to the wall of the artery, often developing protrusions above or below the artery. Intrasellar tumors are subjected to the same forces, which prevent them from being spherical, and the increased pressure within the tumor increases the degree to which the tumor insinuates into surrounding crevices and tissue planes. Separation of these extensions from the main mass of gland or tumor may explain cases in which the tumor and elevated pituitary hormone levels persist or recur after the adenoma is removed.

Intracavernous Venous Connections

Venous sinuses may be found in the margins of the diaphragma and around the gland (8). The intercavernous

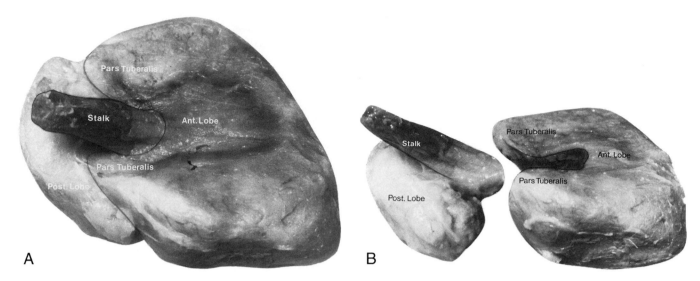

A

B

Figure 3.9.   A. Pituitary gland. Superolateral view. The posterior lobe (*Post. Lobe*) is a lighter color and has a different consistency, being less firm, than the anterior (*Ant.*) lobe. The pars tuberalis partially encircles the stalk. The gland is concave around the stalk. **B.** The anterior and posterior lobes have been separated. The pars tuberalis partially encircles the stalk. (Reprinted with permission from Rhoton AL Jr, Hardy DG, Chambers SM. Microsurgical anatomy and dissection of the sphenoid bone, cavernous sinus and sellar region. Surg Neurol 1979;12: 63–104.)

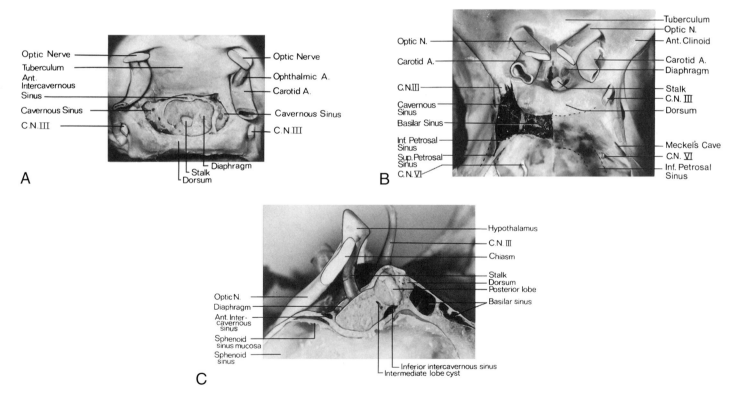

Figure 3.10.   Intercavernous venous connections. A. The ophthalmic artery arises from the superior aspect of the carotid artery and courses laterally beneath the optic nerve to the optic foramen. The dura over the cavernous and anterior (*Ant.*) intercavernous sinuses has been opened to show the venous connection across the midline. *A.,* artery; *C.N.III,* oculomotor nerve. **B.** The basilar sinus connects the posterior portion of the two cavernous sinuses. The dura over the posterior aspect of the left cavernous sinus and the left half of the basilar sinus has been removed. The course of the basilar, inferior (*Inf.*) petrosal, and superior (*Sup.*) petrosal sinuses within the dura is shown by the dotted lines. *C.N.VI,* abducent nerve. **C.** Midsagittal section of the sellar region. The anterior and inferior intercavernous sinuses are small. The basilar sinus, dorsal to the clivus and joining the posterior aspect of the two cavernous sinuses, is the largest connection across the midline. (Reprinted with permission from Renn WH, Rhoton AL Jr. Microsurgical anatomy of the sellar region. J Neurosurg 1975;43:288–298.)

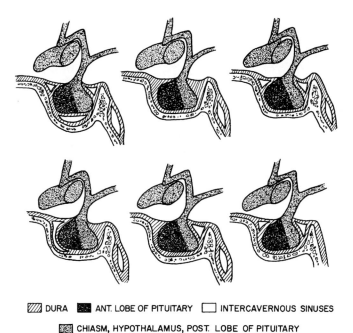

DURA   ANT. LOBE OF PITUITARY   INTERCAVERNOUS SINUSES

CHIASM, HYPOTHALAMUS, POST. LOBE OF PITUITARY

Figure 3.11. Six sagittal sections of the sellar region showing variations in the intercavernous venous connections within the dura. The variations shown include combinations of anterior (*Ant.*), posterior (*Post.*), and inferior intercavernous connections and the frequent presence of a basilar sinus posterior to the dorsum. Either the anterior (*lower center*) or posterior (*lower left*) intercavernous connections or both (*top center*) may be absent. The anterior intercavernous sinus may extend along the whole anterior margin of the gland (*lower left*). The basilar sinus may be absent (*lower right*). (Reprinted with permission from Renn WH, Rhoton AL Jr. Microsurgical anatomy of the sellar region. J Neurosurg 1975;43:288–298.)

connections within the sella are named on the basis of their relationship to the pituitary gland; the anterior intercavernous sinuses pass anterior to the hypophysis, and the posterior intercavernous sinuses pass behind the gland (Figs. 3.10 and 3.11). Actually, these intercavernous connections can occur at any site along the anterior, inferior, or posterior surface of the gland. The anterior sinus is usually larger than the posterior sinus, but either or both may be absent. If the anterior and posterior connections coexist, the whole structure constitutes the "circular sinus." Entering an anterior intercavernous connection that extends downward in front of the gland during transsphenoidal operation may produce brisk bleeding. However, this usually stops with temporary compression of the channel or with light coagulation, which serves to glue the walls of the channel together.

A large intercavernous venous connection called "the basilar sinus" often passes posterior to the dorsum sellae and upper clivus (Figs. 3.10 and 3.11). The basilar sinus connects the posterior aspect of both cavernous sinuses and is usually the largest and most constant intercavernous connection across the midline. The superior and inferior petrosal sinuses join the basilar sinus. The abducent nerve often enters the posterior part of the cavernous sinus by passing through the basilar sinus.

Cavernous Sinus

The cavernous sinus surrounds the horizontal portion of the carotid artery and a segment of the abducent nerve (Figs. 3.5, 3.6, and 3.12). The oculomotor and trochlear nerves and the ophthalmic division of the trigeminal nerve are found in the roof and lateral wall of the sinus (8, 14–16). The lateral wall of the cavernous sinus extends from the superior orbital fissure in front to the apex of the petrous portion of the temporal bone behind. The oculomotor nerve enters the roof of the sinus lateral to the dorsum sellae. The trochlear nerve enters the roof of the sinus posterolateral to the third nerve, and both nerves enter the dura mater immediately below and medial to the free edge of the tentorium. The ophthalmic division enters the low part of the lateral wall of the sinus and runs obliquely upward to pass through the superior orbital fissure. The abducent nerve enters the posterior wall of the sinus by passing through the dura lining the upper clivus and courses forward between the carotid artery medially and the ophthalmic division laterally. It frequently splits into multiple rootlets in its course lateral to the carotid artery.

The branches of the intracavernous portion of the carotid artery are the meningohypophyseal trunk, the artery of the inferior cavernous sinus, and McConnell's capsular arteries (Fig. 3.6). The ophthalmic artery may also take origin from the carotid artery within the sinus in a few patients (8, 15). The most proximal branch of the intracav-

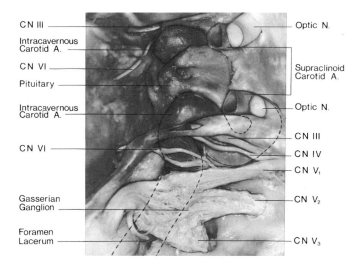

Figure 3.12. Superolateral view of the pituitary gland and right cavernous sinus. The lateral dural wall of the cavernous sinus has been removed. A tortuous carotid artery bulges superiorly. The inferior hypophyseal artery passes to the pituitary gland. Cranial nerves III (*CN III*) and IV (*CN IV*) course in the upper part of the cavernous sinus. Cranial nerve VI (*CN VI*) passes above the trigeminal sensory and motor roots and medial to the first division (*CN V₁*). Further dural removal exposes the trigeminal root and its second (*CN V₂*) and third (*CN V₃*) divisions below the cavernous sinus. The trigeminal root has been displaced laterally to show a second rootlet of cranial nerve VI lateral to the carotid artery. (Reprinted with permission from Harris FS, Rhoton AL Jr. Anatomy of the cavernous sinus: a microsurgical study. J Neurosurg 1976;45:169–180.)

ernous carotid artery, the meningohypophyseal trunk, usually arises below the level of the dorsum sellae near the apex of the curve between the petrous and intracavernous segments of the artery. The three branches of the meningohypophyseal artery are the tentorial artery (of Bernasconi–Cassinari), which courses toward the tentorium; the inferior hypophyseal artery, which courses medially to supply the posterior part of the capsule of the pituitary gland; and the dorsal meningeal artery, which perforates the dura of the posterior wall of the sinus to supply the region of the clivus and the sixth nerve (Figs. 3.4 and 3.6).

The artery of the inferior cavernous sinus, which is also called the inferolateral trunk, originates from the lateral side of the horizontal segment of the carotid artery distal to the origin of the meningohypophyseal trunk (13, 15) (Fig. 3.5C). It passes above the abducent nerve and downward medially to the first trigeminal division to supply the dura of the lateral wall of the sinus. In a few cases it arises from the meningohypophyseal trunk. McConnell's capsular arteries, if present, arise from the medial side of the carotid artery and pass to the capsule of the gland, distal to the point of origin of the artery of the inferior cavernous sinus.

SUPRASELLAR AND THIRD VENTRICULAR REGION

This section deals with neural, arterial, and venous relationships in the suprasellar and third ventricular regions that are important in planning surgery for pituitary adenomas.

Neural Relationships

The third ventricle is located in the center of the head, above the sella turcica, pituitary gland, and midbrain, between the cerebral hemispheres, thalami, and the walls of the hypothalamus and below the corpus callosum and the body of the lateral ventricle (Fig. 3.13). It is intimately related to the circle of Willis and deep venous system of the brain. Manipulation of the walls of the third ventricle may cause hypothalamic dysfunction, as manifested by disturbances of consciousness, temperature control, respiration, and hypophyseal secretion; visual loss owing to damage of the optic chiasm and tracts; and memory loss caused by injury to the columns of the fornix in the walls of the third ventricle (11, 17, 18). The third ventricle is a narrow, funnel-shaped, unilocular, midline cavity with a floor, a roof, and an anterior, posterior, and two lateral walls.

Floor

The floor extends from the optic chiasm anteriorly to the orifice of the aqueduct of Sylvius posteriorly (Figs. 3.13–3.15). The anterior half of the floor is formed by

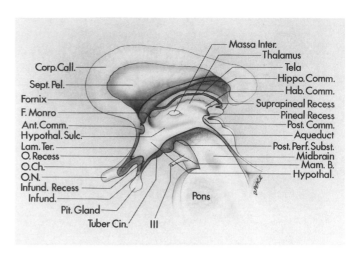

Figure 3.13. Midsagittal section of the third ventricle. The floor extends from the optic chiasm (*O.Ch.*) to the aqueduct of Sylvius and includes the lower surface of the optic chiasm, infundibulum (*Infund.*), infundibular recess (*Infund. Recess*), pituitary gland (*Pit. Gland*), tuber cinereum (*Tuber Cin.*), mamillary bodies (*Mam. B.*), posterior perforated substance (*Post. Perf. Subst.*), and the part of the midbrain anterior to the aqueduct. The anterior wall extends from the optic chiasm to the foramen of Monro (*F. Monro*) and includes the upper surface of the optic chiasm, optic recess (*O. Recess*), lamina terminalis (*Lam. Ter.*), anterior commissure (*Ant. Comm.*), and foramen of Monro. The roof extends from the foramen of Monro to the suprapineal recess and is formed by the fornix and the layers of the tela choroidea (*Tela*), between which course the internal cerebral veins and the medial posterior choroidal arteries. The hippocampal commissure (*Hippo. Comm.*), corpus callosum (*Corp. Call.*), and septum pellucidum (*Sept. Pel.*) are above the roof. The posterior wall extends from the suprapineal recess to the aqueduct and includes the habenular commissure (*Hab. Comm.*), pineal gland, pineal recess, and posterior commissure (*Post. Comm.*). The oculomotor nerve (*III*) exits from the midbrain. The hypothalamic sulcus (*Hypothal. Sulc.*) forms a groove between the thalamic and hypothalamic (*Hypothal.*) surfaces of the third ventricle. *Massa Inter.*, massa intermedia; *O.N.*, optic nerve. (Reprinted with permission from Yamamoto I, Rhoton AL Jr, Peace DA. Microsurgery of the third ventricle: part 1. microsurgical anatomy. Neurosurgery 1981;8:334–356.)

diencephalic structures, and the posterior half is formed by mesencephalic structures.

When viewed inferiorly, the structures forming the floor from anterior to posterior include the optic chiasm, infundibulum of the hypothalamus, tuber cinereum, mamillary bodies, posterior perforated substance, and (most posteriorly) the part of the tegmentum of the midbrain located above the medial aspect of the cerebral peduncles. The optic chiasm is located at the junction of the floor and the anterior wall. The lower surface of the chiasm forms the anterior part of the floor, and the superior surface forms the lower part of the anterior wall. The optic tracts arise from the posterolateral margin of the chiasm and course obliquely away from the floor toward the lateral margin of the midbrain. The infundibulum, tuber cinereum, mamillary bodies, and posterior perforated substance are located in the space limited anteriorly and laterally by the optic chiasm and tracts and posteriorly by the cerebral peduncles.

The infundibulum of the hypothalamus is a hollow, funnel-shaped structure located between the optic chiasm and the tuber cinereum. The pituitary gland (hypophysis) is attached to the infundibulum, and the axons in the infundibulum extend to the posterior lobe of the hypophysis. The tuber cinereum is a prominent mass of hypothalamic gray matter located anterior to the mamillary bodies. The tuber cinereum merges anteriorly into the infundibulum. The tuber cinereum, around the base of the infundibulum, is raised to form a prominence called the median eminence. The mamillary bodies form paired, round prominences posterior to the tuber cinereum. The posterior perforated substance is a depressed, punctated area of gray matter lo-

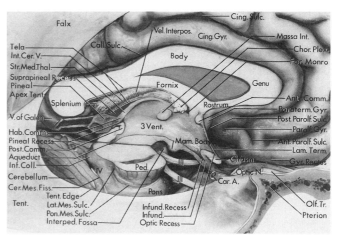

Figure 3.15. Suprasellar and third ventricular (*3 Vent.*) regions. The right cerebral hemisphere has been removed to expose all of the third ventricle. The optic recess extends inferiorly between the optic chiasm and the lamina terminalis (*Lam. Term.*), and the infundibular recess (*Infund. Recess*) extends into the infundibulum behind the chiasm. The layer of tela choroidea that forms the upper wall of the velum interpositum (*Vel. Interpos.*) is adherent to the lower margin of the body and crus of the fornix. The layer of tela choroidea that forms the lower wall of the velum interpositum is attached anteriorly to the striae medullaris thalami (*Str. Med. Thal.*) and posteriorly to the superior margin of the pineal body. The striae medullaris thalami extend forward from the habenular commissure (*Hab. Comm.*) along the superomedial margin of the thalamus. Other structures in the exposure include the interpeduncular fossa (*Interped. Fossa*), tentorial apex (*Apex Tent.*), internal cerebral vein (*Int. Cer. V.*), lateral mesencephalic (*Lat. Mes. Sulc.*) and pontomesencephalic (*Pont. Mes. Sulc.*) sulci, posterior commissure (*Post. Comm.*), vein of Galen (*V. of Galen*), trochlear nerve (*IV*), inferior colliculus (*Inf. Coll.*), cerebellomesencephalic fissure (*Cer. Mes. Fiss.*), and anterior (*Ant. Parolf. Sulc.*) and posterior (*Post. Parolf. Sulc.*) parolfactory sulci. *Chor. Plex.*, choroid plexus; *Massa Int.*, massa intermedia; *Ant. Comm.*, anterior commissure; *For. Monro*, foramen of Monro; *Cing. Sulc*, cingulate sulcus; *Cing. Gyr.*, cingulate gyrus; *Call. Sulc.*, callosal sulcus; *Tent. Edge*, tentorial edge; *Ped.*, peduncle; *Paraterm. Gyr.*, paraterminal gyrus; *Car. A.*, internal carotid artery; *Olf. Tr.*, olfactory tract; *III*, oculomotor nerve; *Parolf. Gyr.*, parolfactory gyrus; *Gyr. Rectus*, gyrus rectus. (Reprinted with permission from Ono M, Ono M, Rhoton AL Jr, Barry M. Microsurgical anatomy of the region of the tentorial incisura. J Neurosurg 1984;60:365–399.)

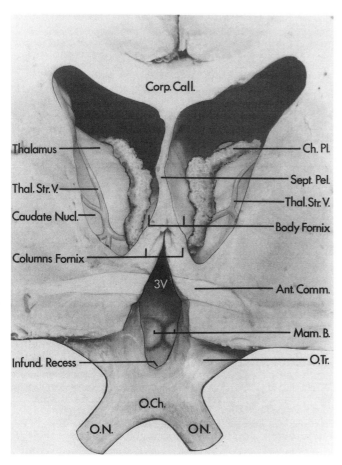

Figure 3.14. Anterosuperior view of the third ventricle. The anterior part of the cerebral hemispheres and part of the anterior wall of the third ventricle have been removed. The optic chiasm (*O.Ch.*) and nerves (*O.N.*) are at the lower margin of the anterior wall. The optic tracts (*O.Tr.*) extend laterally below the floor of the third ventricle (*3V*). The infundibular recess (*Infund. Recess*) extends downward posterior to the optic chiasm and anterior to the mamillary bodies (*Mam. B.*). The midportion of the anterior commissure (*Ant. Comm.*) has been removed to expose the columns of the fornix anterior to the foramina of Monro. The body and columns of the fornix join anterior to the foramina of Monro. The choroid plexus (*Ch.Pl.*) is attached along the cleft between the thalamus and fornix on each side. The thalamostriate veins (*Thal. Str. V.*) course between the caudate nucleus (*Caudate Nucl.*) and the thalamus. Other structures in the exposure include the septum pellucidum (*Sept. Pel.*) and corpus callosum (*Corp. Call.*). (Reprinted with permission from Yamamoto I, Rhoton AL Jr, Peace DA. Microsurgery of the third ventricle: part 1. microsurgical anatomy. Neurosurgery 1981;8:334–356.)

cated in the interval between the mamillary bodies anteriorly and the medial surface of the cerebral peduncles posteriorly. The posterior part of the floor extends posterior and superior to the medial part of the cerebral peduncles and superior to the tegmentum of the midbrain.

When viewed from above and inside the third ventricle, the optic chiasm forms a prominence at the anterior margin of the floor (Figs. 3.14 and 3.15). The infundibular recess extends into the infundibulum behind the optic chiasm. The mamillary bodies form paired prominences on the inner surface of the floor posterior to the infundibular recess. The part of the floor between the mamillary bodies and the aqueduct of Sylvius has a smooth surface, which is concave from side to side. This smooth surface lies above the posterior perforated substance anteriorly and the medial part of the cerebral peduncles and the tegmentum of the midbrain posteriorly.

Anterior Wall

The anterior wall of the third ventricle extends from the foramen of Monro above to the optic chiasm below (Figs. 3.13–3.15). Only the lower two-thirds of the anterior surface is seen on the external surface of the brain; the upper one-third is hidden posterior to the rostrum of the corpus callosum. The part of the anterior wall visible on the surface is formed by the optic chiasm and the lamina terminalis. The lamina terminalis is a thin sheet of gray matter and pia mater that attaches to the upper surface of the chiasm and stretches upward to fill the interval between the optic chiasm and the rostrum of the corpus callosum.

When viewed from within, the boundaries of the anterior wall superiorly to inferiorly are formed by the columns of the fornix, foramen of Monro, anterior commissure, lamina terminalis, optic recess, and optic chiasm. The opening of the foramen of Monro into each lateral ventricle is located at the junction of the roof and the anterior wall of the third ventricle (Figs. 3.13 and 3.16). The foramen is a ductlike canal that opens between the fornix and the thalamus into each lateral ventricle and extends inferiorly below the fornix into the third ventricle as a single channel. The foramen of Monro is bound anteriorly by the junction of the body and the columns of the fornix and posteriorly by the anterior pole of the thalamus.

Posterior Wall

The posterior wall of the third ventricle extends from the suprapineal recess above to the aqueduct of Sylvius below (Figs. 3.13, 3.14, and 3.16). When viewed from anteriorly within the third ventricle, it consists, from above to below, of the suprapineal recess, the habenular commissure, the pineal body and its recess, the posterior commissure, and the aqueduct of Sylvius.

Roof

The roof of the third ventricle forms a gentle upward arch, extending from the foramen of Monro anteriorly to the suprapineal recess posteriorly (Figs. 3.13, 3.15, and 3.16). It is infrequent that pituitary adenomas are approached through the roof of the third ventricle; however, other tumors involving the third ventricle are approached from above. The roof has four layers: one neural layer formed by the fornix, two thin membranous layers of tela choroidea, and a layer of blood vessels between the two sheets of tela choroidea (Figs. 3.15 and 3.16).

The upper, or neural, layer is formed by the fornix. The upper layer of the anterior part of the roof of the third ventricle is formed by the body of the fornix, and the posterior part of the roof is formed by the crura and the hippocampal commissure. The body of the fornix splits into two columns at the anterior margin of the opening of each foramen of Monro into the lateral ventricle. The columns de-

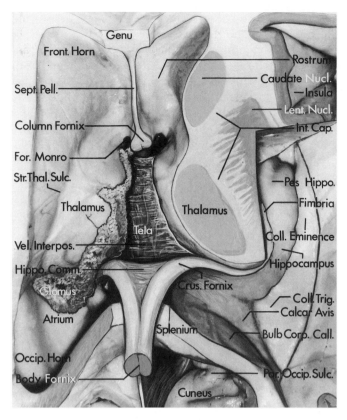

Figure 3.16. Neural relationships. Superior view. The upper part of the cerebral hemispheres have been removed to expose the lateral ventricles and the roof of the third ventricle. The upper part of the roof of the third ventricle is formed by the body and crus of the fornix (*Crus. Fornix*). The columns of the fornix pass anterior and superior to the foramen of Monro (*For. Monro*). The fornix has been divided at the junction of its body and the columns above the foramen of Monro and reflected backward to expose the velum interpositum (*Vel. Interpos.*) located between the layers of tela choroidea (*Tela*) in the roof of the third ventricle. Other structures in the exposure include the pes hippocampus (*Pes Hipp.*), collateral eminence (*Coll. Eminence*), and hippocampal commissure (*Hipp. Comm.*). *Sept. Pell.,* septum pellucidum; *Str. Thal. Sulc.,* striothalamic sulcus; *Occip. Horn,* occipital horn; *Caudate Nucl.,* caudate nucleus; *Lent. Nucl.,* lenticular nucleus; *Bulb Corp. Call.,* bulb of corpus callosum; *Par. Occip. Sulc.,* parieto-ocipital sulcus; *Coll. Trig.,* collateral trigone; *Int. Cap.,* internal capsule. (Reprinted with permission from Ono M, Rhoton AL Jr, Peace DA, et al. Microsurgical anatomy of the deep venous system of the brain. Neurosurgery 1984;15: 621–657.)

scend in the lateral walls of the third ventricle and terminate in the mamillary bodies.

The tela choroidea forms two of the three layers in the roof below the layer formed by the fornix (Figs. 3.15 and 3.16). The tela choroidea consists of two thin, semiopaque membranes derived from pia mater, which are interconnected by loosely organized trabeculae. The final layer in the roof is a vascular layer located between the two layers of tela choroidea. The vascular layer consists of the medial posterior choroidal arteries and their branches and the internal cerebral veins and their tributaries. Parallel strands of choroid plexus project downward on each side of the midline from the inferior layer of tela choroidea into the superior part of the third ventricle.

The velum interpositum is the space between the two layers of tela choroidea in the roof of the third ventricle. The upper layer of the tela choroidea is attached to the lower surface of the fornix and the hippocampal commissure (Figs. 3.15 and 3.16). The lower wall is attached to the teniae thalami, small ridges on the free edge of a fiber tract, the striae medullaris thalami, which extends along the superomedial border of the thalamus from the foramen of Monro to the habenular commissure. The posterior part of the lower wall is attached to the superior surface of the pineal body. The internal cerebral veins arise in the anterior part of the velum interpositum, just behind the foramen of Monro, and they exit the velum interpositum above the pineal body to enter the quadrigeminal cistern and join the great vein. The velum interpositum is usually a closed space that tapers to a narrow apex just behind the foramen of Monro, but it may infrequently have an opening situated between splenium and the pineal body that communicates with the quadrigeminal cistern to form the cisterna velum interpositum.

Lateral Wall

The lateral walls are not visible on the external surface of the brain but hidden between the cerebral hemispheres (Figs. 3.13 and 3.15). They are formed by the hypothalamus inferiorly and the thalamus superiorly. The lateral walls have an outline like the lateral silhouette of a bird's head with an open beak. The head is formed by the oval medial surface of the thalamus; the open beaks, which project anteriorly and inferiorly, are represented by the recesses in the hypothalamus. The pointed upper beak is formed by the optic recess and the lower beak is formed by the infundibular recess. The hypothalamic and thalamic surfaces are separated by the hypothalamic sulcus, a groove that is often ill-defined and extends from the foramen of Monro to the aqueduct of Sylvius. The superior limit of the thalamic surfaces of the third ventricle is marked by narrow, raised ridges, known as the striae medullaris thalami. These striae extend forward from the habenulae along the superomedial surface of the thalamus at the site of the attachment of the lower layer of the tela choroidea.

The massa intermedia projects into the upper one-half of the third ventricle and often connects the opposing surfaces of the thalamus. The massa intermedia was present in 76% of the brains examined and was located 2.5 to 6.0 mm (average, 3.9 mm) posterior to the foramen of Monro (18). The columns of the fornix form distinct prominences in the lateral walls of the third ventricle just below the foramen of Monro, but inferiorly they sink below the surface.

Suprasellar Cisterns and Tentorial Incisura

The suprasellar region is commonly approached through the cisterns surrounding the anterior part of the tentorial incisura (19). The incisura is a triangular space situated between the free edges of the tentorium. The upper part of the brainstem formed by the midbrain sits in the center of the incisura. The area between the midbrain and the free edges is divided into (a) an anterior incisural space located in front of the midbrain, (b) paired middle incisural spaces situated lateral to the midbrain, and (c) a posterior incisural space located behind the midbrain (Fig. 3.15). Pituitary adenomas commonly involve the anterior incisural space.

The anterior incisural space corresponds roughly to the suprasellar area. From the front of the midbrain it extends obliquely forward and upward around the optic chiasm to the subcallosal area. It opens laterally into the sylvian fissure and posteriorly between the uncus and the brainstem into the middle incisural space (Fig. 3.15).

The part of the anterior incisural space located below the optic chiasm has posterior and posterolateral walls. The posterior wall is formed by the cerebral peduncles. The posterolateral wall is formed by the anterior one-third of the uncus, which hangs over the free edge above the oculomotor nerve. The infundibulum of the pituitary gland crosses the anterior incisural space to reach the opening in the diaphragma sellae. The part of the anterior incisural space situated above the optic chiasm is limited superiorly by the rostrum of the corpus callosum, posteriorly by the lamina terminalis, and laterally by the part of the medial surfaces of the frontal lobes located below the rostrum.

The anterior incisural space opens laterally into the part of the sylvian fissure situated below the anterior perforated substance. The anterior limb of the internal capsule, the head of the caudate nucleus, and the anterior part of the lentiform nucleus are located above the anterior perforated substance. The interpeduncular cistern, which sits in the posterior part of the anterior incisural space between the cerebral peduncles and the dorsum sellae, communicates anteriorly with the chiasmatic cistern, which is located below the optic chiasm. The interpeduncular and chiasmatic cisterns are separated by Liliequist's membrane, an arachnoidal sheet extending from the dorsum sellae to the anterior edge of the mamillary bodies. The chiasmatic cistern communicates around the optic chiasm with the cisterna laminae terminalis, which lies anterior to the lamina terminalis.

Cranial Nerves

The optic and oculomotor nerves and the posterior part of the olfactory tracts pass through the suprasellar region and anterior incisural space (Figs. 3.15 and 3.17). Each olfactory tract runs posteriorly and splits just above the anterior clinoid process to form the medial and lateral olfactory striae, which course along the anterior margin of the anterior perforated substance.

The optic nerves and chiasm and the anterior part of the optic tracts cross the anterior incisural space. The optic nerves emerge from the optic canals medial to the attach-

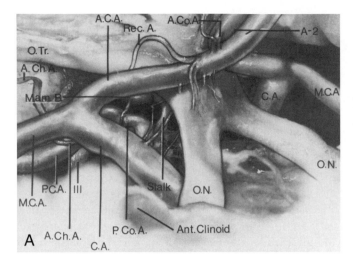

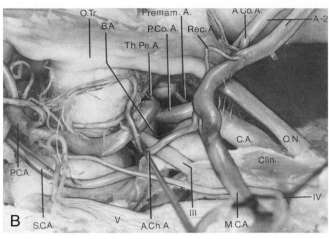

Figure 3.17. Right anterior and lateral views of the suprasellar area. **A.** Right anterolateral view. The anterior clinoid process (*Ant. Clinoid*) and carotid artery (*C.A.*) are lateral to the optic nerve (*O.N.*). Perforating arteries pass from the carotid artery to terminate in the optic chiasm and tract (*O.Tr.*) and the hypothalamus anterior to the mamillary body (*Mam. B.*). The posterior communicating artery (*P.Co.A.*) courses medial to the carotid artery. The anterior choroidal artery (*A.Ch.A.*) arises from the carotid and passes above the posterior cerebral artery (*P.C.A.*). The third nerve (*III*) passes below the posterior cerebral artery. The recurrent artery (*Rec. A.*) arises from the anterior cerebral artery (*A.C.A.*) proximal to the anterior communicating artery (*A.Co.A.*). Other structures in the exposure include the middle cerebral (*M.C.A.*) and distal segment of the anterior cerebral (*A-2*) arteries. **B.** Right lateral view with the temporal lobe removed. The anterior clinoid process (*Clin.*) is lateral to the carotid artery. The premamillary artery (*Premam. A.*) arises from the posterior communicating artery, and the thalamoperforating arteries (*Th. Pe. A.*) arise from the posterior cerebral artery. The third and fourth (*IV*) cranial nerves course between the posterior cerebral and superior cerebellar (*S.C.A.*) arteries. Other structures in the exposure include the trigeminal nerve (*V*) and basilar artery (*B.A.*). (Reprinted with permission from Saeki N, Rhoton AL Jr. Microsurgical anatomy of the upper basilar artery and the posterior circle of Willis. J Neurosurg 1977;46:563–577.)

ment of the free edges to the anterior clinoid processes and are directed posteriorly, superiorly, and medially toward the optic chiasm. From the chiasm, the optic tracts continue in a posterolateral direction around the cerebral peduncles to enter the middle incisural spaces. The optic nerve proximal to its entrance into the optic canal is covered by a reflected leaf of dura mater, the falciform process, which extends medially from the anterior clinoid process across the top of the optic nerve (8). The length of nerve covered by dura only at the intracranial end of the optic canal may vary from less than 1 mm to as great as 1 cm. Coagulation of the dura above the optic nerve just proximal to the optic canal on the assumption that bone separates the dura mater from the nerve could lead to nerve injury. Compression of the optic nerve against the sharp edge of the falciform process may result in a visual field deficit even if the compressing lesion does not damage the nerve enough to cause visual loss. Normally, the optic nerve is separated medially from the sphenoid sinus by a thin layer of bone, but in a few cases this bone is absent and the optic nerves may protrude directly into the sphenoid sinus, separated from the sinus by only mucosa and the dural sheath of the nerve (6, 8).

Optic Chiasm

The relationship of the chiasm to the sella is an important determinant of the ease with which the pituitary fossa can be exposed by the transfrontal surgical route (Fig.

3.18). The normal chiasm overlies the diaphragma sellae and the pituitary gland, the prefixed chiasm overlies the tuberculum sellae, and the postfixed chiasm overlies the dorsum sellae. In approximately 70% of cases, the chiasm is in the normal position. Of the remaining 30%, about half are prefixed and half postfixed (8).

A prominent tuberculum sellae may restrict access to the sellae even in the presence of a normal chiasm. The tuberculum may vary from being almost flat to protruding upward as much as 3 mm, and it may project posteriorly to the margin of a normal chiasm (8).

A prefixed chiasm, a normal chiasm with a small area between the tuberculum and the chiasm, and a superior protruding tuberculum sellae do not limit exposure by the transsphenoidal approach but they limit the access to the suprasellar area provided by the transcranial approach. There are several methods of gaining access to the suprasellar area when these variants are present. One is to expose the sphenoid sinus from above by an opening through the tuberculum and planum sphenoidale, thus converting the approach to a transfrontal–transsphenoidal exposure. If the chiasm is prefixed and the tumor is seen through a thin, stretched anterior wall of the third ventricle, the lamina terminalis may be opened to expose the tumor, but this exposure is infrequently used for pituitary adenomas. If the space between the carotid artery and the optic nerve has been enlarged (e.g., by a lateral or parasellar extension of tumor), the tumor may be removed through this space (11, 17).

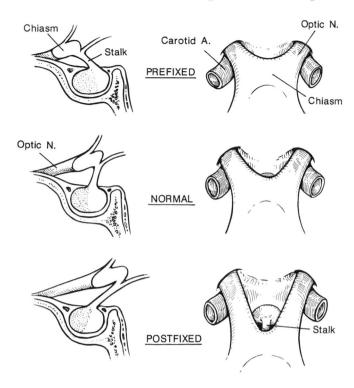

Figure 3.18. Sagittal sections and superior views of the sellar region showing the optic nerve (*Optic N.*) and chiasm and the carotid artery (*Carotid A.*). The prefixed chiasm is located above the tuberculum. The normal chiasm is located above the diaphragma. The postfixed chiasm is situated above the dorsum.

An understanding of the relationship of the carotid artery, optic nerve, and anterior clinoid process is fundamental to all surgical approaches to the sellar and parasellar areas (Fig. 3.18). The carotid artery and the optic nerve are medial to the anterior clinoid process. The artery exits the cavernous sinus beneath and slightly lateral to the optic nerve. The optic nerve pursues a posteromedial course toward the chiasm and the carotid artery pursues a posterolateral course toward its bifurcation into the anterior and middle cerebral arteries.

Arterial Relationships

The arterial relationships in the suprasellar area are among the most complex in the head because this area contains all the components of the circle of Willis (Figs. 3.7, 3.8, and 3.17). Numerous arteries including the internal carotid and basilar arteries and the circle of Willis and its branches may be stretched around tumors in this area. The posterior part of the circle of Willis and the apex of the basilar artery are located in the anterior incisural space below the floor of the third ventricle; the anterior part of the circle of Willis and the anterior cerebral and anterior communicating arteries are intimately related to the anterior wall of the third ventricle; both the anterior and posterior cerebral arteries send branches into the roof of the third ventricle. The internal carotid, anterior choroidal, anterior and posterior cerebral, and anterior and posterior

communicating arteries give rise to perforating branches that reach the walls of the third ventricle and anterior incisional space. All the arterial components of the circle of Willis and the adjacent segments of the carotid and basilar arteries and their perforating branches may be stretched around suprasellar extensions of pituitary tumors (20–24). Arterial lesions at the anterior part of the circle of Willis are more likely to result in disturbances in memory and personality, and those at the posterior part of the circle are more likely to result in disorders of the level of consciousness and are frequently combined with disorders of extraocular motion (23, 24).

Internal Carotid Artery

The internal carotid artery exits the cavernous sinus along the medial surface of the anterior clinoid process to reach the anterior incisural space (Figs. 3.8, 3.9, and 3.18). After entering this space it courses posterior, superior, and lateral to reach the site of its bifurcation below the anterior perforated substance. It is first below and then lateral to the optic nerve and chiasm. It sends perforating branches to the optic nerve, chiasm, and tract and to the floor of the third ventricle. These branches pass across the interval between the internal carotid artery and the optic nerve and may serve as an obstacle to the operative approaches directed through the triangular space between the internal carotid artery, the optic nerve, and the anterior cerebral artery. The internal carotid artery also gives off the superior hypophyseal artery, which runs medially below the floor of the third ventricle to reach the tuber cinereum and joins its mate of the opposite side to form a ring around the infundibulum (21) (Figs. 3.7 and 3.8).

The supraclinoid (C_4) portion of the internal carotid artery is divided into three segments based on the origin of its major branches. The ophthalmic segment extends from the origin of the ophthalmic artery to the origin of the posterior communicating artery; the communicating segment extends from the origin of the posterior communicating artery to the origin of the anterior choroidal artery; and the choroidal segment extends from the origin of the anterior choroidal artery to the bifurcation (21) (Figs. 3.7 and 3.8). Each segment gives off a series of perforating branches with a relatively constant site of termination. The branches arising from the ophthalmic segment pass to the optic nerve and chiasm, the infundibulum, and the floor of the third ventricle. The branches arising from the communicating segment pass to the optic tract and the floor of the third ventricle. The branches arising from the choroidal segment pass upward and enter the brain through the anterior perforated substance.

Ophthalmic Artery

The ophthalmic artery is the first branch of the internal carotid artery above the cavernous sinus (Figs. 3.7 and 3.8). It arises and enters the optic canal below the optic nerve. Its origin and proximal segment may be visible below the optic nerve without retracting the nerve, although elevation of the optic nerve away from the carotid artery is usually required to see the segment proximal to the optic foramen. The artery arises from the supraclinoid segment of the carotid artery in most patients, but it may also arise within the cavernous sinus or be absent (8, 13, 15).

Posterior Communicating Artery

The posterior communicating artery arises from the posterior wall of the internal carotid artery and courses posteromedially below the optic tracts and the floor of the third ventricle to join the posterior cerebral artery (Figs.

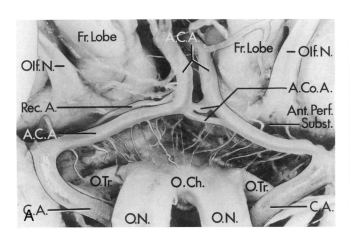

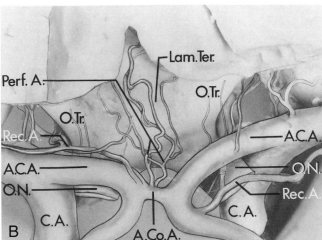

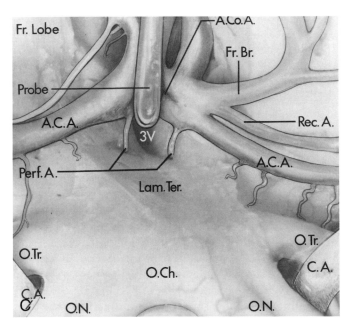

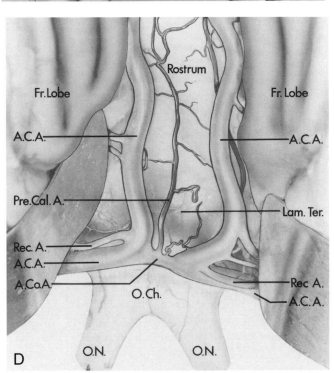

Figure 3.19. Arteries of the anterior wall of the third ventricle. Anterior views. **A.** The anterior cerebral arteries give rise to perforating branches that enter the upper surface of the optic chiasm (*O.Ch.*). The recurrent arteries (*Rec. A.*) arise from the anterior cerebral arteries (*A.C.A.*) near the level of the anterior communicating artery (*A.Co.A.*). Other structures in the exposure include the optic nerves (*O.N.*) and tracts (*O.Tr.*), frontal lobes (*Fr. Lobe*), anterior perforated substance (*Ant. Perf. Subst.*), and olfactory nerves (*Olf.N.*). *C.A.,* carotid artery. **B.** The anterior communicating artery gives rise to a series of perforating arteries (*Perf. A.*) that enter the region of the lamina terminalis (*Lam. Ter.*). **C.** A probe elevates the anterior communicating artery to expose two perforating arteries that pass through the lamina terminalis to reach the walls of the third ventricle (*3V*). The left recurrent artery arises in a common trunk with a branch to the frontal lobe (*Fr. Br.*). **D.** A precallosal artery (*Pre.Cal.A.*) arises from the anterior communicating artery and passes upward on the lamina terminalis to reach the rostrum of the corpus callosum. (Reprinted with permission from Yamamoto I, Rhoton AL Jr, Peace DA. Microsurgery of the third ventricle: part 1. microsurgical anatomy. Neurosurgery 1981;8:334–356.)

3.7, 3.8, and 3.17). Its branches penetrate the floor between the optic chiasm and the cerebral peduncle and reach the thalamus, hypothalamus, subthalamus, and internal capsule. Its posterior course varies depending on whether the artery provides the major supply to the distal posterior cerebral artery. If it is normal, with the posterior cerebral artery arising predominantly from the basilar artery, it is directed posteromedially above the oculomotor nerve toward the interpeduncular fossa (24, 25). If the posterior cerebral artery has a fetal type configuration in which it arises from the carotid artery, the posterior communicating artery is directed posterolaterally below the optic tract. The oculomotor nerve pierces the dura mater of the roof of the cavernous sinus 2 to 7 mm (average 5 mm) posterior to the initial supraclinoid segment of the carotid artery (12, 13).

Anterior Choroidal Artery

The anterior choroidal artery arises from the posterior surface of the internal carotid artery 0.1 to 3.0 mm above the origin of the posterior communicating artery (Figs. 3.7, 3.8, and 3.17). It is directed posterolaterally below the optic tract between the uncus and the cerebral peduncle. It passes through the choroidal fissure behind the uncus to supply the choroid plexus in the temporal horn. It sends branches into the optic tract and the posterior part of the floor that reach the optic radiations, globus pallidus, internal capsule, midbrain, and thalamus (3, 9).

Anterior Cerebral and Anterior Communicating Arteries

The anterior cerebral artery arises from the internal carotid artery below the anterior perforated substance and courses anteromedially above the optic nerve and chiasm to reach the interhemispheric fissure, where it is joined to the opposite anterior cerebral artery by the anterior communicating artery (23, 26) (Figs. 3.7, 3.8, 3.17, 3.19, and 3.20). The junction of the anterior communicating artery with the right and left A$_1$ segments is usually above the chiasm rather than above the optic nerves. In our studies, 70% were above the chiasm and 30% were in a prefixed position above the optic nerves (2, 8). The shorter A$_1$ segments are stretched tightly over the chiasm, and the larger ones pass anteriorly over the nerves. Displacement of the chiasm against these arteries may result in visual loss before that caused by direct compression of the visual pathways by the tumor. The arteries with a more forward course are often tortuous and elongated, and some may course forward and rest on the tuberculum sellae or planum sphenoidale. The anterior cerebral artery ascends in front of the lamina terminalis and the anterior wall of the third ventricle and passes around the corpus callosum.

The anterior cerebral and anterior communicating arteries give rise to perforating branches that terminate in the whole anterior wall of the third ventricle and reach the adjacent parts of the hypothalamus, fornix, septum pellucidum, and striatum (23, 26) (Figs. 3.7, 3.19, and 3.20). A precallosal artery may originate from the anterior cerebral

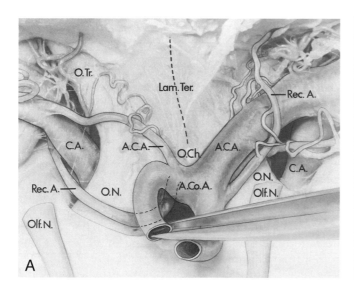
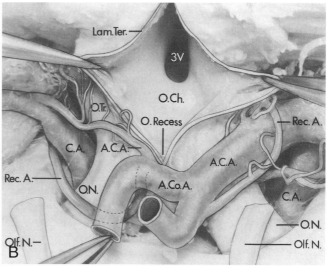

Figure 3.20. Anterior cerebral arteries and the lamina terminalis. **A.** The anterior cerebral (*A.C.A.*), recurrent (*Rec. A.*), and anterior communicating (*A.Co.A.*) arteries have been retracted to expose the lamina terminalis (*Lam. Ter.*). Other structures in the exposure include the optic nerves (*O.N.*), chiasm (*O.Ch.*), and tracts (*O.Tr.*) and the olfactory nerves (*Olf. N.*). The right anterior cerebral artery is hypoplastic. *C.A.,* carotid artery. **B.** The lam- ina terminalis has been opened along the dotted line shown in **A** to expose the cavity of the third ventricle (*3V*). The optic recess (*O. Recess*) extends downward between the lamina terminalis and the superior surface of the optic chiasm. (Reprinted with permission from Yamamoto I, Rhoton AL Jr, Peace DA. Microsurgery of the third ventricle: part 1. microsurgical anatomy. Neurosurgery 1981;8:334–356.)

or the anterior communicating artery, run upward across the lamina terminalis, and send branches into the anterior wall of the third ventricle (Fig. 3.19).

The recurrent branch of the anterior cerebral artery, which is referred to as the recurrent artery of Heubner, is encountered frequently in approaches to the anterior part of the third ventricle (Figs. 3.17, 3.19, and 3.20). It arises from the anterior cerebral artery in the region of the anterior communicating artery, courses laterally above the bifurcation of the internal carotid artery, and enters the anterior perforated substance (23, 27). The recurrent artery courses anterior to the A_1 segment of the anterior cerebral artery and would be seen when elevating the frontal lobe before visualizing the A_1 segment in about two-thirds of cases. Of the remaining one-third, most course superior to A_1. Some of its branches reach the anterior limb and genu of the internal capsule.

Posterior Cerebral Artery

The bifurcation of the basilar artery into the posterior cerebral arteries is located in the posterior part of the suprasellar area below the posterior half of the floor of the third ventricle (24, 25) (Figs. 3.7, 3.8, and 3.17). A high basilar bifurcation may indent the floor. The posterior cerebral artery courses laterally around the cerebral peduncle, above the oculomotor nerve, and passes between the uncus and the cerebral peduncle to reach the quadrigeminal cistern. Its branches reach the floor, roof, and posterior and lateral walls of the third ventricle.

The thalamoperforating arteries are a pair of larger perforating branches that arise from the posterior cerebral artery in the sellar region (Figs. 3.8 and 3.17). The thalamoperforating arteries arise from the proximal part of the posterior cerebral arteries and the posterior part of the posterior communicating arteries and enter the brain through the posterior part of the floor and the lateral walls. Infarction in the distribution of the thalamoperforating branches of the posterior cerebral artery may cause coma and death after the removal of a suprasellar tumor.

The medial posterior choroidal arteries also arise from the proximal portions of the posterior cerebral arteries in the suprasellar area and course around the midbrain to reach the quadrigeminal cistern (3, 9) (Fig. 3.14). They turn forward at the side of the pineal body to reach the velum interpositum and supply the choroid plexus in the roof of the third ventricle and the body of the lateral ventricle.

Venous Relationships

The deep cerebral venous system is intimately related to the walls of the third ventricle (19, 28) (Fig. 3.21). However, the veins do not pose a formidable obstacle to operative approaches to the suprasellar area and anterior third ventricle as they do in the region of the posterior third

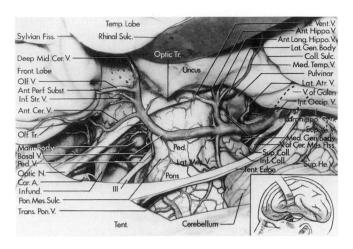

Figure 3.21. Veins in the suprasellar region. Lateral view. Left side. The veins draining the suprasellar area converge on the anterior end of the basal vein (*Basal V.*). The temporal (*Temp. Lobe*) and frontal (*Front. Lobe*) lobes have been elevated, as shown in the inset. The basal vein arises below the anterior perforated substance (*Ant. Perf. Subst.*), passes around the cerebral peduncle (*Ped.*), and joins the vein of Galen (*V. of Galen; dashed lines*). The veins joining the anterior end of the basal vein include the olfactory veins (*Olf. V.*), which pass along the olfactory tract (*Olf. Tr.*); the inferior striate veins (*Inf. Str. V.*), which descend through the anterior perforated substance; the deep middle cerebral veins (*Deep Mid. Cer. V.*), which pass medially from the sylvian fissure (*Sylvian Fiss.*); and the anterior cerebral veins (*Ant. Cer. V.*), which pass across the optic chiasm. Other veins in the exposure include the peduncular (*Ped. V.*), lateral mesencephalic (*Lat. Mes. V.*), inferior ventricular (*Inf. Vent. V.*), anterior hippocampal (*Ant. Hippo. V.*), anterior longitudinal hippocampal (*Ant. Long. Hippo. V.*), medial temporal (*Med. Temp. V.*), lateral atrial (*Lat. Atr. V.*), internal occipital (*Int. Occip. V.*), transverse pontine (*Trans. Pon. V.*), superior vermian (*Sup. Ve. V.*), and superior hemispheric (*Sup. He. V.*) veins and the vein of the cerebellomesencephalic fissure (*V. of Cer. Mes. Fiss.*). Other structures in the exposure include the optic nerve (*Optic N.*) and tract (*Optic. Tr.*); carotid artery (*Car. A.*); lateral geniculate body (*Lat. Gen. Body*); infundibulum (*Infund.*); mamillary bodies (*Mam. Body*); tentorium (*Tent.*); tentorial edge (*Tent. Edge*); oculomotor nerve (*III*); parahippocampal (*Parahippo. Gyr.*), collateral (*Coll. Sulc.*), rhinal (*Rhinal Sulc.*), and pontomesencephalic (*Pon. Mes. Sulc.*) sulci; and superior (*Sup. Coll.*) and inferior (*Inf. Coll.*) colliculi. *Med. Gen. Body*, medial geniculate body. (Reprinted with permission from Ono M, Rhoton AL Jr, Peace DA, et al. Microsurgical anatomy of the deep venous system of the brain. Neurosurgery 1984;15:621–657.)

ventricle because the veins in the suprasellar region are small.

The suprasellar area is drained, almost totally, by tributaries of the basal vein (19, 28). The basal veins are formed by the union of veins draining the suprasellar area and proceed posteriorly between the midbrain and the temporal lobes to empty into the internal cerebral or great vein (Fig. 3.21). The veins joining below the anterior perforated substance to form the basal vein include the olfactory vein, which runs posteriorly in the olfactory sulcus; the fronto-orbital vein, which courses along the orbital surface of the frontal lobe; the deep middle cerebral vein, which receives the veins from the insula and passes medially across the limen insulae; the uncal veins, which course medially from the uncus; and the anterior cerebral vein, which descends on the lamina terminalis and crosses the optic chiasm to reach the basal vein. The paired anterior cerebral veins are joined across the midline above the optic chiasm by the anterior communicating vein and receive the paraterminal veins from the paraterminal and parolfactory gyri and the anterior pericallosal veins from the rostrum and genu of the corpus callosum (Fig. 3.21).

The veins on the surface of the brainstem that form the posterior wall of the anterior incisural space are divided into transversely and vertically oriented groups (19, 28). The transverse veins are the peduncular vein, which passes horizontally around the anterior surface of the cerebral peduncle and terminates in the basal vein, and the vein of the pontomesencephalic sulcus, which courses below the peduncular vein in the pontomesencephalic sulcus.

The vertically oriented veins on the posterior wall of the anterior incisural space are the median anterior pontomesencephalic vein, which courses in the midline and connects the peduncular veins above with the pontine veins below, and the lateral anterior pontomesencephalic veins, which course on the anterolateral surface of the cerebral peduncle and the pons and join the basal vein superiorly and the vein of the pontomesencephalic sulcus below.

The internal cerebral veins course in the roof of the third ventricle and are only infrequently involved in pituitary adenomas (Fig. 3.21). They originate just behind the foramen of Monro and course posteriorly within the velum interpositum. They join above or posterior to the pineal body to form the great vein.

REFERENCES

1. Pait TG, Zeal A, Harris FS, et al. Microsurgical anatomy and dissection of the temporal bone. Surg Neurol 1977;8:363–391.
2. Rhoton AL Jr, Harris FS, Renn WH. Microsurgical anatomy of the sellar region and cavernous sinus. Clin Neurosurg 1977;24:54–85.
3. Rhoton AL Jr, Fujii K, Fradd B. Microsurgical anatomy of the anterior choroidal artery. Surg Neurol 1979;12:171–187.
4. Rhoton AL Jr, Maniscalco J. Microsurgery of the sellar region. Neuroophthalmology 1977;9:106–127.
5. Bergland RM, Ray BS, Torack RM. Anatomical variations in the pituitary gland and adjacent structures in 225 human autopsy cases. J Neurosurg 1968;28:93–99.
6. Fujii K, Chambers SM, Rhoton AL Jr. Neurovascular relationships of the sphenoid sinus: a microsurgical study. J Neurosurg 1978;50:31–39.
7. Hardy J. Transsphenoidal hypophysectomy. J Neurosurg 1971;34:582–594.
8. Renn WH, Rhoton AL Jr. Microsurgical anatomy of the sellar region. J Neurosurg 1975;43:288–298.
9. Fujii K, Lenkey C, Rhoton AL Jr. Microsurgical anatomy of the choroidal arteries: lateral and third ventricles. J Neurosurg 1980;52:165–188.
10. Laws ER, Kern EB. Complications of transsphenoidal surgery. Clin Neurosurg 1976;23:401–416.
11. Rhoton AL Jr. Microsurgical anatomy of the region of the third ventricle. In: Apuzzo M, ed. Surgery of the Third Ventricle. Baltimore: Williams & Wilkins, 1987.
12. Rhoton AL Jr, Hardy DG, Chambers SM. Microsurgical anatomy and dissection of the sphenoid bone, cavernous sinus and sellar region. Surg Neurol 1979;12:63–104.
13. Harris FS, Rhoton AL Jr. Anatomy of the cavernous sinus: a microsurgical study. J Neurosurg 1976;45:169–180.
14. Gudmundsson K, Rhoton AL Jr, Rushton JG. Detailed anatomy of the intracranial portion of the trigeminal nerve. J Neurosurg 1971;35:592–600.
15. Inoue T, Rhoton AL Jr, Theele D, et al. Surgical approaches to the cavernous sinus: a microsurgical study. Neurosurgery 1990;26:903–932.
16. Parkinson D. Transcavernous repair of carotid cavernous fistula: a case report. J Neurosurg 1967;26:420–424.
17. Rhoton AL Jr, Yamamoto I, Peace DA. Microsurgery of the third ventricle: part 2. operative approaches. Neurosurgery 1981;8:357–373.
18. Yamamoto I, Rhoton AL Jr, Peace DA. Microsurgery of the third ventricle: part 1. microsurgical anatomy. Neurosurgery 1981;8:334–356.
19. Ono M, Ono M, Rhoton AL Jr, et al. Microsurgical anatomy of the region of the tentorial incisura. J Neurosurg 1984;60:365–399.
20. Gibo H, Carver CC, Rhoton AL Jr, et al. Microsurgical anatomy of the middle cerebral artery. J Neurosurg 1981;54:151–169.
21. Gibo H, Lenkey C, Rhoton AL Jr. Microsurgical anatomy of the supraclinoid portion of the internal carotid artery. J Neurosurg 1981;55:560–574.
22. Hardy DG, Peace DA, Rhoton AL Jr. Microsurgical anatomy of the superior cerebellar artery. Neurosurgery 1980; 6:10–28.
23. Perlmutter D, Rhoton AL Jr. Microsurgical anatomy of the anterior cerebral-anterior communicating-recurrent artery complex. J Neurosurg 1976;45:259–271.
24. Saeki N, Rhoton AL Jr. Microsurgical anatomy of the upper basilar artery and the posterior circle of Willis. J Neurosurg 1977;46:563–577.
25. Zeal AA, Rhoton AL Jr. Microsurgical anatomy of the posterior cerebral artery. J Neurosurg 1978;48:534–551.
26. Perlmutter D, Rhoton AL Jr. Microsurgical anatomy of the distal anterior cerebral artery. J Neurosurg 1978;49:204–228.
27. Rosner SS, Rhoton AL Jr, Ono M, et al. Microsurgical anatomy of the anterior perforating arteries. J Neurosurg 1984;61:468–485.
28. Ono M, Rhoton AL Jr, Peace DA, et al. Microsurgical anatomy of the deep venous system of the brain. Neurosurgery 1984;15:621–657.

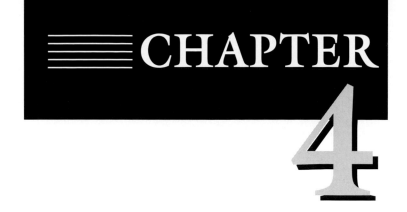

CHAPTER 4

Pathophysiology

Pituitary Adenomas: Perioperative Endocrine Management

Baha M. Arafah, Mary Louise Hlavin,
and Warren R. Selman

INTRODUCTION

Alterations in hormone secretion are frequently observed in patients with secreting or nonsecreting pituitary adenomas. Although some of these changes are relatively minor and not associated with clinical symptoms, most are important and clinically relevant. The alterations in hormone secretion seen in patients with pituitary adenomas are often caused directly by the tumor itself (e.g., excessive hormone secretion) or as a complication of its expansion and compression of surrounding structures, as is often seen in patients with partial or complete hypopituitarism. Alterations in pituitary function also can be caused by surgical procedures (e.g., adenomectomy, hypophysectomy), other forms of treatment (e.g., irradiation), or medications (e.g., dexamethasone) used in the management of patients with pituitary adenomas.

The following review addresses endocrine abnormalities commonly encountered in patients with pituitary adenomas. The focus of the discussion is on the pathophysiologic characteristics and management of alterations in pituitary function seen in patients with pituitary tumors before and, on several occasions, after surgical adenomectomy.

HYPOTHALAMIC-PITUITARY UNIT

Function of the normal pituitary gland depends on the integrity of the hypothalamus, the portal circulation, and the pituitary stalk. Neurohormones produced in cell bodies of the hypothalamus are secreted into the portal circulation. Portal vessels originate in a capillary bed in the median eminence and extend through long portal vessels into the

51

pituitary stalk and to the adenohypophysis. Through this network, releasing and inhibitory hypothalamic hormones or factors control the function of the pituitary gland.

Interruption and/or compression of this network of portal vessels as a result of pressure by any perisellar mass lesion will alter the delivery of hypothalamic factors to the anterior pituitary and cause impairment in its function (1–5). Therefore, the function of the normal pituitary gland can be impaired not only by intrinsic diseases affecting the hypothalamus and the pituitary but also by any mass lesion or disease process involving the sella turcica or the parasellar region.

Synthesis and release of pituitary hormones are primarily regulated by the corresponding releasing and inhibitory hypothalamic hormones. The predominant net hypothalamic regulatory influence is stimulatory for all pituitary hormones except prolactin (PRL), which is under dominant inhibitory control. In addition to hypothalamic regulation, secretion of pituitary hormones is also modulated by hormones secreted by target tissue such as the thyroid or the adrenal gland. Hormones secreted by target tissue (e.g., thyroid hormones) regulate the secretion of hypothalamic hormones (e.g., thyrotropin-releasing hormone) as well as corresponding pituitary hormones (e.g., thyroid-stimulating hormone [TSH]). This regulation is referred to as the classic negative feedback inhibition.

Testing of pituitary function can at times be performed by direct measurement of hormone levels. However, because pituitary hormones are secreted in pulses, single determinations may not accurately represent overall hormone secretion and should therefore be interpreted cautiously. One approach used to overcome this limitation is the use of frequent blood sampling techniques (every 5 to 15 minutes) for a prolonged period (12 to 24 hours). The latter approach is costly and time consuming; therefore, its use for routine clinical studies cannot be justified. The approach is, however, useful in research protocols investigating pulsatile pituitary hormone release. Detailed testing of pituitary function can be accomplished by provocative (stimulation and suppression) tests that can evaluate the dynamics of each hormone. A practical and clinically valuable approach commonly used in evaluating pituitary function is the determination of serum levels of hormones secreted by peripheral glands such as the thyroid. When this is combined with basal pituitary hormone levels, the function of the normal gland can be adequately characterized in most patients (4–6). In some patients, especially those with hypopituitarism, dynamic testing may be necessary to accurately define pituitary function (1, 3, 6, 7).

Pituitary Tumors

These adenomas are the most commonly encountered intracranial neoplasms. Advances in the diagnosis and management of these tumors during the past two decades have resulted in increasing awareness and early detection. Results of recent autopsy studies show that 8 to 20% of humans have pituitary adenomas, and most were unrecognized antemortem. Many of these adenomas are discovered incidentally (8). The current thinking on the pathogenesis of pituitary tumors is that they arise de novo and represent a primary, pituitary disorder. Recent advances in molecular biology have led to newer approaches and studies demonstrating that secreting and nonsecreting adenomas are monoclonal in origin. Thus, the initial event in tumor formation is somatic cell mutation followed by clonal expansion (9).

With the advent of immunocytochemistry, adenomas are now classified according to the hormone-secreting cells present in the tumor. Approximately 85 to 90% of adenomas are functional, i.e., they are composed of cells capable of synthesizing and secreting hormones (e.g., PRL, growth hormone [GH], adrenocorticotropic hormone [ACTH], etc.). A few of these adenomas can secrete part of a hormone molecule, such as the α-subunit. In fact, such tumors were previously classified as nonsecreting until a specific assay became available that could detect these abnormalities. The remaining 10% of adenomas do not secrete or store any known hormone and are labeled nonfunctional or nonsecreting. Frequently, a functioning tumor can produce more than one hormone.

The clinical manifestations of pituitary adenomas are variable but can include (*a*) signs and symptoms caused by excessive hormone secretion (e.g., acromegaly), (*b*) symptoms caused by impairment of normal pituitary function (hypopituitarism), and (*c*) symptoms related to mechanical effects of the tumor mass (headaches, visual field defects).

Management of Pituitary Adenomas: An Overview

Treatment of pituitary tumors depends on several factors, including the associated endocrine abnormalities, the size and extent of the adenoma, and the age and clinical status of the patient. Available therapeutic options include primary medical therapy, external irradiation (proton beam, linear accelerator), and surgical adenomectomy. Some controversy in the literature centers around the treatment choices and the necessity for therapeutic intervention in certain patients, such as those with PRL-secreting microadenomas (10, 11). There is, however, general agreement that surgery is the treatment of choice in patients with ACTH- or GH-secreting pituitary adenomas (10, 12, 13). Although therapy is always individualized, we advocate the use of surgical adenomectomy as the major therapeutic choice in most patients with pituitary adenomas. Several drugs are currently available for the primary treatment of pituitary tumors (10). Dopamine agonists such as bromocriptine, pergolide, and cabergoline represent the variety of drugs used in the medical treatment of PRL-secreting adenomas (10). With such treatment, it is expected that a decrease in adenoma size can be demonstrated in approximately 60 to 70% of patients. These drugs are moderately effective in approximately 25 to 30% of patients with acromegaly. Somatostatin analog was recently shown to be effective in lowering serum GH levels and in ameliorating the symptoms of acromegaly. Results of recent studies show that therapy with this drug can also decrease the size of the adenoma in approximately 35% of patients. It is also reported to be effective in the medical treatment of the rare TSH-secreting adenomas. Furthermore, results of other recent studies suggest that medical treatment of these patients for a defined period of time before surgery might facilitate tumor resection and therefore improve outcome. Proper timing and coordination of efforts between the endocrinologist and the surgeon are important in improving the outcome.

Transsphenoidal microsurgical adenomectomy provides a good chance for complete resection of the tumor, amelioration of clinical symptoms, and resumption of normal hormone secretion without significant morbidity (13, 14). Success with this approach depends to a large degree on the surgeon's expertise and on the size and extent of the adenoma. Patients should be evaluated before and after the procedure for evidence of hormone dysfunction. Patients with preoperative hypopituitarism should be specifically retested after surgery to determine if there was any improvement (or worsening) in pituitary function. In our experience, most such patients show improvement in pituitary function after selective adenomectomy (1–5).

Significant improvement in pituitary function is expected after transsphenoidal adenomectomy. A study conducted at our institution showed that selective adenomectomy in patients with large pituitary adenomas resulted in improved pituitary function in most patients (3). The improvement in pituitary function has provided newer information pertaining to the pathophysiologic mechanisms of hypopituitarism in this setting. Based on detailed dynamic testing data in patients with hypopituitarism, we postulated that the hypopituitarism associated with large pituitary tumors was primarily caused by interruption and compression of the hypothalamic–pituitary portal vessels and the pituitary stalk by the expanding adenoma. An additional factor contributing to pituitary failure in this setting could be the development of ischemia and/or necrosis in the normal gland. Because the pituitary gland cannot regenerate, recovery of pituitary function would not be expected in the latter instance, although the pressure on the portal vessels was relieved. Thus, depending on the presence of viable pituitary tissue, recovery of pituitary function might occur after selective adenomectomy (3). Careful endocrine evaluation in these patients can help identify those likely to recover pituitary function after adenomectomy.

A similar mechanism for hypopituitarism can be seen in patients with other mass lesions in the perisellar region, such as an intracranial aneurysm. In these instances, decompression results in improvement of pituitary function and normalization of the slightly elevated serum PRL levels.

Preoperative Endocrine Assessment and Management

All patients who require surgical removal of perisellar mass lesions should undergo thorough endocrine evaluation before and after the procedure. Particular attention is given to assessment of the integrity of pituitary–adrenal as well as thyroid functions because these have a major impact on outcome of the planned surgery and postoperative management (4–6). Functional integrity of the pituitary–adrenal axis is initially evaluated using basal serum cortisol levels. Patients with clearly high or high-normal levels (>550 nmol/L [>20 g/dL]) who have no clinical symptoms to suggest deficiency will not require further testing of this axis and will not need glucocorticoid replacement therapy. One technical limitation to the latter general rule applies to patients with increased corticosteroid-binding globulin (e.g., those using oral contraceptives or exogenous estrogen supplement). Increased corticosteroid-binding globulin will result in falsely elevated serum cortisol levels. Patients with lower, though normal, basal levels would require dynamic testing to document normal pituitary–adrenal function. In such instances, measurement of basal and stimulated serum cortisol levels following insulin-induced hypoglycemia will be necessary. In patients in whom hypoglycemia is contraindicated, we use metopirone to assess the integrity of the hypothalamic–pituitary–adrenal axis. Cortrosyn stimulation testing in such patients with documented hypopituitarism is not commonly useful because the results are often normal and therefore can be misleading (15, 16). Most patients with pituitary microadenomas have normal adrenal and thyroidal functions. In this group, basal measurements of hormone level are probably sufficient, provided they exceed 410 nmol/L (15 μg/dL). In contrast, patients with macroadenomas are more likely to have abnormalities in normal pituitary function and therefore should undergo thorough testing.

Evaluation of the pituitary–thyroidal axis can be accomplished easily by the simultaneous measurement of TSH and free thyroxine levels (4, 6). Patients with central hypothyroidism usually have a low serum free thyroxine level and a "normal" TSH level. Only rarely will the TSH level be clearly below normal. Pituitary gonadal function can be assessed by measurement of serum gonadotropin levels (follicle-stimulating hormone [FSH], luteinizing hormone [LH]) and the relevant gonadal steroid (testosterone, estradiol). Male patients with hypogonadism typically have low serum testosterone levels and low-normal or low FSH and LH levels (4, 6). Patients with gonadotropin-secreting adenomas often have slightly increased serum FSH and/or LH levels, often associated with low serum testosterone levels (7, 17). In such instances, one should also determine the serum α-subunit level to confirm the finding because similar changes can be seen in patients with primary testicular failure. A similar distinction should be made in postmenopausal women who are normally expected to have elevated serum gonadotropin levels. Evaluation of GH secretion can be achieved by measurement of the hormone serum level during insulin-induced hypoglycemia if the test is already done to assess pituitary–adrenal function (1, 3, 18). In most instances, however, GH secretion can be assessed by measurement of plasma insulin-like growth factor-1 (IGF-1) levels. Patients with excessive GH secretion have clearly elevated plasma IGF-1 levels, whereas those with GH deficiency have low values.

Measurement of the serum PRL level represents one of the most important and frequently obtained tests in patients with hypothalamic–pituitary diseases. Although dynamic testing of PRL secretion can, at times, be helpful, it is often not necessary. Because serum PRL levels are altered by a variety of medications and other medical conditions, its level should be interpreted within the context of the presenting clinical picture (1, 3, 11, 17). PRL-secreting adenomas represent the most common type of pituitary tumor encountered in clinical practice, accounting for approximately 40%. Serum PRL levels in these patients vary greatly; one can occasionally see a patient with a level as low as 35 and others as high as 20,000 μg/L. In general, serum PRL levels correlate with tumor size, and most patients with PRL-secreting adenomas have levels greater than 100 μg/L. Even in patients with pituitary adenomas, other causes of hyperprolactinemia need to be considered in evaluating serum PRL levels. Patients with pituitary adenomas can have hyperprolactinemia through at least three different mechanisms:

1. Secretion by the tumor cell either alone (prolactinomas) or mixed with other hormones (e.g., GH, PRL)

2. Compression of the pituitary stalk and portal vessels by the expanding adenoma, as is seen in patients with large tumors who often present with hypopituitarism

3. Intake of medications or the presence of other diseases known independently to cause hyperprolactinemia

In most patients with large adenomas not secreting PRL, a mild form of hyperprolactinemia is commonly seen. Serum PRL levels in such patients are often mildly increased and range from 20 to 75 μg/L (1, 3, 17). Most patients with mild hyperprolactinemia in this setting have variable degrees of hypopituitarism. Results of studies conducted at our institution show that the hypopituitarism and the hyperprolactinemia observed in these patients are often reversed after surgical removal of the adenoma (3).

Patients with documented ACTH deficiency should be given hydrocortisone replacement therapy as soon as the diagnosis is made. A total of 15 to 30 mg of hydrocortisone, in two or three divided doses, represents adequate physiologic replacement in most patients. Unless severe, thyroid replacement need not be initiated before surgery. Mildly hypothyroid patients can safely undergo pituitary

microsurgery as long as the anesthesiologist, the surgeon, and the endocrinologist are all aware of the diagnosis and coordinate their management (19). However, if surgery is to be delayed for several weeks, replacement therapy with L-thyroxine should be instituted when recognized. Other pituitary hormone deficits, such as GH and gonadotropins, need not be treated before surgery because their management can be addressed after the outcome of surgical adenomectomy is known.

Perioperative Management: Glucocorticoids

Patients with Normal Preoperative Pituitary-Adrenal Function

In most medical centers, patients undergoing transsphenoidal pituitary adenomectomy are still given glucocorticoid therapy during and after the procedure. The rationale for this practice has been the assumption that ACTH secretion is compromised by the trauma of surgery. Our own experience indicates that patients with normal preoperative adrenal function do not require glucocorticoid therapy before or during pituitary microsurgery (1, 3, 20). Results of a study conducted at our institution with a large number of patients demonstrate that patients with normal preoperative adrenal function do well during and after transsphenoidal adenomectomy without receiving exogenous glucocorticoids. Serum cortisol levels in these patients are appropriately elevated and comparable to those reported after other major surgical procedures (Fig. 4.1). Only 1 of 83 such patients had clinical symptoms and biochemical evidence of glucocorticoid deficiency. The diagnosis on the latter patient was made promptly and without associated discomfort. We recommend that patients with normal pre-

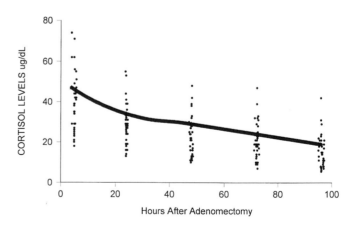

Figure 4.1. Serum cortisol levels in 40 patients with pituitary adenomas measured during the first 4 days after adenomectomy. All patients had normal preoperative pituitary–adrenal function and did not receive glucocorticoids during or after surgery. Each data point represents a single measurement at the specified time. The curve represents the average values on each occasion. The highest levels were noted within 1 hour of surgery. All patients had multiple determinations showing a level of greater than 410 nmol/L (>15 μg/dL). To convert serum cortisol values from μg/dL to nmol/L, multiply by 27.59.

operative adrenal function not receive glucocorticoids during or after selective adenomectomy. Close observation and serial determination of serum cortisol levels in the immediate postoperative period can reliably predict the integrity of pituitary–adrenal function. We recommend measurement of serum cortisol levels twice daily for 2 to 3 days beginning immediately after surgery. Consecutive levels of more than 410 nmol/L (>15 μg/dL) are satisfactory and indicate an intact pituitary–adrenal axis. Patients with intermediate levels (220 to 410 nmol/L [8 to 15 μg/dL]) should be monitored carefully with repeated measurements. Patients with clinical or biochemical evidence of glucocorticoid deficiency (multiple serum cortisol levels <140 nmol/L [<5 μg/dL]) and those suspected of having the deficit can be treated immediately until detailed testing is done later. Plasma ACTH levels also can be monitored in the immediate postoperative period, but they rarely provide information additional to that obtained with serum cortisol levels (3).

Patients with Preoperative ACTH Deficiency

Patients with documented preoperative glucocorticoid deficit should receive replacement before, during, and immediately after surgery. We recommend the use of hydrocortisone because of its predictable effects and duration of action (4, 5). A total of 15 to 30 mg are given in two to three divided oral doses as soon as the diagnosis is established. Oral replacement therapy should continue until the day of surgery, when an intramuscular injection of 50 mg is given early in the morning and an additional 50 mg is also given intramuscularly just before the patient is taken to the operating room. Hydrocortisone, 100 mg, is given in an intravenous drip throughout the procedure, starting with the induction of anesthesia and continuing until closure. Thereafter, hydrocortisone is given in intravenous boluses of 50 mg every 6 hours for 1 day, followed by 25 mg every 6 hours for 2 additional days. Following that, glucocorticoids are given orally in three divided doses totaling 50 mg of hydrocortisone on the fourth day, down to usual replacement doses of 30 mg daily on the fifth postoperative day. Using this protocol, we have had no morbidity or mortality related to glucocorticoid replacement in these patients (3–5). Higher doses of glucocorticoids are associated with more adverse effects and provide no added benefit (21). Results of a recent study conducted in adrenalectomized monkeys undergoing cholecystectomy show that supraphysiologic glucocorticoid replacement is not necessary because hemodynamic stability was similar in those receiving physiologic or supraphysiologic doses of glucocorticoids (22).

The previously described protocol applies in most patients with preoperative ACTH deficiency, particularly in those whose hypopituitarism is judged to be permanent. However, in patients with macroadenomas who are likely to recover function postoperatively, an attempt to evaluate the potential for recovery of function can be made. This can be done by withdrawing glucocorticoid therapy abruptly after the first 36 to 48 hours of the procedure (3). Serum cortisol levels measured 24 hours or longer after glucocorticoid withdrawal reflect endogenous production and can be evaluated accordingly. Serum cortisol levels of 410 nmol/L (15 μg/dL) or more, measured on multiple occasions, support the view that recovery of pituitary–adrenal function already took place and that glucocorticoids need not be given from there on. Patients can then be discharged on schedule without glucocorticoid therapy. In contrast, persistently low serum cortisol levels (<140 nmol/L [<5 gm>/dL]) suggest that recovery from ACTH deficiency did not take place and that replacement therapy needs to be reinstituted. Patients with intermediate values are monitored carefully until a determination is made as to whether they recovered function. Patients who recover pituitary–adrenal function after adenomectomy show clear biochemical evidence for that recovery as early as a few hours postoperatively (3). This approach will allow identification of patients who recover function before they are discharged home and will minimize the chance to give them unnecessary replacement therapy.

An alternative approach to the protocol of rapid discontinuation of glucocorticoid therapy described here is to taper steroids slowly over several weeks and then to assess the patient's pituitary–adrenal axis at a later date. Although both approaches are reasonable, we favor the former method because it avoids the confounding effects of steroids when evaluating the remaining pituitary function as well as the unnecessary use of medication with potential side effects. Furthermore, the former approach of rapid discontinuation of steroids is reliable in that it provides data while patients are still monitored in the hospital.

Perioperative Management of ACTH-Secreting Pituitary Adenomas

Optimal management of patients with ACTH-secreting adenomas during and after pituitary adenomectomy requires close and continued collaboration between the endocrinologist and the neurosurgeon. Glucocorticoid therapy in these patients is variable and depends to a large degree on the experience of the management team. Although some advocate the use of glucocorticoids before, during, and after surgery, others restrict their use to the postoperative period (12, 23). Our approach to the management of these patients is to limit the use of glucocorticoids until clear clinical or biochemical evidence for deficiency is established (12). We therefore do not use any glucocorticoid supplement before or during surgery. Postoperatively, patients are monitored carefully without glucocorticoid therapy and serum cortisol levels are measured two to three times daily, and the results are usually available within 6 to 24 hours. If surgical adenomectomy is complete, signs and symptoms of glucocorticoid deficiency develop within 24 to 48 hours and are always associated with a decrease in serum cortisol levels. Glucocorticoids are given immediately after signs or symptoms are noted or when low serum cortisol levels are demonstrated. This approach provides an immediate assessment of the outcome of surgery (persistent Cushing's versus probable cure) without jeopardizing the patient's clinical management (12). Glucocorticoid replacement can be started with only clinical suspicion of deficiency and without prior biochemical documentation. Blood samples for measuring cortisol and ACTH levels should be drawn before glucocorticoid therapy is initiated. Therapy is initially given intravenously (50 mg every 6 hours for 24 hours), then it is tapered down over 2 days such that by discharge, on the fourth or fifth postoperative day, patients are given 40 to 50 mg of hydrocortisone orally in three divided doses. Patients are monitored and the dose is adjusted depending on clinical symptoms. Evaluation of pituitary–adrenal function is done periodically on all patients, and the glucocorticoid dose is adjusted accordingly. It is anticipated that patients recover pituitary–adrenal function be able to discontinue exogenous glucocorticoid therapy 6 to 24 months after surgery.

Patients with persistently high serum cortisol levels and those with normal values are not given exogenous glucocorticoids unless they have symptoms suggestive of ACTH deficiency. In these patients, additional treatments are given, depending on the findings at the time of surgery and the overall clinical picture.

Perioperative Management of Other Pituitary Hormone Abnormalities

Deficiency of other pituitary hormones need not be addressed in the perioperative period. The only exception to this would be TSH deficiency because the state of hypothyroidism can significantly impact the postoperative course. Hypothyroid patients who were treated before surgery can continue their replacement therapy after surgery. Unless the hypothyroidism is severe, surgery need not be delayed in hypothyroid patients requiring surgery (3–5, 19). It is very important in such instances for the management team to be aware of the disease and its potential impact on the use of anesthesia during the procedure as well as on fluid and pain management. Dosages of all medications, particularly narcotics, need to be decreased in hypothyroid patients because of lower metabolic rate. Continuous communication and feedback from and between members of the management team (endocrinologist, anesthesiologist, surgeon) are extremely important in ensuring the best outcome. Abnormalities in antidiuretic hormone (ADH) secretion can often be seen in the immediate postoperative period. These will be addressed separately.

Postoperative Diabetes Insipidus

Several series have reported the incidence of transient diabetes insipidus (DI) after transsphenoidal surgery to be from 5 to 60%, with most series reporting 10 to 20%. Development of DI is associated with posterior localization of the adenoma, suprasellar extension of the tumor, and operative damage to the proximal portion of the pituitary stalk. DI develops equally in patients with all types of pituitary adenomas (13, 14, 24, 25).

Postoperative DI usually has its onset within 24 to 48 hours of surgery, is usually self-limited, and typically follows one of three patterns. The most common pattern is transient and comprises most cases. It consists of the abrupt onset of polyuria within 24 hours of surgery, with resolution in 1 to 3 days. It may be secondary to the release of bioinactive arginine vasopressin (AVP) precursors, local edema of ADH-producing neurons with a temporary functional impairment, or a disruption of the inferior hypophyseal artery that supplies the ADH transport and storage structures. Proximal damage to the pituitary stalk or hypothalamus can cause a second variant of DI. After previously formed ADH is used up in 1 to 3 days, permanent DI ensues, with a minimal or only partial decrease in urine volume over several days. The partial improvement sometimes seen is likely caused by resolution of edema.

The third pattern of postoperative DI is triphasic in nature. The first phase is marked by the abrupt onset of DI within 24 hours of surgery, which then lasts 1 to 3 days and is thought to be caused by neuronal shock and diminished or absent hormone release. An interphase then follows, during which AVP escapes from degenerating neurons. Urine output slows and urine osmolality rises, making the patient vulnerable to hyponatremia if intravenous fluid administration is not tapered. This interphase may last 1 to 14 days and is followed by a return of DI, which is often permanent owing to the loss of magnocellular neurons by retrograde axonal degeneration.

A urine flow of 150 to 200 mL/h maintained for several hours is highly likely to result from DI, although in any situation in which urine output exceeds fluid intake an abnormal cause of polyuria should be suspected. Differentiating DI from a diuresis of fluids given perioperatively, or diuresis secondary to osmotic or nonosmotic diuretics, can create a confusing clinical picture. Measurement of urine glucose level, specific gravity, and renal function is helpful and should be included on a flow sheet that also has perioperative body weights (taken on the same weighing scale), fluid intake, urine output, urine osmolality, and serum sodium and osmolality. The patient with diuresis of perioperative fluids will have a low urine osmolality in the presence of a low plasma osmolality.

Attention to volume status in the patient with central DI is coupled with administration of ADH, if deemed necessary, to bring polyuria under control. Because polyuria is likely to be transient in the postoperative setting, some clinicians advocate the use of a shorter-acting agent such as aqueous AVP. The latter induces its effects within 1 to 2 hours, which often last for 4 to 6 hours. This relatively short therapeutic time course can be advantageous, particularly when diuresis is short lived. Potential side effects of AVP therapy include nausea, diarrhea, and abdominal cramps. Angina may occasionally be precipitated as a result of the pressor activity of vasopressin and usually responds to the application of topical nitroglycerin. The usual starting dose is 2 to 5 units subcutaneously, with continued surveillance of fluid intake, urine output, body weight, urine osmolality, and serum sodium. A second dose is held until hypotonic polyuria recurs, indicating persistent DI. If the patient's DI resolves, the antidiuretic effect should not be prolonged enough to cause hyponatremia. Alternatively, a more effective and somewhat longer-lasting agent would be desmopressin acetate, particularly when the duration of diuresis is not known. The latter should initially be given parenterally because all patients have intranasal packs at that time. A single dose of 1 or 2 μg of desmopressin acetate can be given intramuscularly or subcutaneously, and its antidiuretic effect often lasts 18 to 24 hours. A practical approach followed at our institution is to give a dose of desmopressin acetate as described previously and to repeat that dose as clinical signs and symptoms, as well as electrolyte and fluid balance, dictate. This approach allows identification of patients whose DI is transient rather than permanent and thus avoids the unnecessary administration of this drug, which potentially has serious side effects (24, 25).

A final note on DI in the postoperative period centers on patients with unrecognized coexistent deficiency of adrenal function, a situation not uncommon in patients with tumors of the sellar region. Glucocorticoid deficiency exerts a nonosmotic stimulus for the release of ADH and creates an ADH-independent impairment in ability to excrete a water load. Thus, patients with primary or secondary adrenal insufficiency may develop hyponatremia from impaired water excretion. An important caveat for patients undergoing hypothalamic–pituitary surgery is that manifestation of DI may be lessened or even abolished by accompanying glucocorticoid deficiency. The polyuria of DI may follow when cortisol is replaced.

Endocrine Management 1 to 2 Weeks Postoperatively

In most patients who undergo pituitary surgery, minimal alterations in pituitary function are expected at 1 to 2 weeks postoperative. Patients are by that time discharged home and are recovering from the surgical procedure. The most significant endocrine abnormalities encountered would be postoperative hyponatremia and adrenal insufficiency.

Postoperative hyponatremia is a relatively common disorder (25, 26). The differential diagnosis and potential causes of hyponatremia vary and depend a great deal on the clinical setting. Decreased sodium concentration can be seen in patients who are hypovolemic and euvolemic, as well as in those with increased plasma volume. Every attempt should be made to classify the patients according to plasma volume status. This will not only help with establishing a cause but will also simplify patient management. In patients with pituitary adenomas, particularly those with large tumors, one needs to consider endocrine factors contributing to hyponatremia in addition to the usual causes. Contributing factors in these patients include hypothyroidism and adrenal insufficiency.

After pituitary surgery, inappropriate ADH may occur in several patterns (25, 26). Excessive ADH release in the interphase of the triphasic response of postoperative DI is the result of damage to the hypothalamic ADH production sites and precedes DI. Another pattern involves the syndrome of inappropriate ADH secretion occurring 5 to 10 days after otherwise uneventful transsphenoidal surgery. Autonomous release of ADH from damaged posterior pituitary cells has been offered as an explanation, and DI does not follow in these cases. This pattern of ADH release is relatively rare, occurring in fewer than 1% of patients who had pituitary surgery. Patients often present with signs and symptoms of hyponatremia 7 to 12 days after uneventful transsphenoidal pituitary surgery. Presenting signs and symptoms include nausea, lethargy, confusion, and headaches. The phenomenon is temporary, and tumor type or size do not help predict its development. Measurement of serum Na$^+$ levels on the seventh through tenth postoperative days, in symptomatic patients, is needed to identify this complication.

Both thyroid and adrenal dysfunction can lead to hyponatremia. Free water clearance is impaired in hypothyroidism. Decreased cardiac output and reduced renal blood flow and glomerular filtration rate are contributory mechanisms. If hypothyroidism is clinically significant, thyroid hormone replacement therapy should be instituted. However, before thyroid hormone replacement is initiated, particular attention should be given to documenting intact adrenal function because hyponatremia often can be seen in patients with glucocorticoid deficiency. Glucocorticoids have a negative feedback effect on vasopressin secretion, which is absent in glucocorticoid deficiency, and results in elevated ADH levels. Also, the reduced cardiac output and renal blood flow in hypocortisolism increases proximal tubular resorption of salt and water and lessens capacity for urinary dilution at the distal nephron. Normal cortisol production must be established before a low sodium concentration can be attributed to the inappropriate release of ADH. Postoperative patients presenting with hyponatremia should be screened with serum cortisol levels to exclude glucocorticoid deficiency as the cause. Patients suspected of having glucocorticoid deficiency can be given immediate supplementation with adequate doses of hydrocortisone and intravenous saline while awaiting the results of cortisol level measurements. This treatment corrects the hyponatremia quickly. Similarly, patients with chronic adrenal insufficiency have hyponatremia that corrects promptly with physiologic replacement doses of glucocorticoids.

Assessment of Pituitary Hormone Secretion 1 to 3 Months After Surgery

Evaluation of pituitary hormone function is an important aspect of patient management at this point. Testing at that time will address the presence or absence of residual tumor as well as assess the function of the normal gland. It is important to document hormone deficiency before long-term replacement therapy is established. As discussed earlier, hormone deficiencies associated with pituitary adenomas are often reversible with surgical resection of the adenoma. Similarly, the surgical procedure itself can, at times, result in partial or complete loss of pituitary hormone function. From a practical standpoint, pituitary function can be assessed easily through outpatient services, and dynamic testing can often be avoided (4–6).

Testing of pituitary function at this time can be done in a similar way to that described earlier. A practical and clinically valuable approach commonly used in evaluating pituitary function is the determination of serum levels of pituitary hormones as well as hormones secreted by peripheral glands such as the thyroid, adrenal, and gonadal steroids. This combination of hormone levels provides reasonably adequate evaluation of pituitary gland function in most patients (4–6). In some patients, especially those with mild adrenal insufficiency, dynamic testing may be necessary to accurately define pituitary function (3).

Patients discharged from the hospital without corticosteroid replacement after adequate documentation of appropriately elevated postoperative cortisol and/or ACTH plasma levels are more likely to continue to have normal pituitary–adrenal function. It is rare and unusual to have a patient acquire adrenal insufficiency so late after pituitary surgery, unless other treatments were given or complications occurred to explain that event. Patients with persistent or acquired glucocorticoid deficiency in the immediate postoperative period are more likely to maintain similar function months after surgery. If ACTH secretion is shown to be abnormal in the immediate postoperative period (i.e., days after surgery), only an unusual patient will show signs of recovery of pituitary–adrenal axis weeks or months later. The only exception to this rule is patients with ACTH-secreting adenomas who develop adrenal insufficiency after complete resection of the adenoma and then recover pituitary–adrenal function in 6 to 24 months.

Patients discharged home with glucocorticoid replacement therapy continue the same physiologic treatment until 2 to 3 days before testing. At that time, replacement is reduced to half of the dose and then discontinued for 24 hours before a blood sample is drawn for measuring the cortisol concentration. A clearly low serum cortisol value (morning level <80 nmol/L [<3 μg/dL]) indicates persistent ACTH deficiency and the need for continued hydrocortisone replacement therapy. A clearly elevated serum cortisol value (morning level >550 nmol/L [>20 μg/dL]) indicates adequate pituitary–adrenal function and should prompt discontinuation of replacement therapy. An intermediate level is indeterminate and requires dynamic testing of pituitary–adrenal function using insulin-induced hypoglycemia or a metopirone test. A cortrosyn stimulation test is unlikely to be helpful because its results are often normal.

Evaluation of pituitary–thyroidal function can be accomplished by measurement of serum-free thyroxine as well as TSH levels. Similarly, pituitary–gonadal function can be assessed by measurement of serum FSH and LH as well as gonadal steroid (testosterone, estradiol) serum levels. Although still controversial, the integrity of GH secretion can be assessed, with reasonable accuracy, in most patients by measurement of plasma IGF-1 levels. A low plasma IGF-1 level, in the absence of major illnesses or malnutrition, suggests but does not establish the diagnosis of GH deficiency.

Residual tumor activity can and should be assessed at this time. Because most tumors are functional, one can use hormone levels of the secreted product as a marker of tumor activity in addition to imaging studies. By that time, the immunocytochemistry of the resected tumor tissue will be available; when this information is combined with preoperative endocrine evaluation, one can interpret postoperative endocrine data more effectively.

Long-Term Hormone Replacement Therapy

Transsphenoidal microsurgical adenomectomy provides a good chance for complete resection of the tumor, amelioration of the clinical symptoms, and resumption of normal hormone secretion without significant morbidity. The success with this approach depends to a large extent on the surgeon's expertise and on the size and extent of the adenoma. Patients should be evaluated before and after the procedure for evidence of hormone dysfunction. Patients with preoperative hypopituitarism should be specifically retested after surgery to determine if there was any improvement (or worsening) in pituitary function. In our experience, most patients show improvement in pituitary function after adenomectomy. The hypopituitarism seen in patients with large adenomas was previously considered to be an irreversible disease process requiring lifelong hormone replacement. Results of recent studies, however, show that the hypopituitarism in this setting is reversible in most patients because it is largely the result of mechanical compression of portal vessels and the pituitary stalk by the expanding adenoma.

Patient education about the disease is an important aspect of the management of hypopituitarism that is often overlooked. Patients should understand the impact of hormone deficit on their daily lives and activities and should be fully aware that treatment may need to be modified in the event of intercurrent illnesses, accidents, or surgical procedures. A medic alert bracelet or necklace, identifying the patient as hypopituitary receiving glucocorticoid replacement therapy, should be worn at all times (4, 5).

Treatment of patients with hypopituitarism should always be individualized, not rigid. Management should take into consideration the patient's age, sex, work schedule, education, original disease process, and clinical history. Either hydrocortisone (cortisol) or cortisone acetate in two or, preferably, three divided doses totaling 15 to 25 mg of the former steroid represent the usual glucocorticoid replacement therapy (27). The dose is titrated individually using primarily clinical symptoms as a guide. Although hyponatremia is seen at times in patients with ACTH deficiency, mineralocorticoid replacement is rarely, if ever, necessary in patients with hypopituitarism. L-thyroxine therapy is the preferred replacement therapy in patients with TSH deficiency. Although measurement of total thyroxine and free thyroxine index serum levels are helpful in determining the optimal dose of L-thyroxine, physicians should rely primarily on clinical symptoms to determine the optimal dose (4, 5).

Treatment of hypogonadism in postpubertal adults can be achieved by giving gonadal steroid replacement in the form of oral estrogen/progestin to women and parenteral testosterone in men. The latter treatment in men is often supraphysiologic when given in the currently used doses of 200 to 300 mg every 2 to 3 weeks. Frequently overlooked complications of testosterone therapy include hyperlipidemia, excessive snoring, prostatism, and progression of previously unrecognized prostate cancer. Every effort, therefore, should be made to give the lowest possible dose to minimize potential side effects. In our experience, most men can be adequately replaced with 125 to 175 mg of testosterone enanthate or cypionate intramuscularly every 2 weeks. Newly introduced testosterone skin patches have been reported to provide a stable and physiologic serum concentration throughout the day. Although this has not been addressed in long-term studies, it is reasonable to speculate that with these preparations, the side effects of testosterone therapy would be less. Fertility can be restored, at least transiently, using exogenous gonadotropin injections. In many patients with hypothalamic gonadotropin-releasing hormone deficiency, fertility can be restored using the pulsatile injection of gonadotropin-releasing hormone through a portable pump.

Treatment of GH deficiency is essential in children with documented deficiency. Although there is extensive experience in the treatment of GH deficiency in children, only limited data are available on its use in adults. Recent preliminary studies demonstrated the beneficial effects of GH treatment in the elderly, in whom an increase in lean body mass, a decrease in body fat, and an improved sense of well-being were shown during short-term therapy (18). Associated side effects included glucose intolerance and arthralgia. It is not clear whether GH deficiency in adults will have any impact on long-term morbidity in patients with hypopituitarism, as was recently suggested. If GH deficiency is confirmed in future studies to contribute to patient morbidity and if treatment can be given without side effects, GH could then be offered to patients with deficit regardless of age (18).

Untreated hypopituitary patients can survive for many years with disease. Survival of untreated patients depends on the severity of the hormone deficit, the axis involved, the cause of hypopituitarism, and other concurrent illnesses. Untreated patients with hypopituitarism have increased morbidity and mortality. Such patients may remain compensated until some stress, trauma, prolonged cold exposure, infection, or medications precipitate an acute life-threatening decompensation (4, 5).

Even with treatment, hypopituitarism can be a major health problem. Patients with this disorder require indefinite and often close medical attention. This is especially true for patients with ACTH deficiency who require monitoring and adjustment of glucocorticoid doses with any intercurrent illnesses, stresses, surgical procedures, and trauma. Despite clinically adequate gonadal, thyroid, and glucocorticoid replacement therapy, results of several studies suggest that hypopituitary patients have increased cardiovascular morbidity and mortality. A recent report implicated myocardial dysfunction in treated adult hypopituitary patients as a possible explanation for increased cardiovascular mortality. In some studies, the persistence of GH deficiency in hypopituitary patients was suggested as a possible contributing factor for the increased cardiovascular mortality in these patients. Currently available data do not provide adequate explanation for the cause of increased morbidity or mortality in these patients. One should, however, attempt to provide optimal replacement therapy that is as close to being physiologic as humanly possible. It is also important to always think about the potential reversibility of hypopituitarism in many patients who can be spared lifelong replacement therapy.

ACKNOWLEDGMENTS

We thank the staff of the Clinical Research Center at The University Hospitals of Cleveland, Cleveland, OH, for their help with the clinical studies and Robert Meyers for preparing the manuscript.

REFERENCES

1. Arafah BM. Reversible hypopituitarism in patients with large nonfunctioning pituitary adenomas. J Clin Endocrinol Metab 1986;62: 1173–1181.
2. Anonymous. Reversible hypopituitarism. Lancet 1991;337:276. Editorial.
3. Arafah BM, Kailani S, Nekl KE, et al. Immediate recovery of pituitary function after transsphenoidal resection of pituitary macroadenomas. J Clin Endocrinol Metab 1994;79:348–354.
4. Arafah BM, Gold R, Selman WR. Clinical manifestations and management of hypopituitarism. Contemp Neurosurg 1995;17:1–6.
5. Arafah BM. Hypopituitarism. In: Rakel RE, ed. Conn's Current Therapy. Philadelphia: WB Saunders, 1997:629–633.
6. Vance ML. Hypopituitarism. N Engl J Med 1994;330:1651–1662.
7. Daneshdoost L, Gennarelli TA, Bashey HM, et al. Recognition of gonadotroph adenomas in women. N Engl J Med 1991;324: 589–594.

8. Molitch ME, Russell EJ. The pituitary "incidentaloma." Ann Intern Med 1990;112:925–931.

9. Alexander JM, Biller BMK, Bikkal H, et al. Clinically non-functioning pituitary tumors are monoclonal in origin. J Clin Invest 1990; 86:336–340.

10. Klibanski A, Zervas NT. Diagnosis and management of hormone secreting pituitary adenomas. N Engl J Med 1991;324:822–831.

11. Feigenbaum SL, Downey DE, Wilson CB, et al. Extensive personal experience: transsphenoidal pituitary resection for preoperative diagnosis of prolactin-secreting pituitary adenoma in women: long term follow-up. J Clin Endocrinol Metab 1995;81(5):1711–1719.

12. Arafah BM, Pearson OH. Cushing's syndrome. In: Rakel RE, ed. Conn's Current Therapy. Philadelphia: WB Saunders, 1985;482–488.

13. Landolt AM. Transsphenoidal surgery of pituitary tumors: its pitfalls and complications. Prog Neurol Surg 1990;13:1–30.

14. Zervas NT. Surgical results for pituitary adenomas: results of an international survey. In: Black Z, Ridgway M, eds. Secretory Tumors of the Pituitary Gland. New York: Raven Press, 1984:377–385.

15. Borst GC, Michenfelder HJ, O'Brian JT. Discordant cortisol response to exogenous ACTH and insulin-induced hypoglycemia in patients with pituitary disease. N Engl J Med 1982;307: 1462–1464.

16. Cunningham SK, Moore A, McKenna TS. Normal cortisol response to corticotropin in patients with secondary adrenal failure. Arch Intern Med 1983;143:2276–2279.

17. Young WF, Scheithauer BW, Kovacs KT, et al. Gonadotroph adenoma of the pituitary gland: a clinicopathologic analysis of 100 cases. Mayo Clin Proc 1996;71:649–656.

18. De Boer H, Blok GJ, Van Der Veen E. Clinical aspects of growth hormone deficiency in adults. Endocr Rev 1995;16:63–86.

19. Markin JM. Anesthesia and hypothyroidism: a review of thyroxine physiology, pharmacology, and anesthetic implications. Anesth Analg 1982;61:371–383.

20. Hout WM, Arafah BM, Salazar R, et al. Evaluation of the hypothalamic pituitary adrenal axis immediately after pituitary adenomectomy: is perioperative steroid therapy necessary? J Clin Endocrinol Metab 1988;66:1208–1212.

21. Munck A, Guyre PM. Glucocorticoid physiology, pharmacology, and stress. Adv Exp Med Biol 1986;196:81–96.

22. Udelsman R, Ramp J, Gallucci WT, et al. Adaptation during surgical stress: reevaluation of the role of glucocorticoids. J Clin Invest 1986; 77:1377–1381.

23. Tsigos C, Papanicolau DA, Chrousos GP. Advances in the diagnosis and treatment of Cushing's syndrome. Bailliere's Clin Endocrinol Metab 1995;9(2):315–336.

24. Obert KP. Diabetes insipidus. Crit Care Clin 1991;7:109–125.

25. Vokes TJ, Robertson GL. Disorders of antidiuretic hormone. Endocrinol Metab Clin North Am 1988;17:281–299.

26. Sterns RH. The treatment of hyponatremia: first, do no harm. Am J Med 1990;88:557–560.

27. Esteban NV, Loughlin T, Vergey AL, et al. Daily cortisol production rate in man determined by stable isotope dilution/mass spectrometry. J Clin Endocrinol Metab 1991;71:39–45.

Molecular Pathogenesis of Human Pituitary Tumors

Joseph M. Alexander

INTRODUCTION

Pituitary adenomas are the most common adult intracranial neoplasms. They compose approximately 10% of diagnosed brain tumors. Although basic research investigating the causes of pituitary tumors is ongoing, and a great deal of descriptive information regarding tumor phenotype has been published, the molecular events leading to their formation are largely unknown. Historically, pituitary tumors have been categorized by the hormones they secrete, the resulting syndromes of clinical hormone excess, and the pituitary cell type of origin. Prolactinomas, the most common pituitary tumor type, are lactotroph derived. Patients with these tumors typically present with symptoms of galactorrhea and amenorrhea that are associated with clinical hyperprolactinemia. Growth hormone (GH)–secreting pituitary adenomas are somatotroph derived and cause acromegaly, with clinical features of acral enlargement, altered facial characteristics, visual field defects, and hypogonadism. Corticotroph tumors synthesize and secrete excess adrenocorticotropic hormone (ACTH), leading to clinical symptoms of Cushing's disease caused by hypercortisolemia. Thyrotroph-derived adenomas are rare. Their clinical manifestations of secondary hyperthyroidism arise from overproduction of thyroid-stimulating hormone (TSH). Endocrine-inactive pituitary adenomas are considered to be of gonadotroph cell origin because, although they do not cause a recognized syndrome of excess hormone overproduction, they often secrete intact gonadotropins and/or their free subunits (1, 2). Such tumors are slow-growing macroadenomas with extrasellar extension, and patients often present with symptoms of mass effect, including headache, visual field deficits, cranial nerve palsies, and associated hypopituitarism.

THE GENETIC BASIS OF HUMAN PITUITARY TUMORIGENESIS

Many studies have used molecular genetic assessments of X chromosome inactivation and tumor clonality to establish the mutational basis of human pituitary adenomas.

Historically, two theories of pituitary tumorigenesis have been proposed: hormone regulatory dysfunction versus somatic mutation. Until recently there was little evidence to support either theory, and both relied on inferential tumor histologic findings and serum hormone data. Because of the complex and highly regulated nature of the hypothalamic axis and its known effects on pituicyte hormonal phenotype, hypothalamic dysregulation has long been considered an obvious candidate for the primary pathogenetic mechanism of pituitary adenoma formation. Indeed, several studies have demonstrated that hypothalamic and circulating regulatory peptides probably play a critical role as pituitary cell growth factors to stimulate not only hormone secretion but also tumor proliferation (3–6). However, X-inactivation studies have repeatedly shown that most benign and malignant human tumors are monoclonal in origin. Based on these data, human pituitary tumors are considered to result from genomic mutations that facilitate a selective growth advantage to a single cell. Although pituitary adenomas have pathogenetic mechanisms similar to those of other human tumors and seem to arise de novo as a result of genomic mutation, ultimately their growth and phenotype may be influenced by hypothalamic or hormonal dysregulation. Thus, two theories that at first were diametrically opposed may be incorporated into a more cohesive and realistic model of human pituitary tumorigenesis.

The Hypothalamic Theory of Pituitary Neoplasia

This hypothesis of pituitary tumorigenesis states that pituitary adenomas are caused by hypothalamic or hormonal dysregulation, and that dysregulation of a specific endocrine axis stimulates the growth of many normal pituitary cell subtypes. This chronic pituitary hypertrophy results in a heterogeneous population of mitogenic cells that ultimately give rise to what is viewed both pathologically and medically as a discrete pituitary adenoma. Therefore, an extended period of pituitary hypertrophy/hyperplasia would be required for tumor development. Several lines of evidence support this theory. First, both the histologic appearance and the production of multiple pituitary hormones (demonstrated by immunocytochemical staining within single tumor sections) can be variable within a single tumor, consistent with a multicellular origin of proliferating pituitary cells (7–10). Second, ectopic biosynthesis of hypothalamic-releasing factors by ectopic endocrine tumors (specifically, corticotropin-releasing hormone [CRH] and growth hormone-releasing hormone [GHRH]) often creates multifocal pituitary hyperplasia and syndromes of clinical hormone excess (11–14). Third, results of transgenic studies and in vitro data strongly support the role of hypothalamic-releasing peptides as pituitary cell growth factors and identify excessive hypothalamic stimulation as a contributor to pituitary adenoma formation (3–6, 15). These data suggest that adenomas are not the result of spontaneous genetic alterations in pituitary cells but instead arise from hypothalamic dysregulation or other as yet unidentified imbalances in endocrine regulatory mechanisms.

The Mutational Theory of Pituitary Neoplasia

The sporadic mutation hypothesis states that an oncogenic mutation within a single pituitary cell offers a selective growth advantage over normal pituicytes. This mutated proliferating cell then establishes a monoclonal neoplasm with a homogeneous genetic makeup. Several clinical and pathologic observations support this theory. First, chronic primary endocrine end organ failure (i.e., hypothyroidism from autoimmune thyroid disease or premature ovarian failure) rarely gives rise to adenoma development. Second, pituitary neoplasms seldom contain the regions of cellular hyperplasia that would be expected if an extended period of multifocal cellular growth preceded neoplastic transformation (10). Third, the recurrence rates of pituitary tumors following surgical resection are low (16). Fourth, pituitary tumors in patients with multiple endocrine neoplasia type I have been detected in a number of documented kindreds with the disease (17). Multiple endocrine neoplasia type I (MEN-1) is caused by an altered tumor suppressor allele at 11q13 that exhibits an autosomal-dominant pattern of genetic inheritance. Presumably, this genomic alteration underlies development of MEN-1–associated pituitary tumors. Collectively, these observations infer that tumor formation begins with a genetic lesion in a single pituitary cell.

CLONALITY STUDIES IN PITUITARY TUMORS

Gonadotroph Adenomas

Clonality studies of clinically nonfunctioning adenomas were the first to demonstrate the monoclonal origins of pituitary adenomas (18, 19). Protein and mRNA analysis have shown that most clinically nonfunctioning adenomas synthesize and secrete intact free α- and β-gonadotropin subunits and that many actively secrete follicle-stimulating hormone (FSH) but not luteinizing hormone (LH), preferentially (1, 20). Nonfunctioning pituitary tumors may exhibit TSH-β biosynthesis and/or TSH secretion, but they rarely secrete ACTH, prolactin (PRL), or GH (20). Many clinically nonfunctioning adenomas exhibit immunocytochemical heterogeneity of gonadotropin subunit protein synthesis, with diverse secretory phenotypes observed within the same pathologic section in some tumors. Despite this apparent heterogeneity, molecular genetic analyses of X-inactivation patterns in these tumors have verified their origin from a single cell (18, 19, 21). Later tumorigenic events, such as differential expression of hormonal cell-surface receptors or synthesis of autocrine/paracrine regulatory factors, may foster the observed heterogeneous tumor phenotype (22–26).

GH- and PRL-Secreting Adenoma

Hypothalamic and hormonal factors may promote extensive proliferative responses in both somatotroph and lactotroph cells. For example, transgenic mouse models of GHRH overproduction and constitutively activated GHRH cytoplasmic signaling pathways (27–29), as well as a case report of an acromegalic patient with ectopic GHRH-producing tumor (14), have demonstrated GHRH to be a potent proliferative agent that can promote somatotroph hyperplasia. In addition, a transgenic mouse model of GHRH overproduction has demonstrated that continuous GHRH exposure for 10 to 12 months promotes pathologically confirmed adenoma formation (15). Similarly, in lactotrophs, chronic estrogen (E_2) administration induces proliferation that leads to hyperplasia and hyperprolactinemia in animal models (30–32). These proliferative effects of hypothalamic-releasing factors inferred that these pituitary tumor subtypes arise from polyclonal proliferation of pituitary cells. However, the clonal origins of pituitary hyperplasia and associated adenomas in animals is not known. Human tumor X-inactivation studies have demonstrated that sporadic somatotroph and lactotroph adenomas are monoclonal in origin (33). Therefore, hypothalamic or hormonal stimulation of proliferation must occur either early in tumorigenesis or before oncogenic transformation if it is to contribute to the onset of human pituitary tumorigenesis. Alternatively, these factors may affect clonal tumor growth via oncogenic changes in receptor status and/or intracellular signaling pathways.

Corticotroph Adenoma

Several observations suggest that hypothalamic stimulation may produce corticotroph tumors and Cushing's disease (9), including (*a*) tumor recurrence after surgical cure (34), (*b*) the diffuse corticotroph hyperplasia found in surgical specimens (7, 8), and (*c*) cases of ectopic CRH-producing tumors producing Cushing's disease and corticotroph hyperplasia (11, 12, 35). The effects of chronic CRH excess on corticotroph proliferation and secretion have been tested in animal models, only to yield conflicting results. Frank corticotroph hyperplasia has been observed in rats injected daily with CRH (5). However, transgenic mice that chronically overproduce CRH exhibit symptoms of Cushing's disease without concomitant corticotroph proliferation (36). There are also several lines of evidence implicating a primary pituitary oncogenic mutation as the underlying cause of corticotroph adenomas. Most patients with Cushing's disease are cured surgically by adenomectomy (16). The typical persistence of hypoadrenalism several months after surgery suggests that there is no chronic source of excess CRH (37). Subsequently, patients may reestablish normal hypothalamic–pituitary–adrenal axis

function. Clinical hypercortisolism was not reversed by pituitary stalk section in a patient with Cushing's disease; this is also consistent with intrinsic pituitary, rather than hypothalamic, pathogenesis (38).

Data aggregated from four separate studies show that 87% (27/31) of pituitary adenomas from patients with either Cushing's disease or Nelson's syndrome are monoclonal in origin (33, 35, 39, 40). One of the four polyclonal tumor specimens had interspersed normal tissue within the tumor specimen (33). The remaining three (two macroadenoma and one microadenoma) were examined for contaminating normal cells, but none were detected (39). Another study analyzed the clonality of human corticotroph hyperplasia in a patient with an ectopic CRH-producing bronchial carcinoid and Cushing's disease (35). Polymerase chain reaction–based determination of X-inactivation patterns showed a polyclonal pattern, consistent with a multicellular proliferative response to excess levels of circulating CRH. Thus, most corticotroph adenomas result from spontaneous mutations in a single cell. However, a few Cushing's tumors may develop from a multicellular field of proliferating cells.

Although almost all types of human tumors are monoclonal in origin, there are a few notable exceptions. Some neurofibromas (41) and trichoepitheliomas (42) are polyclonal. In addition, MT1/GHRH transgenic mice that have constitutively high levels of GHRH develop adenomas in foci of hyperplasia (15). However, the clonal origin of GHRH-induced somatotroph hyperplasia has not been documented. In summary, molecular genetic techniques permit analysis of X-inactivation patterns in genomic DNA from human pituitary tumors. This analysis demonstrates that almost all pituitary tumors are monoclonal in origin and arise de novo from oncogenic transformation of a single pituitary cell.

SOMATIC GENETIC MUTATIONS IN HUMAN PITUITARY ADENOMAS

Despite the monoclonal nature of human pituitary adenomas, the specific genetic alterations that give rise to a monoclonal pituitary neoplasm remain elusive. The foremost example of linkage of a specific molecular defect to pituitary tumorigenesis is the characterization of Gsα-activating mutations. These mutations were discovered based on observations that a subset of human somatotroph tumors had constitutive activation of GHRH-stimulated pathways in primary tumor cell culture (43). To date, activating mutations have been localized to two sites within Gsα, codons 201 and 227. Both mutations result in a constitutively activated stimulatory G-protein trimeric complex that leads to increased adenylyl cyclase activity and elevated intracellular cyclic adenosine monophosphate (cAMP) levels. This activation of G-protein signaling pathways results in GH hypersecretion in somatotroph adenomas and/or increased cellular proliferation. The effects of these mutations on somatotroph cell proliferative rates have been verified by several transgenic mouse models in which activated cAMP pathways cause marked somatotroph hyperplasia and, in older transgenic animals, discrete adenoma formation (6, 15).

Modern molecular cancer genetic studies have defined two broad classes of genes responsible for increased proliferative and oncogenic transformation of normal cells (44). Candidate class I oncogenes and tumor suppressor genes are those that are stably mutated or deleted in many characterized human neoplasms. These include activating mutations of oncogenes such as *ras*, which has been shown to be constitutively activated by genetic mutation in up to 40% of human cancers (45). Conversely, allelic loss and subsequent inactivation of tumor suppressor genes such as retinoblastoma and p53 have been demonstrated in several human tumors (46). Molecular genetic studies by several groups analyzing these candidate class I oncogenes and tumor suppressor genes have consistently demonstrated that they are not mutated in human pituitary adenomas (Table 5.1). Other studies examining inactivation of the MEN-1 gene at chromosome 11q13 have found the rate of allelic loss of this important endocrine tumor suppressor gene to be relatively rare in sporadic human pituitary tumors (47–51). Thus, although pituitary tumors are conclusively monoclonal in origin, and therefore harbor a somatic genetic defect that confers a selective growth advantage, the elucidation of such mutations has not been straightforward. Indeed, because pituitary adenomas rarely progress to malignancy and form metastases, their underlying genetic defects may be subtle. Therefore, candidate class I cancer genes that are demonstrated to be important in the pathogenesis of more aggressive human neoplasms may be of limited use in addressing the genetic basis of human pituitary adenoma formation.

Rather than being mutated at the DNA level and affecting cellular neoplasia, class II cancer genes affect tumor phenotype and progression by virtue of their altered patterns of gene expression during tumorigenesis. An alternate paradigm for studying the molecular basis of human pituitary tumorigenesis is to concentrate on downstream events in the neoplastic process by studying tumor-specific

changes in gene expression of growth-related genes. This method of investigation is termed "expression genetics" and is a fundamentally different strategy for studying human tumorigenesis. Using this approach, there has been substantial progress made in elucidating the molecular pathogenesis of human pituitary tumors. Genes that are not mutated in human pituitary adenomas and that have stably altered tumor-specific gene expression patterns may offer insights into the mechanisms of human pituitary tumorigenesis. Most important, because these class II genes are not mutated in human tumors but instead have altered expression in neoplastic tissue, they may be candidates for novel medical therapies and even future genetic therapies as that technology becomes more sophisticated and efficacious. Several candidate class II neoplastic genes have been identified in human pituitary tumors, including transcription factors that exhibit altered levels of tumor-specific gene expression, such as c-*myc*. Tumor-specific patterns of mRNA splicing and phosphorylation have been demonstrated for transcription factors Pit-1 and CREB, respectively (52–55). Human pituitary tumors also exhibit altered endogenous expression of several growth-related factors, such as fibroblast growth factors -2 and -4 as well as activin, a member of the transforming growth factor (TGF)–β superfamily of antiproliferative cytokines (22, 56–61).

Because cell-surface and cytosolic receptors are critical signaling molecules that may have profound effects on tumor growth rates and phenotype, they are also considered candidate class II cancer genes. Alterations in the gene expression and/or mRNA/protein structure of several cell-surface receptors have also been documented in human pituitary tumors. For example, GHRH receptor mRNA have been shown to exhibit tumor-specific alternative splicing, resulting in receptor isoforms with severely truncated cytoplasmic domains (62). In the remainder of this chapter I discuss studies from our laboratory that investigate tumor-specific patterns of gene expression and alternate mRNA splicing of three types of class II cancer genes that encode cell-surface or cytosolic receptors. Each of these class II genes may have potent proliferative effects on pituicytes and therefore tumor-specific changes in their expres-

Table 5.1. *Molecular Alterations in Human Pituitary Tumors*

Class I Gene	References	Class II Gene	References
Gsp mutations	43, 47, 147–154	CREB activation	52
11q13 chromosome loss	47–51	GHRH receptor alternative splicing	62, 155
13q14 chromosome loss	48, 120, 156–159	GnRH-Rc	86
H-*ras* mutations	160–162	Activin type I receptor alternative splicing	57
Protein kinase C mutations	163	ER alternative splicing	24
10q26	48	Pit-1 alternative splicing	53–55
13q12–14	48, 157	c-*myc*	164
		nm23	165
		hst/fibroblast growth factor-4/fibroblast growth factor-2	59–61, 166
		TGFα	167

sion and/or structure that could potentially mediate the pathogenesis of a clonal human pituitary neoplasm.

THE ROLE OF CELL-SURFACE AND CYTOSOLIC RECEPTORS IN THE PATHOGENESIS OF PITUITARY ADENOMAS

Human pituitary tumors typically have been classified by secretory phenotype. Hormone secretion by pituitary adenomas has been studied at several levels, from initial radioimmunoassays that measure serum hormone levels to more recent molecular biology techniques that measure tumor-specific hormone mRNA biosynthesis in vitro by northern hybridization and reverse transcriptase–polymerase chain reaction (RT-PCR) as well as at the single-cell level by in situ hybridization and immunocytochemistry. In recent years, several studies have begun to elucidate critical cell-surface and cytosolic receptors that control the biosynthesis and secretion of pituitary hormones from neoplastic pituicytes. Indeed, one overarching strategy for investigating pituitary tumorigenesis is to understand the molecular basis of secretory hormone imbalances in neoplastic pituicytes. This paradigm was elegantly used in the discovery of Gsp mutations in somatotroph tumors, although the genetic alteration was in the α-subunit of a receptor-linked stimulatory G-protein and not in the receptor itself. Many of the steroid and hypothalamic peptide receptors are important regulators of cell proliferative rates as well as hormone secretion, and therefore may be of potential interest when considering candidate class II cancer gene targets for future therapeutic avenues for the treatment of human pituitary tumors.

Medical therapies that act to arrest pituitary tumor cell growth have proven to be efficacious in reducing hormone secretion and tumor mass in a subset of patients with secretory tumors. These treatments began with a basic biochemical understanding of relevant pituitary cell-surface receptor expression and intracellular signaling pathways involved in pituitary tumor growth and hormone secretion. For example, bromocriptine, a dopamine agonist, has been useful in controlling both PRL hypersecretion and prolactinoma growth in patients with lactotroph adenomas. In somatotroph tumors, the normalization in serum GH levels with the somatostatin analog Octreotide is paralleled by a significant decrease in tumor mass in approximately half of treated patients (63). Therefore, one strategy for characterizing candidate class II cancer genes is to focus on receptors that influence cell proliferative rates as well as hormone biosynthesis and secretion.

Gonadotropin-Releasing Hormone (GnRH) Receptors

In contrast to the intact LH and intact FSH produced by normal gonadotrophs, uncombined FSHβ- or α-sub-

units are frequently secreted by neoplastic gonadotrophs (64–69). The well-documented hypersecretion of free FSHβ-subunit is commonly observed in vivo as well as in primary tissue culture of gonadotroph tumors and has been estimated to occur in up to one-third of patients with gonadotroph adenomas (65). Gonadotroph tumors may also secrete excessive intact bioactive FSH and, rarely, LH (70). Significantly, in contrast to normal pituitary or placental tissue in which α-subunit is synthesized in excess of either β-gonadotropin subunit, men with FSH-producing tumors have elevated levels of serum FSHβ relative to α-subunit compared with normal or hypogonadal men (67). Another study that examined gonadotropin gene expression found that FSHβ steady state mRNA levels were constitutively higher than levels of α-subunit mRNA in up to 33% of human gonadotroph tumors (65). These data demonstrate that pituitary adenomas have imbalanced gonadotropin subunit steady state mRNA levels, and FSHβ hypersecretion may reflect on the biosynthesis of gonadotropin subunit abnormalities in neoplastic gonadotrophs.

Cells from human gonadotroph tumors studied in primary tissue culture display similar abnormalities of gonadotropin biosynthesis and secretion found in the intact tumor. Therefore, this secretory phenotype would seem to be autonomous and is maintained in the absence of hypothalamic and hormone stimuli. A substantial subset of gonadotroph adenomas continue to secrete FSHβ-subunit in excess of α-subunit in primary tissue culture (71–73), and in vitro production of LHβ in excess of α-subunit at both mRNA and protein levels rarely occurs (70). These data suggest that underlying gonadotropin biosynthetic defects result in aberrant gonadotropin gene expression and subunit secretion in neoplastic human pituitary cells. The factors responsible for these abnormalities of control of gonadotropin biosynthesis and secretion may also comprise the downstream events of a primary genetic lesion and be caused by dysregulation of class II cancer genes.

One critical regulator of the production of LH and FSH by normal pituitary gonadotrophs and thus serum LH and FSH levels is the amplitude and frequency of hypothalamic pulsatile GnRH. Administration of GnRH antagonist to normal human (74) and normal rat pituitary cells in vitro (75) consistently decreases intact gonadotropin and α-subunit secretion without a stimulatory agonist phase. Several studies demonstrate that only a subset of human gonadotroph tumors are GnRH responsive in vitro. For example, GnRH induces mobilization of intracellular Ca^{++} and subunit secretion culture cells of pituitary tumors (71, 76, 77). Although these experiments confirm in vivo clinical studies documenting GnRH responsiveness of a subset of human gonadotroph adenomas, they do not address the physiologic regulation of neoplastic gonadotrophs by pulsatile GnRH. In addition, the mechanisms underlying the documented GnRH nonresponsiveness in a significant percentage of neoplastic gonadotrophs are unknown.

The clinical and in vitro data demonstrating that some gonadotroph tumors are unresponsive to GnRH despite their gonadotroph secretory phenotype may reflect a fundamental dysregulation of GnRH-receptor (GnRH-Rc) biosynthesis and/or cell signaling pathways. The cloning of human hypothalamic-releasing peptide receptors opens new opportunities for investigating receptor expression and function in human neoplastic gonadotroph cells (78–80). Gonadotropin-releasing hormone–receptor biosynthesis is regulated by both gonadal steroids and GnRH itself (81, 82). Investigation of neoplastic GnRH-Rc gene expression may reveal cell signaling defects that offer an increase in the cellular proliferative index in human gonadotroph tumors. Sequence analysis of the human GnRH-Rc shows that it is a G-protein coupled receptor (78). The conserved structure of the cloned GnRH-Rc confirms biochemical data that its stimulation of phospholipase C and phosphatidyl-inositol hydrolysis is mediated by its interactions with $Gq\alpha$ guanosine triphosphate–binding proteins (83, 84). Constitutive activation of this cell signaling pathway has mitogenic and transforming effects in NIH3T3 mouse fibroblasts (85). Therefore, dysregulation of GnRH-Rc gene expression may modulate tumor growth as well as gonadotropin biosynthesis and secretion.

Studies examining human gonadotroph tumor responsiveness to GnRH in perifused gonadotroph adenomas with evidence of gonadotropin biosynthesis and secretion found that 9 of 13 tumors were unresponsive to pulsatile GnRH (86). No significant differences were found in the mean baseline secretion of intact gonadotropins or α-subunit between responders and GnRH. However, FSHβ was undetectable in all GnRH unresponsive tumors. Mean secretory rates of LH, FSH, and α-subunit ranged from < 0.8 to 4.2 IU (< 0.8 to 4.2 IU/L[min^{-1}]), 1.1 to 5.1 IU (1.1 to 5.1 IU/L[min^{-1}]), and 0.2 to 0.6 IU (0.2 to 0.6 μg/L[min^{-1}]), respectively. Secretory profiles and GnRH receptor gene expression in representative responsive and unresponsive tumors are shown in Figure 5.1. A membrane-depolarizing pulse of 60 mmol of potassium chloride was administered to four of the nine GnRH-unresponsive tumors to confirm that lack of response was not caused by absence of intracellular gonadotropins. In each case, a significant transient secretory burst of gonadotropins and/or free subunits occurred. Gonadotropin-releasing hormone–receptor mRNA was detected in all GnRH-responsive tumors and was comparable with that seen in normal human pituitary tissue. In contrast, gonadotroph tumors unresponsive to pulsatile GnRH had no detectable GnRH-Rc mRNA. Responsiveness of perifused tumors to exogenous GnRH could be predicted by the presence of GnRH-Rc mRNA expression. GnRH-Rc is thus critically dependent on GnRH-Rc mRNA expression. These data indicate that GnRH-Rc biosynthesis is deficient in most human gonadotroph adenomas.

Alterations in GnRH-Rc biosynthesis in neoplastic gonadotrophs may, in turn, reflect defects in cell signaling pathways. In one model of constitutive activation of GnRH pathways, continuous in vitro administration of GnRH to normal rat pituitary cells decreased pituitary GnRH-Rc

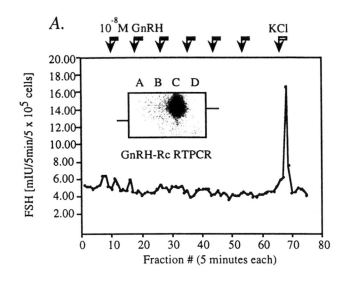

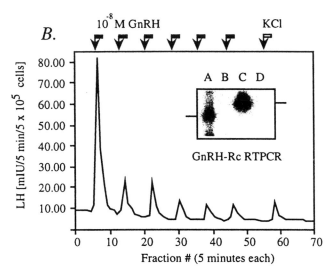

Figure 5.1. Gonadotropin-releasing hormone receptor biosynthetic defects in human gonadotroph tumors. Secretion of FSH and LH in perifusion by GnRH-unresponsive (**A**) and GnRH-responsive (**B**) pituitary tumors, respectively. Results of RT-PCR are shown for GnRH-Rc mRNA. *Lane A,* GnRH-RC (+reverse transcriptase); *lane B,* GnRH-RC (-reverse transcriptase); *lane C,* GapDH (+reverse transcriptase); and *lane D,* GapDH (-reverse transcriptase). Note the lack of GnRH-Rc mRNA in *Lane A* of the unresponsive tumor. Ten-minute GnRH pulses were given every 45 minutes, followed by a single 10-minute pulse of 60 mmol potassium chloride at the conclusion of the experiment. *Arrows* indicate the timing and duration of each GnRH pulse.

mRNA levels (82). This suggests that long-term desensitization of GnRH responses following application of GnRH agonists results from down-regulation of constitutive GnRH-Rc gene expression and steady state mRNA levels. Therefore, mutations that activate gonadotroph-specific GnRH second-messenger pathways can chronically down-regulate GnRH-Rc biosynthesis and desensitize neoplastic gonadotrophs to GnRH stimulation. It is unknown whether mutations that activate downstream second-messenger systems stimulate cell proliferation as well as desensitize the GnRH signaling pathways that modulate gonadotropin biosynthesis and secretion. However, studies using a GnRH antagonist have now clearly shown that despite long-term suppression of gonadotropin secretion, tumor mass is completely unaffected. This dissociation between hormone secretion and tumor proliferation strongly suggests that GnRH signaling pathways do not influence the proliferative index of neoplastic pituitary cells in gonadotroph tumors in which the GnRH receptor is expressed. However, it is unknown if GnRH signaling pathways are dysregulated in the 50 to 67% of gonadotroph tumors that do not exhibit measurable GnRH receptor gene expression. An important unanswered question in this class of gonadotroph tumor is whether the Gq/phospholipase C/protein kinase C pathway is up-regulated, either by primary genetic mutation or by dysregulation of class II cancer gene expression.

Activin/TGFβ Receptors

Activins are sulfhydryl-linked dimers comprising two distinct protein subunits (βA and βB) that are encoded by separate genes and are structurally related to a diverse family of antiproliferative factors in the TGFβ gene family (87, 88). Locally secreted activin potently and selectively induces differentiation in pituitary cells and regulates FSHβ biosynthesis and secretion (89, 90). Activin binds to a heterotetromeric transmembrane receptor complex with serine/threonine (Ser/Thr) kinase activity (91). The activin signaling pathway modulates the expression and activity of several nuclear factors important in gene regulation and cell cycling, such as the immediate early gene junB (92) and the tumor suppressor protein retinoblastoma (93). Growth inhibition by activin occurs in several cell types, including human K562 erythroleukemic cells (93), human fetal adrenal cells (94), and epidermal growth factor–stimulated hepatocytes (95). However, activins can stimulate cell proliferation in some endocrine cells, including human granulosa cells (96, 97), a testicular tumor cell line (98), and fetal rat osteoblast cells (99).

Model systems have offered insight into activin effects on cellular growth and phenotype in normal pituitary. Activin inhibits basal and GHRH-stimulated GH secretion and intracellular cAMP levels and has an antimitogenic action on rat somatotroph cells (100). Activin-A also inhibits propiomelanocortin mRNA biosynthesis, ACTH secretion, and cell proliferation in AtT20 cells, an established mouse corticotroph cell line (101). In normal pituitary gonadotrophs, activin increases several FSH-producing cells, although its effects on gonadotroph proliferative rates are unknown. Therefore, autocrine biosynthesis of activin may regulate proliferation of both normal and neoplastic cells. Human pituitary tumors synthesize activin mRNAs and secrete bioactive activin (22, 56). The effects of activin are down-regulated by follistatin (89), a monomeric glycoprotein that binds activin and is expressed in normal rat pituitary (102, 103). Endogenous follistatin mRNA has been identified in gonadotroph adenomas (22, 58), but tumor-specific follistatin biosynthesis has not been found in any other secretory pituitary tumor subtype.

In contrast to the uniform growth arrest and hormone regulation effects by activin observed in animal model systems, a subset of human pituitary tumors do not respond to exogenous activin (73). Alterations in cell-surface receptor gene expression by pituitary adenomas have been hypothesized to be an underlying cellular mechanism modulating cell proliferation in responsive versus nonresponsive human pituitary tumors (25, 26, 86). For example, disruption of tumor-specific expression of activin receptor subtypes by a large percentage of human gonadotroph tumors may facilitate resistance to the antiproliferative effects of activin, as has been shown for TGFβ in human lymphoid (104), breast, and colorectal tumors (105) as well as Hep2B and Mv1Lu cell lines (106). Whether the observed nonresponsive phenotype in gonadotroph tumors is caused by dysregulation of activin receptor gene expression, as has been shown for other human tumors, is unknown.

Recent cloning of the activin family of cell-surface receptors has revealed a novel family of receptor complexes with transmembrane Ser/Thr kinase activity and varying affinities for TGFβ and its related cytokines (91). The activin receptor family consists of two classes, designated type I and type II receptor Ser/Thr kinases. Recent studies have hypothesized a series of noncovalent molecular interactions between type I and type II receptors that give rise to active signaling receptor complexes (107). Human type I receptors, Alk1–5 (activinlike receptor kinases), primarily function as intracellular signal transducers, whereas binding specificity for TGFβ or activin resides in the type II receptors, TβRII (TGFβ) or ActRIIA and ActRIIB (107). Therefore, receptor complexes composed of both receptor classes are required for functional activin or TGFβ signaling. For both activin and TGFβ signaling, type I receptor is activated by ligand-bound type II receptor cross-phosphorylation at intracellular Ser and Thr residues. This activated complex then stimulates specific intracellular signaling cascades via type I receptor-specific Ser/Thr kinase activity (107). The identification of these receptors for TGFβ-related cytokines such as activin in human neoplastic pituitary tissue is a first step in investigating their role as signal transducers in tumor pathogenesis, hormone secretory phenotype, and cellular growth arrest. In addition, pituitary tumors may be an important model in elucidating activin effects in some human endocrine neoplasms.

The human type I activin receptor Alk4 (ActRIB) is the key receptor that modulates activin signaling (108). Functional complementation studies in mink lung epithelial (Mv1Lu) cell lines that lack type I or type II receptor expression have demonstrated that specific heteromeric complexes mediate intracellular signaling in response to activin and TGFβ. The type I activin receptor Alk4 is unique in its ability to up-regulate an activin-responsive reporter gene construct (3TPlux) when coexpressed with ActRII in Mv1Lu cells treated with activin (109, 110). In

Table 5.2. *Expression of TGFβ/Activin Receptors by Normal and Neoplastic Human Pituitary*

Activin/TGFβ Receptor Type	Somatotroph Adenomas	Corticotroph Adenomas	Prolactinomas	Nonfunctioning Adenomas	Normal Pituitaries
Type I-Rcs					
Alk1	5/8	1/8	7/9	5/9	5/5
Alk2	5/8	0/8	4/9	0/9	0/5
Alk3	7/8	7/8	8/9	8/9	5/5
Alk4-1	8/8	7/8	9/9	8/9	1/5
Alk4-2	7/8	2/8	8/9	6/9	0/5
Alk4-3	8/8	3/8	9/9	6/9	0/5
Alk4-4	8/8	7/8	9/9	9/9	2/5
Alk4-5	8/8	2/8	8/9	6/9	0/5
Alk5	7/8	1/8	7/9	3/9	0/5
Type II-Rcs					
ActRII	8/8	8/8	7/9	9/9	5/5
ActRIIB	7/8	7/8	9/9	9/9	2/5
TSRII	7/8	7/8	7/9	5/9	5/5

this system, coexpression of TβRII and Alk4 did not confer responsiveness when cells were treated with TGFβ, confirming that this type I receptor is activin specific. Similarly, the TGFβ specificity of Alk5 has been demonstrated, and Alk3 and Alk6 have been shown to be bone morphogenetic protein (BMP-2/4)–specific type I receptors (111, 112). Alk1 does not confer signaling to any known TGFβ-related ligand but has been implicated in the rare heritable syndrome hemorrhagic telangiectasia type 2 (113).

Table 5.2 shows the frequency of mRNA expression for type I and type II activin/TGFβ receptor mRNAs by human pituitary adenomas (57). Alk2 and Alk5, specific mediators of activin and TGFβ signals, respectively, are expressed in tumors but not in normal human pituitary cells. Alk2 receptor mRNA expression was further restricted to mammosomatotroph tumors. In contrast, mRNA encoding Alk1, a type I orphan receptor, is present in all normal human pituitaries studied and is highly prevalent in all tumor types except corticotroph adenomas. Alk3 mRNA is prevalent in both neoplastic and normal pituitary. Type II receptor mRNAs encoding ActRII and TβRII are found in both normal and neoplastic pituitary tissue. In contrast, ActRIIB mRNA is highly prevalent in all tumors but is scarce in normal human pituitary tissues.

Recently, detailed functional studies have delineated critical domains of the Alk4 receptor intracellular region that are important for type II receptor interactions as well as activation of downstream signaling pathways. A highly conserved glycine/Ser–rich juxtamembrane region termed the GS domain was found to be critical for downstream activation of the 3TPlux reporter in Mv1Lu cells (108). Site-specific mutagenesis studies have demonstrated that alterations in the GS domain and adjacent residues can render Alk4 either signaling deficient or constitutively active, depending on the exact location and nature of the amino acid substitution. For example, substitutions of nonpolar alanine residues for critical Sers in the GS domain render Alk4 signaling deficient, whereas glutamic acid substitutions in the same region exhibit wild-type activity with re-

spect to both basal and activin-stimulated levels of reporter 3TPlux activity (108). Similar mutational analysis of Thr residues immediately carboxyl to the GS domain showed that although alanine substitutions failed to support activin-induced luciferase activity, Thr to glutamic acid at residue 206 yielded a constitutively active Alk4. Together, these data strongly support the hypothesis that the GS domain, although lacking inherent kinase activity, is important for downstream signaling by type I receptors.

In addition to the juxtamembrane GS domain of Alk4, the intracellular kinase region is critical for proper activin signaling. Phylogenetic mapping of conserved Ser/Thr kinase catalytic domains predicts that the cytoplasmic domain of Alk4 consists of 11 kinase subdomains that are critical for modulating receptor function and intracellular signaling (114, 115). The carboxyl kinase catalytic domain, and the region with maximum conservation, resides within subdomains VI through XI. Subdomains VI and VII are involved in adenosine triphosphate binding in those kinases that use adenosine triphosphate as a phosphate donor. Subdomain VIII is thought to play a role in recognition of the correct hydroxylamino acids, as its residues are specifically conserved in either Ser/Thr or tyrosine kinase members. Subdomains IX and X, although highly conserved, have not been functionally defined by mutagenesis studies. However, phosphorylation of c-jun by c-jun amino-terminal kinase (JNK2) has been shown to be mediated via carboxyl terminus subdomains in mutagenesis studies, demonstrating that these subdomains are critical in kinase function (116). Finally, subdomain XI at the carboxyl terminus of the kinase domain has been implicated as playing a critical role in transphosphorylation of type I receptor by type II receptor (117). A missense mutation of Pro525 to Leu in human TβR-II type II receptor disrupts transphosphorylation of TβR-I and subsequent downstream signaling by type I receptor. In addition, a truncated form of type II receptor lacking kinase subdomains X and XI has been shown to abolish either TGFβ or activin-induced signaling in transfected cell lines (115). Interestingly, kinase subdomain XI is highly variable among Ser/Thr kinase receptor subtypes and, given its demonstrated functional role in transphosphorylation by type II receptors, may play a critical role in kinase substrate specificity (114). Because subdomains VIII through XI are critical for Ser/Thr kinase activity, as well as intracellular substrate specificity, they are hypothesized to play a critical role in type I receptor signaling in response to activin.

Structure/function analyses of activin type I receptors in model systems all point toward Alk4 as the critical mediator of activin signaling. When appropriately expressed, full-length Alk4 has the capacity to generate a specific intracellular signaling cascade in response to extracellular activin. Therefore, Alk4 intracellular domains that specifically interact with second-messenger pathways are hypothesized to be a critical link in cellular activin responses. One hypothesis is that kinase-deficient activin receptor complexes are unable to transmit signal via type I cytoplasmic Ser/Thr kinase domains and therefore act as dominant-negative receptors. Candidates for such a dominant-negative receptor phenotype are Alk4 receptor forms that lack full-length Ser/Thr kinase domains at their carboxyl terminus. Recently, Vale et al. have demonstrated that Alk4 receptors that lack both the GS domain and the entire kinase domain block activin-induced transcriptional activity in both CHO and K562 erythroleukemic cell lines (118). This effect can be rescued by the addition of excess full-length normal Alk4, indicating that the truncated Alk4 receptor isoform acts as a dominant-negative receptor.

Because functional studies with cloned kinase-deficient Alk4 demonstrate that it can function as a dominant negative to block activin signaling, one hypothesis that would account for activin-nonresponsive pituitary tumors is that truncated forms of Alk4 are expressed in human neoplastic pituicytes. The Alk4 gene region has been characterized extensively, and its genomic structure predicts four alternatively spliced mRNAs that alter the cytoplasmic structure of the Alk4 Ser/Thr kinase domain (119). The cytoplasmic domain of Alk4 mRNA can undergo alternate splicing to generate several truncated forms of the receptor that lack specific carboxyl kinase subdomains (119). The most limited truncation excludes subdomain XI, whereas the most extensive truncation excludes the kinase subdomains VIII through XI. All these forms retain the GS domain yet lack the critical kinase subdomains X and XI. Such truncated type I receptor forms may have several potential roles, including activation of other proliferative signaling pathways

and uncoupling of transcriptional versus proliferative responses to activin by separate carboxyl kinase subdomains.

We have recently identified four truncated forms of the intracellular carboxyl terminus of the Alk4 receptor in human pituitary adenomas, designated Alk4–2 through Alk4–5, which lack some or all of kinase subdomains VIII through X-XI, respectively (Fig. 5.2). Of importance, these truncated forms are specific to human pituitary tumors and are not detected in nonneoplastic human pituitary tissue (Table 5.3). By forming inactive type I/type II signaling complexes, truncated forms of the Alk4 cytoplasmic domain may attenuate activin signal transduction and have a dominant-negative phenotype for growth arrest by activin. The full-length Alk4 receptor mRNA as well as three truncated Alk4 mRNA variants generated by alternate splicing of the cytoplasmic Ser/Thr kinase occur in most pituitary tumors of all types. Two of these mRNA variants (Alk4–2 and –3) occur only in tumors and not in normal pituitary tissue. Another Alk4 splice variant (Alk4–5) generated by alternate splicing that eliminates exon 9 is also found only in tumors (Fig. 5.3).

Experiments examining the mechanisms underlying activin-induced cellular growth arrest have been reported in erythroleukemic K562 cells, which differentiate and upregulate globin expression in response to activin. These studies have demonstrated that activin causes a transient hypophosphorylation of the retinoblastoma protein and blocks the cell cycle at G1. Later studies examining the phenotype of a retinoblastoma knock-out mouse demonstrated marker pituitary hyperplasia associated with loss of retinoblastoma function (120). Retinoblastoma phosphorylation is mediated via at least three cyclin-cyclin dependent kinases (CDKs), CDK2-cyclinE/A, CDK4-cyclinD, and CDK6-cyclinD. Each of these CDK complexes can be inhibited by the nucleoproteins p27^{kip1} and p15^{ink4B}. Down-regulation of various CDKs through the cooperative action of an Ink4 CDK inhibitor and a Cip/Kip CDK inhibitor may be a potent mechanism for hypophosphorylation of retinoblastoma and resultant cell cycle arrest (121).

Recent studies from three separate laboratories have demonstrated that knock-out mice lacking p27^{kip1} exhibit marked pituitary hyperplasia and pituitary tumorigenesis, a phenotype similar to the retinoblastoma knock-out mouse (122–124). Because activin is a member of the TGFβ family of antiproliferative cytokines, its signaling pathway may ultimately use the same nuclear mechanisms to cause its antiproliferative effect in normal and responsive neoplastic

Table 5.3. *Expression of Activin Type I Receptor Isoforms by Normal and Neoplastic Human Pituitary*

Activin Type I Receptor Isoform	Somatotroph Adenomas	Corticotroph Adenomas	Prolactinomas	Nonfunctioning Adenomas	Normal Pituitaries
Alk4-1	8/8	7/8	9/9	8/9	1/5
Alk4-2	7/8	2/8	8/9	6/9	0/5
Alk4-3	8/8	3/8	9/9	6/9	0/5
Alk4-4	8/8	7/8	9/9	9/9	2/5
Alk4-5	8/8	2/8	8/9	6/9	0/5

Figure 5.2. Genomic and protein structure of Alk4 normal and truncated receptor forms. **A.** Predicted protein structure of each Alk4 isoform. *Asterisk* (*) indicates novel Ser/Thr residues encoded by unique COOH termini of each Alk4 isoform. Each truncated isoform is missing some or all of the critical kinase subdomains X-XI. **B.** Peptide sequence of each Alk isoform. *Underlines* indicate novel COOH termini of alternately spliced Alk4. Residues critical for FNTA phosphorylation are in the box. Kinase subdomains are in *roman numerals.* **C.** Genomic structure of exons 7 through 11 encoding the COOH-Ser/Thr kinase domains. Ser/Thr kinase subdomains are listed in *roman numerals* above each exon. Ser or Thr (*) and tyrosine (o) residues are also shown above each exon. *Black boxes* indicate coding sequence; *stippled areas,* novel coding sequences generated by alternate splicing of Alk4.

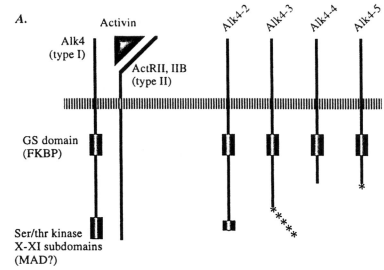

A.

B.

```
       residue 362
           │
           ▼                          VIII              IX
Alk4-2  VTDTIDIAPN QRVGTKRYMA PEVLDETINM KHFDSFKCAD IYALGLVYWE
Alk4-4  VTDTIDIAPN QRVGTKR... .......... .......... ..........
Alk4-5  VTDTIDIAPN QRVGTKRSP. .......... .......... ..........
 Alk4   VTDTIDIAPN QRVGTKRYMA PEVLDETINM KHFDSFKCAD IYALGLVYWE
Alk4-3  VTDTIDIAPN QRVGTKRYMA PEVLDETINM KHFDSFKCAD IYALGLVYWE

                                    X
Alk4-2  IARRCNSGGV HEEYQLPYYD LVPSDPSIEE MRKVVCDQKL RPNIPNWWQS
Alk4-4  .......... .......... .......... .......... ..........
Alk4-5  .......... .......... .......... .......... ..........
 Alk4   IARRCNSGGV HEEYQLPYYD LVPSDPSIEE MRKVVCDQKL RPNIPNWWQS
Alk4-3  IARRCNSGG. .TFLFCLCS YLPFQDAGSP KAVLLPPFFL QPVGCLLPEP

                    XI
Alk4-2  YEVRSWPPAA FPSA...... .......... .......... ..........
Alk4-4  .......... .......... .......... .......... ..........
Alk4-5  .......... .......... .......... .......... ..........
 Alk4   YEALRVMGKM MRECWYANGA ARLTALRIKK TLSQLSVQED VKI...
Alk4-3  ESSFKVAIKG VEVAVLRVRL FFRDQFVE.. .......... ......
```

C.

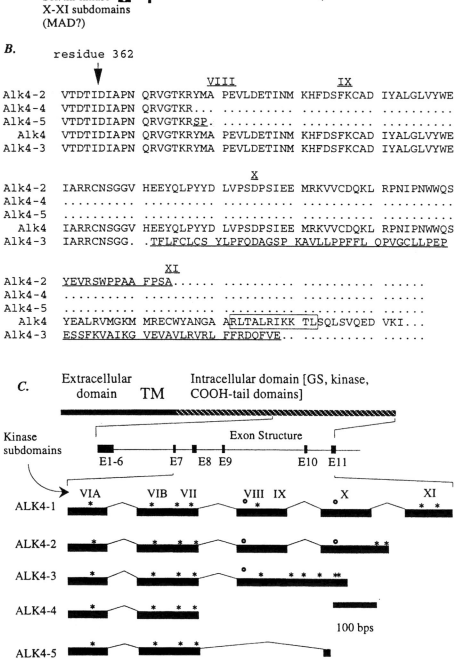

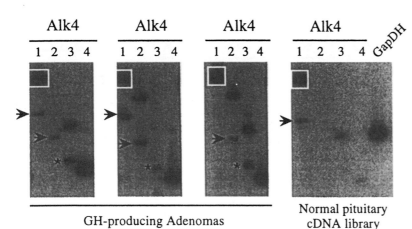

Figure 5.3. Results of RT-PCR of Alk4 receptor isoforms in normal and neoplastic pituitary adenomas. Amplified products were visualized by incorporation of 32P-dCTP and were size-fractionated by PAGE. The expected PCR product sizes are Alk4-1 (lane 1, white box), 530 bp; Alk4-2 (lane 2), 453; Alk4-3 (lane 3), 346; and Alk4-4 (lane 4), 248. *Arrows* indicate Alk4-5 in lanes 1 and 2. The 265-bp product in lane 3 of all tumors (*) is a nonspecific PCR product and does not hybridize to any Alk4 probe.

GH-producing Adenomas

Normal pituitary cDNA library

pituicytes. If truncated Alk4 type I receptor isoforms are dominant-negative agents and abrogate growth arrest by activin, a transgenic model of Alk4 truncated receptor expression may display the same phenotype as the reported p27^{kip1} knock-out mice. The identification of truncated type I receptors for activin in human neoplastic pituitary tissue is a first step in investigating their potential role as dominant-negative receptors that abrogate signal transduction in human pituitary tumors and the concomitant effects on tumors pathogenesis, hormone secretory phenotype, and neoplastic cell proliferation.

E$_2$ Receptors

The gonadal steroid E$_2$ regulates the biosynthesis and secretion of many anterior pituitary hormones. It also selectively stimulates proliferation of both normal and transformed lactotrophs and gonadotrophs (125–127). Up to 30% of women with macroadenomas (> 1 cm) experience symptomatic pituitary tumor enlargement during pregnancy because of elevated E$_2$ levels (128). In addition, studies in experimental animals have shown that prolonged administration of E$_2$ induces pituitary tumors, particularly prolactinomas (129, 130). E$_2$, therefore, seems to be a potent mitogen of a specific subset of pituitary cells. The documented mitogenic and regulatory effects of E$_2$ are mediated by its nuclear receptor (ER), a ligand-activated transcriptional factor of the steroid receptor superfamily. The ER is encoded by eight exons and is composed of at least four functional domains important for transcriptional activation function as well as DNA and ligand binding (131, 132). Sequence analysis of the ER gene reveals strong homology to the viral v-*erb*-A oncogene, suggesting that ER is a cellular homolog of this oncogene (133). In addition to its well-characterized role as an E$_2$-activated transcription factor, ER has recently been shown to interact directly with peptide growth factors, independent of E$_2$ (134, 135). Because ER mediates pituitary cell proliferation through several intracellular mitogenic signaling pathways, its dysregulation, either in terms of biosynthesis or

structure, may qualify it as a class II cancer gene in some subtypes of human pituitary adenomas.

In other hormone-dependent tumors, such as breast cancer, ER isoforms generated by alternative mRNA splicing (termed ER variants) have recently been identified (Fig. 5.4) (136–138). Some of these ER variants have differential effects on E$_2$-responsive gene expression. For example, an exon-5 ER spliced variant (Δ5ER) that lacks most of the hormone binding domain of the receptor has been shown to constitutively activate E$_2$-responsive genes (139). Coexpression of this variant with the wild-type ER in MCF-7 human breast cancer cells confers resistance to the E$_2$ antagonist tamoxifen (136, 137). Furthermore, an ER isoform lacking most of the hormone binding domain that is structurally similar to Δ5ER has been shown to activate c-*fos* promoter independent of E$_2$ administration (140). Therefore, this variant may stimulate cell proliferation independent of E$_2$ and may also contribute to clinical antiestrogen resistance. In contrast, an exon-3 ER spliced variant (Δ3ER) that lacks a portion of DNA binding domain has been shown to have a dominant-negative effect on wild-type receptor transcriptional activation when cotransfected with wild-type receptor in HeLa cells (141) and may decrease E$_2$ sensitivity in tumor cells. Results of these studies strongly suggest that differential exon alternative splicing of the ER gene can give rise to a variety of variant receptor isoforms that may potentiate the diverse actions of E$_2$ through a single receptor gene.

In the pituitary, wild-type ER mRNA has been demonstrated recently in normal and adenomatous lactotrophs and gonadotrophs (142, 143). Altered ER gene expression in E$_2$-sensitive pituitary adenomas may modulate normal ER function affecting both neoplastic cell proliferation and hormone secretion. Therefore, we investigated the expression of all potential exon alternate splice variant mRNAs, designated Δ2ER to Δ7ER, in 40 human pituitary adenomas of different phenotypes and normal pituitary tissues using RT-PCR, dideoxy sequencing, and Southern blot analyses. We identified differential ER isoform expression in human pituitary tumors of various phenotypes and found

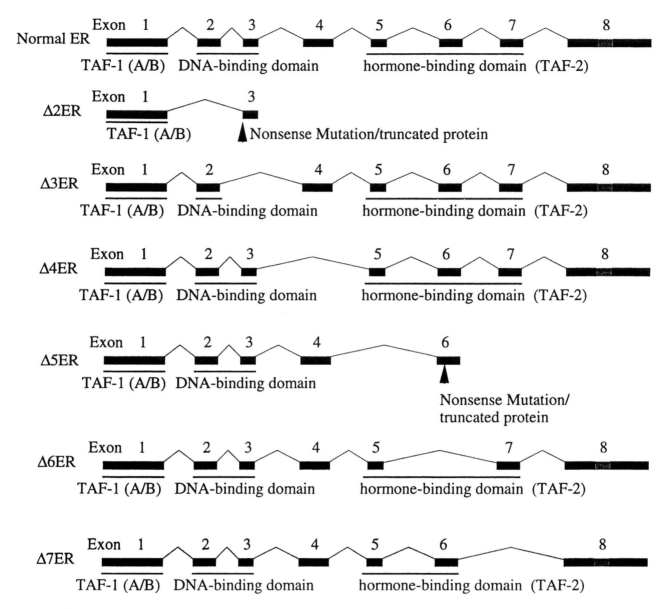

Figure 5.4. Structure of the human ER gene and alternatively spliced ER variant mRNAs. **A.** Schematic representation of a human ER gene consisting of eight exons (*closed boxes*) with a coding sequence from nucleotide 233 to 2020. Exon 1 encodes for the hormone-independent transcriptional activation function *(TAF-1)*, whereas exons 2 and 3 encode for the DNA binding domain and exons 4 through 8 for the hormone binding domain of the receptor. **B.** The expected size of the full-length ER as well as each alternatively spliced ER, designated Δ2ER to Δ7ER.

that multiple forms of alternatively spliced ER mRNA except Δ6ER were coexpressed with wild-type ER mRNA in a tumor phenotype–specific manner (Table 5.4). Prolactinomas displayed the greatest diversity of variant ER mRNA expression, including Δ2, Δ3, Δ4, Δ5, and Δ7ER, although Δ3ER mRNA was expressed at much lower levels. Glycoprotein hormone (GPH)–producing tumors that synthesized FSH also expressed multiple ER spliced variants (Δ2ER, Δ5ER, and Δ7ER), particularly Δ2ER, which expressed at levels comparable with those of wild-type ER mRNA. Variant and normal ER were not found in any other tumor subtypes except mixed GH/PRL and ACTH/PRL tumors in which low levels of both normal and variant ER were also detected. Only Δ4ER and Δ7ER were uni-

formly expressed in normal pituitaries at levels comparable with those detected in human pituitary tumor specimens. Δ2ER and Δ5ER, which were abundantly expressed in lactotroph and gonadotroph tumors, were nearly undetectable in normal tissues. No multiple exon deletion of more than a single exon was identified using Southern blot analysis. These data demonstrate that the expression of certain alternatively spliced ER variants in human pituitary tumors is both tumor specific and tumor phenotype specific. Furthermore, the wide array of ER isoforms detected are restricted in their expression to PRL- and GPH-producing tumors.

Although multiple isoforms of ER variants are coexpressed with wild-type ER in human pituitary tumors of

Table 5.4.   *Expression of ER Isoforms by Normal and Neoplastic Human Pituitary*

Tumor Type	Normal ER	Δ2ER	Δ3ER	Δ4ER	Δ5ER	Δ6ER	Δ7ER
Prolactinoma	11/11	9/11	6/11	9/11	9/11	0/11	11/11
Gonadotroph	4/7	4/7	0/7	1/7	4/7	0/7	3/7
Somatotroph							
Mammosomatotroph	4/4	0/4	1/4	2/4	2/4	0/4	4/4
Pure somatotroph	0/5	0/5	0/5	0/5	0/5	0/5	0/5
Corticotroph	1/10	0/10	0/10	1/10	0/10	0/10	0/10
Null cell	0/3	0/3	0/3	0/3	0/3	0/3	0/3

lactotroph and gonadotroph origins, their functional consequences are unknown. Because full-length ER is composed of several functional domains important for DNA binding, hormone binding, and maximal transcription activation, a deletion of a specific domain because of alternative mRNA splicing may give rise to a variant receptor with altered receptor activity. Variants of ER may have differential biologic effects at several levels by (*a*) competing with the ability of wild-type ER to bind with high affinity to E_2, (*b*) affecting the formation of stable ER homodimers following E_2 binding, or (*c*) altering the *trans*-activation of ER at E_2-responsive gene promoters. Therefore, differential exon alternative splicing of the ER gene can give rise to a variety of variant receptor isoforms that may potentiate the diverse actions of E_2 through a single receptor gene.

Little is known about the Δ2ER variant that encodes only the A/B domain of hormone-independent transcriptional activation function. Sequence analysis indicates that the protein product encoded by this variant is severely truncated and lacks domains critical for binding E_2-response elements or E_2. However, the A/B domain of the receptor has been demonstrated to stimulate transcription from certain E_2-responsive genes such as pS2 (131), c-*fos* (144), and C3 (145) and is requisite for growth factor interactions with ER signaling pathways (146). Moreover, functional analysis of an ER mutant containing only the A/B domain similar to Δ2ER has been shown to be highly effective in repressing Fos-mediated transcription in HeLa cells. Fos protein is known to antagonize transcription of the c-*fos* gene promoter induced by ER (144). Therefore, the Δ2ER truncated receptor may retain selective transcriptional activity and act as coactivator or repressor of wild-type ER. It may also play a role in nuclear receptor cross-coupling with other growth signal transduction pathways.

Δ5ER was also found to be expressed in PRL- and GPH-producing tumors and not readily detected in most normal pituitary tissues studied, including a normal pituitary cDNA library obtained from nine men and women. This variant has been shown to have constitutive transcriptional activity on E_2 response elements and to confer tamoxifen-resistant growth in human breast cancer MCF-7 cells (137, 139). A mutagenesis-generated ER isoform lacking most of the hormone binding domain structurally similar to Δ5ER-encoded protein also has been shown to activate c-*fos* pro-

moter independent of E_2 administration (140). Therefore, Δ5ER might also have constitutive activity and function to up-regulate growth factor–induced transcriptional response in human pituitary tumors. However, whether this ER variant possesses similar transcriptional activity in pituitary cells remained to be determined.

Prolactinomas and gonadotroph tumors coexpress multiple alternatively spliced ER variant mRNAs lacking a single exon along with wild-type ER in a tumor phenotype–specific manner. Most prolactinomas, as well as a subset of GPH-producing adenomas that synthesized FSH, expressed Δ2ER, Δ4ER, Δ5ER, and Δ7ER. Coexpression of variant and wild-type receptors is compatible with potential interactions between ER and its variant isoforms in E_2-sensitive pituitary cell types. For example, specific ER variants may have a role in modulating E_2 sensitivity in normal and adenomatous cells, whereas others may be involved in promoting aberrant cell growth and abnormal hormone production in the tumors. Given their potential as class II neoplasia genes, the identification of ER variant mRNAs in human pituitary tumors is a first step in investigating their functional significance in the pituitary as well as their potential role in modulating pituitary neoplastic cell growth and hormone biosynthesis.

CONCLUSIONS

The transformation from normal cells to neoplastic cells is a multistep process in most human tumor models (46). This additive effect of both genetic (class I gene mutation) and epigenetic (class II gene expression) alterations invokes a number of genomic mutations, including allelic loss of tumor suppressor genes, changes in DNA methylation patterns, faulty DNA editing and repair enzymes, and oncogene activation at many points along intracellular signaling and mitogenic pathways. Pathogenetic studies using modern molecular genetic tools will continue to concentrate on documenting the genomic changes that are associated with pituitary tumor formation. However, although somatic mutation is clearly a primary causative pathogenetic mechanism in most pituitary tumors, as clearly shown by clonality studies, there remain many important unanswered issues regarding the molecular pathogenetic mechanisms of human pituitary neoplasia with regard to both class I and class II neoplasia genes. Do epigenetic changes in endocrine systems potentiate pituitary adenoma formation? For example, does a period of hyperplasia invoke pituitary cells to acquire genetic lesions or do they truly arise spontaneously from mitotically quiescent pituitary cells? Similarly, dysregulated expression of autocrine/paracrine factors, such as the loss of TGFβ-related antiproliferative pathways, that increase rates of pituitary cell growth may concomitantly affect the frequency of oncogenic mutations. Are changes in hormone cell-surface receptor gene expression, such as GnRH receptors, causal or coincidental events in the pathogenesis of these tumors? What is the role of alternate splicing in the pathogenesis of human pituitary adenomas? Is the demonstrated alternate splicing of a number of receptor types in pituitary neoplasia a pathogenetic mechanism by which tumors arise or is alternate splicing a resultant (and perhaps reinforcing) event in human pituitary neoplasia? Future studies will need to investigate both the genetic and the epigenetic mechanisms that give rise to pituitary tumors, and this undoubtedly will lead to a greater understanding of the multistep process of pituitary neoplasia.

REFERENCES

1. Jameson JL, Klibanski A, Black PM, et al. Glycoprotein hormone genes are expressed in clinically nonfunctioning pituitary adenomas. J Clin Invest 1987;80:1472–1478.
2. Black PM, Hsu DW, Klibanski A, et al. Hormone production in clinically nonfunctioning pituitary adenomas. J Neurosurg 1987; 66:244–250.
3. Billestrup N, Swanson LW, Vale W. Growth hormone-releasing factor stimulates proliferation of somatotrophs in vitro. Proc Natl Acad Sci USA 1986;83:6854–6857.
4. Billestrup N, Mitchell RL, Vale W, et al. Growth hormone-releasing factor induces c-fos expression in cultured primary pituitary cells. Mol Endocrinol 1987;1:300–305.
5. Gertz BJ, Contreras LN, McComb DJ, et al. Chronic administration of corticotropin-releasing factor increases pituitary corticotroph number. Endocrinology 1987;120:381–388.
6. Mayo KE, Hammer RE, Swanson LW, et al. Dramatic pituitary hyperplasia in transgenic mice expressing a human growth hormone-releasing factor gene. Mol Endocrinol 1988;2:606–612.
7. Schnall AM, Kovacs K, Brodkey JS, et al. Pituitary Cushing's disease without adenoma. Acta Endocrinol 1980;94:297–303.
8. Saeger W, Ludecke DK. Pituitary hyperplasia: definition, light and electron microscopical structures and significance in surgical specimens. Virchows Arch 1983;399:277–287.
9. McNicol AM. Patterns of corticotropic cells in the adult human pituitary in Cushing's disease. Diagn Histopathol 1981;4: 335–341.
10. Kovacs K, Horvath E. Pathology of pituitary tumors. Endocrinol Metab Clin North Am 1987;16:529–551.
11. Belsky JL, Cuello B, Swanson LW, et al. Cushing's syndrome due to ectopic production of corticotropin-releasing factor. J Clin Endocrinol Metab 1985;60:496–500.
12. Carey RM, Varma SK, Drake CR Jr, et al. Ectopic secretion of corticotropin-releasing factor as a cause of Cushing's syndrome: a clinical, morphologic, and biochemical study. N Engl J Med 1984; 311:13–20.
13. Caselitz J, Saeger W. The ultrastructure of the pituitary gland under chronic stimulation of the ACTH-cells in human pathology and animal experiments. Endokrinologie 1979;74:163–176.
14. Thorner MO, Perryman RL, Cronin MJ, et al. Somatotroph hyperplasia: successful treatment of acromegaly by removal of a pancreatic islet tumor secreting a growth hormone-releasing factor. J Clin Invest 1982;70:965–977.
15. Stefaneanu L, Kovacs K, Horvath E, et al. Adenohypophysial changes in mice transgenic for human growth hormone-releasing factor: a histological, immunocytochemical, and electron microscopic investigation. Endocrinology 1989;125:2710–2718.
16. Laws ER Jr. Pituitary surgery. Endocrinol Metab Clin North Am 1987;16:647–665.
17. Brandi ML, Marx SJ, Aurbach GD, et al. Familial multiple endocrine neoplasia type I: a new look at pathophysiology. Endocr Rev 1987;8:391–405.
18. Alexander JM, Biller BM, Bikkal H, et al. Clinically nonfunctioning pituitary tumors are monoclonal in origin. J Clin Invest 1990;86: 336–340.
19. Jacoby LB, Hedley-Whyte ET, Pulaski K, et al. Clonal origins of pituitary adenomas. J Neurosurg 1990;73:731–735.
20. Snyder P. Gonadotroph cell adenomas of the pituitary. Endocr Rev 1985;6:552.
21. Herman V, Fagin J, Gonsky R, et al. Clonal origin of pituitary adenomas. J Clin Endocrinol Metab 1990;71:1427–1433.
22. Alexander JM, Swearingen B, Tindall GT, et al. Human pituitary adenomas express endogenous inhibin subunit and follistatin messenger ribonucleic acids. J Clin Endocrinol Metab 1995;80: 147–152.
23. Alexander JM, Klibanski A. Gonadotropin-releasing hormone receptor mRNA expression by human pituitary tumors in vitro. J Clin Invest 1994;93:2332–2339.
24. Chaidarun SS, Klibanski A, Alexander JM. Tumor-specific expression of alternatively spliced estrogen receptor mRNA variants in human pituitary adenomas. J Clin Endocrinol Metab 1997;82: 1058–1065.
25. Greenman Y, Melmed S. Heterogeneous expression of two somatostatin receptor subtypes in pituitary tumors. J Clin Endocrinol Metab 1994;78:398–403.
26. Miller GM, Alexander JM, Bikkal HA, et al. Somatostatin receptor subtype gene expression in pituitary adenomas. J Clin Endocrinol Metab 1995;80:1386–1392.
27. Struthers RS, Vale WW, Arias C, et al. Somatotroph hypoplasia and dwarfism in transgenic mice expressing a non-phosphorylatable CREB mutant. Nature 1991;350:622–624.
28. Sutcliffe JG, Travis GH, Danielson PE, et al. Molecular approaches to genes of the CNS. Epilepsy Res Suppl 1991;4:213–223.
29. Burton FH, Hasel KW, Bloom FE, et al. Pituitary hyperplasia and gigantism in mice caused by a cholera toxin transgene. Nature 1991;350:74–77.
30. Chaidarun SS, Eggo MC, Steward PM, et al. Role of growth factors and estrogen as modulators of growth, differentiation, and expression of gonadotropin subunit genes in primary cultured sheep pituitary cells. Endocrinology 1994;134:935–944.
31. El-Azouzi M, Hsu DW, Black PM, et al. The importance of dopamine in the pathogenesis of experimental prolactinomas. J Neurosurg 1990;72:273–281.
32. Gooren LJ, Assies J, Asscheman H, et al. Estrogen-induced prolactinoma in a man. J Clin Endocrinol Metab 1988;66:444–446.
33. Herman V, Fagin J, Gonsky R, et al. Clonal origin of pituitary adenomas. J Clin Endocrinol Metab 1990;71:1427–1433.
34. Bigos ST, Somma M, Rasio E, et al. Cushing's disease: management by transsphenoidal pituitary microsurgery. J Clin Endocrinol Metab 1980;50:348–354.
35. Biller BM, Alexander JM, Zervas NT, et al. Clonal origins of adrenocorticotropin-secreting pituitary tissue in Cushing's disease. J Clin Endocrinol Metab 1992;75:1303–1309.
36. Stenzel-Poore MP, Cameron VA, Vaughan J, et al. Development of Cushing's syndrome in corticotropin-releasing factor transgenic mice. Endocrinology 1992;130:3378–3386.
37. Fitzgerald PA, Aron DC, Findling JW, et al. Cushing's disease: transient secondary adrenal insufficiency after selective removal of pituitary microadenomas: evidence for a pituitary origin. J Clin Endocrinol Metab 1982;54:413–422.

38. Liddle GW. The George M. Kober Lecture: "Cushing's syndrome—1980." Trans Assoc Am Physicians 1980;93:40–51.
39. Schulte HM, Oldfield EH, Allolio B, et al. Clonal composition of pituitary adenomas in patients with Cushing's. J Clin Endocrinol Metab 1991;73:1302–1308.
40. Gicquel C, Le-Bouc Y, Luton JP, et al. Monoclonality of corticotroph macroadenomas in Cushing's disease. J Clin Endocrinol Metab 1992;75:472–475.
41. Fialkow PJ, Sagebiel RW, Gartler SM, et al. Multiple cell origin of hereditary neurofibromas. N Engl J Med 1971;284:298–300.
42. Gartler SM, Ziprkowski L, Krakowski A. Glucose-6-phosphate dehydrogenase mosaicism as a tracer in the study of hereditary multiple trichoepithelioma. Am J Hum Genet 1966;18:282–287.
43. Landis CA, Masters SB, Spada A, et al. GTPase inhibiting mutations activate the alpha chain of Gs and stimulate adenylyl cyclase in human pituitary tumours. Nature 1989;340:692–696.
44. Sager R. Expression genetics in cancer: shifting the focus from DNA to RNA. Proc Natl Acad Sci USA 1997;94:952–955.
45. Bos JL. Ras oncogenes in human cancer: a review. Cancer Res 1989;49:4682–4689.
46. Fearon ER, Voglestein B. A genetic model for colorectal tumorigenesis. Cell 1990;61:759–767.
47. Boggild MD, Jenkinson S, Pistorello M, et al. Molecular genetic studies of sporadic pituitary tumors. J Clin Endocrinol Metab 1994;78:387–392.
48. Bates AS, Farrell WE, Bicknell EJ, et al. Allelic deletion in pituitary adenomas reflects aggressive biological activity and has potential value as a prognostic marker. J Clin Endocrinol Metab 1997;82:818–824.
49. Herman V, Drazin NZ, Gonsky R, et al. Molecular screening of pituitary adenomas for gene mutations and rearrangements. J Clin Endocrinol Metab. 1993;77:50–55.
50. Bystrom C, Larsson C, Blomberg C, et al. Localization of the MEN1 gene to a small region within chromosome 11q13 by deletion mapping in tumors. Proc Natl Acad Sci U S A 1990;87:1968–1972.
51. Thakker RV, Pook MA, Wooding C, et al. Association of somatotrophinomas with loss of alleles on chromosome 11 and with gsp mutations. J Clin Invest 1993;91:2815–2821.
52. Bertherat J, Chanson P, Montminy M. The cyclic adenosine 3′,5′-monophosphate-responsive factor CREB is constitutively activated in human somatotroph adenomas. Mol Endocrinol 1995;9:777–783.
53. Friend KE, Chiou YK, Laws ER Jr, et al. Pit-1 messenger ribonucleic acid is differentially expressed in human pituitary adenomas. J Clin Endocrinol Metab 1993;77:1281–1286.
54. Hamada K, Nishi T, Kuratsu J, et al. Expression and alternative splicing of Pit-1 messenger ribonucleic acid in pituitary adenomas. Neurosurgery 1996;38:362–366.
55. Pellegrini I, Barlier A, Gunz G, et al. Pit-1 gene expression in the human pituitary and pituitary adenomas. J Clin Endocrinol Metab 1994;79:189–196.
56. Haddad G, Penabad JL, Bashey HM, et al. Expression of activin/inhibin subunit messenger ribonucleic acids by gonadotroph adenomas. J Clin Endocrinol Metab 1994;79:1399–1403.
57. Alexander JM, Bikkal HA, Zervas NT, et al. Tumor-specific expression and alternate splicing of mRNAs encoding activin/transforming growth factor-beta receptors in human pituitary adenomas. J Clin Endocrinol Metab 1996;81:783–790.
58. Penabad JL, Bashey HM, Asa SL, et al. Decreased follistatin gene expression in gonadotroph adenomas. J Clin Endocrinol Metab 1996;81:3397–3403.
59. Zimering MB, Brandi ML, deGrange DA, et al. Circulating fibroblast growth factor-like substance in familial multiple endocrine neoplasia type 1. J Clin Endocrinol Metab 1990;70:149–154.
60. Zimering MB, Katsumata N, Sato Y, et al. Increased basic fibroblast growth factor in plasma from multiple endocrine neoplasia type 1: relation to pituitary tumor. J Clin Endocrinol Metab 1993;76:1182–1187.
61. Zimering MB, Riley DJ, Thakker-Varia S, et al. Circulating fibroblast growth factor-like autoantibodies in two patients with multiple endocrine neoplasia type 1 and prolactinoma. J Clin Endocrinol Metab 1994;79:1546–1552.
62. Tang J, Lagace G, Castagne J, et al. Identification of human growth hormone-releasing receptor splicing variants. J Clin Endocrinol Metab 1995;80:2381–2387.
63. Wynick D, Bloom SR. Clinical review 23: the use of the long-acting somatostatin analog octreotide in the treatment of gut neuroendocrine tumors. J Clin Endocrinol Metab 1991;73:1–3.
64. Demura R, Jibiki K, Kubo O, et al. The significance of alpha-subunit as a tumor marker for gonadotropin-producing pituitary adenomas. J Clin Endocrinol Metab 1986;63:564–569.
65. Katznelson L, Alexander JM, Bikkal HA, et al. Imbalanced follicle-stimulating hormone beta-subunit hormone biosynthesis in human pituitary adenomas. J Clin Endocrinol Metab 1992;74:1343–1351.
66. Ridgway EC, Klibanski A, Ladenson PW, et al. Pure alpha-secreting pituitary adenomas. N Engl J Med 1981;304:1254–1259.
67. Snyder PJ, Johnson J, Muzyka R. Abnormal secretion of glycoprotein alpha subunit and follicle-stimulating (FSH) hormone beta subunit in men with pituitary adenomas and FSH hypersecretion. J Clin Endocrinol Metab 1980;51:579–584.
68. Snyder PJ, Muzyka R, Johnson J, et al. Thyrotropin-releasing hormone provokes abnormal follicle-stimulating hormone (FSH) and luteinizing hormone responses in men who have pituitary adenomas and FSH hypersecretion. J Clin Endocrinol Metab 1980;51:744–748.
69. Snyder PJ, Bashey HM, Kim SU, et al. Secretion of uncombined subunits of luteinizing hormone by gonadotroph cell adenomas. J Clin Endocrinol Metab 1984;59:1169–1175.
70. Klibanski A, Deutsch PJ, Jameson JL, et al. Luteinizing hormone-secreting pituitary tumor: biosynthetic characterization and clinical studies. J Clin Endocrinol Metab 1987;64:536–542.
71. Lamberts SW, Verleun T, Oosterom R, et al. The effects of bromocriptine, thyrotropin-releasing hormone, and gonadotropin-releasing hormone on hormone secretion by gonadotropin-secreting pituitary adenomas in vivo and in vitro. J Clin Endocrinol Metab 1987;64:524–530.
72. Yamada S, Asa SL, Kovacs K, et al. Analysis of hormone secretion by clinically nonfunctioning human pituitary adenomas using the reverse hemolytic plaque assay. J Clin Endocrinol Metab 1989;68:73–80.
73. Alexander JM, Jameson JL, Bikkal HA, et al. The effects of activin on follicle-stimulating hormone secretion and biosynthesis in human glycoprotein hormone-producing pituitary adenomas. J Clin Endocrinol Metab 1991;72:1261–1267.
74. Mansfield JM, Beardsworth DE, Loughlin JS. Long-term treatment of central precocious puberty with a long-acting analogue of luteinizing hormone-releasing hormone: effects on somatic growth and skeletal maturation. N Engl J Med 1983;309:1286–1291.
75. Danforth DR, Williams RF, Gordon K, et al. Inhibition of pituitary gonadotropin secretion by the gonadotropin-releasing hormone antagonist antide, I: in vitro studies on mechanism of action. Endocrinology 1991;128:2036–2040.
76. Kwekkeboom DJ, De Jong FH, Lamberts SWJ. Gonadotropin release by clinically nonfunctioning and gonadotroph pituitary adenomas in vivo and in vitro: relation to sex and effects of thyrotropin-releasing hormone, gonadotropin-releasing hormone, and bromocriptine. J Clin Endocrinol Metab 1989;68:1128–1135.
77. Spada A, Reza-Elahi F, Lania A, et al. Hypothalamic peptides modulate cytosolic free Ca2+ levels and adenylyl cyclase activity in human nonfunctioning pituitary adenomas. J Clin Endocrinol Metab 1991;73:913–918.
78. Chi L, Zhou W, Prikhozhan A, et al. Cloning and characterization of the human GnRH receptor. Mol Cell Endocrinol 1993;91:R1–6.
79. Gaylinn BD, Harrison JK, Zysk JR, et al. Molecular cloning and expression of a human anterior pituitary receptor for growth hormone-releasing hormone. Mol Endocrinol 1993;7:77–84.
80. Mayo KE. Molecular cloning and expression of a pituitary-specific receptor for growth hormone-releasing hormone. Mol Endocrinol 1992;6:1734–1744.
81. Bauer-Dantoin AC, Weiss J, Jameson JL. Roles of estrogen, progesterone, and gonadotropin-releasing hormone (GnRH) in the control of pituitary GnRH receptor gene expression at the time of the preovulatory gonadotropin surges. Endocrinology 1995;136:1014–1019.
82. Kaiser UB, Jakubowiak A, Steinberger A, et al. Regulation of rat pituitary gonadotropin-releasing hormone receptor mRNA levels in vivo and in vitro. Endocrinology 1993;133:931–934.
83. Kaiser UB, Katzenellenbogen RA, Conn PM, et al. Evidence that

signalling pathways by which thyrotropin-releasing hormone and gonadotropin-releasing hormone act are both common and distinct. Mol Endocrinol 1994;8:1038–1048.

84. Hsieh K-P, Martin TFJ. Thyrotropin-releasing hormone and gonadotropin-releasing hormone receptors activate phospholipase C by coupling to the guanosine triphosphate-binding proteins Gq and G11. Mol Endocrinol 1992;6:1673–1681.

85. Kalinec G, Nazarali AJ, Hermouet S, et al. Mutated alpha subunit of the Gq protein induces malignant transformation in NIH 3T3 cells. Mol Cell Biol 1992;12:4687–4693.

86. Alexander JM, Klibanski A. Gonadotropin-releasing hormone receptor mRNA expression by human pituitary tumors in vitro. J Clin Invest 1994;93:2332–2339.

87. Mason AJ, Hayflick JS, Ling N, et al. Complementary DNA sequences of ovarian follicular fluid inhibin show precursor structure and homology with transforming growth factor-β. Nature 1985; 318:659–663.

88. Ling N, Ying S-Y, Ueno N, et al. Pituitary FSH is released by a heterodimer of the β-subunits from the two forms of inhibin. Nature 1986;321:779–782.

89. Carroll RS, Corrigan AZ, Gharib SD, et al. Inhibin, activin, and follistatin: regulation of follicle-stimulating hormone messenger ribonucleic acid levels. Mol Endocrinol 1989;3:1969–1976.

90. Carroll RS, Corrigan AZ, Vale W, et al. Activin stabilizes follicle-stimulating hormone-beta messenger ribonucleic acid levels. Endocrinology 1991;129:1721–1726.

91. Mathews LS. Activin receptors and cellular signaling by the receptor serine kinase family. Endocr Rev 1994;15:310–325.

92. Hashimoto M, Gaddy-Kurten D, Vale W. Protooncogene junB as a target for activin actions. Endocrinology 1993;133:1934–1940.

93. Sehy DW, Shao LE, Yu AL, et al. Activin A-induced differentiation in K562 cells is associated with a transient hypophosphorylation of RB protein and the concomitant block of cell cycle at G1 phase. J Cell Biochem 1992;50:255–265.

94. Spencer SJ, Rabinovici J, Jaffe RB. Human recombinant activin-A inhibits proleiferation of human fetal adrenal cells in vitro. J Clin Endocrinol Metab 1990;71:1678–1680.

95. Yasuda H, Mine T, Shibata H, et al. Activin A: an autocrine inhibitor of initiation of DNA synthesis in rat hepatocytes. J Clin Invest 1993;92:1491–1496.

96. Rabinovici J, Spencer SJ, Jaffe RB. Recombinant human activin-A promotes proliferation of human luteinized preovulatory granulosa cells in vitro. J Clin Endocrinol Metab 1990;71:1396–1398.

97. Gonzalez-Manchon C, Vale W. Activin-A, inhibin and transforming growth factor-beta modulate growth of two gonadal cell lines. Endocrinology 1989;125:1666–1672.

98. Roberts V, Meunier H, Sawchenko PE, et al. Differential production and regulation of inhibin subunits in rat testicular cell types. Endocrinology 1989;125:2350–2359.

99. Centrella M, McCarthy TL, Canalis E. Activin-A binding and biochemical effects in osteoblast-enriched cultures from fetal-rat parietal bone. Mol Cell Biol 1991;11:250–258.

100. Billestrup N, Gonzalez-Manchon C, Potter E, et al. Inhibition of somatotroph growth and growth hormone biosynthesis by activin in vitro. Mol Endocrinol 1990;4:356–362.

101. Bilezikjian LM, Blount AL, Campen CA, et al. Activin-A inhibits proopiomelanocortin messenger RNA accumulation and adrenocorticotropin secretion of AtT20 cells. Mol Endocrinol 1991;5: 1389–1395.

102. DePaolo LV, Mercada M, Guo Y, et al. Increased follistatin (activin-binding protein) gene expression in rat anterior pituitary tissue after ovariectomy may be mediated by pituitary activin. Endocrinology 1993;132:2221–2228.

103. Kaiser UB, Chin WW. Regulation of follistatin messenger ribonucleic acid levels in the rat pituitary. J Clin Invest 1993;91: 2523–2531.

104. Kadin ME, Cavaille-Coll MW, Gertz R, et al. Loss of receptors for transforming growth factor beta in human T-cell malignancies. Proc Natl Acad Sci USA 1994;91:6002–6006.

105. Markowitz S, Wang J, Myeroff L, et al. Inactivation of the type II TGF-beta receptor in colon cancer cells with microsatellite instability. Science 1995;268:1336–1338.

106. Park K, Kim SJ, Bang YJ, et al. Genetic changes in the transforming growth factor beta (TGF-beta) type II receptor gene in human gastric cancer cells: correlation with sensitivity to growth inhibition by TGF-beta. Proc Natl Acad Sci USA 1994;91:8772–8776.

107. Wrana JL, Attisano L, Wieser R, et al. Mechanism of activation of the TGF-beta receptor. Nature 1994;370:341–347.

108. Willis SA, Zimmerman CM, Li L, et al. Formation and activation by phosphorylation of activin receptor complexes. Mol Endocrinol 1996;10:367–379.

109. Attisano L, Carcamo J, Ventura F, et al. Identification of human activin and TGF beta type I receptors that form heteromeric kinase complexes with type II receptors. Cell 1993;75:671–680.

110. Carcamo J, Weis FM, Ventura F, et al. Type I receptors specify growth-inhibitory and transcriptional responses to transforming growth factor beta and activin. Mol Cell Biol 1994;14: 3810–3821.

111. Koenig BB, Cook JS, Wolsing DH, et al. Characterization and cloning of a receptor for BMP-2 and BMP-4 from NIH 3T3 cells. Mol Cell Biol 1994;14:5961–5974.

112. ten Dijke P, Yamashita H, Sampath TK, et al. Identification of type I receptors for osteogenic protein-1 and bone morphogenetic protein-4. J Biol Chem 1994;269;16985–16988.

113. McAllister KA, Grogg KM, Johnson DW, et al. Endoglin, A TGF-beta binding protein of endothelial cells, is the gene for hereditary haemorrhagic telangiectasia type 1. Nat Genet 1994;8:345–351.

114. Hanks SK, Quinn AM, Hunter T. The protein kinase family: conserved features and deduced phylogeny of the catalytic domains. Science 1988;241:42–52.

115. Wieser R, Attisano L, Wrana JL, et al. Signaling activity of transforming growth factor beta type II receptors lacking specific domains in the cytoplasmic region. Mol Cell Biol 1993;13: 7239–7247.

116. Kallunki T, Su B, Tsigelny I, et al. JNK2 contains a specificity-determining region responsible for efficient c-Jun binding and phosphorylation. Genes Dev 1994;8:2996–3007.

117. Carcamo J, Zentella A, Massague J. Disruption of transforming growth factor beta signaling by a mutation that prevents transphosphorylation within the receptor complex. Mol Cell Biol 1995;15: 1573–1581.

118. Tsuchida K, Vaughan JM, Wiater E, et al. Inactivation of activin-dependent transcription by kinase-deficient activin receptors. Endocrinology 1995;136:5493–5503.

119. Xu J, Matsuzaki K, McKeehan K, et al. Genomic structure and cloned cDNAs predict that four variants in the kinase domain of serine/threonine kinase receptors arise by alternative splicing and poly (A) addition. Proc Natl Acad Sci USA 1994;91:7957–7961.

120. Jacks T, Fazeli A, Schmitt EM, et al. Effects of an Rb mutation in the mouse. Nature 1992;359:295–300.

121. Reynisdottir I, Polyak K, Lavarone A, et al. Kip/Cip and Ink4 Cdk inhibitors cooperate to induce cell cycle arrest in response to TGF-beta. Genes Dev 1995;9:1831–1845.

122. Fero ML, Ribkin M, Tasch M, et al. A syndrome of multiorgan hyperplasia with features of gigantism, tumorigenesis, and female sterility in p27kip1-deficient mice. Cell 1996;85:733–744.

123. Kiyokawa H, Kineman RD, Manova-Todorova KO, et al. Enhanced growth of mice lacking the cyclin-dependent kinase inhibitor function of p27kip1. Cell 1996;85:721–732.

124. Nakayama K, Ishida N, Shirane M, et al. Mice Lacking p27kip1 display increased body size, multiple organ hyperplasia, retinal dysplasia, and pituitary tumors. Cell 1996;85:707–720.

125. Chaidarun SS, Eggo MC, Stewart PM, et al. Role of growth factors and estrogen as modulators and growth, differentiation and expression of gonadotropin subunit genes in primary cultured sheep pituitary cells. Endocrinology 1994;134:935–944.

126. Lieberman ME, Maurer RA, Claude P, et al. Regulation of pituitary growth and prolactin gene expression by estrogen, hormones and cancer. In: Leavitt WW, ed. Hormones and Cancer. New York: Plenum Press, 1980:151–163.

127. Shupnik MA, Gharib SD, Chin WW. Divergent effects of estradiol on gonadotropin gene transcription in pituitary fragments. Mol Endocrinol 1989;3:474–480.

128. Holmgren U, Bergstrand G, Hagenfeldt K, et al. Women with prolactinoma-effect of pregnancy and lactation on serum prolactin and on tumor growth. Acta Endocrinol (Copenh) 1986;111: 452–459.

129. Furth J. Experimental pituitary tumors. Recent Prog Horm Res 1955;11:221–249.

130. Lloyd RV. Estrogen-induced hyperplasia and neoplasia in the rat anterior pituitary gland. Am J Pathol 1983;113:198–206.

131. Kumar V, Green S, Stack G, et al. Functional domains of the human estrogen receptor. Cell 1987;51:941–951.
132. Ponglikitmongkol M, Green S, Chambon P. Genomic organization of the human estrogen receptor gene. Embo J 1988;7:3385–3388.
133. Green S, Walter P, Kumar V, et al. Human estrogen receptor cDNA: sequence, expression and homology to v-erbA. Nature 1986;320:134–139.
134. Ignar-Trowgridge DM, Pimentel M, Teng CT, et al. Cross talk between peptide growth factor and estrogen receptor signalling systems. Environ Health Perspect 1995;103(Suppl 7):35–38.
135. Newton CJ, Buric R, Trapp T, et al. The unliganded estrogen receptor (ER) transduces growth factor signals. J Steroid Biochem Mol Biol 1994;48:481–486.
136. Fuqua SAW, Allred DC, Auchus RJ. Expression of estrogen receptor variants. J Cell Biochem 1993;17G:194–197.
137. Fuqua SAW. Estrogen receptor mutagenesis and hormone resistance. Cancer 1994;74:1026–1029.
138. Gotteland M, Desauty G, Delarue JC, et al. Human estrogen receptor messenger RNA variants in both normal and tumor breast tissues. Mol Cell Endocrinol 1995;112:1–13.
139. Fuqua SAW, Fitzgerald SD, Chamness GC, et al. Variant human breast tumor estrogen receptor with constitutive transcriptional activity. Cancer Res 1991;51:105–109.
140. Weisz A, Rosales R. Identification of an estrogen response element upstream of the human c-fos gene that binds the estrogen receptor and the AP-1 transcription factor. Nucleic Acids Res 1990;18:5097–5105.
141. Wang Y, Miksicek RJ. Identification of a dominant negative form of the human estrogen receptor. Mol Endocrinol 1991;5:1707–1715.
142. Friend KE, Chiou YK, Lopes MBS, et al. Estrogen receptor expression in human pituitary: correlation with immunohistochemistry in normal tissue, and immunohistochemistry and morphology in macroadenomas. J Clin Endocrinol Metab 1994;78:1497–1504.
143. Zafar M, Ezzat S, Ramyar L, et al. Cell-specific expression of estrogen receptor in the human pituitary and its adenomas. J Clin Endocrinol Metab 1995;80:3621–3627.
144. Ambrosino C, Cicatiello L, Cobellis G, et al. Functional antagonism between the estrogen receptor and Fos on the regulation of c-fos protooncogene transcription. Mol Endocrinol 1993;7:1472–1483.
145. McDonnell DP, Lieberman BA, Norris J. Development of tissue-selective estrogen receptor modulators. In: Baird DT, Schutz G, Krattenmacher R, eds. Organ-Selective Actions of Steroid Hormones. New York: Springer-Verlag, 1995:1–28.
146. Ignar-Trowbridge DM, Pimentel M, Parker MG, et al. Peptide growth factor cross-talk with estrogen receptor requires the A/B domain and occurs independently of protein kinase C or estradiol. Endocrinology 1996;137:1735–1744.
147. Clementi E, Malgaretti N, Meldolesi J, et al. A new constitutively activating mutation of the Gs protein alpha subunit-gsp oncogene is found in human pituitary tumours. Oncogene 1990;5:1059–1061.
148. Lyons J, Landis CA, Harsh G, et al. Two G protein oncogenes in human endocrine tumors. Science 1990;249:655–659.
149. Landis CA, Harsh G, Lyons J, et al. Clinical characteristics of acromegalic patients whose pituitary tumors contain mutant Gs protein. J Clin Endocrinol Metab 1990;71:1416–1420.
150. Spada A, Vallar L, Faglia G. G-protein oncogenes in pituitary tumors. Trends Endocrinol Metab 1992:3–5.
151. Spada A, Arosio M, Bochicchio D, et al. Clinical biochemical, and morphological correlates in patients bearing growth hormone-secreting pituitary tumors with or without constitutively active adenylyl cyclase. J Clin Endocrinol Metab 1990;71:1421–1426.
152. Williamson EA, Ince PG, Harrison D, et al. G-protein mutations in human pituitary adrenocorticotrophic hormone-secreting adenomas. Eur J Clin Invest 1995;25:128–131.
153. Williamson EA, Daniels M, Foster SFKW, et al. Gs-alpha and Gi2-alpha mutations in clinically non-functioning pituitary tumours. Clin Endocrinol 1994;41:815–820.
154. Tordjman K, Stern N, Ouaknine G, et al. Activating mutations of the Gs alpha-gene in nonfunctioning pituitary tumors. J Clin Endocrinol Metab 1993;77:765–769.
155. Hashimoto K, Koga M, Motomura T, et al. Identification of alternatively spliced messenger ribonucleic acid encoding truncated growth hormone-releasing hormone receptor in human pituitary adenomas. J Clin Endocrinol Metab 1995;80:2933–2939.
156. Cryns VL, Alexander JM, Klibanski A, et al. The retinoblastoma gene in human pituitary tumors. J Clin Endocrinol Metab 1993;77:644–646.
157. Pei L, Melmed S, Scheithauer B, et al. Frequent loss of heterozygosity at the retinoblastoma susceptibility gene (RB) locus in aggressive pituitary tumors: evidence for a chromosome 13 tumor suppressor gene other than RB. Cancer Res 1995;55:1613–1616.
158. Woloschak M, Roberts JL, Post KD. Loss of heterozygosity at the retinoblastoma locus in human pituitary tumors. Cancer 1994;74:693–696.
159. Zhu J, Leon SP, Beggs AH, et al. Human pituitary adenomas show no loss of heterozygosity at the retinoblastoma gene locus. J Clin Endocrinol Metab 1994;78:922–927.
160. Cai WY, Alexander JM, Hedley-Whyte ET, et al. Ras mutations in human prolactinomas and pituitary carcinomas. J Clin Endocrinol Metab 1994;78:89–93.
161. Karga HJ, Alexander JM, Hedley-Whyte ET, et al. Ras mutations in human pituitary tumors. J Clin Endocrinol Metab 1992;74:914–919.
162. Pei L, Melmed S, Scheithauer B, et al. H-ras mutations in human pituitary carcinoma metastases. J Clin Endocrinol Metab 1994;78:842–846.
163. Alvaro V, Levy L, Dubray C, et al. Invasive human pituitary tumors express a point-mutated alpha-protein kinase-C. J Clin Endocrinol Metab 1993;77:1125–1129.
164. Woloschak M, Roberts JL, Post K. c-myc, c-fos, and c-myb gene expression in human pituitary adenomas. J Clin Endocrinol Metab 1994;79:253–257.
165. Takino H, Herman V, Weiss M, et al. Purine-binding factor (nm23) gene expression in pituitary tumors: marker of adenoma invasiveness. J Clin Endocrinol Metab 1995;80:1733–1738.
166. Gonsky R, Herman V, Melmed S, et al. Transforming DNA sequences present in human prolactin secreting pituitary tumors. Mol Endocrinol 1991;5:1687–1695.
167. McAndrew J, Paterson AJ, Asa SL, et al. Targeting of transforming growth factor-alpha expression to pituitary lactotrophs in transgenic mice results in selective lactotroph proliferation and adenomas. Endocrinology 1995;136:4479–4488.

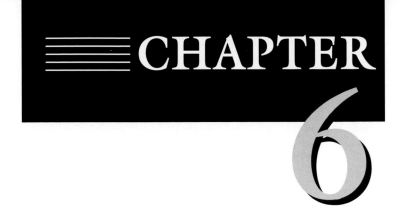

CHAPTER 6

The Antidiuretic Hormone: Physiology and Pathophysiology

W. Brian Reeves and Thomas E. Andreoli

INTRODUCTION

Water is the most plentiful substance within the body, composing 50 to 60% of the total body weight. The ratio of total body solute to total body water defines the osmolality of body fluids. Sudden alterations in body fluid osmolality may have lethal consequences as the result of abrupt changes in the volume of the central nervous system (CNS) that occur when the osmotic disturbance is acute: brain shrinkage in the hypertonic syndromes and brain swelling in the hypotonic syndromes. Not surprisingly, the osmolality of body fluids is regulated within a narrow range, usually 280 to 295 mOsm/L. Maintenance of a near constant body fluid osmolality is achieved primarily through the regulation of water balance rather than solute balance. Both the intake of water and the renal excretion of water are controlled, in large part, by the hypothalamic–neurohypophyseal system. Indeed, dysfunction of the neurohypophysis is most apparent clinically as a failure to regulate the osmolality of body fluid. This chapter reviews the coordinated responses involving vasopressin (also called antidiuretic hormone [ADH]), thirst, and the kidney, which maintain osmotic homeostasis.

Anatomy

The neurohypophysis consists of a set of hypothalamic nuclei that house the perikarya of the magnocellular neurons responsible for synthesis of ADH; the axonal processes of these neurons, which form the supraopticohypophyseal tract; and the axonal terminations of these neurons within the posterior lobe of the pituitary.

The supraoptic nucleus (SON) consists almost entirely of magnocellular neurons, all which project to the posterior pituitary (1); the paraventricular nucleus (PVN) contains magnocellular neurons that project to the posterior pituitary as well as parvocellular neurons that project to the median eminence or to autonomic centers in the brainstem (2). Results of immunocytochemical staining have demonstrated cells containing ADH in both nuclei (3, 4). In several species, including humans, ADH-containing magnocellular neurons occupy the more ventral aspects of the SON and are located more centrally within the PVN (5). ADH is also found in certain parvocellular neurons in the PVN and in some magnocellular neurons near the organum vasculosum of the lamina terminalis (6). ADH secretion by parvocellular neurons, which terminate in the hypophy-

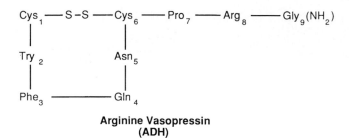

**Arginine Vasopressin
(ADH)**

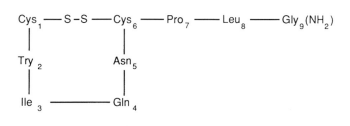

Oxytocin

**1-deamino-8-D-arginine Vasopressin
(dDAVP)**

Figure 6.1. Chemical structures of the major posterior pituitary hormones and desmopressin, a commonly used synthetic vasopressin analog.

seal–portal capillary bed, accounts for the high concentration of ADH in portal blood (7, 8).

Chemistry

Figure 6.1 shows the structure of ADH and that of a commonly used analog, 1-deamino-8-D-arginine vasopressin (desmopressin [DDAVP]). ADH is a nonapeptide with a molecular mass of approximately 1.1 kd. A sulfhydryl bond between the cysteine residues at positions 1 and 6 forms a single cystine moiety, yielding a ring comprising 20 atoms. At least nine neurohypophyseal octapeptides have been isolated from vertebrates (9).

There are many synthetic analogs of ADH. Most of these agents possess various degrees of antidiuretic, vasopressor, and uterotonic activities. Analogs also exist that function as competitive antagonists of both the vasopressor and the antidiuretic action of the hormone. ADH acts via tissue receptors classified as V_1 receptors in smooth muscle and V_2 receptors in renal epithelia; only the latter receptors activate adenylate cyclase (10). Antidiuretic activity in the intact animal depends on the ability of a peptide to bind

to the renal receptor, to stimulate the adenylate cyclase system, and to resist metabolic degradation.

The Neurophysins

The neurophysins are sulfur-rich proteins with molecular masses of 9 to 10 kd that form insoluble, ionic complexes with neurohypophyseal hormones (11). Neurophysins contain 92 to 95 amino acid residues with conservation of the central portion of molecules from all species (11); a high content of cysteine residues results in extensive disulfide binding within the molecule.

Separate hormone-specific neurophysins exist for vasopressin and oxytocin in each species (12). The vasopressin-associated neurophysin is designated NpII, and the oxytocin-associated neurophysin is designated NpI. As is discussed below, neurophysin plays an important role in the processing and secretion of vasopressin. Indeed, mutations in the prepro-neurophysin II gene have been identified in humans with familial central diabetes insipidus (CDI), a condition in which vasopressin secretion is impaired.

Hormone Biosynthesis

Figure 6.2 summarizes the cardinal steps in hormone biosynthesis. Results of in vivo pulse labeling studies (13–16) indicate that ADH and neurophysin are derived from a common precursor. Further proof has come from analysis of the ADH gene (17, 18). The organization of the ADH precursor peptide and the ADH gene of the rat is illustrated in Figure 6.3. The hormone precursor contains three peptide regions: a signal peptide and ADH at the NH_2 terminus, a neurophysin II region, and a COOH-terminal glycoprotein region of unknown significance (19). Each of these regions of the precursor protein is, in turn, coded for by one of three exons of the ADH precursor gene. The human ADH gene is on chromosome 20 (20).

The main steps in the biosynthesis of ADH are as follows: transcription of the ADH precursor messenger RNA (mRNA); translation of the mRNA to a preprohormone of 166 amino acids; removal of the signal peptide sequence while the peptide is still attached to the ribosome to yield the prohormone; and conversion of the prohormone pep-

Form	Molecular Weight	Synthetic Step
Preprohormone	≈ 21,000	Protein synthesis; magnocellular neuron ribosomes
↓		
Prohormone	≈ 23,000	Glycosylation and membrane packaging; Magnocellular neuron Golgi apparatus
↓		
Neurosecretory Granule (NSG)	$(23,000)_n$	Transport down supraopticohypophyseal tract as osmotically inactive granules
Neurophysin	≈ 10,000	
+		Storage in posterior pituitary; cleavage within NSG
Hormone	≈ 1,100	

Figure 6.2. Flow diagram for the pathway of posterior pituitary hormone biosynthesis.

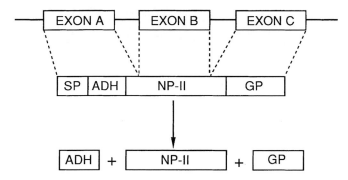

Figure 6.3. A schematic representation of the organization of the ADH gene and its relation to the preprohormone and final peptide products. *GP*, glycoprotein; *NP-II*, neurophysin II; *SP*, signal peptide. (Reprinted with permission from Reeves WB, Bichet DG, Andreoli TE. The posterior pituitary and water metabolism. In: Wilson JD, Foster DW, eds. Williams Textbook of Endocrinology. 9th ed. Philadelphia: WB Saunders, 1997.)

tide into ADH and neurophysin II. This final step occurs within the neurosecretory granules during transport to the neurohypophysis (21). The extrahypothalamic mRNA is shorter than the hypothalamic mRNA because of differences in the length of the poly (adenylic acid) tail.

THE CONTROL OF ADH RELEASE

To maintain plasma osmolality at a constant level, ADH secretion from the posterior pituitary must vary in response to small changes in plasma osmolality. However, ADH may also be released when the plasma osmolality is less than normal, if the effective circulating volume is decreased.

Osmotic Regulation of ADH Release

Verney postulated the presence of osmoreceptors, located in the distribution of the internal carotid arteries, that stimulate ADH release when plasma osmolality is raised by solutes to which osmoreceptors are impermeable (22).

The precise location of the osmoreceptors is still debated. Evidence suggests that the osmoreceptor is separate from the SON. First, results of studies by McKinley and colleagues (23) and Thrasher et al. (24) indicate that the osmoreceptor lies outside the blood-brain barrier. Second, the observation that neurotransmitter antagonists block osmotically induced ADH release (25) suggests a need for neural afferents in the process. Third, lesions of the organum vasculosum of the lamina terminalis, which reside outside of the blood-brain barrier (see earlier), impair ADH secretion (25). Finally, interruption of the pathways between the region of the anteroventral aspect of the third ventricle, which includes the organum vasculosum of the lamina terminalis, and the SON produces hypernatremia in rats (26, 27). Thus, afferent fibers, probably from the organum vasculosum of the lamina terminalis, play an important role in the osmotic stimulation of ADH secretion.

Nonosmotic Regulation of ADH Release

Volume-mediated release of ADH may occur as a consequence of stimuli arising from "volume receptors," or baroreceptors. The electrical activity of the baroreceptor is related to the degree of stretch in the vessel wall. Increases in pressure and wall tension cause an increase in the rate of firing of the receptor. Conversely, decreases in blood pressure or blood volume result in a decrease in the electrical activity of the baroreceptor (28).

The afferent pathways for the atrial and carotid bifurcation baroreceptors seem to be the vagus and glossopharyngeal nerves, respectively. Following synapses in the nucleus tractus solitarius, noradrenergic projections relay baroreceptor input to the PVN and the SON (28, 29). Baroreceptors exert an inhibitory influence on ADH secretion under resting conditions, and severing of all baroreceptor afferents results in a marked increase in plasma ADH levels. In addition, stimulation of baroreceptors by balloon distension of either the left atrium or the carotid bifurcation inhibits electrical activity in the SON (29). This inhibitory influence is abolished by section of the vagus nerve or local anesthesia of the carotid bifurcation.

In humans, an acute reduction in arterial blood pressure exceeding 5 to 10% causes an exponential rise in ADH secretion (30). Likewise, volume depletion in humans (31) and in a variety of animal species (32–34) produces little elevation in plasma ADH levels until blood volume decreases by more than 8 to 10%. Further volume depletion results in exponential increases in plasma ADH levels (Fig. 6.4).

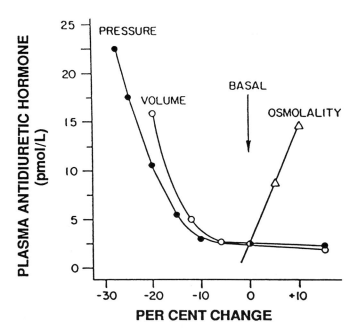

Figure 6.4. The relationship between plasma ADH and changes in plasma osmolality, blood volume, and mean arterial pressure in humans. To convert ADH values to picomoles per liter, divide by 1.1. (Adapted from Robertson GL, Berl T. Water metabolism. In: Brenner BM, Rector FCJ, eds. The Kidney. Philadelphia: WB Saunders, 1986:385–432.)

An interplay exists between osmotic and nonosmotic stimuli for ADH release (33). Decreases in left atrial pressure reduce the osmotic threshold and increase the sensitivity for osmotic ADH release, whereas increases in left atrial pressure raise the threshold and dampen the sensitivity for osmotic ADH release (Fig. 6.5).

Chemical Mediators of ADH Release

Another dimension of complexity to understanding nonosmotic mechanisms for ADH release has been added with the recognition that ADH release can also be modulated by agents that have either systemic hemodynamic effects or CNS actions. Table 6.1 lists some drugs, neurotransmitters, and other chemical agents that modulate the regulation of ADH release via either peripheral nervous system or CNS effects.

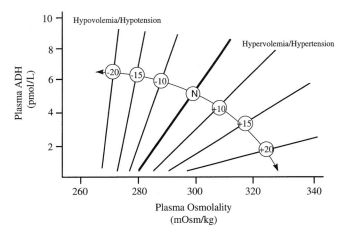

Figure 6.5. The effect of changes in blood volume or arterial pressure on the relation between plasma osmolality and plasma ADH activity. To convert ADH values to picomoles per liter, divide by 1.1. (Modified from Robertson GL, Berl T. Water metabolism. In: Brenner BM, Rector FCJ, eds. The Kidney. Philadelphia: WB Saunders, 1986:385–432.)

Table 6.1. Agents That Modulate ADH Release

Agents That Enhance Release	Agents That Suppress Release
Prostaglandin E2	Phenytoin
Nicotine	Alcohol
β-Adrenergic agents	α-Adrenergic agents
Angiotensin II	Atrial natriuretic peptide
Anesthetic agents	Narcotine analogs
Hypoxia	
Hypercapnia	
Vincristine	
Cyclophosphamide	
Clofibrate	
Barbiturates	
Acetylcholine	
Histamine	
Metoclopramide	

THE RENAL CONTRIBUTION TO OSMOTIC HOMEOSTASIS

The ability of the kidney to excrete either a dilute or concentrated urine depends on the integrity of the countercurrent multiplication system, driven by active NaCl transport from the thick ascending limb, and on the water permeability of the collecting duct. As we shall see, ADH is the principal physiologic regulator of both processes.

The Collecting Tubule

The major contribution of ADH to the renal antidiuretic response is to increase the water permeability of terminal nephron segments, specifically, the cortical collecting duct, the outer medullary collecting duct, and the papillary collecting duct. The increase in the water permeability of these nephron segments augments osmotic water flow from tubular lumen into a hypertonic medullary interstitium, thus providing for maximal urine concentration during antidiuresis. A second action of ADH in the collecting duct is to increase the permeability of the terminal portion of the inner medullary collecting duct to urea. This provides a pathway for urea to be recycled from the medullary urine back into the papillary interstitium for enrichment of the interstitial osmolality.

ADH increases the water permeability of apical plasma membranes in hormone-responsive epithelia (35, 36). Grantham and Burg (37) observed that freshly dissected rabbit cortical collecting duct segments have a high initial water permeability that declines temporarily and reaches a minimum in approximately 180 minutes; when ADH is introduced into the bathing solution, the water permeability rises to its initial high value.

Intracellular Mediators of Vasopressin Action

Two scientific breakthroughs in the past few years have advanced our understanding of the cellular actions of vasopressin and have provided diagnostic and therapeutic insights into disorders of water metabolism. These two achievements are the cloning and characterization of the vasopressin V_2 receptor (38, 39) and the discovery of a family of water channel proteins, the aquaporins (AQPs) (40). These elements constitute the initial and final events in vasopressin action in the collecting duct cell—i.e., the binding of the hormone to its receptor at the basolateral membrane—and the movement of water across the apical membrane through water channels.

The effects of ADH on transport processes in renal epithelia are mediated primarily by the intracellular second messenger cyclic adenosine monophosphate (cAMP) (41). ADH binds to specific receptors, the V_2 receptors, on basolateral membrane surfaces of hormone-responsive epithelial cells and activates membrane-associated adenylate cyclase to catalyze cAMP generation from adenosine triphosphate.

Results of recent studies of the distribution of V_2 receptors along the nephron using either immunolocalization (42) or reverse transcriptase–polymerase chain reaction analysis of microdissected nephron segments (43) are consistent with those of previous biochemical and hormone binding studies. Namely, V_2 receptors are expressed at high levels throughout the collecting duct and at lower levels in the thick ascending limb of Henle's loop (43).

The biophysical characteristics of water flow in renal proximal tubules and collecting ducts suggested that transmembrane water movement in these cells occurred through pores, or channels, rather than by diffusion across the lipid bilayer. The first demonstration of a membrane protein that served as a water channel came in 1992 when Preston et al. (44) expressed CHIP28, a protein purified from red blood cells, in *Xenopus* oocytes. The injection of CHIP28 cRNA into the oocytes produced a dramatic increase in the water permeability of the oocyte membrane. Using a polymerase chain reaction–based approach, Fushimi et al. (45) identified a second water channel, AQP2, that shares 42% amino acid identity with AQP1. It is now known that AQP2 is the vasopressin-regulated collecting duct water channel (45–51). The expression of AQP2 is increased by dehydration and by vasopressin (47, 48). Thus, vasopressin regulates collecting duct water permeability acutely through the translocation and, perhaps, the phosphorylation (see below) of AQP2 channels and chronically by increasing the expression of AQP2 channels.

Morphologic Studies of the Vasopressin Response

The final site of ADH action on water permeability is at the apical epithelial surface. Results of structural studies of ADH-responsive anuran epithelia (principally toad and frog urinary bladders) led to the hypothesis that ADH-responsive water channels (AQP2) are shuttled between a cytoplasmic pool and the apical membrane in response to ADH. The validity of the shuttle hypothesis (Fig. 6.6) for the regulated insertion and retrieval of water channels at the apical membrane of the collecting duct is supported by results of recent immunolocalization studies of the vasopressin-regulated water channel (40, 45, 46).

In summary, ADH, working via cAMP and protein kinase, alters water transport in hormone-responsive epithelia by causing the microtubule-dependent insertion of specialized membrane units within the apical plasma membranes of these cells.

Effects of ADH on Urea Transport

The production of a concentrated urine is dependent on the presence of a corticomedullary gradient of increasing tissue osmolality, which drives the osmotic extraction of water from the collecting duct (52). Urea is the most abundant solute in the inner medulla, accounting for approximately 50% of the interstitial osmolality (53). Urea accumulates in the inner medulla as a result of the resorption of hypertonic urea across the terminal portions of the

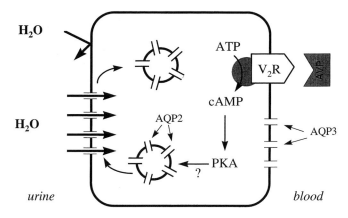

Figure 6.6. A schematic model of the shuttle mechanism for the action of ADH in the collecting tubule. In the absence of ADH, AQP2 water channels are located in vesicles, or endosomes, beneath the apical membrane. On stimulation by ADH, these endosomes fuse with the apical membrane delivering water channels to the cell surface. Water channels are retrieved from the cell surface by endocytosis of clathrin-coated vesicles. AQP3 water channels in the basolateral membrane facilitate the exit of water from the collecting duct cell. V_2R, vasopressin antidiuretic (V_2) receptor; *CDI*, central diabetes insipidus; *PKA*, protein kinase A; *cAMP*, cyclic adenosine monophosphate. (Reprinted with permission from Reeves WB, Bichet DG, Andreoli TE. The posterior pituitary and water metabolism. In: Wilson JD, Foster DW, eds. Williams Textbook of Endocrinology. 9th ed. Philadelphia: WB Saunders, 1997.)

inner medullary collecting duct. ADH, via cAMP (54, 55), stimulates passive urea transport (53) in the inner medullary collecting duct. Finally, although the transport of urea per se in the inner medulla may be passive, the generation of the high concentration of urea in the tubule fluid depends ultimately on the active transport of NaCl by the thick ascending limb with the consequent creation of a hypertonic outer medullary interstitium. Therefore, any process that interferes with active salt transport by the thick ascending limb (e.g., loop diuretics) will diminish urea recycling, deplete medullary interstitial urea, and blunt urinary concentrating ability.

The Medullary Thick Ascending Limb of Henle (mTALH)

Figure 6.7 presents a general model for net NaCl absorption in the mTALH based on current experimental data on this nephron segment in mammalian species, notably the mouse and the rabbit. Luminal salt entry into cells is mediated by an electroneutral $Na^+,K^+,2Cl^-$ cotransport mechanism (56, 57).

The apical membrane also contains K^+ channels (56, 58) that constitute the route for the active K^+-secretory pathway in renal tubular diluting segments (59, 60). Most K^+ that is secreted from cells to lumen is recycled into cells via the $Na^+,K^+,2Cl^-$ cotransport process.

Cl^- exit from the cell across the basolateral membrane of the TALH appears to be mediated primarily through Cl^- conductive channels (61, 62). A Cl^- channel belonging to the ClC family of Cl⁻ channels has been cloned from the kidneys of rats, humans, and rabbits (63–65). Staining of kidney sections with an antibody to the rabbit Cl⁻ channel (rbClC-Ka) localized the channel to the basolateral membrane of medullary and cortical thick ascending limbs.

The Effect of Vasopressin on Net Salt Absorption

ADH increases the net rate of salt absorption in isolated mouse mTAL segments (66, 67). This stimulating effect on net salt absorption occurs at peritubular hormone concentrations found in the plasma of mammalian species during ordinary antidiuresis, and cAMP analogs produce the same effect on mouse mTAL segments (67).

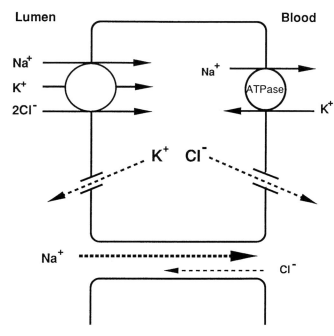

Figure 6.7. A model for salt absorption in mouse mTALH. The *solid lines* denote conservative (primary or secondary) processes; the *dashed lines* denote dissipative processes.

The effects of ADH on salt and water transport in the mTAL and collecting duct, respectively, are modulated by several factors (Table 6.2).

Integration of the Actions of ADH on the Urinary Concentrating Mechanism

Figure 6.8 depicts some of the major effects of ADH on the components of the urinary concentrating mechanism and the interplay between those components. As summarized in the preceding sections, direct effects of ADH on renal epithelial cells include stimulation of active salt absorption by the mTAL, enhancement of the water permeability of the cortical and medullary collecting ducts, and increase in the urea permeability of the terminal inner medullary collecting duct. Active salt absorption by the TAL is the "single effect" that drives countercurrent multiplication in the outer medulla. The ADH-induced increase in salt absorption leads to an increase in the osmolality of the outer medullary interstitium, which, in conjunction with the ADH-induced increase in collecting duct water permeability, results in water absorption and concentration of the tubular fluid in the collecting duct. The high result-

Table 6.2. *Agents That Alter Renal Tubular Responsiveness to Vasopressin*

Agents that increase ADH effects
Chlorpropamide
Carbamazepine
Chronic dehydration
Nonsteroidal anti-inflammatory agents
Agents that decrease ADH effects
α-Adrenergic agents
Atrial natriuretic peptide
Prostaglandin E2
Hypokalemia
Hypercalcemia
Protein kinase C
Lithium
Demeclocycline

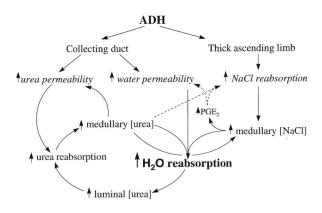

Figure 6.8. Effects of antidiuretic hormone (*ADH*) on the urinary concentrating mechanism. *PGE₂*, prostaglandin E2.

ing concentration of urea in the tubular fluid, together with the ADH-induced increase in urea permeability, drives urea resorption into the papillary interstitium. This high interstitial urea content, in turn, provides for passive countercurrent multiplication in the inner medulla. Thus, ADH acts in an integrated fashion at several sites along the nephron to promote maximal antidiuresis. In addition to the direct effects of ADH on renal epithelial cells, the urinary concentrating mechanism features multiple layers of feedback control. The dashed lines in Figure 6.8 denote negative feedback loops. The increase in interstitial osmolality that occurs during antidiuresis directly inhibits further NaCl absorption by the TAL, thereby blunting concentrating ability (68). In addition, the ADH-induced increase in interstitial NaCl content also inhibits both TAL NaCl absorption and collecting duct water transport indirectly by stimulating prostaglandin E2 release from interstitial cells (69). Prostaglandin E2, in turn, reduces ADH-induced cAMP production in both segments (70–72). The net effect is a negative feedback loop on ADH-dependent urinary concentration. In contrast, ADH-induced increases in interstitial osmolality may increase urea transport by the inner medullary collecting duct, thereby promoting urinary concentration (73).

SELECTED CLINICAL DERANGEMENTS OF WATER BALANCE

The control of plasma osmolality and its primary determinant, the plasma sodium concentration, is achieved through ADH-mediated water conservation and thirst-induced water acquisition. Therefore, abnormal plasma osmolality, i.e., hyponatremia or hypernatremia, is generally the result of a derangement in water balance rather than salt balance. The integrated actions of the two effector limbs of the water balance are required: water conservation and water intake.

The principal physiologic stimulus for ADH secretion is plasma osmolality (74). At low plasma osmolalities, ADH secretion is suppressed; however, when plasma osmolality exceeds the threshold value, usually about 280 mmol/kg H_2O, ADH secretion increases in a linear fashion. ADH, in turn, produces urine concentration. At a plasma osmolality of 290 mmol/kg H_2O, 10 mmol/kg H_2O above the ADH threshold, the plasma ADH concentration, approximately 4 to 5 pmol/L (4 to 5 ng/L), is sufficient to cause maximal urine concentration. Conversely, at a plasma osmolality of 280 mmol/kg H_2O, the plasma ADH level is completely suppressed, and the urine is maximally dilute. In other words, a 3% increase in plasma osmolality converts a normal individual from a state of maximal diuresis to one of maximal antidiuresis.

The urine flow rate varies inversely with the urine osmolality. Thus, when plasma ADH is suppressed to levels that allow maximal urine dilution, the rate of water excretion

Table 6.3. *Major Causes of Hypernatremia*

Impaired thirst
Coma
Essential hypernatremia
Excessive water losses
Renal
Central diabetes insipidus
Nephrogenic diabetes insipidus
Impaired medullary hypertonicity
Extrarenal
Sweating
Osmotic diarrhea
Burns
Solute diuresis
Uncontrolled diabetes
Mannitol administration
Glycerol administration
Sodium excess
Administration of hypertonic NaCl
Administration of hypertonic NaHCO$_3$

increases dramatically. At solute excretion rates of 800 to 900 mmol/day, for example, the free water clearance can approach 20 L/day. That is, a normal individual can ingest up to 20 L of water daily and not risk water intoxication.

The osmotic threshold for thirst is roughly 290 mmol/kg H_2O, 10 mmol/kg H_2O above the ADH threshold. Small increases in plasma osmolality above the thirst threshold result in intense thirst and a large increase in water intake. Thus, the thresholds for ADH and thirst form the lower and upper boundaries, respectively, for plasma osmolality. A fall in plasma osmolality toward the ADH threshold causes a large water diuresis with a subsequent increase in plasma osmolality. An increase in plasma osmolality past the thirst threshold, conversely, causes a large increase in water intake with a subsequent fall in plasma osmolality. It should also be apparent that, within the range defined by these thresholds, the plasma osmolality is determined primarily by ADH-mediated changes in urine concentration.

The Hypertonic Syndromes

The hypertonic syndromes are defined by an increased ratio of an effectively impermeable solute to water in the extracellular fluid (ECF) and are directly associated with cellular dehydration and shrinkage. Because body fluids are in osmotic equilibrium, the plasma osmolality is determined by the ratio of total body solutes to total body water. The major extracellular and intracellular solutes are salts of sodium and potassium, respectively. Accordingly, hypertonicity can result from an increase in total body sodium or potassium, or both, or from a decrease in total body water.

Failure of water homeostasis may result from inadequacy of either ADH-dependent water conservation or thirst-mediated water acquisition. On the basis of the underlying pathophysiologic mechanisms, the clinical circumstances that lead to hypernatremia may be grouped into the general categories that are given in Table 6.3.

Total deficiency of renal concentrating mechanisms will not lead to hypertonicity if free access to water is ensured. Most commonly, clinically significant hypertonic volume depletion is seen in the very young or the very old, in whom either physical immaturity or debility prevents the translation of thirst into water-acquiring behavior, and in individuals who are unable to communicate thirst, for example, trauma victims and comatose patients. In a small group of patients, those with essential hypernatremia, the osmoregulatory centers are diseased, and osmotic stimulation of both ADH release and thirst is impaired.

CDI

CDI is a polyuric syndrome that results from a lack of sufficient ADH to concentrate the urine for water conservation. The disease is identified by three primary findings: the persistence of an inappropriately dilute urine in the presence of strong osmotic or nonosmotic stimuli for ADH secretion; the absence of intrinsic renal disease; and a rise in urine osmolality on the administration of ADH.

Etiologic Factors

The spectrum of etiologic factors causing CDI (Table 6.4) has changed over time. In 1928, Fink (75) reviewed

Table 6.4.   Causes of CDI

Congenital CDI
  Familial (autosomal dominant)
  Septo-optic dysplasia
  Familial hypopituitarism
  Congenital cytomegalovirus infection

Acquired CDI
  Idiopathic
  Trauma
  Postsurgical
  Neoplastic
    Craniopharyngioma
    Pineal tumors
    Pituitary tumors
    Lymphoma
    Meningioma
    Metastatic tumors
  Ischemic
    Sheehan's syndrome
    Brain death
  Granulomatous
    Sarcoidosis
    Histiocytosis
    Wegener's granulomatosis
    Bronchocentric granulomatosis
  Infections
    Tuberculosis
    Blastomycosis
    Syphilis
    Viral encephalitis
    Bacterial meningitis
  Autoimmune

CDI, central diabetes insipidus.

necropsy data from 107 recorded cases of CDI and found 63% of cases to be associated with tumors of the basilar surface of the brain, 11% to be secondary to head trauma, and 25% to be associated with inflammation of the basal meninges; of the last group, half were syphilitic and one-fifth were tuberculous. In contrast, of 92 patients with CDI who were studied by Moses and Notman (76) from 1972 to 1980, 30% of cases were idiopathic, 25% were related to malignant or benign tumors of either the brain or the pituitary fossa, 16% were secondary to head trauma, and 20% followed cranial surgery for tumor or hypophysectomy. A recent retrospective study of the causes of CDI in children found brain tumors to be the most common cause (60%), followed by cerebral malformations (25%) (77).

Primary intracranial tumors that are associated with diabetes insipidus are often craniopharyngiomas or pineal tumors (78), and metastatic tumors are most often from lung or breast, although many primary sites have been reported (79–82). The appearance of local hypothalamic disease may be delayed up to 10 years after the onset of diabetes insipidus (83, 84). Periodic follow-up of patients who are diagnosed as having idiopathic CDI is recommended to detect delayed intracranial lesions. Finally, histiocytosis (either eosinophilic granuloma or Hand-Schüuller-Christian disease), encephalitis or meningitis, granulomatous diseases such as sarcoidosis or Wegener's granulomatosis, lymphocytic hypophysitis, and intraventricular hemorrhage can cause CDI (76, 85–90).

Two features associated with the development of diabetes insipidus after injury to the neurohypophyseal system are noteworthy: the first relates to the site and degree of injury necessary to reduce ADH levels to levels lower than those that are required for normal water homeostasis; the second is the characteristic triphasic response of neurohypophyseal function to injury.

Removal of the posterior pituitary gland does not necessarily lead to diabetes insipidus (91). Rather, persistent polyuria develops only after an injury that is sufficiently high in the supraopticohypophyseal tract to cause bilateral neuron degeneration in the SON and PVN (92). In fact, roughly 90% of the magnocellular neurons in the SON and PVN have to be lost before diabetes insipidus develops (93, 94). In short, although transient diabetes insipidus may accompany any injury to the neurohypophysis, permanent diabetes insipidus usually follows damage that is high and proximal in the pituitary stalk.

Diabetes insipidus after surgery to the pituitary or hypothalamus may exhibit one of three patterns: transient, permanent, or triphasic. Transient diabetes insipidus usually has an abrupt onset within the first postoperative day and resolves within several days. This is the most common pattern (50 to 60%) of postsurgical diabetes insipidus and typically occurs after transsphenoidal resections of pituitary adenomas. Permanent or prolonged diabetes insipidus also has an abrupt and early onset but persists for weeks or may be permanent. This form of diabetes insipidus follows either damage to the neurohypophyseal stalk or hypothalamus or wide resection of the pituitary for large masses with extrasellar extension (95). The triphasic pattern, shown in Figure 6.9, is characterized by an immediate postinjury increase in urine volume and a concomitant fall in urine osmolality, which lasts 4 to 5 days; an intervening period of 5 to 7 days (the interphase), during which urine flow falls abruptly and urine osmolality rises; and a final phase consisting of permanent, hyposthenuric polyuria.

The initial diuresis of the triphasic response has been assumed to be caused by an injury-related neuronal shock, during which time no hormone release occurs (85, 96). The interphase seems to be caused by the leak of hormone from degenerating neurons because the urinary excretion of water cannot be altered either by water loading or by hypotonic saline infusions (97) and because complete removal of the posterior pituitary together with hypothalamic nuclei of the neurohypophyseal system prevents the appearance of an interphase (85).

Patients who develop CDI postoperatively can osmoregulate effectively despite these extreme fluctuations in ADH levels as long as they control water intake through thirst. However, severe water intoxication can develop during the phase of autonomous ADH release if infusion of hypotonic fluids, which is often initiated during the initial polyuric phase, is continued. Urine and serum osmolalities should be monitored carefully in patients after surgery in the area of the neurohypophysis. Moreover, if hormone replacement is needed in the early postoperative period, short-acting agents, i.e., aqueous vasopressin, should be used to minimize the risk of subsequent hyponatremia should a phase of autonomous ADH release develop.

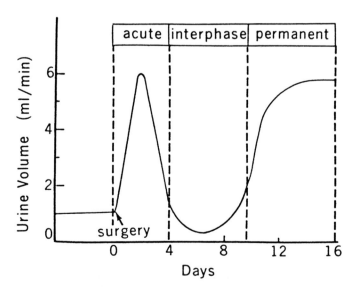

Figure 6.9. Triphasic response of urine volume after injury to the supraopticohypophyseal system. (Reprinted with permission from Fisher C, Ingram WR. The effect of interruption of the supra-optico-hypophyseal tracts on the antidiuretic, pressor and oxytocic activity of the posterior lobe of the hypophysis. Endocrinology 1936;20:762–768.)

Clinical Manifestations

The primary symptoms of diabetes insipidus are persistent polyuria and its constant companions, thirst and polydipsia. The volume of urine excreted may vary from only a few liters per day, in the case of a partial hormone deficiency, to a maximum of about 18 L/day, the average volume of glomerular filtrate that is delivered to collecting ducts, in the case of a total absence of ADH. Thus, patients with partial CDI may be so little inconvenienced as to ignore their symptoms, with the disorder being noticed only when they are deprived of water. Nocturia is almost invariably present in patients with diabetes insipidus, as opposed to patients with primary polydipsia, in whom nocturia is uncommon.

Patients with CDI usually show a particular predilection for cold or iced drinks to quench thirst. The most striking clinical manifestations occur if access to water is interrupted and hypertonic volume depletion develops. This condition is characterized by CNS manifestations beginning with irritability, followed by mental dullness, and progressing to coma with secondary signs of ataxia, hyperthermia, and hypotension. Finally, in patients with diabetes insipidus caused by intracranial lesions, neurologic symptoms of the primary lesion may be prominent.

Laboratory Manifestations

Persistent hyposthenuria, with a urine specific gravity of 1.005 or less and a urine osmolality less than 200 mmol/kg H_2O, is the hallmark of diabetes insipidus (76, 85). Partial deficiency of ADH may be recognized only as an inappropriately dilute urine in the face of an elevated serum osmolality (98). In euvolemic patients, the glomerular filtration rate (GFR) is normal (76, 85). Because patients with diabetes insipidus ingest water in response to plasma hypertonicity, random plasma osmolality determinations in these patients are, on average, above the usual normal value of 287 mmol/kg H_2O (99). The serum sodium concentrations are also elevated and account for the increases in plasma osmolality. In contrast, individuals with primary polydipsia have a primary aberration of the thirst mechanism and ingest water independent of physiological stimuli. These patients often have mild dilutional hyponatremia (99). In patients in whom diabetes insipidus, either central or nephrogenic in origin, begins in childhood, considerable dilation of the urinary bladder, ureters, and renal pelvis may lead to renal damage (100, 101).

Diagnosis

With reference to Table 6.3, CDI must be separated from other polyuria states, such as solute diuresis, impaired renal concentrating ability, or nephrogenic diabetes insipidus (NDI). Measurement of serum and urine solute concentrations should disclose osmotic diuretics (glucose, mannitol, urea), and measurement of serum creatinine and serum electrolyte levels identifies GFR reductions, hypokalemia, and hypercalcemia. A history of recent head trauma,

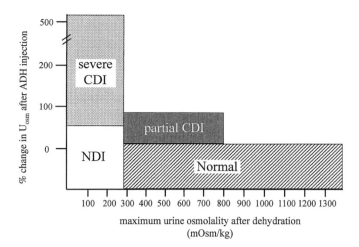

Figure 6.10. Response of urine osmolality to water deprivation and subsequent ADH (vasopressin) injection. *NDI*, nephrogenic diabetes inspidus; *U$_{osm}$*, urine osmolality. (Reprinted with permission from Miller M, Dalakos T, Moses AM, et al. Recognition of partial defects in antidiuretic hormone secretion. Ann Intern Med 1970;73:721–729.)

intracranial surgery, or neurologic deficits (bitemporal hemianopsia) that suggest midline tumors obviously points to CDI as a cause of the polyuric state.

A more difficult diagnostic problem is the separation of patients with partial or complete deficiency of ADH from those with primary polydipsia (98, 99, 102). Certain factors suggest the most likely diagnosis. For example, a 24-hour urine volume greater than 18 L, a random plasma osmolality determination lower than 285 mmol/kg H$_2$O, and a history of episodic polyuria all suggest compulsive water drinking as the underlying disorder. A history of head trauma or neoplasm, a history of sudden onset of unrelenting polyuria, and a random plasma osmolality determination higher than 290 mmol/kg H$_2$O suggest CDI. These distinguishing features depend on the fact that patients with CDI ingest water only in response to appropriate physiologic stimuli and therefore do not ingest water to the point of becoming hyponatremic.

The basis of all tests for CDI rests on the ability of the kidney to excrete a hypertonic urine after an osmotic stimulus. The simplest maneuver is to produce hypertonicity of body fluids by water deprivation. The maximal urine osmolality that is achieved with water deprivation depends on maximal degrees of endogenous ADH release in response to dehydration. Therefore, in individuals with intact ADH production and release, the administration of exogenous vasopressin does not produce an increase in the maximal urine osmolality that is achieved via water deprivation. This rationale forms the framework for a test scheme (76, 98), which is illustrated in Figure 6.10, for distinguishing complete or partial CDI from other polyuria syndromes.

In patients with mild polyuria, water deprivation may begin the night preceding the test; patients with severe polyuria should have water restricted during the day to allow for close observation. The test begins with paired measurements of osmolality of urine and plasma. All water intake is then withheld, and hourly measurements of urine osmolality and body weight are made. When two sequential urine osmolality values vary by less than 30 mmol/kg H$_2$O, or when 3 to 5% of body weight is lost, 5 units of aqueous vasopressin is injected subcutaneously. A final urine osmolality measurement is taken 60 minutes later. It is particularly important that this test be carried out under careful supervision to avoid water intoxication in patients with primary polydipsia related to continued ingestion of water in association with parenteral vasopressin administration.

In normal individuals, the water deprivation results in a urine osmolality two to four times greater than that of plasma. More important, the subsequent administration of exogenous vasopressin results in less than 9% further increase in urine osmolality. Patients with primary polydipsia, who have reduced medullary interstitial tonicity as a result of prolonged water diuresis, may concentrate urine only slightly after water deprivation. However, they too have maximally enhanced endogenous ADH release and exhibit a less than 9% rise in urine osmolality with supplemental vasopressin use.

Patients with complete CDI do not increase urine osmolality above plasma osmolality in response to water deprivation but do show a greater than 50% increase in urine osmolality in response to injection of vasopressin (76, 98). Patients with partial CDI may concentrate the urine to some degree in response to water deprivation, but they also increase urine osmolality by at least 10% after vasopressin injection (76, 98). Patients with partial CDI often show a peak urine osmolality that decreases with further water restriction, which suggests a limited reserve of neurohypophyseal hormone that becomes depleted after an initial secretory burst. Finally, deprivation of water in patients with NDI fails to increase urine osmolality above plasma osmolality even when exogenous vasopressin is given.

When a diagnosis of CDI is made, a careful evaluation for neoplasms involving the hypothalamus or the neurohypophyseal tract is mandatory. Magnetic resonance imaging is the preferred imaging technique. A curious observation, in this regard, is that T1-weighted images of the normal posterior pituitary yield a hyperintense signal. This hyperintense signal is presumed to be caused by some constituent of the vasopressin-containing neurosecretory granules. In patients with CDI, the hyperintense signal in the posterior pituitary is almost always absent (103, 104). An exception may be the rare patient with familial CDI in whom the hyperintense signal may persist. In contrast, patients with primary polydipsia and NDI have normal posterior pituitary hyperintensity (103). In addition to the loss of the hyperintense signal, magnetic resonance images in patients with CDI may reveal thickening of the pituitary stalk or masses resulting from primary or metastatic tumors (104). Thus, although not replacing traditional biochemical and physiologic approaches to the diagnosis of polyuria, magnetic resonance imaging may be a useful adjunct, particularly in differentiating patients with primary polydipsia from those with CDI (103).

Levels of circulating ADH have heretofore been measured by radioimmunoassay only for research purposes. A commercial assay is marketed for clinical use, but its general applicability is undefined. Zerbe and Robertson (102) compared the diagnostic accuracy of the indirect test for ADH release described earlier with actual measurements of plasma ADH levels by radioimmunoassay. These authors concluded that direct measurement of plasma ADH levels can improve the diagnostic accuracy of indirect tests for diagnosis of the polyuria syndromes, but care must be taken in interpreting results from currently available radioimmunoassays (102, 105).

Therapy

Estimation of Free Water Deficit. Patients with diabetes insipidus, either central pituitary or nephrogenic, may require emergency treatment for hypertonic encephalopathy consequent to polyuria and inadequate water intake. The goal in treating hypertonic encephalopathy is to replenish body water, thereby restoring osmotic homeostasis and repleting cell volume at a rate that avoids significant complications. Because the brain adjusts to hypertonicity, at least in part, by increasing the intracellular solute content via the accumulation of "idiogenic osmoles" (106, 107), the rapid repletion of body water with ECF dilution causes translocation of water into cells to achieve osmotic equilibrium. The result of this water movement is cell swelling and cerebral edema. If slower water repletion is undertaken, brain cells lose the accumulated intracellular solutes, and osmotic equilibration can occur without cell swelling. Consequently, a good rule of thumb is to administer fluids at a rate that reduces the serum sodium concentration by about 1 mmol/L every 2 hours.

The magnitude of acute water loss in disorders such as CDI or NDI, in which hypernatremia is caused by water loss exclusively, can be estimated by using the following equation:

$$Water\ Deficit = 0.6 \times Body\ Weight\ ([Na^+]/140 - 1)$$

The choice of fluid to be administered to patients with diabetes insipidus depends on three factors: the extent to which circulatory collapse may be present, the rate at which hypernatremia has developed, and the magnitude of the hypernatremia. Hypotonic NaCl solutions or oral fluids are best used as initial therapy in patients with modest volume contraction and only modest elevations of serum sodium concentrations, that is, less than 160 mmol/L. However, in patients with more advanced hypernatremia, particularly if the hypernatremia has developed gradually, that is, over a period of more than 24 hours, and is accompanied by circulatory collapse, a more prudent initial therapy is to administer normal saline solutions. The reasons for this choice are twofold: in advanced hypernatremia, a normal saline solution is dilute relative to body fluid osmolality and thus will dilute the latter while minimizing the risk of iatrogenic cerebral swelling; at the same time, normal saline provides an effective means of volume expansion.

Finally, 5% glucose solutions may be used to replenish body water in patients with acute hypernatremia in the absence of significant circulatory collapse. However, the glucose infusion rate must be less than the rate of glucose metabolism to avoid glycosuria. Otherwise, the resulting osmotic diuresis will thwart attempts to replenish body free water.

Chronic Therapy. Because the most troublesome effects of CDI are persistent polyuria, inevitable nocturia, and constant thirst, the goal of treatment is to reduce the daily volume of urine excretion. Patients with partial hormonal deficiency and urine volumes of 2 to 6 L daily may require no treatment as long as they are assured access to water. The specific therapy for patients with CDI is some form of vasopressin replacement.

A synthetic analog of vasopressin, desmopressin, provides antidiuretic activity for 8 to 20 hours with negligible pressor effect, can be taken as a nasal formulation, and is the drug of choice for both adults and children (76, 85, 108). The drug is best started at night to find the lowest dose that prevents nocturia. This dose, usually 5 to 10 μg, can be given twice daily or can be doubled as a single morning dose. A nasal catheter is calibrated for convenient dosing in the 5 to 20 μg range. Headache and flushing may be troublesome side effects of taking large doses, but these side effects usually disappear with a reduction of dosage (109). A parenteral formulation is available for patients who are unable to take the drug by nasal insufflation. The parenteral route is also used when desmopressin is used for its hemostatic effects in patients with uremia or von Willebrand disease. Desmopressin also can be effective when administered orally (110, 111). The bioavailability of oral desmopressin is much lower than when administered intranasally or parenterally, necessitating higher doses than are required for the nasal route (110). An oral preparation of desmopressin is now available in the United States. The recommended starting dose of the drug is 0.05 mg twice a day, with subsequent dose adjustment to achieve optimal water balance.

For patients with some residual ADH production, use of the oral hypoglycemic agent chlorpropamide may provide adequate amelioration of symptoms. There is now general agreement (76, 85, 112, 113) that chlorpropamide therapy enhances the action of small amounts of ADH on renal tubules to augment urine-concentrating ability. Doses of 250 to 750 mg of chlorpropamide daily are sufficient to reduce polyuria in most patients with partial CDI (85). The side effect of hypoglycemia, which is especially common in children and in patients taking more than 500 mg daily of the drug, limits its usefulness.

Therapy with the hypolipidemic agent clofibrate (114) and the anticonvulsant carbamazepine (115) may also curtail polyuria in patients with partial CDI. Both drugs seem

Table 6.5. *Causes of Nephrogenic Diabetes Insipidus (NDI)*

Familial NDI
  X linked
  Autosomal recessive (rare)
Acquired NDI
  Tubulointerstitial renal disease
    Sickle cell disease or trait
    Amyloidosis
    Polycystic kidney disease
    Obstructive uropathy
    Medullary sponge kidney
  Electrolyte disorders
    Hypokalemia
    Hypercalcemia
  Drugs
    Lithium
    Demeclocycline
    Methoxyflurane
    Amphotericin B
    Vincristine
  Pregnancy

to work by directly stimulating the release of ADH from the hypothalamus. In addition, carbamazepine therapy may increase the sensitivity of the kidney to ADH (115). Combination therapy with clofibrate and chlorpropamide is useful for some patients (85).

Finally, use of thiazide diuretics may reduce the volume of urine in patients with any form of diabetes insipidus, that is, either central or nephrogenic, by causing mild salt depletion. The effect is produced by taking 50 to 100 mg of hydrochlorothiazide daily, is sustained by salt restriction, and can be abolished by salt loading even with continued diuretic administration (116).

Also, patients with diabetes insipidus, either central or nephrogenic, should carry some form of identification, such as a Medic Alert bracelet, to alert physicians and emergency workers to their condition in the event of an accident or hypertonic encephalopathy.

NDI

NDI is a polyuric disorder that is identified by the presence of normal rates of renal filtration and solute excretion, persistently hypotonic urine, normal or high levels of plasma ADH, and a failure of exogenous vasopressin therapy to raise urine osmolality or to reduce urine volume. Some of the conditions that are associated with failure of the renal tubule to respond to vasopressin therapy are noted in Table 6.5.

Familial NDI

Familial NDI, a rare form of NDI, can be transmitted as either an X-linked or an autosomal-recessive trait.

The lack of response to vasopressin therapy in these patients seems to be restricted to the responses mediated by the V_2 receptor. V_1 receptor–mediated effects, such as vasoconstriction and enhancement of corticotropin release and renal prostaglandin production, are preserved in patients with familial NDI (117, 118).

In familial NDI, the renal collecting ducts are resistant to the antidiuretic action of arginine vasopressin or to its antidiuretic analog desmopressin (119–121). This rare, but now well-described, entity results from mutations in either the *AVPR2* gene that codes for the vasopressin antidiuretic (V_2) receptor or mutations in the *AQP2* gene (51, 119–121) that codes for the vasopressin-dependent water channel (49, 122). Of 75 families with congenital NDI referred to a medical center in Montreal, 71 families had *AVPR2* mutations and 4 had *AQP2* mutations (51).

Isolation of the human gene encoding the V_2 receptor (38, 39) and its assignment to the X chromosome were important steps toward identification of the molecular defects in patients with X-linked NDI. The availability of the genomic sequence allowed the synthesis of primers suitable for amplification of the entire transcriptional unit (2 kb) or portions of it by polymerase chain reaction analysis. Using this approach, approximately 72 different *AVPR2* mutations have been reported in 102 unrelated families with X-linked NDI (119, 123–131).

On the basis of desmopressin infusion studies and phenotypic characteristics of both males and females affected with NDI, a non–X-linked form of NDI with a postreceptor (post-cAMP) defect was suggested (132–135). Mutations in the *AQP2* gene, encoding the ADH-sensitive water channel, have now been identified in several patients with autosomal-recessive NDI (49, 122). Results of functional expression studies show that *Xenopus* oocytes injected with mutant cRNA had abnormal water permeability, whereas *Xenopus* oocytes injected with both mutant and normal cRNAs had water permeability similar to those of normal constructs alone (49, 122). These findings provide conclusive evidence that NDI can be caused by homozygosity for mutations in the *AQP2* gene.

Pregnancy

Diabetes insipidus is a rare complication of pregnancy (136–139). This disorder, which has features of both CDI and NDI, is thought to be caused by the degradation of circulating ADH by the enzyme vasopressinase (136–138, 140, 141). The polyuria usually begins in the third trimester and resolves spontaneously after delivery. Plasma ADH levels are low, but the polyuria may not respond to exogenous vasopressin. In contrast, desmopressin promptly controls the polyuria (136, 138). The serum contains high levels of vasopressinase (136). This enzyme, which is a cysteine aminopeptidase, degrades ADH but not desmopressin, which accounts for the difference in therapeutic efficacy. Serum vasopressinase activity falls after delivery. In pregnant women, the turnover rate of ADH normally increases during the later stages of pregnancy, presumably because of the high activity of vasopressinase in the placenta

Table 6.6. The Hypotonic Syndromes

Excessive water ingestion

Decreased water excretion
  Decreased solute delivery to diluting segments
    Starvation
    Beer potomania
  ADH excess
    SIADH
  ADH excess with decreased distal solute delivery
    Congestive heart failure
    Cirrhosis
    Nephrotic syndrome
    Adrenal insufficiency
    Hypothyroidism
    Diuretic use
  Renal failure

SIADH, syndrome of inappropriate ADH secretion.

(142). Some women with subclinical forms of CDI may develop symptomatic polyuria during pregnancy because of the increased rate of metabolism of vasopressin (140).

True NDI has also been reported during pregnancy. This condition, which is characterized by high plasma ADH levels and no response to therapy with either exogenous vasopressin or desmopressin, also remits after delivery. The pathogenesis is not known (143).

Women with preexisting diabetes insipidus are generally treated with desmopressin. Because this drug is not metabolized by placental vasopressinase, the drug dosage does not need to be adjusted. A review of the use of desmopressin during pregnancy did not detect any increase in fetal morbidity or mortality (144).

The Hypotonic Syndromes

The hypotonic syndrome results when free water is not excreted at a rate sufficient to maintain the serum sodium concentration and the body fluid osmolality at normal rather than subnormal values. Such a circumstance might occur for any of the following reasons: (a) ingestion of a quantity of water that exceeds the capacity of the normal kidney to excrete it (primary polydipsia); (b) diminished capacity to excrete a water load because of inadequate solute delivery to the diluting segment; and (c) diminished capacity to excrete a water load because of sustained, nonosmotic release of ADH. A pathophysiologic classification of the hypotonic syndromes, with some clinical examples, is presented in Table 6.6.

The Clinical Syndromes

Adrenal Insufficiency

Hyponatremia may complicate untreated adrenal insufficiency. In patients with mineralocorticoid deficiency, the combination of ECF volume contraction, GFR reduction, enhanced proximal tubular salt absorption, and volume-

mediated, nonosmotic ADH release seems to be responsible for an inability to handle water loads (145, 146). Glucocorticoid treatment is also required for complete correction of the defect in water excretion in patients with adrenal insufficiency (145, 146). A glucocorticoid-mediated impairment of cardiac function also contributes to the reduction in effective circulating volume in patients with adrenal insufficiency (145).

Finally, nonosmotic ADH release may contribute to water retention (147). Glucocorticoid-deficient rats have inappropriately high plasma ADH levels and an inability to excrete a water load (147, 148). Use of specific ADH antagonists largely corrects the deficit in water excretion (149). As noted earlier, ADH and corticotropin-releasing hormone are coproduced by certain parvocellular neurons in the PVN (6), and both hormones are under negative feedback controlled by cortisol. After adrenalectomy, the number of cells in this region that contain immunoreactive ADH increases dramatically (150). In situ hybridization with probes for the ADH mRNA confirms that ADH synthesis is increased in the absence of glucocorticoids (151).

Hypothyroidism

The cause of the hyponatremia that is occasionally seen in hypothyroid patients is not clear. Hyponatremia in myxedema might occur because of sustained ADH release (152) or because of a "reset osmostat" (145), that is, normal modes for regulating plasma osmolality but at reduced plasma osmolality levels. Alternatively, DeRubertis and coworkers (153) inferred that salt delivery to the loop of Henle is reduced in patients with hypothyroidism and that this effect accounted for the defect in free water excretion. Regardless of the mechanism involved, appropriate treatment of myxedema is accompanied by the restoration of renal concentrating and diluting capacities (154).

Syndrome of Inappropriate Antidiuretic Hormone (SIADH): Vasopressin Excess

The sustained release of ADH in the absence of either osmotic or nonosmotic stimuli is a common cause of hyponatremia. In general, a primary excess of ADH occurs in two settings: in SIADH and as a consequence of drugs that enhance ADH release or action. Measurements of ADH levels in patients with hyponatremia indicate that SIADH is the single most common cause of hyponatremia in hospitalized and, particularly, postoperative patients (155–157). Overall, excessive, nonosmotic release of ADH is present in more than 95% of hospitalized patients with hyponatremia (155, 156, 158).

In most patients with SIADH, there is persistent production of ADH or an ADH-like peptide despite body fluid hypotonicity and an expanded effective circulating volume (146, 159, 160). Zerbe and colleagues (159) documented four kinds of responses of serum ADH levels to osmotic and nonosmotic stimuli in patients with SIADH:

1. The most common derangement (40%) is wide fluctuations of ADH levels independent of osmotic or nonosmotic control.

2. About one-third of patients have an abnormally low osmotic threshold for ADH release, but at higher osmolalities a normal correlation exists between plasma ADH levels and plasma osmolality. These patients can produce maximally dilute urine if they are sufficiently hyponatremic.

3. In one-fifth of patients, ADH release is sustained ("ADH leak") below serum osmolality values of 278 mmol/kg H_2O, and ADH release is normal in response to osmotic stimuli.

4. Approximately one-sixth of patients have no detectable abnormality of ADH levels but a failure to dilute urine maximally. This type of SIADH, therefore, has a poorly understood pathogenesis.

As a result of the sustained release of ADH or ADH-like substances, patients retain ingested water and become hyponatremic and modestly volume expanded and generally increase body weight by 5 to 10%. The volume expansion results in reduced rates of proximal tubular sodium absorption and consequently in natriuresis, albeit at a total expansion of total body weight. Increased levels of atrial natriuretic peptide also contribute to natriuresis. Because aldosterone secretion is stimulated by hyponatremia, secretion of this mineralocorticoid may also contribute to reducing renal sodium losses in volume-expanded hyponatremic patients. There are also increased urinary losses of substances like uric acid, whose excretion rates vary directly with effective circulating volume and with rates of sodium excretion. Consequently, hypouricemia is common in patients with SIADH. The GFR is normal, as is adrenal and thyroid function.

Diagnosis

The diagnosis of hyponatremia is most commonly made from routine laboratory findings. Hyponatremia also should be considered whenever there is a sudden deterioration in CNS function, particularly in circumstances such as intractable heart failure, hepatic cirrhosis with ascites, or the administration of large volumes of intravenous fluids.

The history and physical examination are generally adequate for recognizing disorders such as compulsive water ingestion and for noting the ingestion of drugs that stimulate ADH release or enhance ADH action. The presence of edema is characteristic of individuals in whom hyponatremia occurs because of a reduced effective circulating volume coupled with ECF volume expansion. In patients with hypothyroidism and adrenal insufficiency, typical clinical and laboratory findings are generally present.

The most difficult differential diagnosis among hyponatremic disorders involves the distinction between patients who are modestly volume contracted and those who have SIADH. In both circumstances, the serum sodium level and the serum osmolality are reduced, and the urine osmolality is inappropriately high with respect to the reduced serum osmolality. Nonosmotic water conservation in SIADH and in volume contraction is recognized by the presence of a urine osmolality value higher than 120 to 150 mmol/kg H_2O in association with a reduced serum osmolality.

Patients who are volume contracted may provide a history of volume losses or of diuretic ingestion and exhibit the signs of ECF volume contraction. When the volume losses are the result of extrarenal causes, the urine sodium concentration is less than 10 to 15 mmol/L, and the fractional excretion of sodium is generally less than 1%. The presence of hyperuricemia and azotemia is also a useful index to ECF volume contraction. In contrast, patients with SIADH are generally normovolemic or slightly volume expanded and therefore exhibit none of the signs of volume contraction. The serum blood urea nitrogen and creatinine values are normal, and the serum uric acid level is generally reduced. The urine sodium concentration usually exceeds 30 mmol/L, and the fractional excretion of sodium is greater than 1%. Results of adrenal function tests are normal.

The above-mentioned studies usually discriminate between SIADH and extrarenal volume contraction. However, when ECF volume contraction is caused by renal salt wasting, urine sodium losses generally persist unless volume contraction is profound. A useful diagnostic and therapeutic maneuver in this situation is to observe the results of water restriction. When water intake is restricted to 600 to 800 mL daily, patients with SIADH exhibit a highly characteristic response: a 2- to 3-kg weight loss accompanied by correction of hyponatremia and cessation of salt wasting, usually over a period of 2 to 3 days. If weight loss fails to correct both hyponatremia and urine sodium wasting simultaneously, the diagnosis of SIADH is doubtful. Rather, renal sodium wasting with ECF volume contraction, related to adrenal insufficiency or the other renal salt-losing disorders listed in Table 6.6, is the more probable diagnosis.

Therapy

The goal of treatment is to correct body water osmolality and to restore cell volume to normal by raising the ratio of sodium to water in the ECF. The increase in ECF osmolality draws water from cells and therefore reduces their volume. The therapeutic approach, as well as whether net sodium and water balance is adjusted to be positive or negative during therapy, depends on the serum sodium concentration, the rate at which hyponatremia has developed, the clinical status, and the underlying disorder.

Symptomatic Hyponatremia. Severe hyponatremia that is associated with a serum sodium concentration below 120 to 125 mmol/L and CNS manifestations requires immediate therapy. In volume-contracted states, the treatment of choice is to raise the serum sodium level to 125 mmol/L by administering hypertonic (3 to 5%) saline. Because the desired effect is to correct body water osmolality, the amount of sodium that is administered must be sufficient to raise total body water osmolality to approximately 250 mmol/kg H_2O, that is, to approximately twice the desired serum sodium concentration. A convenient formula for calculating this sodium requirement is as follows:

$$[125 - measured\ serum\ Na] \times 0.6\ body\ weight = required\ mmol\ of\ Na$$

The serum sodium concentration is in millimoles per liter and the body weight is in kilograms. Because 60% of body weight is water, the formula allows an estimate of the amount of sodium required to raise body water osmolality to 250 mmol/kg H_2O.

The administration of hypertonic saline is hazardous in volume-expanded, salt-retaining states such as congestive heart failure. Furthermore, in patients with SIADH that is associated with volume expansion and sodium wasting, the administration of hypertonic saline alone may be ineffective in correcting hyponatremia because the administered salt is excreted promptly in a relatively concentrated urine. In such circumstances, normal saline or hypertonic saline solutions may be used in combination with furosemide (161). The diuretic induces urine salt loss and therefore reduces the risk of ECF volume expansion. Moreover, the diuresis that is induced by furosemide is characterized by the excretion of urine with an osmolality that is lower than the plasma osmolality. Consequently, the combination of intravenously administered normal or hypertonic saline, coupled with a furosemide-induced diuresis of urine that is dilute with respect to plasma, provides an effective way of raising the serum sodium level in SIADH or other volume-expanded states.

The rapid elevation of serum sodium concentrations to levels higher than 125 mmol/L is potentially hazardous. Because loss of brain solute represents one of the compensatory mechanisms for preserving brain cell volume in dilutional states (162–164), a serum sodium level of 140 mmol/L is relatively hypertonic to brain cells that have become partially depleted of solute as a result of hyponatremia. Consequently, raising the serum sodium level rapidly to higher than 120 to 125 mmol/L can cause CNS damage such as central pontine myelinolysis (165–168). Moreover, raising the serum sodium concentration to higher than 120 mmol/L is not only hazardous but unnecessary.

The major, and still unresolved, controversy surrounding the treatment of hyponatremia concerns the rate at which hyponatremia should be corrected (169, 170). Advocates of rapid correction point to the high mortality rate among patients with hyponatremia, as high as 86% in one series. Advocates of slow correction caution that the rapid correction of hyponatremia itself may produce central pontine myelinolysis.

Mortality rates for severe hyponatremia of 33 to 86% have been cited in support of prompt correction of hyponatremia. These estimates, however, derive largely from single case reports and small, often selective, series of patients. Thus, these data may overestimate the mortality from hyponatremia. In a prospective study of 33 patients with symptomatic hyponatremia, no deaths occurred (171). Likewise, two studies of patients with severe hyponatremia (serum sodium level < 110 mmol/L) found a mortality rate of only 8%, with most deaths attributed to underlying diseases (168, 172). Slow or delayed correction of hyponatremia was not associated with higher mortality or with neurologic complications. Indeed, the risk of developing neurologic complications was greatest in patients whose serum sodium concentrations were corrected at a rate greater than 0.6 mmol/L per hour (14 mmol/day) (168, 172). In part, the discrepant mortality rates may relate to differences in the patient populations under study. Arieff (169) and others (171, 173–175) reported on more than 80 healthy young women who developed symptomatic hyponatremia after elective surgery and subsequently died or suffered permanent brain damage. Although women do not seem to be any more prone than men to develop postoperative hyponatremia, they have a 25-fold increased risk of death or permanent neurologic damage as a result of the hyponatremia (175). Children also seem to be at increased risk of death or permanent neurologic damage from hyponatremia (176). The gender and age differences are also seen in animal models of hyponatremia (177–180). Finally, the imposition of a hypoxic cerebral insult in the setting of hyponatremia increases the mortality rate dramatically (181). Animal studies indicate that hypoxia or ischemia impair the adaptive mechanisms to hyponatremia and result in greater cerebral edema than occurs in uncomplicated hyponatremia (181). This may have clinical relevance because many of the young women described by Arieff and others (174, 175) suffered respiratory arrests in the course of their hyponatremia. In contrast, the patients reported in the prospective studies tend to be older men and have underlying illnesses or are receiving diuretics. In these patients, the hyponatremia does not carry as grave a prognosis as in young women.

On the basis of available data, it seems prudent to correct the sodium concentration at a rate of 0.5 mmol/L per hour until the serum sodium concentration reaches 120 to 125 mmol/L. However, young women with acute symptomatic hyponatremia are at risk for respiratory arrest, severe neurologic sequelae, and death. It is reasonable to treat these patients with hypertonic saline to raise the serum sodium concentration to 125 mmol/L at a rate of 1 to 2 mmol/L per hour (168, 182). At this point, the patient should be asymptomatic and the serum sodium concentration can be returned to normal gradually over several days with water restriction. Overcorrection of the serum sodium concentration (to higher than 130 mmol/L) is unnecessary and potentially harmful. Even in patients with acutely developing hyponatremia, symptoms and CNS signs are uncommon until the serum sodium concentration falls below 120 mmol/L. Patients with chronic hyponatremia may tolerate well even greater degrees of hyponatremia (170, 183).

Asymptomatic Hyponatremia. Mild, asymptomatic chronic hyponatremia is generally managed by correction of the underlying disorder when the hyponatremia occurs in volume contraction or in salt-regaining states such as congestive heart failure or hepatic cirrhosis with ascites. Chronic hyponatremia in SIADH may be easily corrected by restricting water intake to 800 to 1000 mL daily, provided that patients can adhere to the program of water restriction.

An alternative approach involves the use of agents such as lithium or demeclocycline, which interfere with the renal tubular effects of ADH. However, the response to lithium is variable, and lithium itself causes multiple side effects, including renal tubular acidosis, cardiotoxicity, and thyroid dysfunction (184–188). In contrast, demeclocycline re-

producibly inhibits renal concentrating ability in patients with SIADH (188, 189). However, demeclocycline should be used cautiously in patients with coexisting liver disease because of the risk of toxic nephropathy produced by accumulation of the drug (190). As another alternative, some researchers (191) have recommended reducing renal concentrating ability by administering oral urea loads that are sufficient to produce osmotic diuresis. A maneuver that is effective in patients who are not edematous, hypertensive, or in congestive heart failure is to administer oral furosemide in association with a high-salt diet. Finally, competitive antagonists of vasopressin may prove to be useful in the treatment of acute and chronic water intoxication. A nonpeptide vasopressin antagonist, OPC-31260, can be administered orally and was effective in increasing free water excretion in rats with either cirrhosis (192) or SIADH (193). The short-term use of this agent in humans seems to be safe (194), but the therapeutic efficacy of this agent in the treatment of hyponatremia in humans has not yet been established.

REFERENCES

1. Morris JF. Organization of neural inputs to the supraoptic and paraventricular nuclei: anatomical aspects. Prog Brain Res 1983; 60:3–18.
2. Sawchenko PE, Swanson LW. The organization and biochemical specificity of afferent projections to the paraventricular and supraoptic nuclei. Prog Brain Res 1983;60:19–29.
3. Vandesande F, Dierickx K. Identification of the vasopressin producing and of the oxytocin producing neurons in the hypothalamic magnocellular neurosecretory system of the rat. Cell Tissue Res 1975;164:153–162.
4. Zimmerman EA, Robinson AG. Hypothalamic neurons secreting vasopressin and neurophysin. Kidney Int 1976;10:12–24.
5. Zimmerman EA, Defendi R. Hypothalamic pathways containing oxytocin, vasopressin and associated neurophysins. In: Moses AM, Share L, eds. Neurohypophysis. Basel: Karger, 1977:22–29.
6. Sawchenko PE, Swanson LW, Vale WW. Co-expression of corticotropin-releasing factor and vasopressin immunoreactivity in parvocellular neurosecretory neurons of the adrenalectomized rat. Proc Natl Acad Sci USA 1984;81:1883–1887.
7. Zimmerman EA, Silverman AJ. Vasopressin and adrenal cortical interactions. Prog Brain Res 1983;60:493–504.
8. Whitnall MH, Mezey E, Gainer H. Co-localization of corticotropin-releasing factor and vasopressin in median eminence neurosecretory vesicles. Nature 1985;317:248–252.
9. du Vigneaud V. Hormones of the mammalian posterior pituitary gland and their naturally occurring analogues. Johns Hopkins Med J 1969;124:53–65.
10. Sawyer WH. Evolution of neurohypophyseal hormones and their receptors. Fed Proc 1977;36:1842–1847.
11. Pickering BT, Jones CW. Neurophysins. In: Li CH, ed. Hormonal Proteins and Peptides. New York: Academic, 1978;5:103–158.
12. Robinson AG. The neurophysins. In: Reichlin S, ed. The Neurohypophysis: Physiological and Clinical Aspects. New York: Plenum, 1984:65–93.
13. Takabatake Y, Sachs H. Vasopressin biosynthesis, III: in vitro studies. Endocrinology 1964;75:934–942.
14. Sachs H, Fawcett P, Takabatake Y, et al. Biosynthesis and release of vasopressin and neurophysin. Recent Prog Horm Res 1969;25:447–484.
15. Brownstein MJ, Russell JT, Gainer H. Synthesis, transport and release of posterior pituitary hormones. Science 1980;207:373–378.
16. Russell JT, Brownstein MJ, Gainer H. Time course of appearance

and release of [35S]cysteine labelled neurophysins and peptides in the neurohypophysis. Brain Res 1981;205:299– 311.
17. Land H, Schuetz G, Schmale H, et al. Nucleotide sequence of cloned cDNA encoding bovine arginine vasopressin–neurophysin II precursor. Nature 1982;295:299–303.
18. Schmale H, Heinsohn S, Richter D. Structural organization of the rat gene for the arginine vasopressin–neurophysin II precursor. EMBO J 1983;2:763–767.
19. Schmale H, Fehr S, Richter D. Vasopressin biosynthesis: from gene to peptide hormone. Kidney Int 1987;32:S8–S13.
20. Riddell DC, Mallonee R, Phillips JA, et al. Chromosomal assignment of human sequences encoding arginine vasopressin–neurophysin II and growth hormone releasing factor. Somat Cell Mol Genet 1985;11:189–195.
21. Gainer H, Sarne Y, Brownstein MJ. Neurophysin biosynthesis: conversion of a putative precursor during axonal transport. Science 1977;195:1354–1356.
22. Verney EB. The antidiuretic hormone and the factors which determine its release. Proc R Soc Lond B Biol Sci 1947;135:25–105.
23. McKinley MJ, Denton DA, Weisinger RS. Sensors for antidiuresis and thirst: osmoreceptors or CSF sodium detectors? Brain Res 1978;141:89–103.
24. Thrasher TN, Brown CJ, Keil LC, et al. Thirst and vasopressin release in the dog: an osmoreceptor or sodium receptor mechanism? Am J Physiol 1980;238:R333–R339.
25. Thrasher TN, Keil LC, Ramsay DJ. Lesions of the organum vasculosum of the lamina terminalis (OVLT) attenuate osmotically-induced drinking and vasopressin secretion in the dog. Endocrinology 1982;110:1837–1839.
26. Bealer SL, Crofton JT, Share L. Hypothalamic knife cuts alter fluid regulation, vasopressin secretion and natriuresis during water deprivation. Neuroendocrinology 1983;36:364– 370.
27. Honda K, Negoro H, Higuchi T, et al. Activation of neurosecretory cells by osmotic stimulation of anteroventral third ventricle. Am J Physiol 1987;252:R1039–R1045.
28. Sved AF. Central neural pathways in baroreceptor control of vasopressin secretion. In: Schrier RW, ed. Vasopressin. New York: Raven Press, 1985:443–453.
29. Poulain DA, Wakerley JB. Electrophysiology of hypothalamic magnocellular neurones secreting oxytocin and vasopressin. Neuroscience 1982;7:773–808.
30. Robertson GL, Berl T. Water metabolism. In: Brenner BM, Rector FCJ, eds. The Kidney. Philadelphia: WB Saunders, 1986:385–432.

31. Caillens H, Pruszczynski W, Meurier A, et al. Relationship between change in volemia at constant osmolality and plasma antidiuretic hormone. Miner Electrolyte Metab 1980;4:161–171.

32. Stricker EM, Verbalis JG. Interaction of osmotic and volume stimuli in regulation of neurohypophyseal secretion in rats. Am J Physiol 1986;250:R267–R275.

33. Quillen EW, Cowley AW. Influence of volume changes on osmolality-vasopressin relationships in conscious dogs. Am J Physiol 1983;244:H73–H79.

34. Ross MG, Ervin MG, Leake RD, et al. Continuous ovine fetal hemorrhage: sensitivity of plasma and urine arginine vasopressin response. Am J Physiol 1986;251:E464–E469.

35. Hebert SC, Schafer JA, Andreoli TE. The effects of antidiuretic hormone (ADH) on solute and water transport in the mammalian nephron. J Membr Biol 1981;58:1–19.

36. Hebert SC, Andreoli TE. Water permeability of biological membranes: lessons from antidiuretic hormone–responsive epithelia. Biochim Biophys Acta 1982;650:267–280.

37. Grantham JJ, Burg MB. Effect of vasopressin and cyclic AMP on permeability of isolated collecting tubules. Am J Physiol 1966; 211:255–259.

38. Lolait SJ, O'Carroll AM, McBride OW, et al. Cloning and characterization of a vasopressin V_2 receptor and possible link to nephrogenic diabetes insipidus. Nature 1992;357:336–339.

39. Birnbaumer M, Seibold A, Gilbert S, et al. Molecular cloning of the receptor for human antidiuretic hormone. Nature 1992;357: 333–335.

40. Nielsen S, Agre P. The aquaporin family of water channels in kidney. Kidney Int 1995;48:1057–1068.

41. Dousa TP. Cyclic nucleotides in the cellular action of neurohypophyseal hormones. Fed Proc 1977;36:1867–1871.

42. Fahrenholz F, Jurzak M, Gerstberger R, et al. Renal and central vasopressin receptors: immunocytochemical localization. Ann N Y Acad Sci 1993;689:194–206.

43. Firsov D, Mandon B, Morel A, et al. Molecular analysis of vasopressin receptors in the rat nephron, evidence for alternative splicing of the V_2 receptor. Pflugers Arch 1994;429:79–89.

44. Preston BM, Carroll TP, Guggino WB, et al. Appearance of water channels in *Xenopus* oocytes expressing red cell CHIP28 protein. Science 1992;256:385–387.

45. Fushimi K, Uchida S, Hara Y, et al. Cloning and expression of apical membrane water channel of rat kidney collecting tubule. Nature 1993;361:549–552.

46. Nielsen S, Digiovanni SR, Christensen EI, et al. Cellular and subcellular immunolocalization of vasopressin-regulated water channel in rat kidney. Proc Natl Acad Sci USA 1993;90:11663–11667.

47. Digiovanni SR, Nielsen S, Christensen EI, et al. Regulation of collecting duct water channel expression by vasopressin in Brattleboro rat. Proc Natl Acad Sci USA 1994;91:8984–8988.

48. Yamamoto T, Sasaki S, Fushimi K, et al. Localization and expression of a collecting duct water channel, aquaporin, in hydrated and dehydrated rats. Exp Nephrol 1995;3:193–201.

49. Deen PMT, Verdijk MA, Knoers NVAM, et al. Requirement of human renal water channel aquaporin-2 for vasopressin-dependent concentration of urine. Science 1994;264:92–95.

50. Deen PMT, Croes H, vanAubel RAMH, et al. Water channels encoded by mutant Aquaporin-2 genes in nephrogenic diabetes insipidus are impaired in their cellular routing. J Clin Invest 1995; 95:2291–2296.

51. Reeves WB, Bichet DG, Andreoli TE. The posterior pituitary and water metabolism. In: Wilson JD, Foster DW, eds. Williams Textbook of Endocrinology. 9th ed. Philadelphia: WB Saunders, 1997.

52. Knepper MA, Rector FCJ. Urine concentration and dilution. In: Brenner BM, ed. The Kidney. 5th ed. Philadelphia: WB Saunders, 1996:532–570.

53. Bankir L. Urea and the kidney. In: Brenner BM, ed. The Kidney. 5th ed. Philadelphia: WB Saunders, 1996:571–606.

54. Sands JM, Nonoguchi H, Knepper MA. Vasopressin effects on urea and H_2O transport in inner medullary collecting duct subsegments. Am J Physiol 1987;253:F823–F832.

55. Star RA, Nonoguchi H, Balaban R, et al. Calcium and cyclic adenosine monophosphate as second messengers for vasopressin in the rat inner medullary collecting duct. J Clin Invest 1988;81: 1879–1888.

56. Greger R, Schlatter E. Properties of the lumen membrane of the cortical thick ascending limb of Henle's loop of rabbit kidney. Pflugers Arch 1983;396:315–324.

57. Molony DA, Reeves WB, Andreoli TE. $Na^+:K^+:2Cl^-$ cotransport and the thick ascending limb. Kidney Int 1989;36:418–426.

58. Hebert SC, Andreoli TE. Effects of antidiuretic hormone on cellular conductive pathways in mouse medullary thick ascending limbs of Henle, II: determinants of the ADH-mediated increases in transepithelial voltage and in net Cl- absorption. J Membr Biol 1984; 80:221–233.

59. Hebert SC, Friedman PA, Andreoli TE. The effects of antidiuretic hormone on cellular conductive pathways in mouse medullary thick ascending limbs of Henle, I: ADH increases transcellular conductance pathways. J Membr Biol 1984;80:201–219.

60. Stokes JB. Consequences of potassium recycling in the renal medulla: effects on ion transport by the medullary thick ascending limb of Henle's loop. J Clin Invest 1982;70:219–229.

61. Hebert SC, Andreoli TE. Control of NaCl transport in the thick ascending limb. Am J Physiol 1984;15:F745–F756.

62. Reeves WB, Andreoli TE. Cl- transport in basolateral renal medullary vesicles, II: Cl- channels in planar lipid bilayers. J Membr Biol 1990;113:57–65.

63. Adachi S, Uchida S, Ito H, et al. Two isoforms of a chloride channel predominantly expressed in thick ascending limb of Henle's Loop and collecting ducts of rat kidney. J Biol Chem 1994;269: 17677–17683.

64. Kieferle S, Fong P, Bens M, et al. Two highly homologous members of the ClC chloride channel family in both rat and human kidney. Proc Natl Acad Sci USA 1994;91:6943–6947.

65. Zimniak L, Winters CJ, Reeves WB, et al. Cl- channels in basolateral renal medullary vesicles, X: cloning of a basolateral mTAL Cl- channel. Kidney Int 1995;48:1828–1836.

66. Molony DA, Reeves WB, Hebert SC, et al. ADH increases apical $Na^+,K^+,2Cl^-$ entry in mouse medullary thick ascending limbs of Henle. Am J Physiol 1987;252:F177–F187.

67. Hebert SC, Culpepper RM, Andreoli TE. NaCl transport in mouse medullary thick ascending limbs, I: functional nephron heterogeneity and ADH-stimulated NaCl cotransport. Am J Physiol 1981; 241:F412–F431.

68. Hebert SC, Culpepper RM, Andreoli TE. NaCl transport in mouse medullary thick ascending limbs, III: modulation of the ADH effect by peritubular osmolality. Am J Physiol 1981;241: F443–F451.

69. Craven PA, DeRubertis FR. Effects of vasopressin and urea on Ca^{2+}-calmodulin-dependent renal prostaglandin E. Am J Physiol 1981;241:F649–F658.

70. Nadler SP, Hebert SC, Brenner BM. PGE2, forskolin, and cholera toxin interaction in rabbit cortical collecting tubule. Am J Physiol 1986;250:F127–F135.

71. Culpepper RM, Andreoli TE. PGE2, forskolin, and cholera toxin interactions in modulating NaCl transport in mouse mTALH. Am J Physiol 1984;247:F784–F792.

72. Culpepper RM, Andreoli TE. Interactions among prostaglandin E2, antidiuretic hormone, and cyclic adenosine monophosphate in modulating Cl- absorption in single mouse medullary thick ascending limbs of Henle. J Clin Invest 1983;71:1588–1601.

73. Sands JM, Schrader DC. An independent effect of osmolality on urea transport in rat terminal IMCDs. J Clin Invest 1991;88: 137–142.

74. Robertson GL, Athar S, Shelton RL. Osmotic control of vasopressin function. In: Andreoli TE, Grantham JJ, Rector FC, eds. Disturbances in Body Fluid Osmolality. Bethesda: American Physiological Society, 1977:125–148.

75. Fink EB. Diabetes insipidus. Arch Pathol Lab Med 1928;6: 102–120.

76. Moses AM, Notman DD. Diabetes insipidus and syndrome of inappropriate antidiuretic hormone secretion (SIADH). Adv Intern Med 1973;27:73–100.

77. Wang LC, Chohen ME, Duffner PK. Etiologies of central diabetes insipidus in children. Pediatr Neurol 1994;11:276–277.

78. Tarng DC, Huang TP. Diabetes insipidus as an early sign of pineal tumor. Am J Nephrol 1995;15:161–164.

79. Genka S, Soeda H, Takahashi M, et al. Acromegaly, diabetes insipidus, and visual loss caused by metastatic growth hormone-releasing hormone-producing malignant pancreatic endocrine tumor in the pituitary gland. J Neurosurg 1995;83:719–723.

80. Kawamura J, Tsukamoto K, Yamakawa K, et al. Diabetes insipidus

due to pituitary metastasis from bladder cancer. Urol Int 1991; 46(2):217–220.

81. Tham LC, Millward MJ, Lind MJ, et al. Metastatic breast cancer presenting with diabetes insipidus. Acta Oncol 1992;31:679–680.

82. Koshiuyama H, Ohgaki K, Hida S, et al. Metastatic renal cell carcinoma to the pituitary gland presenting with hypopituitarism. J Endocrinol Invest 1992;15:677–681.

83. Sherwood MC, Stanhope R, Preece MA, et al. Diabetes insipidus and occult intracranial tumours. Arch Dis Child 1986;61: 1222–1224.

84. Randall RV, Clark EC, Bahn RC. Classification of the causes of diabetes insipidus. Mayo Clin Proc 1959;34:299–302.

85. Weitzman RE, Kleeman CR. The clinical physiology of water metabolism, part II: renal mechanisms for urinary concentration; diabetes insipidus. West J Med 1979;131:486–515.

86. Imura H, Nakao K, Shimatsu A, et al. Lymphocytic infundibuloneurohypophysitis as a cause of central diabetes insipidus. N Engl J Med 1993;329:683–689.

87. Ashmed SR, Aiello DP, Page R, et al. Necrotizing infundibulohypophysitis: a unique syndrome of diabetes insipidus and hypopituitarism. J Clin Endocrinol Metab 1993;76:1499–1504.

88. Czarnechi EJ, Spickler EM. MR demonstration of Wegener granulomatosis of the infundibulum, a cause of diabetes insipidus. Am J Neurorad 1995;16:968–970.

89. Rossi GP, Pavan E, Chiesura-Corona M, et al. Bronchocentric granulomatosis and central diabetes insipidus successfully treated with corticosteroids. Eur Respir J 1994;7:1893–1898.

90. Matsumot AT, Sanno K, Osamura Y. Lymphocytic hypophysitis: case report. Neurosurgery 1995;36:1016–1019.

91. Camus J, Roussy G. Experimental researches on the pituitary body. Endocrinology 1920;4:507–522.

92. Fisher C, Ingram WR. The effect of interruption of the supraoptico-hypophyseal tracts on the antidiuretic, pressor and oxytocic activity of the posterior lobe of the hypophysis. Endocrinology 1936;20:762–768.

93. Heinbecker P, White HL. Hypothalamico-hypophysial system and its relation to water balance in the dog. Am J Physiol 1944;133: 582–593.

94. Rasmussen AT, Gardner WJ. Effects of hypophysial stalk resection on the hypophysis and hypothalamus of man. Endocrinology 1940;27:219–226.

95. Bononi PL, Robinson AG. Central diabetes insipidus: management in the postoperative period. The Endocrinologist 1996;1: 180–185.

96. Lipsett MB, MacLean JP, West CD, et al. An analysis of the polyuria induced by hypophysectomy in man. J Clin Endocrinol Metab 1956;16:183–195.

97. Mudd RH, Dodge HW, Clark EC, et al. Experimental diabetes insipidus: a study of the normal interphase. Proc Staff Meet Mayo Clin 1957;32:94–108.

98. Miller M, Dalakos T, Moses AM, et al. Recognition of partial defects in antidiuretic hormone secretion. Ann Intern Med 1970;73: 721–729.

99. Barlow E, deWardener HE. Compulsive water drinking. Q J Med 1959;28:235–258.

100. Manson AD, Yalowitz PA, Randall RV, et al. Dilatation of the urinary tract associated with pituitary and nephrogenic diabetes insipidus. J Urol 1970;103:327–331.

101. Streitz JMJ, Streitz JM. Polyuric urinary tract dilatation with renal damage. J Urol 1988;139:784–785.

102. Zerbe RL, Robertson GL. A comparison of plasma vasopressin measurements with a standard indirect test in the differential diagnosis of polyuria. N Engl J Med 1981;305:1539–1546.

103. Moses AM, Clayton B, Hochhauser L. Use of T1-weighted MR imaging to differentiate between primary polydipsia and central diabetes insipidus. Am J Neurorad 1992;13:1273–1277.

104. Tien R, Kucharczyk J, Kucharczyk W. MR imaging of the brain in patients with diabetes insipidus. Am J Neurorad 1991;12: 533–542.

105. Robertson GL. The use of vasopressin assays in physiology and pathophysiology. Semin Nephrol 1994;14:368–383.

106. Arieff AI, Guisado R, Lazarowitz VC. The pathophysiology of hyperosmolar states. In: Andreoli TE, Grantham JJ, Rector FC, eds. Disturbances in Body Fluid Osmolality. Bethesda: American Physiological Society, 1977:227–250.

107. Chan PH, Fishman RA. Elevation of rat brain amino acids and idiogenic osmoles induced by hyperosmolality. Brain Res 1979; 161:293–301.

108. Robertson GL, Harris A. Clinical use of vasopressin analogues. Hosp Pract 1989;24:114–139.

109. Cobb WE, Spare S, Reichlin S. Neurogenic diabetes insipidus: management with dDAVP (1-desamino-8-D arginine vasopressin). Ann Intern Med 1978;88:183–188.

110. Fjellestad-Paulson A, Paulsen O, D'Agay-Abensour L, et al. Central diabetes insipidus: oral treatment with dDAVP. Regul Pept 1993;45:303–307.

111. Cunnah D, Ross G, Besser GM. Management of cranial diabetes insipidus with oral desmopressin (dDAVP). Clin Endocrinol 1986; 24:253–257.

112. Pokracki FJ, Robinson AG, Seif SM. Chlorpropamide effect: measurement of neurophysin and vasopressin in humans and rats. Metabolism 1981;30:72–78.

113. Kusano E, Braun-Werness JL, Vick DJ, et al. Chlorpropamide action on renal concentrating mechanism in rats with hypothalamic diabetes insipidus. J Clin Invest 1983;72:1298–1313.

114. Moses AM, Howanitz J, van Gemert M, et al. Clofibrate-induced antidiuresis. J Clin Invest 1973;52:535–542.

115. Gold PW, Robertson GL, Ballenger JC, et al. Carbamazepine diminishes the sensitivity of the plasma arginine vasopressin response to osmotic stimulation. J Clin Endocrinol Metab 1983;57: 952–957.

116. Crawford JD, Kennedy GC. Clinical results of treatment of diabetes insipidus with drugs of the chlorothiazide series. N Engl J Med 1960;262:737–742.

117. Orr FR, Filipich RL. Studies with angiotensin in nephrogenic diabetes insipidus. Can Med Assoc J 1967;97:841–845.

118. Moses AM, Scheinman SJ, Schroeder ET. Antidiuretic and PGE2 responses to AVP and dDAVP in subjects with central and nephrogenic diabetes insipidus. Am J Physiol 1985;248:F354–F359.

119. Fujiwara TM, Morgan K. Molecular biology of diabetes insipidus. Ann Rev Med 1995;46:331–343.

120. Knoers N, Monnens LAH. Nephrogenic diabetes insipidus: clinical symptoms, pathogenesis, genetics and treatment. Pediatr Nephrol 1992;6:476–482.

121. Holtzman EJ, Kolakowski LF, Ausiello DA. The molecular biology of congenital nephrogenic diabetes insipidus. In: Bonventre J, ed. Molecular Nephrology. New York: M. Dekker, 1994:887–912.

122. van Lieburg AF, Verdijk MAJ, Knoers NVAM, et al. Patients with autosomal nephrogenic diabetes insipidus homozygous for mutations in the aquaporin 2 water-channel gene. Am J Hum Genet 1994;55:648–652.

123. Knoers NVAM, van den Ouweland AMW, Verdijk M, et al. Inheritance of mutations in the V₂ receptor gene in thirteen families with nephrogenic diabetes insipidus. Kidney Int 1994;46: 170–176.

124. Bichet DG, Birnbaumer M, Lonergan M, et al. Nature and recurrence of AVPR2 mutations in X-linked nephrogenic diabetes insipidus. Am J Hum Genet 1994;55:278–286.

125. Tsukaguchi H, Matsubara H, Taketani S, et al. Binding-, intracellular transport-, and biosynthesis-defective mutants of vasopressin type 2 receptor in patients with X-linked nephrogenic diabetes insipidus. J Clin Invest 1995;96:2043–2050.

126. Wildin RS, Antush MJ, Bennett RL, et al. Heterogeneous AVPR2 gene mutations in congenital nephrogenic diabetes insipidus. Am J Hum Genet 1994;55:266–277.

127. Oksche A, Dickson J, Schhlein R, et al. Two novel mutations in the vasopressin V₂ receptor gene in patients with congenital nephrogenic diabetes insipidus. Biochem Biophys Res Comm 1994; 205:552–557.

128. Yuasa H, Ito M, Kurokawa M, et al. Novel mutations in the V₂ vasopressin receptor gene in two pedigrees with congenital nephrogenic diabetes insipidus. J Clin Endocrinol Metab 1994;79: 361–365.

129. Jinnouchi H, Araki E, Miyamura N, et al. Analysis of vasopressin receptor type II (V₂R) gene in three Japanese pedigrees with congenital nephrogenic diabetes insipidus: identification of a family with complete deletion of the V₂R gene. Eur J Endocrinol 1996; 143:689–698.

130. Yokoyama K, Yamauchi A, Izumi M, et al. A low-affinity vasopressin V₂-receptor gene in a kindred with X-linked nephrogenic diabetes insipidus. J Am Soc Nephrol 1996;7:410–414.

131. Tajima T, Nakae J, Takekoshi Y, et al. Three novel AVPR2 muta-

tions in three Japanese families with X-linked nephrogenic diabetes insipidus. Pediatr Res 1996;39:522–526.

132. Brenner B, Seligsohn U, Hochberg Z. Normal response of factor VIII and von Willebrand factor to 1-deamino-8D-arginine vasopressin in nephrogenic diabetes insipidus. J Clin Endocrinol Metab 1988;67:191–193.

133. Knoers N, Monnens AH. A variant of nephrogenic diabetes insipidus: V$_2$ receptor abnormality restricted to the kidney. Eur J Pediatr 1991;150:370–373.

134. Langley JM, Balfe JW, Selander T, et al. Autosomal recessive inheritance of vasopressin-resistant diabetes insipidus. Am J Med Genet 1991;38:90–94.

135. Lonergan M, Birnbaumer M, Arthus MF, et al. Non-X-linked nephrogenic diabetes insipidus: phenotype and genotype features. J Am Soc Nephrol 1993;4:264. Abstract.

136. Durr JA, Hoggard JG, Hunt JM, et al. Diabetes insipidus in pregnancy associated with abnormally high circulating vasopressinase activity. N Engl J Med 1987;316:1070–1074.

137. Barron WM, Cohen LH, Ulland LA, et al. Transient vasopressin-resistant diabetes insipidus of pregnancy. N Engl J Med 1984;310:442–444.

138. Hughes JM, Barron WM, Vance ML. Recurrent diabetes insipidus associated with pregnancy: pathophysiology and therapy. Obstet Gynecol 1989;73:462–464.

139. Shah SV, Thakur V. Vasopressinase and diabetes insipidus of pregnancy. Ann Intern Med 1988;109:435–436.

140. Lindheimer MD, Davison JM. Osmoregulation, the secretion of arginine vasopressin and its metabolism during pregnancy. Eur J Endocrinol 1995;132:133–143.

141. Gordge MP, Williams DJ, Huggett NJ, et al. Loss of biological activity of arginine vasopressin during its degradation by vasopressinase from pregnancy serum. Clin Endocrinol 1995;42:51–58.

142. Davison JM, Sheills EA, Barron WM, et al. Changes in the metabolic clearance of vasopressin and in plasma vasopressinase throughout human pregnancy. J Clin Invest 1989;83:1313–1318.

143. Ford SMJ. Transient vasopressin-resistant diabetes insipidus of pregnancy. Obstet Gynecol 1986;68:288–289.

144. Kallen BA, Carlsson SS, Bengtsson BK. Diabetes insipidus and use of desmopressin (Minirin) during pregnancy. Eur J Endocrinol 1995;132:144–146.

145. Fanestil DA. Hyposmolar syndromes. In: Andreoli TE, Grantham JJ, Rector FC, eds. Disturbances in Body Fluid Osmolality. Bethesda: American Physiological Society 1977:267–284.

146. Weitzman RE, Kleeman CR. The clinical physiology of water metabolism, III: the water depletion (hyperosmolar) and water excess (hyposmolar) syndromes. West J Med 1980;132:16–38.

147. Raff H. Glucocorticoid inhibition of neurohypophysial vasopressin secretion. Am J Physiol 1987;252:R635–R644.

148. Linas SL, Berl T, Robertson GL, et al. Role of vasopressin in the impaired water excretion of glucocorticoid deficiency. Kidney Int 1980;18:58–67.

149. Ishikawa S-E, Kim JK, Schrier RW. Effects of arginine vasopressin antidiuretic and vasopressor antagonists in glucocorticoid and mineralocorticoid deficient rats. In: Schrier RW, ed. Vasopressin. New York: Raven Press, 1985:171–180.

150. Kiss JZ, Mezey E, Skirboll L. Corticotropin-releasing factor–immunoreactive neurons of the paraventricular nucleus become vasopressin-positive after adrenalectomy. Proc Natl Acad Sci USA 1984;81:1854–1858.

151. Davis LG, Arentzen R, Reid JM, et al. Glucocorticoid sensitivity of vasopressin mRNA levels in the paraventricular nucleus of the rat. Proc Natl Acad Sci USA 1986;83:1145–1149.

152. Chinitz A, Turner FL. The association of primary hypothyroidism and inappropriate secretion of the antidiuretic hormone. Arch Intern Med 1965;l116:871–874.

153. DeRubertis FR, Mechelis MF, Bloom ME, et al. Impaired water excretion in myxedema. Am J Med 1971;51:41–53.

154. DiScala VA, Kinney MJ. Effects of myxedema on the renal diluting and concentrating mechanism. Am J Med 1971;50:325–335.

155. Anderson RJ, Chung H-M, Kluge R, et al. Hyponatremia: a prospective analysis of its epidemiology and the pathogenetic role of vasopressin. Ann Intern Med 1985;102:164–168.

156. Chung H-M, Kluge R, Schrier RW, et al. Postoperative hyponatremia: a prospective study. Arch Intern Med 1986;146:333–336.

157. Gross PA, Pehrisch H, Rascher W, et al. Pathogenesis of clinical hyponatremia: observations of vasopressin and fluid intake in 100 hyponatremic medical patients. Eur J Clin Invest 1987;17:123–129.

158. Gross P, Pehrisch H, Rascher W, et al. Vasopressin in hyponatremia: what stimuli? J Cardiovasc Pharmacol 1986;8:S92–S95.

159. Zerbe R, Stropes L, Robertson AG. Vasopressin function in the syndrome of inappropriate diuresis. Annu Rev Med 1980;31:315–327.

160. Goldberg M. Abnormalities in the renal excretion of water. Med Clin North Am 1963;47:915–933.

161. Hantman D, Rossier B, Zohlman R, et al. Rapid correction of hyponatremia in the syndrome of inappropriate secretion of antidiuretic hormone. Ann Intern Med 1973;78:870–875.

162. Pollock AS, Arieff AI. Abnormalities of cell volume regulation and the functional consequences. Am J Physiol 1980;239:F195–F205.

163. Sterns RH, Baer J, Ebersol S, et al. Organic osmolytes in acute hyponatremia. Am J Physiol 1993;264:F833–F836.

164. Sterns RH, Thomas DJ, Herndon RM. Brain dehydration and neurologic deterioration after rapid correction of hyponatremia. Kidney Int 1989;35:69–75.

165. Kleinschmidt-DeMasters BK, Norenberg MD. Rapid correction of hyponatremia causes demyelination: relation to central pontine myelinolysis. Science 1981;211:1068–1070.

166. Telfer AB, Miller EM. Central pontine myelinolysis following hyponatremia, demonstrated by computerized tomography. Ann Neurol 1979;6:455–456.

167. Norenberg MD, Leslie KO. Correction of hyponatremia and central pontine myelinolysis. Am J Med 1982;73:882.

168. Sterns RH, Cappucio JD, Silver SM, et al. Neurologic sequelae after treatment of severe hyponatremia: a multicenter perspective. J Am Soc Nephrol 1994;4:1522–1530.

169. Arieff AI. Hyponatremia associated with permanent brain damage. Adv Intern Med 1987;32:325–344.

170. Berl T. Treating hyponatremia: damned if we do and damned if we don't. Kidney Int 1990;37:1006–1018.

171. Ayus JC, Krothapalli RK, Arieff AI. Treatment of symptomatic hyponatremia and its relation to brain damage: a prospective study. N Engl J Med 1987;317:1190–1195.

172. Sterns R. Severe symptomatic hyponatremia: treatment and outcome. Ann Intern Med 1987;107:656–664.

173. Fraser CL, Arieff AI. Fatal central diabetes mellitus and insipidus resulting from untreated hyponatremia: a new syndrome. Ann Intern Med 1990;112:113–119.

174. Arieff AI. Hyponatremia, convulsions, respiratory arrest, and permanent brain damage after elective surgery in healthy women. N Engl J Med 1986;314:1529–1535.

175. Ayus JC, Wheeler JM, Arieff AI. Postoperative hyponatremic encephalopathy in menstruant women. Ann Intern Med 1992;117:891–897.

176. Arieff AI, Ayus JC, Fraser CL. Hyponatraemia and death or permanent brain damage in healthy children. Br Med J 1992;304:1218–1222.

177. Ayus JC, Krothapalli RK, Arieff AI. Sexual difference in survival with severe symptomatic hyponatremia. Kidney Int 1988;33:180.

178. Fraser CL, Kucharczyk J, Arieff AI, et al. Sex differences result in increased morbidity from hyponatremia in female rats. Am J Physiol 1989;256:R880–R885.

179. Arieff AI, Kozniewska E, Roberts TP, et al. Age, gender, and vasopressin affect survival and brain adaptation in rats with metabolic encephalopathy. Am J Physiol 1995;268:R1143–R1152.

180. Kozniewska E, Roberts TP, Vexler ZS, et al. Hormonal dependence of the effects of metabolic encephalopathy on cerebral perfusion and oxygen utilization in the rat. Circ Res 1995;76:551–558.

181. Vexler ZS, Ayus JC, Roberts TP, et al. Hypoxic and ischemic hypoxia exacerbate brain injury associated with metabolic encephalopathy in laboratory animals. J Clin Invest 1994;93:256–264.

182. Sterns RH. The management of hyponatremic emergencies. Crit Care Clin 1991;7:127–142.

183. Sterns RH. Neurological deterioration following treatment for hyponatremia. Am J Kidney Dis 1989;13:434–437.

184. Singer I, Forrest JN. Drug-induced states of nephrogenic diabetes insipidus. Kidney Int 1976;10:82–95.

185. Jackson BA, Edwards RM, Dousa TP. Lithium-induced polyuria: effect of lithium on adenylate cyclase and adenosine 3′,5′-monophosphate phosphodiesterase in medullary ascending limb of Henle's loop and in medullary collecting tubules. Endocrinology 1980;107:1693–1698.

186. Libber S, Harrison H, Spector D. Treatment of nephrogenic diabetes insipidus with prostaglandin synthesis inhibitors. J Pediatr 1986;108:305–311.

187. Kosten TR, Forrest JN. Treatment of severe lithium-induced polyuria with amiloride. Am J Psychiatry 1986;143:1563–1568.

188. Forrest JNJ, Cox M, Hong C, et al. Superiority of demeclocycline over lithium in the treatment of chronic syndrome of inappropriate secretion of antidiuretic hormone. N Engl J Med 1978;298:173–177.

189. Dias N, Hocken AG. Oliguric renal failure complicating lithium carbonate therapy. Nephron 1972;10:246–249.

190. Schrier RW. New treatments for hyponatremia. N Engl J Med 1978;298:214–215.

191. Decaux G, Brimioulle S, Genette F, et al. Treatment of the syndrome of inappropriate secretion of antidiuretic hormone by urea. Am J Med 1980;69:99–106.

192. Tsuboi YS, Ishikawa S, Fujisawa G, et al. Therapeutic efficacy of the non-peptide AVP antagonist OPC-31260 in cirrhotic rats. Kidney Int 1994;46:237–244.

193. Fujisawa G, Ishikawa S, Tsuboi Y, et al. Therapeutic efficacy of non-peptide ADH antagonist OPC-31260 in SIADH rats. Kidney Int 1993;44:19–23.

194. Ohnishi A, Orita Y, Okahara R, et al. Potent aquaretic agent: a novel nonpeptide selective vasopressin 2 antagonist (OPC-31260) in men. J Clin Invest 1993;92:2653–2659.

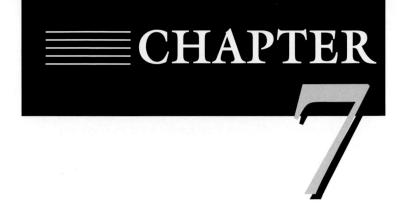

CHAPTER 7

Pathology of Sellar and Parasellar Tumors

Ali F. Krisht and Muhammad Husain

INTRODUCTION

The region of the sella turcica is a crossroad of several anatomic structures, including vascular elements, neural elements, glandular elements, and osseous elements. This fact, and the fact that the sellar and parasellar region is formed as a result of an intricate and complex array of embryological developments, provide the substrate for a large number of pathophysiologic processes that lead to the formation of a variety of pathologic entities. This chapter is a review of the various pathologic and neoplastic entities involving the sellar and parasellar region. The first part describes pathologic entities related to the pituitary gland itself and, specifically, the anterior lobe. The second part of the chapter discusses the nonadenomatous lesions involving the sellar and parasellar regions.

PATHOLOGIC FEATURES OF THE PITUITARY GLAND (ADENOMATOUS LESIONS)
The Normal Pituitary Gland

In humans, the pituitary gland is formed by two anatomic structures—the anterior lobe (adenohypophysis) and the posterior lobe (neurohypophysis)—which have different functions and different embryological backgrounds. The anterior lobe (adenohypophysis) is subdivided into three components—the pars distalis, the pars tuberalis, and the pars intermedia. The pars distalis is the largest in humans and it is the main component of the anterior lobe of the pituitary gland. The pars intermedia is more developed in lower animals, and the pars tuberalis is the upward extension of the anterior lobe along the pituitary stalk. Grossly, the anterior lobe is yellowish-orange, with moderate to high vascularity. It is firm in consistency, especially compared with the posterior lobe (neurohypophysis), which is less vascular and much softer and similar to the brain white matter. A detailed account of the gross anatomy of the pituitary gland and its relationship to the surrounding sellar and parasellar structures is given in Chapter 3.

At the cellular level, the pituitary gland is formed by five cell types (gonadotrophs, lactotrophs, somatotrophs, corticotrophs and thyrotrophs), the distribution and density of which is thought to have a somewhat topographical arrangement within the gland. The function of the different cell types of the pituitary gland is the secretion of the various pituitary hormones. These hormones are secreted as a result of a delicate balance of positive and negative feedbacks arising from the hypothalamus and the target organs. The prolactin (PRL)-producing cells tend to accumulate in the posterior-lateral aspect of the gland, whereas the growth hormone (GH)-producing cells tend to aggregate in the anterior-lateral aspect of the gland. The corticotrophs are thought to be more concentrated in a central wedge and just anterior to the posterior lobe. Thyroid-stimulating hormone (TSH)–producing cells are thought to aggregate in the anterior portion of the central wedge, and the gonadotrophs are thought to have a diffuse distribution throughout the gland with no specific aggregation areas (1) (Fig. 7.1). The microscopic architecture of the pituitary gland is that of glandular acinar architecture, with cells arranged in circular aggregates around a central lumen and surrounded by a fibrovascular stroma (Fig. 7.2). It is the disruption of this architecture that helps differentiate a normal pituitary gland from pituitary adenomas (2).

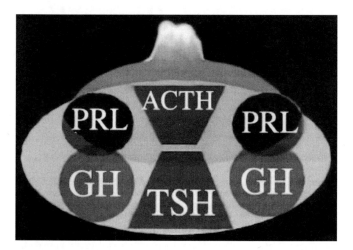

Figure 7.1. Distribution of pituitary cells in the gland. *ACTH,* adrenocorticotropic hormone; *PRL,* prolactin; *GH,* growth hormone; *TSH,* thyroid-stimulating hormone.

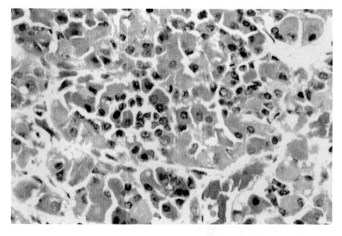

Figure 7.2. Microscopy of a normal pituitary gland.

Pituitary Hyperplasia

Hyperplasia of the pituitary gland can result from a normal physiologic response under certain conditions. Such an example is PRL cell hyperplasia that occurs during pregnancy. This leads to an increase in the size of the pituitary gland. PRL serum levels increase up to 10 times normal toward the end of pregnancy (3). Hyperplasia of the adenohypophysis can also occur as a compensatory mechanism. An example is prolonged hypothyroidism that leads to thyrotroph cell hyperplasia (4). Hyperplasia was thought to be the prelude to the formation of pituitary neoplasia. The recent advances in molecular biologic techniques have shown that most pituitary tumors are monoclonal and not polyclonal. This fact does not support the role of hyperplasia as a cause of neoplasia. However, evidence exists that prolonged hyperplasia may lead to adenoma formation, and this evidence is more experimental than clinical.

Growth Hormone Cell Hyperplasia

Hyperplasia of GH-producing cells was first recognized in patients harboring ectopic growth hormone–releasing hormone (GHRH)–producing tumors (5). The ectopic GHRH-producing cells are usually part of endocrine tumors of the pancreas, gastrointestinal tract, and lungs. In an experimental model of GHRH transgenic mice, mammosomatotroph and GH cell hyperplasia was found by 8 months of age (6). When the same group of mice were further followed they developed mammosomatotroph cell adenomas between 16 and 24 months of age (7).

Prolactin Cell Hyperplasia

PRL cell hyperplasia leading to PRL cell adenoma is well-known to occur in rats as a result of high exposure to an estrogenic environment. Although this is the case experimentally, no evidence exists of PRL cell hyperplasia leading to the formation of PRL cell adenomas in humans. During pregnancy, a high estrogen period, PRL cell hyperplasia occurs as early as the second month of gestation. It can progress to resemble a pituitary adenoma by the time of delivery (8). Despite this hyperplastic state, the incidence of PRL cell adenomas is unchanged in pregnant and postpartum women compared with age-matched nonpregnant women.

Corticotroph Cell Hyperplasia

Corticotroph cell hyperplasia is a more common disease entity than the other pituitary-related hyperplasias. It is usually secondary to corticotropin-releasing hormone (CRH) secretion by ectopic CRH-producing tumors (9). Such tumors include malignancies of the lung, pancreas, and prostate, as well as other tumors such as hypothalamic gangliocytomas. Although corticotroph cell hyperplasia is clinically encountered, very little evidence exists of its role in the pathogenesis of adrenocorticotropic hormone (ACTH)–producing adenomas in most patients with Cushing's disease. Hyperplastic corticotroph cells have ultrastructural features very similar to those of corticotroph adenoma cells with well-developed rough endoplasmic reticulum (RER) and golgi complexes and the occurrence of Crook's hyaline changes. Corticotroph cell hyperplasia can complicate the surgical excision of microadenomas because of the difficulty in distinguishing between these disease entities. This is especially so when dealing with a microadenoma of the pituitary gland (10–12).

Thyrotroph Cell Hyperplasia

The relationship between thyrotroph cell hyperplasia and pituitary adenomas is better established. It is suggested that 50% of thyrotroph cell adenomas are encountered in patients with a history of hypothyroidism (13). Prolonged untreated hypothyroidism results in thyrotroph cell hyperplasia and enlargement of the pituitary gland, with possible formation of pituitary adenomas (14, 15). In experimental studies, rats exposed to a thyroidectomy developed large thyrotroph cells (thyroidectomy cells) in their pituitary gland associated with significant hyperplasia (10, 16).

Gonadotroph Cell Hyperplasia

Gonadotroph cell hyperplasia is rare. It has been seen in patients with primary hypogonadism (17) and has been reported in association with gonadotroph cell adenomas in some patients (18). Although this is the case, it is not established that primary hypogonadism leads to the formation of gonadotroph cell adenomas. In gonadectomized rats, gonadotroph cell hyperplasia is manifested by the "gonadectomy cells," which have a signet ringlike appearance as a result of the remarkable enlargement of the cytoplasm because of marked dilatation of the RER (16).

Although experimental studies of chronic hyperplasia suggest its role in the formation of pituitary adenomas, the clinical manifestation of such an occurrence is extremely rare.

Pituitary Adenomas

The potential pathophysiologic mechanisms that lead to the formation of pituitary adenomas are well covered in Chapter 5. The annual incidence of pituitary adenomas varies from 2 to 7 per 100,000 population (19). They are considered among the most common intracranial tumors and account for up to 10 to 15% of all intracranial neoplasia. They are most commonly seen in patients between the third and sixth decades of life, with a higher tendency to occur in females and an increased risk during the childbearing years.

Most pituitary adenomas are histologically benign and have a low growth rate. Pituitary adenomas are usually surrounded by a pseudocapsule composed of compressed adenohypophyseal tissue. Although most small adenomas remain confined to the sella turcica, it is not unusual to witness cavernous sinus infiltration in small-sized tumors. This fact, and the fact that a good number of patients with such infiltrative tumors can go on for a long period of time with minimal or no growth in the size of the tumor, suggests that infiltration of the adjacent anatomic structures is not always an indicator of the aggressive potential of a tumor. It could mean that the tumor grew into the naturally opened planes such as incompetent sellar borders. However, invasive adenomas have a more aggressive course and tend to have a rapid growth rate and invade the surrounding suprasellar and parasellar anatomic structures. A detailed account of invasive pituitary adenomas is given in Chapter 20.

Classification of Pituitary Adenomas

Several classifications were used to describe different pituitary adenomas. They are classified on the basis of their radiological appearance, the endocrine functions of the different tumors, the size and extent of the tumor, the morphological features of the tumor, and the cytogenesis. The morphological classification is among the oldest and most rapidly changing classifications. Pituitary adenomas were originally grouped based on their staining characteristics into acidophilic, basophilic, and chromophobic adenomas. This classification is very nonspecific and has very limited clinical application. The introduction of immunohistochemical staining techniques and electron microscopy led to a more pertinent classification that is based on the hormonal properties of the tumor cells and their ultrastructural features (19–21). This classification is shown in Table 7.1. Advances in cell culture and molecular biological tech-

Table 7.1. *Pituitary Gland Pathologic Classification*[a]

Pituitary hyperplasia
  GH cell
  PRL cell
  Corticotroph cell
  Thyrotroph cell
  Gonadotroph cell
Pituitary adenomas
  GH cell adenomas
  PRL cell adenomas
  GH cell–PRL cell adenomas
    Mixed-cell adenomas
    Mammosomatotroph cell adenomas
    Acidophil–stem cell adenomas
  ACTH cell adenomas
  Thyrotroph cell adenomas
  Gonadotroph cell adenomas
  Nonfunctioning adenomas
    Silent cell adenomas
    Null-cell and oncocytoma
Pituitary carcinoma
Plurihormonal adenomas

[a] GH indicates growth hormone; PRL, prolactin; ACTH, adrenocorticotropic hormone.

niques further enhanced our understanding of these tumors, especially those that were initially considered nonfunctional tumors and were later found to be gonadotroph adenomas, in their majority.

Growth Hormone Cell Adenomas

On light microscopy, GH cell adenomas are either acidophilic or chromophobic, and they are usually PAS negative (Fig. 7.3) (19, 21, 22). On electron microscopy they are either densely granulated or sparsely granulated (23). Densely granulated GH adenomas account for up to 50% of all GH-producing tumors. The cells have normal ultrastructural features similar to normal GH-producing cells. They correspond to the acidophilic subpopulation of cells as seen by light microscopy. The cytoplasm of such cells is strongly immunopositive to staining with the avidin–biotin–peroxidase complex method (24–26). Electron microscopy shows well-developed cells (Fig. 7.4) with well-visualized RER, prominent golgi complexes, and intracytoplasmic secretory granules, most being between 400 and 500 nm in diameter (19–25). Many densely granulated GH cells show immunopositivity with PRL and one or more of the glycoprotein hormones, especially the α-subunit (26–29).

The sparsely granulated GH cell adenomas correspond to the chromophobic cells as seen by light microscopy. The immunopositivity for GH with the avidin–biotin–peroxidase complex method is not as pronounced in the cytoplasm, and it is usually manifested by streaks or crescentlike densities that are diffusely noticed in the cytoplasm. On electron microscopy, the sparsely granulated GH cell adenomas are different from the normal GH cells in that they have less differentiated features (Fig. 7.5) with conspicuous golgi complexes and irregular nuclei surrounded by widely dispersed RER. When present, the secretory granules are very small. The cytoplasm has a high frequency of fibrous bodies that are made of spherically arranged type II filaments (19–21, 24, 25, 27, 30, 31) (Fig. 7.6). The fibrous bodies correspond with positive immunostaining with cytokeratin.

Up to 10% of GH cell adenomas show both densely granulated and sparsely granulated cells at the same time. No correlation exists between the ultrastructural features of GH cell adenomas and the serum GH levels or the response to GHRH. However, a significant clinical difference exists in the behavior of these tumors. The densely granulated GH cell adenomas have a more benign course. They usually have a slower growth rate and tend to remain confined to the sella and have a higher chance of being cured surgically. Sparsely granulated GH cell adenomas have a more aggressive clinical course and tend to present at a younger age. They are more likely to be invasive macroadenomas and have a lower surgical cure rate (19, 31, 32). Dopaminergic agonists (bromocriptine) and long-acting somatostatin analogs (SMS-202-995) have been used in the treatment of GH-producing tumors. Such therapy re-

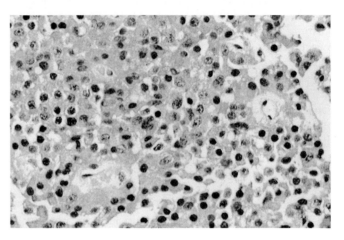

Figure 7.3. Light microscopy of a pituitary adenoma. Notice the uniformity of the cells and the loss of the normal pituitary gland architecture.

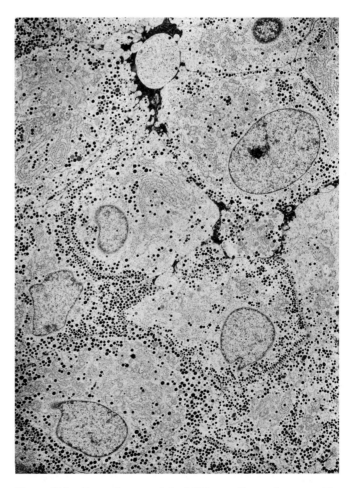

Figure 7.4. Densely granulated GH-secreting adenoma. The intracellular organelles are well differentiated.

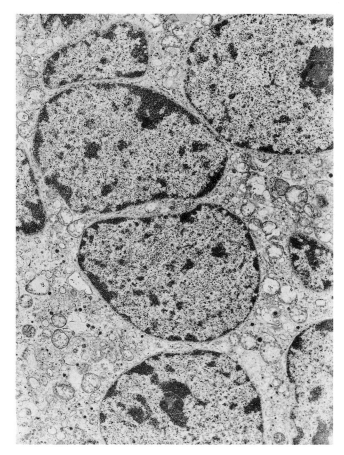

Figure 7.5. Sparsely granulated GH cell adenoma. Notice the poorly developed intracellular organelles and the paucity of the secretory granules in the cytoplasm.

sulted in an increase in the density of intracytoplasmic granules without a significant morphological change in the tumor and its size. This result suggests that the ultrastructural changes are not caused by suppression of hormonal synthesis and are more related to posttranslational inhibition of the secretory process (33–39).

Prolactin Cell Adenomas

PRL cell adenomas can also be either densely granulated or sparsely granulated at the ultrastructural level. The secretory granule density correlates with neither the serum PRL level nor the clinical course in either subtype. Most PRL cell adenomas are sparsely granulated, and the densely granulated type is very rare. Similar to GH cell adenomas, densely granulated PRL cell adenomas have more differentiated features at the ultrastructural level, with well-developed RER, prominent golgi complexes, and numerous cytoplasmic secretory granules measuring between 600 and 700 nm in diameter (19, 40). Some of the granules undergo what is described as misplaced exocytosis (19, 24, 41) (Fig. 7.7).

Histologically, the densely granulated adenomas correlate with the acidophilic cells seen under light microscopy.

The more common sparsely granulated PRL cell adenomas are either chromophobic or slightly acidophilic on light microscopy. The strong positivity of the immunohistochemical staining of the sparsely granulated PRL cell adenomas is predominantly caused by the strong immunostaining of the golgi complexes and not the few intracytoplasmic granules. This is why the immunopositive pattern is that of either ringlike or crescent-shaped streaks (19, 21, 23, 40, 42, 43). At the ultrastructural level, sparsely granulated PRL cell adenomas resemble stimulated nontumorous cells and reveal conspicuous RER that tends to form whorls (Nebenkens). They also have prominent golgi complexes and sparsely distributed cytoplasmic granules measuring 150 to 300 nm in diameter (Fig. 7.8). Misplaced exocytosis is the extrusion of the cytoplasmic secretory granules from the lateral aspect of the cell membrane, and it is characteristic of PRL cell adenomas. Calcification and amyloid deposition can be seen within PRL cell adenomas. On rare occasions, the calcification is extensive, leading to the formation of a hard tumor (pituitary stone) (44).

The histopathologic changes that occur in PRL cell adenomas secondary to bromocriptine treatment are worth mentioning. Bromocriptine therapy results in remarkable morphological changes, including significant reduction in

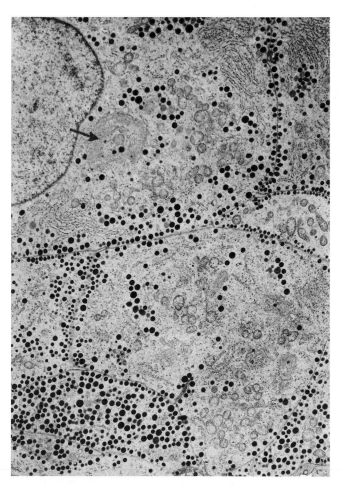

Figure 7.6. An intracytoplasmic fibrous body (*arrow*).

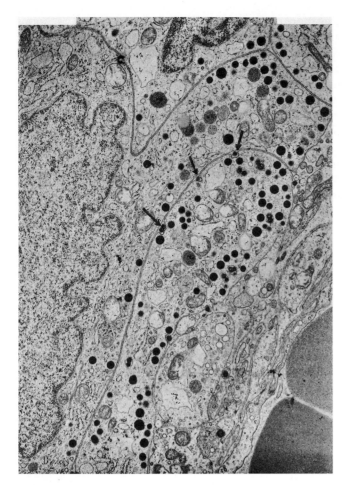

Figure 7.7. Displaced exocytosis in a PRL cell adenoma (*arrows*).

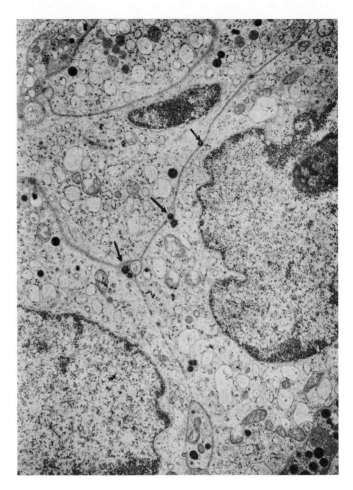

Figure 7.8. Sparsely granulated PRL cell adenoma. Notice the poorly differentiated intracellular structures with misplaced exocytosis (*arrows*).

the cytoplasmic volume and the density of golgi complexes and endoplasmic reticulum. These changes are consistent with its effect at the transcriptional level, leading to shrinkage in the tumor volume secondary to reduction in cell size. These effects are usually reversible once bromocriptine use is stopped. Occasionally, the effects of bromocriptine therapy persist in focal areas (40, 45–52). Long-term treatment with bromocriptine may result in significant fibrosis (Fig. 7.9) that may change the consistency of the tumor, which can effect its surgical removal (53–56).

Growth Hormone-Prolactin Cell Adenomas

In 30% of GH cell adenomas, a high PRL level is detected. This comprises most of what is described as plurihormonal adenomas (57, 58). This percentage is increased to 50% when immunohistochemical staining techniques are used. This means that up to 50% of GH cell adenomas have positive immunostaining with PRL (59). Using molecular biological techniques and messenger RNA analysis, a higher positivity of PRL is encountered in these tumors compared with immunohistochemical techniques (60, 61). These tumors were subdivided into three morphologically

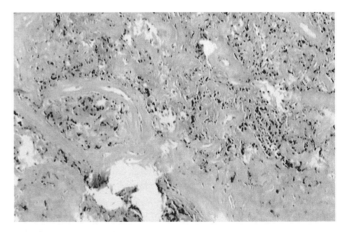

Figure 7.9. Light microscopy of prolactinoma after treatment with bromocriptine. Notice the clumping of the cells over a fibrous background. Compare with Figure 7.3.

distinct groups: (*a*) mixed GH cell–PRL cell adenoma, (*b*) mammosomatotroph cell adenoma, and (*c*) acidophil–stem cell adenomas.

Mixed Growth Hormone-Prolactin Cell Adenoma

Mixed GH-PRL cell adenomas usually present with acromegaly and elevated GH levels. They are associated with varying levels of hyperprolactinemia. The tumor is made up of two populations of cells—GH cells and PRL cells. The immunohistochemical study results are usually positive for both GH and PRL in different cells. At the ultrastructural level, either cell population can be densely or sparsely granulated, with the most common combination being densely granulated GH cells and sparsely granulated PRL cells (19, 21, 62–65).

Mammosomatotroph Cell Adenomas

Unlike the mixed-cell adenomas, mammosomatotroph cell adenomas are monomorphous. The tumor cells are usually mature mammosomatotroph cells that are well differentiated and secrete both GH and PRL from the same cell. These tumors are usually very acidophilic, and in a good number of patients a long history of gigantism or acromegaly is noted, with or without hyperprolactinemia. Unlike stem cell adenomas, which have a rapid growth rate, mammosomatotroph cell adenomas are slow growing and have a benign course. The ultrastructural features are similar to those of the well-differentiated, densely granulated GH adenoma cells. The cytoplasmic secretory granules measure between 200 and 2000 nm in diameter, and they are differentiated from GH cell adenomas by the presence of exocytosis and extracellular secretory particles (19, 21, 22, 66–69).

Acidophil-Stem Cell Adenomas

These tumors are similar to the mammosomatotroph cell adenoma in being monomorphous tumors and bihormonal. They are thought to be derived from less differentiated progenitor cells that have the capability to differentiate into GH-producing cells, PRL-producing cells, and/or cells that produce both GH and PRL. They clinically present with symptoms related to hyperprolactinemia, although their PRL serum level is not as high compared with that of PRL cell adenomas of the same size. These tumors have a more aggressive clinical course and tend to invade the surrounding structures. On light microscopy they are less acidophilic and more chromophobic than the mammosomatotroph cell adenomas. This is thought to be caused by intracytoplasmic oncocytic changes that are commonly seen in these tumors. The immunohistochemical study results are positive for both GH and PRL in the same cells. Occasionally, GH immunoreactivity is absent. At the ultrastructural level, electron microscopic features include rather elongated cells, large cytoplasm, and less differentiated features, including scattered RER and poorly devel-

oped golgi complexes. The secretory granules are small, 100 to 300 nm in diameter, and occasional. Misplaced exocytosis is occasionally found. They also contain fibrous bodies, centrioles, and cilia. Oncocytic changes with enlargement of cytoplasmic mitochondria are characteristic of these tumors and correlate with the cytoplasmic vacuolization seen on light microscopy (19, 21, 70, 71).

Adrenocorticotropic Hormone Cell Adenomas

Corticotroph cell adenomas are the classic basophilic adenomas as seen by light microscopy. The immunohistochemical staining of these tumors is usually positive for ACTH and other peptide derivatives from the proopiomelanocortin hormone, such as beta-lipotropin, endorphins, and others. The ultrastructural features on electron microscopy show well-differentiated, densely granulated cells with abundant cytoplasmic RER and prominent golgi complexes. The cytoplasmic secretory granules are seen more on the periphery of the cytoplasm and measure 200 to 450 nm in diameter. Intracytoplasmic type I filaments can be very abundant and tend to displace other intracytoplasmic organelles to the periphery (Fig. 7.10). The deposits of the type I filaments are equivalent to the Crooke's hyalinization seen at the light microscopy level in which a clear ringlike halo is seen in the perinuclear area (21, 22, 72–78).

In Nelson's syndrome, the loss of the negative corticosteroid feedback leads to the rapid proliferation of the adenoma, which continues to secrete ACTH and other related peptides, including beta-lipotropin or beta-melanocyte–stimulating hormone, leading to hyperpigmentation. The light microscopic and electron microscopic features of

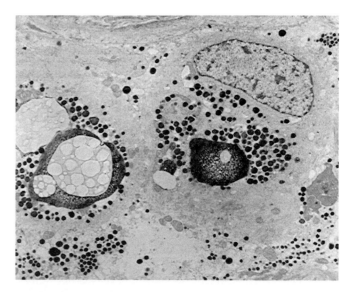

Figure 7.10.   Electron microscopy of Crooke's cell. Notice the type I microfilaments filling the cytoplasm. (These changes were seen in nontumorous portions of a pituitary gland harboring corticotroph cell adenoma.) (Modified from Kovacs K, Horvath E. Tumors of the Pituitary Gland. Washington, DC: Armed Forces Institute of Pathology, 1986.)

the tumor cells in Nelson's syndrome are similar to cortico-troph cell adenomas. The main difference is in the absence of type I filaments and the lack of the Crooke's hyaliniza-tion equivalent. This led to the suggestion that the presence of Crooke's hyalinization correlates with the level of the negative feedback mechanism. In the absence of the corti-costeroid negative feedback, Crooke's hyalinization be-comes absent (13, 19, 21, 73, 79).

Thyrotroph Cell Adenomas

Thyrotroph cell adenomas are usually encountered in patients with a long history of hypothyroidism. They are rare, and that is the reason they are not well defined com-pared with other pituitary adenomas. At the light micro-scopic level, thyrotroph cell adenomas are usually well-vas-cularized, chromophobic tumors. Immunohistochemical staining usually shows weak positivity to TSH and the α-subunit. The ultrastructural features are important to verify to make a better diagnosis of these tumors. They usually show well-differentiated cells similar to thyrotroph cells, with elongated cytoplasmic processes, irregular nuclei, and abundant RER with prominent golgi complexes. The se-cretory granules are 150 to 250 nm in diameter. Secretory granules tend to accumulate in the cytoplasmic processes. Sometimes the cells have poorly differentiated features sim-ilar to those of null-cell adenomas (13, 19, 21, 22, 31, 80–83).

Gonadotroph Cell Adenomas

Most gonadotroph cell adenomas are chromophobic at the light microscopy level and may show slight positivity with PAS staining. The cells are rather elongated and part of a sinusoidal pattern, with the tendency to form pseudo-rosettes around blood vessels. The sinusoidal spaces con-tain a homogenous material that is PAS positive, especially in tumors that tend to have follicular formations (13, 19, 21, 22, 84–89). In general, gonadotroph cell adenomas do not show strong positivity on immunohistochemical studies. They usually show diffuse, rather weak, positive staining to the α-subunit, follicle-stimulating hormone, and luteinizing hormone, as well as TSH. The immunopos-itivity could be caused by a combination of one or more of these hormones. Some gonadotroph cell adenomas are negative on immunohistochemical studies, and these tu-mors were recently recognized as gonadotrophs using mes-senger RNA analysis in cell culture studies (refer to Chapter 5). However, the poor staining with immunohistochemical studies has been the subject of several speculations. The most accepted explanation is the fact that the gonadotroph tumor cells are inefficient secretors, unlike other tumor cells, such as PRL cell adenoma cells. At the ultrastructural level, gonadotroph cell adenomas show different features in men and women. In women, the cells are more differen-tiated, and the cytoplasmic organelles are similar to the nontumorous gonadotroph cells. The golgi complexes

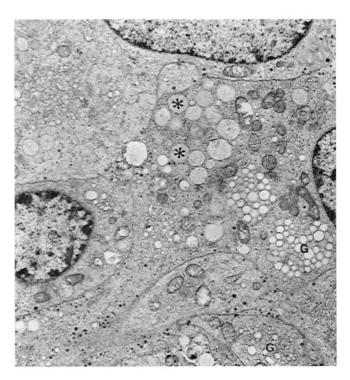

Figure 7.11. Electron microscopy of gonadotroph cell ade-noma, "female type." Notice the large and well-differentiated golgi complexes (*G*) with the distinctive honeycomb appear-ance. (Modified from Kovacs K, Horvath E. Tumors of the Pituitary Gland. Washington, DC: Armed Forces Institute of Pathology, 1986.)

continue to have the remarkably dilated honeycomb ap-pearance, and the RER are slightly dilated with occasional cytoplasmic secretory granules that are small and usually located in the cell processes (50–150 nm in diameter) (Fig. 7.11). In men, the cells are less differentiated and the cyto-plasm contains poorly developed golgi complexes and sparse RER and secretory granules. Some of the poorly differentiated cells are reminiscent of the null-cell adeno-mas (13, 19, 21, 22, 84–89).

Nonfunctioning Adenomas

Until recently the functional adenomas were thought to arise from two main cell groups—null-cell adenomas and oncocytomas. More recent studies have shown that non-functional adenomas are made up of a morphologically het-erogenous group of tumors based on immunohistochemi-cal and ultrastructural characteristics (19, 21, 22). To better understand the clinically nonfunctioning group of adenomas, they are classified into two main subgroups. One group comprises the clinically silent adenomas. The immunohistochemical and ultrastructural features in this group of tumors are equivalent to those of one of the bio-chemically active adenomas, such as corticotroph, thyro-troph, somatotroph, and gonadotroph cell adenomas. The other subgroup comprises tumors that are clinically non-functioning and have no ultrastructural or immunohistochemical resemblance to any of the adenohypophyseal cells. This subgroup includes null-cell adenomas and oncocytomas.

Silent Cell Adenomas

The silent cell adenomas are clinically nonfunctioning tumors. They usually present with headaches, visual disturbances, and other symptoms related to the tumor mass effect. Patients with silent somatotroph cell adenomas may have normal or slightly elevated serum GH levels and no clinical evidence of acromegaly. Their diagnosis is established by the combination of the results of the immunohistochemical studies and electron microscopic ultrastructural features. They resemble the sparsely granulated GH adenomas. Silent corticotroph cell adenomas usually present with normal ACTH and cortisol serum levels. These tumors are further subdivided into subtype-I silent corticotroph cell adenomas, which are usually basophilic and strongly immunoreactive to ACTH and related peptides, and subtype-II silent corticotroph cell adenomas, which are usually chromophobic or slightly basophilic. The ultrastructural characteristics of subtype-I cells are similar to those of well-differentiated corticotroph cell adenomas, whereas subtype-II silent cell adenomas are not as similar and lack the presence of the type I filaments.

Silent gonadotroph cell adenomas have ultrastructural features similar to those of gonadotroph cell adenomas. They usually have some immunoreactivity with follicle-stimulating hormone, luteinizing hormone, and/or the α-subunit (19, 21, 90–96).

The absence of clinical symptoms in patients with silent cell adenomas is not well answered. In silent somatotroph cell adenomas, it was suggested that the cause of the clinical silence of these tumors is the lack of bioactivity in the secreted GH or insulinlike growth factor molecules (93). In silent corticotroph cell adenomas, a posttranslational step was suggested as a cause of the abnormality that leads to the production of hormones lacking the ACTH bioactivity but continues to preserve their immunopositivity (13). In silent gonadotroph cell adenomas, the very small amount of hormone secreted by these tumors was suggested as the possible cause of their clinical silence (96).

Null-Cell Adenomas and Oncocytomas

Null-Cell Adenomas

On light microscopy, null-cell adenomas are usually chromophobic and have a sinusoidal pattern with the tendency to form pseudorosettes. At the ultrastructural level the null-cells show poorly developed cytoplasm with scattered RER and poorly or moderately developed golgi complexes. Small secretory granules (100–250 nm in diameter) are occasionally seen scattered in the cytoplasm and frequently line up along the cell membrane (19, 21, 97, 98).

Results of recent in vitro studies, including RNA analysis and cell culture techniques, revealed that null-cell adeno-

mas and oncocytomas have the potential to secrete some of the adenohypophyseal hormones and most commonly gonadotropin hormones. Results of these studies suggest that null-cell adenomas and gonadotroph adenomas may share a cell origin and could both be derived from multipotential progenitor cells (96, 98).

Oncocytomas

Oncocytic cells differ from null cells in abundance of cytoplasmic mitochondria. It has even been suggested that oncocytomas are the result of oncocytic transformations of null-cell adenomas (13, 19, 21). On light microscopy the tumor is rather acidophilic, and its immunohistochemical staining characteristics are similar to those of null-cell adenomas. Electron microscopy is essential in diagnosing this subtype of pituitary tumor, and it usually reveals the characteristic abundance of cytoplasmic mitochondria (Fig. 7.12).

Pituitary Carcinoma

Pituitary carcinoma is a diagnosis that is best made based on both pathologic and clinical criteria because although

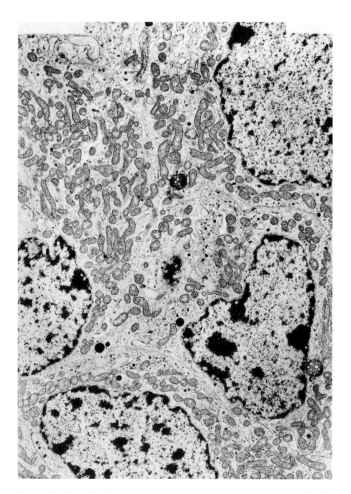

Figure 7.12. Electron microscopy of an oncocytoma. Notice the abundance of mitochondria in the cytoplasm.

histologic features may show cellular pleomorphism, mitotic figures, and nuclear atypia, which are suggestive of a high proliferating potential, the clinical course may still be more benign (19, 21, 99). Conversely, pituitary adenomas with benign histologic features may show potential of invasiveness and have a more aggressive clinical course. For this reason, the diagnosis of pituitary carcinoma has been reserved to tumors that show cerebrospinal and/or extracranial metastasis. This diagnosis has previously been reported with nonfunctioning adenomas (100), PRL-producing tumors (101–103), GH-producing tumors (104), and ACTH-producing tumors (105–107). Immunohistochemical staining in pituitary carcinoma is important to differentiate these tumors from other metastatic carcinomas to the pituitary gland. Invasive pituitary adenomas are not considered pituitary carcinomas. A detailed account of giant and invasive pituitary adenomas is given in Chapter 20.

Plurihormonal Adenomas

The term plurihormonal refers to tumors that are capable of producing more than one hormone. The recent introduction of molecular biological techniques suggests that the number of adenomas that express more than one messenger RNA for the different pituitary hormones is much higher than the number of adenomas that stain with more than one hormone on immunohistochemical studies (60, 108–110).

These findings suggest several explanations that are probably related to the pathophysiologic process related to adenoma formation. Tumors expressing more than one hormone may have arisen from multipotential progenitor cells that could differentiate into different cells capable of expressing different hormones. The expression of these hormones may be changed or adjusted by the local microenvironment influenced by the different hypothalamic and target organ factors that may influence the phenotypic expression of these tumors. Also, dedifferentiation or mutational changes may further contribute to this process. It is expected that the introduction of more sensitive techniques in the diagnostic process of pituitary adenomas is going to yield an increase in the diagnosis of plurihormonal adenomas. It is not unlikely that in the few coming years the whole classification scheme of pituitary adenomas may drastically change.

At this stage, the plurihormonal adenomas are classified into two groups—monomorphous adenomas and polymorphous adenomas. Monomorphous adenomas are best represented by mammosomatotroph adenomas and acidophilic–stem cell adenomas in which the same cell expresses more than one hormone. Polymorphous plurihormonal adenomas are best represented by mixed GH cell–PRL cell adenomas in which two populations of cells each expressing a different hormone are found in the same tumor. The most common bihormonal production is that of GH and PRL. The α-subunit is frequently expressed in plurihormo-

nal adenomas. They are more commonly seen with GH cell adenomas with its immunopositivity found in the same cells expressing the GH (28, 108, 111). Occasionally, GH cell adenomas, especially the densely granulated type, show immunopositivity with TSH (108, 112, 113). TSH positivity has also been encountered in combination with gonadotroph adenomas (114, 115).

An interesting type of plurihormonal tumor is the rare silent subtype-III adenoma, a tumor that was previously classified under the silent corticotroph cell adenoma subtypes. This rare adenoma has monomorphous cells with well-differentiated ultrastructural features. Although these tumors have immunopositivity to the ACTH- and proopiomelanocortin-derived peptides, it is clinically silent in this respect. Some of these patients present clinically with acromegaly or hyperprolactinemia. The most common immunoreactivity is that of GH and ACTH (114, 115).

PITUITARY PATHOLOGIC FEATURES OF THE SELLAR AND PARASELLAR REGIONS (NONADENOMATOUS LESIONS)

Both neoplastic and nonneoplastic mass lesions involve the sellar and parasellar regions. Tumors of these regions include those that arise specifically from sellar and suprasellar structures as well as those that are typically found in other sites of the central nervous system (CNS) and happen to be in proximity with the sellar region. Besides the neoplastic lesions, various vascular, inflammatory, and hamartomatous malformations are also found in this region. These malformations either arise primarily from structures present in the region or encroach on the sellar/parasellar region from adjacent structures. Craniopharyngioma and Rathke's cleft cyst are the two neoplastic lesions that are unique to this region, and they will be described in detail. For the other lesions, only factors relevant to parasellar involvement are discussed.

CRANIOPHARYNGIOMAS

Craniopharyngiomas are the second most frequently occurring tumors in the region of the sella and constitute 2 to 3% of intracranial neoplasms. Occasionally they arise outside the sellar region. Craniopharyngiomas are common in children, and their incidence has two peaks—one in the middle of the second decade of life and the other between the sixth and seventh decades of life. They comprise approximately 9% of childhood intracranial tumors.

Origin

The histogenesis of craniopharyngiomas is not well understood and remains controversial. They are thought to arise from the remnants of Rathke's pouch, the embryonic superior evagination from the roof of the primitive oral cavity or stomodeum. The superior end of this pouch gives origin to the cells of the anterior pituitary. The occurrence of squamous epithelial clumps along the route of migration of Rathke's pouch was the basis of the proposal by Erdheim that craniopharyngiomas arise from these epithelial nests (116). However, these cell nests are not commonly found in childhood but are more common in adults and increase with age. These epithelial cells arise as a result of metaplasia of adenohypophyseal cells (117). The marked histologic similarity of craniopharyngiomas with odontogenic tumors of the jaw, such as ameloblastoma (adamantinoma) and calcifying odontogenic cyst, is consistent with their common embryogenesis and raises the question of whether craniopharyngiomas originate from misplaced odontogenic epithelial cells (118).

Clinical Features

Most craniopharyngiomas, 80 to 90%, are suprasellar in location, and almost half of these also have an intrasellar component. About 20% of craniopharyngiomas are only intrasellar. The suprasellar tumors produce symptoms by virtue of their compressive effects on the adjacent structures, such as the optic apparatus, the third ventricle, the hypothalamus, the infundibulum, and the pituitary gland. Headache and visual disturbances are the most common manifestations. Other signs and symptoms include hydrocephalus, mental changes, nausea, vomiting, papilledema, somnolence, autonomic disturbances, abnormal reflexes, anosmia, choreiform movements, and decerebrate rigidity (119). Craniopharyngiomas have rarely been described in ectopic locations like the optic chiasm, pharynx, cerebellopontine angle, and pineal region (120–125). Neonatal craniopharyngiomas have also been reported (126). About 4% of suprasellar craniopharyngiomas extend to the posterior fossa (127).

Visual disturbances are more common in adults than in children. Diabetes insipidus (DI), short stature, and obesity secondary to hyperphagia are common manifestations in children. In adults, headache and visual disturbances are common, and one-third of patients have associated endocrine dysfunction, usually related to hypogonadism or hyperprolactinemia (128). Aseptic meningitis from spontaneous rupture of craniopharyngioma cyst and purulent meningitis from bacterial abscess formation in craniopharyngioma have been described (129, 130). Occasionally, craniopharyngiomas extend from the suprasellar region to the region of the foramen magnum (131).

Histopathologic Features

In addition to the classic adamantinomatous craniopharyngiomas, a distinct variety called papillary craniopharyngiomas have recently been described. The clinical, radiological, and pathological features of the two variants are diverse enough to merit considering them as distinct varieties.

Adamantinomatous Craniopharyngiomas

Ninety percent of all craniopharyngiomas are of the classic adamantinomatous variant. Most of these tumors are cystic. About 35% have both solid and cystic components. Most childhood craniopharyngiomas are of this variety. Their average size is 3 to 4 cm, but they may be large enough to cover a substantial part of the base of the brain. Generally well circumscribed but not capsulated, they insinuate themselves into the adjacent structures and sometimes firmly adhere to them, which makes their complete surgical resection a challenge. The solid tumors have a pale granular appearance with a rubbery texture. The cysts vary in size from microscopic to the entire tumor being a large cyst. Occasionally, multiple small cysts give the tumor a spongy appearance. The cyst content is a mixture of variably calcified desquamated debris and cholesterol crystals, giving its fluid content a yellow or dark brown appearance that has been likened to machine oil or motor oil. The cyst wall varies in thickness, and its cut surface is reddish gray mixed with irregular, hard, white areas of calcification. The calcification may vary from microscopic foci to large, grossly visible concretions with bonelike formations. Calcification in craniopharyngiomas should not be considered an indication of inactivity of the tumor; instead, reappearance of calcium after tumor removal is a reliable sign of recurrence (132).

A typical adamantinomatous craniopharyngioma is very characteristic in histologic appearance and, when fully expressed, can be recognized at a glance at low power. However, diagnostic difficulty arises when the tumor is made up of a large single cyst. In its typical appearance, the tumor shows multinodular cloverleaf lobules of solid and cystic squamous epithelium joined by trabeculae of epithelium in a background of connective tissue matrix (Fig. 7.13).

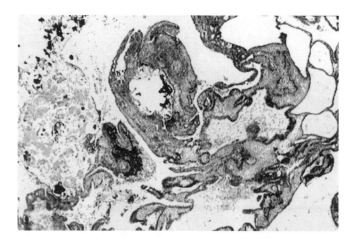

Figure 7.13. Craniopharyngioma. Adamantinomatous pattern. Loosely arranged stellate cells marginated by palisading columnar cells. Note cysts and soft keratin. Calcification and ossification may occur in the soft keratin.

The cells at the periphery of the lobules and trabeculae are columnar, with darker cytoplasm and nuclei arranged in a palisading pattern. The centrally located squamous cells have lighter cytoplasm and a variable degree of loose reticulated texture, giving a stellate myxoid appearance. Complete degeneration of these cells produces cystic spaces that are also marginated by palisaded cells. In other areas, more typical squamous epithelial cells with intercellular bridges and keratinization are seen. More typical and of diagnostic significance is the presence of "wet keratin." These are nodules of squamous cells with an eosinophilic, pale necrotic appearance containing ghost nuclei. Calcium deposition is frequent in wet keratin. In addition to the epithelial components, chronic inflammation with foci of lymphocytic infiltration, a variable degree of fibrosis, and cholesterol clefts with or without foreign body giant cell reaction are found (Fig. 7.14). Craniopharyngiomas are locally invasive, with infiltrating tumor columns seen extending to the brain. This elicits an extensive glial reaction, with formation of Rosenthal fibers in the immediate vicinity of the tumor, which, to the unwary, may be mistaken for pilocytic astrocytoma. Predominantly cystic craniopharyngiomas may sometimes mimic epidermoid cysts, or papillary craniopharyngioma when the cystic spaces are not apparent.

Because of the distinctive histologic appearance of craniopharyngioma, ultrastructural studies and immunohistochemical stains are seldom necessary. Ultrastructurally, the epithelial cells show bundles of tonofilaments and well-formed desmosomes. The epithelium is covered by a basal lamina at its interface with the stroma (133). Blood vessels with fenestrated endothelial cells are seen in the stroma. Immunohistochemically, the epithelial cells are keratin positive, as expected. The significance of recently demonstrated estrogen receptors in craniopharyngiomas is uncertain (134). Progesterone receptor gene expression has also been demonstrated (135). Rapid recurrence of a craniopharyngioma during pregnancy has been reported (136).

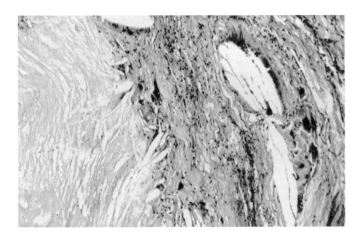

Figure 7.14. Craniopharyngioma. Cholesterol crystals with foreign body giant cell reaction.

Papillary Craniopharyngiomas

Papillary craniopharyngiomas comprise about 10% of all craniopharyngiomas. In contrast to adamantinomatous craniopharyngiomas, papillary craniopharyngiomas occur almost exclusively in adults. They are suprasellar and often arise from the third ventricle (137, 138). They are mostly solid and encapsulated. The discrete masses have a smooth surface and can readily be separated from the surrounding brain tissue. Papillary craniopharyngiomas also lack the calcification and cholesterol-rich (machine oil) content seen in adamantinomatous craniopharyngiomas. When cysts are present, their content is clear.

Histologically, papillary craniopharyngiomas are composed of epithelial cells that have a less complex pattern than the adamantinomatous variant. Solid sheets of well-differentiated epithelial cells are intercepted by cores of fibrovascular stroma. They lack the peripheral columnar palisading. Cholesterol clefts, keratin pearls, wet keratin, calcification, and the inflammatory response characteristic of adamantinomatous craniopharyngiomas are absent here. Presence of focal goblet and ciliated cells indicate histogenetic relationship to Rathke's cleft cyst (139, 140). The prognosis for patients with papillary craniopharyngiomas is better than for those with adamantinomatous craniopharyngiomas (137, 141, 142).

RATHKE'S CLEFT CYST

Microscopic asymptomatic epithelial cysts can be seen in most pituitary glands at the interface between anterior and posterior lobes. These cysts are considered remnants of Rathke's pouch, which in the embryo arises from the epithelial lining of the cranial end of the craniopharyngeal duct, which gives rise to the anterior pituitary. Macroscopic asymptomatic enlargement of these Rathke's cleft cysts can be seen in 20% of pituitaries. Symptomatic enlargement of these cysts can occur presumably by progressive accumulation of cyst contents.

Symptomatic Rathke's cleft cysts are usually 1 cm or more in diameter and mostly affect adults. The cysts are mostly intrasellar, with possible suprasellar components. Occasionally they are entirely suprasellar (143, 144). Headache, disturbances of vision, and endocrine dysfunctions (hypopituitarism, hyperprolactinemia, and, rarely, DI) are the common clinical presentations.

Grossly, Rathke's cleft cysts are thin-walled, uniloculate, fluid-filled structures. The cyst contents vary from watery to mucoid. Microscopically, the cysts are lined by cuboidal or columnar epithelium with cilia and mucin-producing goblet cells (Fig. 7.15). Adenohypophyseal cells can also be found in small numbers. Calcification is rare. Squamous metaplasia of the lining cells may occur and may result in loss of superficial columnar cells and may mimic papillary craniopharyngioma. Rathke's cleft cyst may rarely occur in association with a pituitary adenoma (145, 146). Some of these cases demonstrate a transition between the cells of

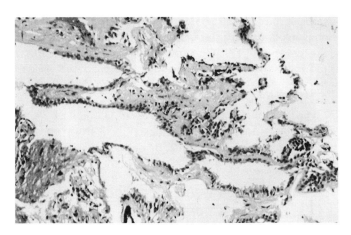

Figure 7.15. Light microscopic features of the wall of a Rathke's cleft cyst.

the cyst and those of the adenoma and have been termed "transitional cell tumor of the pituitary"; this entity remains controversial (146, 147). Recurrence of Rathke's cleft cysts after surgical treatment is very rare.

MENINGIOMAS

Approximately 10% of intracranial meningiomas involve the sellar and parasellar structures. The dural origin of these meningiomas include the tuberculum sellae, planum sphenoidale, diaphragma sellae, olfactory groove, medial sphenoid wing, optic nerve sheath, or anterior fossa floor above the orbital roof (128). Rarely, the tumor may be entirely intrasellar (148–150). Intrasellar meningiomas closely mimic pituitary adenomas. Most meningiomas involving the sellar region are large, well-circumscribed lesions that compress the basal brain structures. The cavernous sinus may be involved. Symptoms are usually caused by the tumor mass effect, with visual disturbances being the most common. DI, or hypopituitarism, is common, with meningiomas arising from the inferior leaf of the diaphragma sellae (151). Despite compression of the pituitary stalk, pituitary insufficiency is not common with meningiomas.

The pathologic features of meningiomas involving the sellar region are similar to those of meningiomas arising from other intracranial sites. All variants of meningiomas may be represented.

Dural hemangiopericytomas, previously classified as a variant of meningioma but now considered a nonmeningoepithelial neoplasm, have rarely been reported in the sellar region (152–154). Their distinction from meningiomas is important being a malignant neoplasm with the capacity to metastasize.

GERM CELL TUMORS

Besides migration to the developing gonads, the primordial germ cells also disseminate in extragonadal sites, fre-

quently in the mediastinum and midline central neuraxis. The pineal and hypothalamic regions are the most frequent sites in the CNS. Other rare intracranial sites reported in the literature include the fourth ventricle, intrasellar, occipital, basal ganglia, thalamus, and cauda equina (155). Synchronous or metachronous involvement of the pineal and suprasellar regions have also been reported (156). A double suprasellar and cerebellar localization of a germinoma have been reported in a 9-year-old female (157). The incidence of germ cell tumors is approximately 0.3 to 5% of all intracranial tumors. The pineal region is affected more frequently than the suprasellar region. Of the five major types of germ cell tumors—germinoma, teratoma, embryonal carcinoma, endodermal sinus tumor (yolk sac tumor), and choriocarcinoma—germinomas are most frequently encountered.

Suprasellar germinomas are infiltrative lesions and involve a variety of structures, including the floor of the third ventricle, hypothalamus, pituitary stalk, neurohypophysis, and optic nerve, chiasm, and tracts. The exact anatomic site of origin may be difficult to establish. Clinically, visual disturbance, DI, and hypopituitarism occur to a varying degree. In contrast to pineal germ cell tumors, which have a male predominance, a female predominance is seen in suprasellar germ cell tumors.

Except for mature teratomas, which are noninfiltrative and discrete lesions, all other germ cell tumors infiltrate the surrounding neural structures and tend to obstruct cerebrospinal fluid pathways, leading to hydrocephalus. Germinomas are soft and have a gray-tan, homogeneous appearance that mimics the appearance of lymphoma. They may have focal small areas of hemorrhage. However, the presence of significant hemorrhage and necrosis is generally indicative of more high-grade malignancy, such as embryonal carcinoma, endodermal sinus, and choriocarcinoma. Teratomas frequently have solid and cystic components; the mature variant may be recognized by its content of teeth, hair, bone, cartilage, etc. The different types of germ cell tumors express various biochemical markers, such as human chorionic gonadotropin, placental alkaline phosphatase, and α-fetoprotein, which can be demonstrated in blood or cerebrospinal fluid immunohistochemically in the tumors.

The reader is referred to other texts for detailed microscopic and immunohistochemical appearances of germ cell tumors of the neuraxis (158, 159).

GLIOMAS

Glial tumors should be considered in the differential diagnosis of suprasellar masses, particularly in the pediatric population in which pilocytic astrocytomas can arise from the hypothalamus, the optic nerves and chiasm, and the third ventricle. Other tumors of ventricular origin, such as ependymomas and choroid plexus papillomas, may descend to the suprasellar region. Clinically, parasellar gliomas generally manifest by endocrine dysfunction, hydrocephalus, or visual symptoms. Fibrillary astrocytomas arising from cerebral hemispheres and the basal ganglia region may secondarily involve hypothalamic structures and rarely invade the sella or infiltrate the pituitary gland.

Rare gliomas, termed infundibulomas and pituicytomas, have been described to arise from the infundibulum and the posterior pituitary, respectively (160–163). Histologically, these are pilocytic astrocytomas. The small numbers of these reported cases preclude any generalization about their clinicopathologic entity.

CHORDOMAS

Chordomas are tumors of the bone arising from remnants of the notochord. Any part of the axial skeleton may be the site of origin, but 50% arise from the sacrum and 15% arise from the rest of the spinal column. Intracranial chordomas arise almost exclusively from the clivus and comprise 15% of chordomas. Involvement of sellar and suprasellar structures are secondary to the extension of chordomas arising from the upper clivus and dorsum sellae. Chordomas arising exclusively in the intrasellar region have rarely been described (164).

HAMARTOMAS AND GANGLIOGLIOMAS

Tumors composed of neurons can form masses in the sellar region. They are considered hamartomatous lesions in view of their benign course and slow growth rate. Their histologic appearance resembles mature hypothalamic tissue. A confusing array of nomenclatures has been applied to them, such as ganglioglioma, gangliocytoma, neuronal hamartoma, gangliocytoma-pituitary adenoma, etc. Based on their locations either in the hypothalamus or the sella, two lesions are recognized, namely, hypothalamic neuronal hamartoma and adenohypophyseal-neuronal choristoma or intrasellar gangliocytoma.

Hypothalamic Neuronal Hamartomas

Minute foci of clinically insignificant ectopic hypothalamic tissue are occasionally found at autopsies at the base of the brain attached to the ventral hypothalamus, on the adjacent pia mater, or on the surface of posterior cerebral arteries (165). On rare occasions, such nodules may undergo symptomatic enlargement and compress the adjacent structures. They may retain their attachment to the hypothalamus, tuber cinereum, or mamillary bodies or may form a solitary mass. Well-known clinical manifestations are precocious puberty in a young male (166) and inappropriate and uncontrollable episodes of laughing (gelastic epilepsy). Childhood and neonatal cases have been described (167, 168). The tumor is firm and has a homogene-

ous cut surface. Microscopically, the tumor is composed of neurons of varying sizes, shapes, and numbers arranged in clusters among a background of axons and glial stroma. Immunopositivity has been variously demonstrated for gonadotropin-releasing hormone, GHRH, and CRH in these neurons (169).

Hypothalamic hamartomas also occur, along with many extracranial malformations, as Pallister-Hall syndrome, inherited as an autosomal-dominant pattern (170, 171).

Adenohypophyseal Gangliocytomas (Choristomas)

Also known as adenohypophyseal neuronal choristomas, adenohypophyseal gangliocytomas are histologically similar to hypothalamic neuronal hamartomas but are not attached to the hypothalamus and are intrasellar. They are commonly associated with endocrinologically functional pituitary adenomas. The lesion consists of islands of neurons and associated neuropil within the substance of adenoma.

Rare neoplasms composed of both adenohypophyseal cells and ganglionlike cells are encountered within the sella. Despite the similarity of the ganglion cell component of these neoplasms to the hypothalamic hamartoma, they are not attached to the hypothalamus and are endocrinologically functional. They have been designated "pituitary adenoma–neuronal choristoma" by Horvath et al. and "mixed pituitary adenoma–gangliocytoma" by Towfighi et al. (172, 173).

The tumor is an admixture of pituitary adenoma and ganglion cells in varying proportions. GHRH or CRH has been demonstrated in the gangliocytomatous neurons and is associated with GH-producing adenomas or corticotroph adenomas, respectively. Rarely, they are prolactinoma or nonfunctioning adenomas (173–175).

EPIDERMOID AND DERMOID CYSTS

These cysts represent 0.2 to 1% of all intracranial tumors. Epidermoid cysts are 10 times more frequent than dermoid cysts. Although most of the epidermoid cysts occur in the cerebellopontine angle, occasional cases are found in the sellar or chiasmal region. Dermoid cysts, because of their propensity for midline sites, are more common than epidermoid cysts in the sellar region.

Slowly growing, epidermoid cysts tend to surround and envelop, instead of displace or infiltrate, the regional structures. Depending on the extent of the lipid content, variable signal intensity is given by magnetic resonance imaging. Grossly, they have a pearly white appearance because of thin wall and keratin content. The cyst content has a thick, viscid, soft, gray-white appearance. Microscopically, the cyst wall is composed of well-differentiated squamous epithelium containing keratohyaline granules; the interior of the cyst has multiple layers of acellular desquamated keratin.

Dermoid cysts are similar to epidermoid cysts, with an added feature related to the presence of cutaneous adnexa.

INFLAMMATORY LESIONS

Although rare, various inflammatory lesions, both infectious and autoimmune, involve the sellar region. Nonspecific clinical and radiological profiles of these lesions may prompt a diagnosis of nonfunctioning pituitary tumor and subject patients to surgical intervention. Of the inflammatory lesions, an array of bacterial, mycobacterial, fungal, or protozoal infections may occur. They may be intrasellar, extrasellar, or both and usually represent extension of an infectious process from adjacent structures (176–180).

Lymphocytic Hypophysitis

Lymphocytic hypophysitis is well known among the noninfectious inflammatory lesions involving the pituitary gland that are considered to be autoimmune. It affects mostly young females, usually during late pregnancy or the first postpartum year. Sellar enlargement is common, sometimes with extrasellar extension. Clinically and radiologically, the lesion resembles pituitary adenoma. An elevated PRL level secondary to pituitary stalk compression is common, and this, with occurrence in females during childbearing years, clinically may mimic a prolactinoma. A variable pituitary hormone deficiency may occur, but DI is uncommon. Histologically, lymphocytic hypophysitis is characterized by diffuse infiltration of the adenohypophysis by lymphocytes, plasma cells, eosinophils, and macrophages, often punctuated by lymphoid follicle formation. Destruction of the architecture of the gland occurs. Both T and B lymphocytes participate in the inflammatory process (181–184).

GIANT CELL GRANULOMAS

Giant cell granuloma of the pituitary is a rare condition that affects the anterior lobe. Involvement of the posterior pituitary or hypothalamus is very rare. The predilection is for females, but no association with pregnancy is noted. This lesion also typically mimics pituitary adenoma with suprasellar extension. Clinically, hormonal deficiency and DI are common. Histologically, sarcoidlike noncaseating granulomatous inflammation involves the anterior pituitary. Pathogenesis is not known but may be autoimmune in nature (185).

GRANULAR CELL TUMORS

Tumors of the posterior pituitary are very rare. Granular cell tumor is the better known of the two entities of tumors of the posterior pituitary, the other being glioma (infundibuloma or pituicytoma). Other designations used to describe granular cell tumor are choristoma or granular cell myoblastoma.

Small microscopic clumps of granular cells can incidentally be found in the posterior pituitary or infundibulum in autopsy cases. These clusters of granular cells as well as the much larger symptomatic granular cell tumor of the pituitary and suprasellar region most likely arise from cells of the posterior pituitary (pituicytes) (186–188). Thus, histogenetically, they are different from granular cell tumors at extracranial sites, which are presumed to be of Schwann cell origin. Most granular cell tumors of the posterior pituitary represent incidental autopsy findings in adults.

Grossly, the granular cell tumor is a rubbery, lobulated, well-demarcated but nonencapsulated mass. Frequently adherent to the surrounding structures, they may incite marked fibrillary gliosis in the adjacent brain. Microscopically, the tumor is highly characteristic and is composed of large, polygonal-shaped cells containing abundant pale eosinophilic, PAS-positive granules. Electron microscopically, the granules represent lysosomes.

METASTATIC TUMORS

Most metastatic tumors to the pituitary are asymptomatic and have an incidence of 1 to 2% in autopsy findings of patients with widespread cancer. The posterior lobe is more commonly involved, and this is why many of the symptomatic metastases present with DI. This is thought to be the result of the hematogenous spread by the direct arterial blood supply of the posterior lobe, which is not the case in the anterior lobe. Carcinomas of the breast, lung, and gastrointestinal tract are the most frequent primary lesions (189). Metastatic carcinoma to a pituitary adenoma has also been described (190).

LANGERHANS' CELL HISTIOCYTOSIS

Langerhans' cell histiocytosis includes a spectrum of disorders ranging from relatively benign, solitary eosinophilic granuloma of bone to the lethal form of generalized, fulminant Letterer-Siwe disease. These conditions represent proliferation of histiocytes mixed with eosinophils and mononuclear cells.

Involvement of the CNS by Langerhans' cell histiocytosis is usually part of disseminated disease but rarely precedes or occurs in the absence of disease elsewhere (191). The hypothalamus, posterior pituitary, and pituitary stalk are the preferred sites of involvement. In most cases, involvement of these sites represents extension from nearby bony lesions or leptomeningeal involvement from disseminated disease. Very rarely, isolated and localized hypothalamic and neurohypophyseal involvement have been recognized, which historically had been termed "Gagel's granuloma" or "Ayala's disease" (192, 193). The most common clinical manifestation is DI. Histologically, the lesion is characterized by histiocytes mixed with eosinophils and lymphocytes. The diagnostic feature is the presence of Langerhans' cells, large mononuclear histiocytic cells containing deeply indented nuclei. These cells express S-100

protein and CD1 antigen. Ultrastructurally, a tennis racket–shaped pentalaminar tubular structure—Birbeck granules—is diagnostic (194).

ACKNOWLEDGMENTS

Our special thanks go to Robert Mrak, MD, PhD, for his contribution of electron microscopic illustrations to this chapter.

REFERENCES

1. Kovacs K, Horvath E. Cytology. In: Hartmann WH, Sobin LH, eds. Tumors of the Pituitary Gland. Washington, DC: Armed Forces Institute of Pathology, 1986:16–50.
2. Kovacs K, Horvath E. Pituitary adenomas. In: Hartmann WH, Sobin LH, eds. Tumors of the Pituitary Gland. Washington, DC: Armed Forces Institute of Pathology, 1986:57–69.
3. Friesen HG, Fournier P, Desjardins P. Pituitary prolactin in pregnancy and normal and abnormal lactation. Clin Obstet Gynecol 1973;16:25–45.
4. Pioro EP, Scheithauer BW, Laws ER Jr, et al. Combined thyrotroph and lactotroph cell hyperplasia simulating prolactin-secreting pituitary adenoma in long-standing primary hypothyroidism. Surg Neurol 1988;29:218–226.
5. Sana T, Asa SL, Kovacs K. Growth hormone-releasing hormone-producing tumors: clinical, biochemical, and morphological manifestations. Endocr Rev 1988;9:357–373.
6. Stefaneanu L, Kovacs K, Horvath E, et al. Adenohypophyseal changes in mice transgenic for human growth hormone-releasing factor: a histological, immunocytochemical, electron microscopic investigation. Endocrinology 1989;125:2710–2718.
7. Asa SL, Kovacs K, Stefaneanu L, et al. Pituitary mammosomatotroph adenomas develop in old mice transgenic for growth hormone-releasing hormone. Proc Soc Exp Biol Med, 1990;193:232–235.
8. Scheithauer BW, Sano T, Kovacs KT, et al. The pituitary gland in pregnancy: a clinicopathologic and immunohistochemical study of 69 cases. Mayo Clin Proc 1990;65:461–474.
9. Carey RM, Varma SK, Drake CR Jr, et al. Ectopic secretion of corticotropin-releasing factor as a cause of Cushing's syndrome. N Engl J Med 1984;311:13–20.
10. Horvath E, Kovacs K. Pituitary gland. Pathol Res Pract 1988;183:129–142.
11. McKeever PE, Koppelman MCS, Metcalf D, et al. Refractory Cushing's disease caused by multinodular ACTH-cell hyperplasia. J Neuropathol Exp Neurol 1982;41:490–499.
12. Scheithauer BW, Kovacs K, Randall RV. The pituitary gland in untreated Addison's disease. Arch Pathol Lab Med 1983;107:484–487.
13. Scheithauer BW. Surgical pathology of the pituitary: the adenomas. Pathol Annu 1984;19(Part II):269–329.
14. Scheithauer BW, Kovacs K, Randall RV, et al. Pituitary gland in hypothyroidism: histologic and immunocytologic study. Arch Pathol Lab Med 1985;109:499–504.
15. Samaan NA, Osborne BM, Mackay B, et al. Endocrine and morphologic studies of pituitary adenomas secondary to primary hypothyroidism. J Clin Endocrinol Metab 1977;45:903–911.
16. Horvath E, Kovacs K. Fine structural cytology of the adenohypophysis in rat and man. J Electron Microsc Tech 1988;8:401–432.
17. Snyder PJ. Gonadotroph cell pituitary adenomas. In: Molitch ME, ed. Pituitary Tumors: Diagnosis and Management. Philadelphia: WB Saunders, 1987;16:755–764.
18. Woolf PD, Schnenk EA. A FSH-producing pituitary tumor in a patient with hypogonadism. J Clin Endocrinol Metab 1974;38:561–568.
19. Kovacs K, Horvath E. Tumors of the pituitary gland. In: Hartman WH, ed. Atlas of Tumor Pathology. Fascicle 21, 2nd series. Washington, DC: Armed Forces Institute of Pathology, 1986:1–269.
20. Horvath E, Kovacs K. Ultrastructural classification of pituitary adenomas. Can J Neurol Sci 1976;3:9–21.
21. Horvath E, Kovacs K. Pathology of the hypothalamus and pituitary gland. In: Mendelsohn G, ed. Diagnosis and Pathology of Endocrine Diseases. Philadelphia: Lippincott, 1988:379–412.
22. Horvath E, Kovacs K. The adenohypophysis. In: Kovacs K, Asa SL, eds. Functional Endocrine Pathology. Boston: Blackwell Scientific Publications, 1990:245–281.
23. Scheithauer BW. Surgical pathology of the pituitary: the adenomas. Pathol Annu 1984;19(Part I):313–374.
24. Landolt AM. Ultrastructure of human sella tumors: correlations of clinical findings and morphology. Acta Neurochir Suppl (Wien) 1975;27:1–167.
25. Halmi NS. Immunostaining of growth hormone and prolactin in paraffin embedded and stored or previously stained materials. J Histochem Cytochem 1978;26:486–495.
26. Kovacs K, Horvath E, Ryan N. Immunocytology of the human pituitary. In: Delellis RA, ed. Diagnostic Immunohistochemistry. New York: Mason, 1981:17–35.
27. Landolt AM, Heitz PU, Zenklusen HR. Production of the α-subunit of glycoprotein hormones by pituitary adenomas. Pathol Res Pract 1988;183:610–612.
28. Osamura RY, Watanabe K. Immunohistochemical colocalization of growth hormone (GH) and subunit in human GH secreting pituitary adenomas. Virchows Arch [A] 1987;411:323–330.
29. Riedel M, Saeger W, Ludecke DK. Grading of pituitary adenomas in acromegaly: comparison of light microscopical, immunocytochemical, and clinical data. Virchows Arch [A] 1985;407:83–95.
30. McNicol AM. Pituitary adenomas (invited review). Histopathology 1987;11:995–1011.
31. Robert F. Electron microscopy of pituitary tumors. In: Tindall GT, Collins WF, eds. Clinical Management of Pituitary Disorders. New York: Raven Press, 1979:113–131.
32. Smallman LA, Dunn PTS, Curran RC, et al. Pituitary adenomas producing growth hormone in acromegalic patients. J Clin Pathol 1984;37:382–389.
33. Ho KY, Weissberger AJ, Marbach P, et al. Therapeutic efficacy of the somatostatin analog SMA 201-995 (Octreotide) in acromegaly: effects of dose and frequency and long-tem safety. Ann Intern Med 1990;112:173–181.
34. Melmed S. Acromegaly. N Engl J Med 1990;322:966–977.
35. Popovic V, Nesovic M, Micic D, et al. A comparison among the effectiveness of growth hormone suppression in active acromegaly of bromocriptine and long acting somatostatin analogue (SMS 201-995). Exp Clin Endocrinol 1990;95:251–257.
36. George SR, Kovacs K, Asa SL, et al. Effect of SMS 201-905, a long acting somatostatin analog on the secretion and morphology of a pituitary growth hormone cell adenoma. Clin Endocrinol (Oxf) 1987;26:395–405.
37. Landolt AM, Osterwalder V, Stuckmann G. Preoperative treatment of acromegaly with SMS 201-995: surgical and pathological observations. In: Ludecke DK, Tolis G, eds. Growth Hormone, Growth Factors, and Acromegaly. New York: Raven Press, 1987:229–244.
38. Beckers A, Stevenaert A, Kovacs K, et al. The treatment of acromegaly with SMA 201-995. Adv Biosci 1988;69:227–228.
39. McComb DJ, Kovacs K, Horvath E. Correlative ultrastructural

morphometry of human prolactin-producing adenomas. Acta Neurochir (Wien) 1980;53:217–223.

40. Horvath E, Kovacs K. Pathology of prolactin cell adenomas of the human pituitary. Semin Diagn Pathol 1986;3:4–17.

41. Landolt AM. Progress in pituitary adenoma biology: results of research and clinical applications. Adv Tech Stand Neurosurg 1978; 5:3–49.

42. Kameya T, Tsumuraya M, Adachi I, et al. Ultrastructure, immunohistochemistry and hormone release of pituitary adenomas in relation to prolactin production. Virchows Arch [A] 1980;387:31–46.

43. Esiri MM, Bevan JS, Burke CW, et al. Pituitary adenomas: immunohistology and ultrastructural analysis of 118 tumors. Acta Neuropathol (Berl) 1983;62:1–14.

44. Rasmussen C, Larsson SG, Bergh T. The occurrence of macroscopial pituitary calcifications in prolactinomas. Neuroradiology 1990; 31:507–511.

45. Anniko M, Wersall J. Morphological changes in bromocriptine-treated pituitary tumours. Acta Otolaryngol (Stockh) 1983;96: 337–353.

46. Bassetti M, Spada A, Pezzo G, et al. Bromocriptine treatment reduces the cell size in human macroprolactins: a morphometric study. J Clin Endocrinol Metab 1984;58:268–273.

47. Duffy AE, Asa SL, Kovacs K. Effect of bromocriptine on secretion and morphology of human prolactin cell adenomas in vitro. Horm Res 1988;30:32–38.

48. Hassoun J, Jacquel P, Devictor B, et al. Bromocriptine effects on cultured human prolactin-producing pituitary adenomas: in vitro, ultrastructural, morphometric and immunoelectron microscopic studies. J Clin Endocrinol Metab 1985;61:686–692.

49. Landolt A, Minder H, Osterwalder V, et al. Bromocriptine reduces the size of cells in prolactin-secreting pituitary adenomas. Experientia 1983;39:625–626.

50. Rengachary SS, Tomita T, Jefferies BF, et al. Structural changes in human pituitary tumor after bromocriptine therapy. Neurosurgery 1982;10:242–252.

51. Saitoh Y, Mori S, Arta N, et al. Cytosuppressive effect of bromocriptine on human prolactinomas: stereological analysis of ultrastructural alterations with special reference to secretory granules. Cancer Res 1986;46:1507–1512.

52. Tindall GT, Kovacs K, Horvath E, et al. Human prolactin-producing adenoma and bromocriptine: a histological, immunocytochemical, ultrastructural and morphometric study. J Clin Endocrinol Metab 1982;55:1178–1183.

53. Landolt AM, Osterwalder V. Perivascular fibrosis in prolactinomas: is it increased by bromocriptine? J Clin Endocrinol Metab 1984; 58:1179–1183.

54. Gen M, Uozumi T, Ohta M, et al. Necrotic changes in prolactinomas after long term administration of bromocriptine. J Clin Endocrinol Metab 1984;59:463–470.

55. Esiri MM, Bevan JS, Burke C, et al. Effect of bromocriptine treatment on the fibrous tissue component of prolactin-secreting and nonfunctioning macroadenomas of the pituitary gland. J Clin Endocrinol Metab 1987;63:383–388.

56. Bevan JS, Adams CBT, Burke CW, et al. Factors in the outcome of transsphenoidal surgery for prolactinoma and nonfunctioning pituitary tumors, including pre-operative bromocriptine therapy. Clin Endocrinol (Oxf) 1987;26:541–556.

57. Lamberts SWJ, Liuzzi A, Chiodini PG, et al. The value of plasma prolactin levels in the prediction of the responsiveness of growth hormone secretion to bromocriptine and TRH in acromegaly. Eur J Clin Invest 1982;12:151–155.

58. Serri O, Comtois R, Jilwan N, et al. Distinctive features of prolactin secretion in acromegalic patients with hyperprolactinemia. Clin Endocrinol (Oxf) 1987;27:429–436.

59. Bassetti M, Arosio M, Spada A, et al. Growth hormone and prolactin secretion in acromegaly: correlation between hormonal dynamics and immunocytochemical findings. J Clin Endocrinol Metab 1988;67:1195–1204.

60. Lloyd RV, Cano M, Chandler WF, et al. Human growth hormone and prolactin secreting pituitary adenomas analyzed by in situ hybridization. Am J Pathol 1989;134:605–613.

61. Nagaya T, Seo H, Kuwayama A, et al. Prolactin gene expression in human growth hormone-secreting adenomas. J Neurosurg 1990;72:879–882.

62. Bendayan M, Maestracci ND. Pituitary adenomas: patterns of hPrl and hGH secretion as revealed by high resolution immunocytochemistry. Biol Cell 1984;52:129–138.

63. Corenblum B, Sirek AMT, Horvath E, et al. Human mixed somatotrophic and lactotrophic pituitary adenomas. J Clin Endocrinol Metab 1976;42:857–863.

64. Kanie N, Kagayama N, Kuwayama N, et al. Pituitary adenomas in acromegalic patients: an immunohistochemical and endocrinological study with special reference to prolactin-secreting adenoma. J Clin Endocrinol Metab 1983;57:1093–1101.

65. Lloyd RV, Gikes RV, Changler WF. Prolactin and growth hormone-producing pituitary adenomas: an immunohistochemical and ultrastructural study. Am J Surg Pathol 1983;7:251–260.

66. Felix IA, Horvath E, Kovacs K, et al. Mammosomatotroph adenoma of the pituitary associated with gigantism and hyperprolactinemia: a morphological study including immunoelectron microscopy. Acta Neuropathol (Berl) 1986;71:76–82.

67. Hom R, Nesland JM, Attramadal A, et al. Mixed growth hormone- and prolactin-cell adenomas of the pituitary gland: an immunoelectron microscopic study. J Submicrosc Cytol Pathol 1989;21: 339–350.

68. Horvath E, Kovacs K, Josse R. Pituitary corticotroph cell adenoma with marked abundance of microfilaments. Ultrastruct Pathol 1983;5:249–255.

69. Robert F, Pelletier G, Serri O, et al. Mixed growth hormone and prolactin-secreting human pituitary adenomas: a pathologic, immunocytochemical, ultrastructural, and immunoelectron microscopic study. Hum Pathol 1988;19:1327–1334.

70. Horvath E, Kovacs K, Singer W, et al. Acidophil stem cell adenoma of the human pituitary. Arch Pathol Lab Med 1977;101:594–599.

71. Horvath E, Kovacs K, Singer W, et al. Acidophil stem cell adenoma of the human pituitary: clinicopathological analysis of 15 cases. Cancer 1981;47:761–771.

72. Charpin C, Hassoun J, Oliver C, et al. Immunohistochemical and immunoelectron-microscopic study of pituitary adenomas associated with Cushing's disease: a report of 13 cases. Am J Pathol 1982;109:1–7.

73. Felix IA, Horvath E, Kovaks K. Massive Crooke's hylinization in corticotroph cell adenomas of the human pituitary: a histological, immunocytological, and electron microscopic study of three cases. Acta Neurochir (Wien) 1982;58:235–243.

74. Horvath E, Kovacs K, Josse R. Pituitary corticotroph cell adenoma with marked abundance of microfilaments. Ultrastruct Pathol 1983;5:249–255.

75. Lloyd RV, Chandler WF, McKeever PE, et al. The spectrum of ACTH-producing pituitary lesions. Am J Surg Pathol 1986;10: 618–626.

76. McNicol AM. Current topics in neuropathology: Cushing's disease. Neuropathol Appl Neurobiol 1985;II:485–498.

77. Robert F, Hardy J. Human corticotroph cell adenomas. Semin Diagn Pathol 1986;3:34–41.

78. Saeger W. Morphology of ACTH-producing pituitary tumors. In: Fahlbusch R, Von Werder K, eds. Treatment of Pituitary Adenomas. Stuttgart: Thieme, 1978:122–130.

79. Findling JW, Aron DC, Tyrrell JB. Cushing's disease. In: Imura H, ed. The Pituitary Gland. New York: Raven Press, 1985:441–466.

80. Girod C, Trouillas J, Claustrat B. The human thyrotropic adenoma: pathologic diagnosis in five cases and critical review of the literature. Semin Diagn Pathol 1986;3:58–68.

81. Katz MS, Gregerman RI, Horvath E, et al. Thyrotroph cell adenoma of the human pituitary gland associated with primary hypothyroidism: clinical and morphological features. Acta Endocrinol (Copenh) 1980;95:41–48.

82. Mashiter K, Van Noorden S, Fahlbusch R, et al. Hyperthyroidism due to TSH secreting pituitary adenoma: case report, treatment and evidence for adenoma TSH by morphological and cell culture studies. Clin Endocrinol (Oxf) 1983;18:473–483.

83. Saeger W, Ludecke DK. Pituitary adenomas with hyperfunction of TSH: frequency, histological classification, immunohistochemistry and ultrastructure. Virchows Arch [A] 1982;394:255–267.

84. Borges JLC, Ridgway EC, Kovacs K, et al. Follicle-stimulating hormone-secreting pituitary tumor with concomitant elevation of serum α-subunit levels. J Clin Endocrinol Metab 1984;58: 937–941.

85. Horvath E, Kovacs K. Gonadotroph adenomas of the human pituitary: sex related fine-structural dichotomy: a histologic, immuno-

cytochemical and electron microscopic study of 30 tumors. Am J Pathol 1984;117:429–440.

86. Kovacs K, Horvath E, Van Look GR, et al. Pituitary adenomas associated with elevated blood follicle-stimulating hormone levels: a histologic, immunocytologic, and electron microscopic study of two cases. Fertil Steril 1978;29:622–628.

87. Kovacs K, Horvath E, Rewcastle NB, et al. Gonadotroph cell adenoma of the pituitary in a woman with long-standing hypogonadism. Arch Gynecol 1980;229:57–65.

88. Trouillas J, Girod C, Sassolas G, et al. Human pituitary gonadotrophic adenoma: histological, immunocytochemical, and ultrastructural and hormonal studies in eight cases. J Pathol 1981;135:315–336.

89. Trouillas J, Girod C, Sassolas G, et al. The human gonadotropic adenoma: pathologic diagnosis and hormonal correlations in 26 tumors. Semin Diagn Pathol 1986;3:42–57.

90. Hassoun J, Charpin C, Jacquet P, et al. Corticolipotropin immunoreactivity in silent chromophobe adenomas: a light and electron microscopic study. Arch Pathol Lab Med 1982;106:25–30.

91. Horvath E, Kovacs K, Killinger DW, et al. Silent corticotrophic adenomas of the human pituitary gland. Am J Pathol 1980;98:617–638.

92. Kovacs K, Horvath E, Bayley JA, et al. Silent corticotroph cell adenoma with lysosomal accumulation and crinophagy. Am J Med 1977;64:492–499.

93. Klibanski A, Zervas NT, Kovacs K, et al. Clinically silent hypersecretion of growth hormone in patients with pituitary tumors. J Neurosurg 1987;66:806–811.

94. Randall R, Scheithauer BW, Laws ER Jr. Hormone-containing, non-secreting pituitary tumors: clinically silent monohormonal pituitary adenomas. Trans Am Clin Climatol Assoc 1984;92:98–103.

95. Snyder PJ. Gonadotroph cell adenomas of the pituitary. Endocr Rev 1985;6:552–563.

96. Asa SL, Gerrie BM, Singer W, et al. Gonadotropin secretion in vitro by human pituitary null cell adenomas and oncocytomas. J Clin Endocrinol Metab 1986;62:1011–1019.

97. Kovacs K, Horvath E, Ryan N, et al. Null cell adenomas of the human pituitary gland. Virchows Arch [A] 1980;387:165–174.

98. Yamada S, Sylvia SL, Kovacs K, et al. Analysis of hormone secretion by clinically nonfunctioning human pituitary adenomas using the reverse hemolytic plaque assay. J Clin Endocrinol Metab 1989;68:73–79.

99. Scheithauer BW, Kovacs K, Laws ER Jr, et al. Pathology of invasive pituitary tumors with special reference to functional classification. J Neurosurg 1986;65:733–744.

100. Luzi R, Miracco C, Lio R, et al. Endocrine inactive pituitary carcinoma metastasizing to cervical lymph nodes: a case report. Hum Pathol 1987;18:90–92.

101. Martin NA, Hales M, Wilson CB. Cerebellar metastasis during treatment with bromocriptine. J Neurosurg 1981;55:615–619.

102. Cohen DL, Diengdoh JV, Thomas DGT, et al. An intracranial metastasis from a Prl secreting pituitary tumour. Clin Endocrinol (Oxf) 1983;18:259–264.

103. USH, Johnson C. Metastatic prolactin-secreting pituitary adenomas. Hum Pathol 1984;15:94–96.

104. Ogilvy KM, Jukabowski J. Intracranial dissemination of pituitary adenomas. J Neurol Neurosurg Psychiatry 1973;36:199–205.

105. Facnie JD, Zafar MS, Mellinger RC, et al. Pituitary carcinoma mimics the ectopic adrenocorticotropin syndrome. J Clin Endocrinol Metab 1980;50:1062–1065.

106. Gabrilove JL, Anderson PJ, Halmi NS. Pituitary proopiomelanocortin-cell carcinoma occurring in conjunction with glioblastoma in a patient with Cushing's disease and subsequent Nelson's syndrome. Clin Endocrinol (Oxf) 1986;25:117–126.

107. Queiroz LS, Facure NO, Facure JJ, et al. Pituitary carcinoma with liver metastases and Cushing syndrome. Arch Pathol 1975;99:32–35.

108. Giannattasio G, Bassetti M. Human pituitary adenomas: recent advances in morphological studies. J Endocrinol Invest 1990;13:435–454.

109. Kovacs K, Horvath E, Asa SL, et al. Pituitary cells producing more than one hormone: human pituitary adenomas. TEM 1989;Nov/Dec:104–107.

110. Scheithauer BW, Horvath E, Kovacs K, et al. Plurihormonal pituitary adenomas. Semin Diagn Pathol 1986;3:69–82.

111. Beck-Peccoz P, Bassetti M, Spada A, et al. Glycoprotein hormone α-subunit response to growth hormone (GH)-releasing hormone in patients with active acromegaly: evidence for a α-subunit and GH coexistence in the same tumoral cells. J Clin Endocrinol Metab 1985;61:541–546.

112. Assadian H, Shimatsu A, Koshiyama H, et al. Secretion of alpha and TSH-beta subunits in patients with acromegaly: an in vivo study. Acta Endocrinol (Copenh) 1990;122:729–734.

113. Beck-Peccoz P, Piscitelli G, Amr S, et al. Endocrine, biochemical, and morphological studies of a pituitary adenoma secreting growth hormone, thyrotropin (TSH), and α-subunit: evidence for secretion of TSH with increased bioactivity. J Clin Endocrinol Metab 1986;62:704–711.

114. Horvath E, Kovacs K, Smyth HS, et al. A novel type of pituitary adenomas: morphological features and clinical correlations. J Clin Endocrinol Metab 1988;66:1111–1118.

115. Osamura RY, Watanabe K. Immunohistochemical studies of human FSH producing pituitary adenomas. Virchows Arch [A] 1988;413:61–68.

116. Erdheim J. Ueber hypophysengangsgeshwulste und hirnscholesteatome: sitzungsbericht det kaiselichen akademie der wissenchaften. Mathematisch-naturwissen-schaftliche Classe 1904;113:537–726.

117. Asa SL, Kovacs K, Bilbao, JM. The pars tuberalis of the human pituitary: a histologic, immunohistochemical, ultrastructural and immunoelectron microscopic analysis. Virchows Arch [A] 1983;399:49–59.

118. Bernstein ML, Buchino JJ. The histologic similarity between craniopharyngioma and odontogenic lesions: a reappraisal. Oral Surg Oral Med Oral Pathol 1983;56:502–511.

119. Kovacs K, Horvath E. Tumors of the Pituitary Gland: Atlas of Tumor Pathology (Fascicle 21). Washington, DC: Armed Forces Institute of Pathology, 1983.

120. Altinors N, Senveli E, Erdogan A, et al. Craniopharyngioma of the cerebellopontine angle: case report. J Neurosurg 1984;60:842–844.

121. Cooper PR, Ransohoff J. Craniopharyngioma originating in the sphenoid bone: case report. J Neurosurg 1972;36:102–106.

122. Solarski A, Panke ES, Panke TW. Craniopharyngioma in the pineal gland (letter). Arch Pathol Lab Med 1978;102:490–491.

123. Sangiovanni G, Tancioni F, Tartara F, et al. Ectopic craniopharyngioma: presentation of a case arising from the corpus callosum. Acta Neurochirurgica 1997;139:379–380.

124. Bashir EM, Lewis PD, Edwards MR. Posterior fast craniopharyngioma. Br J Neurosurg 1996;10:613–615.

125. Kanungo N, Just N, Black M, et al. Nasopharyngeal craniopharyngioma in an unusual location. AJNR Am J Neuroradiol 1995;16:1372–1374.

126. Kultursay N, Gelal F, Mutluer S, et al. Antenatally diagnosed neonatal craniopharyngioma. J Perinatol 1995;15:426–428.

127. Connolly ES Jr, Winfree CJ, Carmel PW. Giant posterior fossa cystic craniopharyngiomas presenting with hearing loss: report of three cases and review of the literature. Surg Neurol 1997;47:291–299.

128. Thapar K, Kovacs K. Neoplasms of the sellar region. In: Bigner DD, McLendon RE, Bruner JM, eds. Russell and Rubinstein's Pathology of Tumors of the Nervous System. 6th ed. London: Edward Arnold, 1998:561–677.

129. Patrick BS, Smith RR, Baily TO. Aseptic meningitis due to spontaneous rupture of craniopharyngioma cyst: case report. J Neurosurg 1974;41:387–390.

130. Obrador S, Blazquez MG. Pituitary abscess in a craniopharyngioma: case report. J Neurosurg 1972;36:785–789.

131. Sener RN, Kismali E, Akyar S, et al. Large craniopharyngioma extending to the posterior cranial fossa. Magn Reson Imaging 1997;15:1111–1112.

132. Pang D. Surgical management of craniopharyngioma. In: Sekhar L, Janecka I, eds. Surgery of Cranial Bone Tumors. New York: Raven Press, 1993:787–808.

133. Ghatak NR, Hirano A, Zimmerman HM. Ultrastructure of a craniopharyngioma. Cancer 1971;27:1465–1475.

134. Thapar K, Stefaneanu L, Kovacs K, et al. Estrogen receptor gene expression in craniopharyngiomas: an in situ hybridization study. Neurosurgery 1994;35:1012–1017.

135. Honegger J, Renner C, Fahlbusch R, et al. Progesterone receptor

gene expression in craniopharyngiomas and evidence for biological activity. Neurosurgery 1997;41:1359–1363.

136. Maniker AH, Krieger AJ. Rapid recurrence of craniopharyngioma during pregnancy with recovery of vision: a case report. Surg Neurol 1996;45:324–327.

137. Crotty T, Scheithauer BW, Young WF, et al. Papillary craniopharyngiomas: a morphological and clinical study of 46 cases. Endocr Pathol 1992;3(Suppl 1):S6.

138. Giangaspero F, Burger PC, Osborne DR, et al. Suprasellar papillary squamous epithelioma ("papillary craniopharyngioma"). Am J Surg Pathol 1984;8:57–64.

139. Oka H, Kawano N, Yagishita S, et al. Ciliated craniopharyngioma indicates histogenetic relationship to Rathke cleft epithelium. Clin Neuropathol 1997;16:103–106.

140. Oka H, Kawano N, Yagishita S, et al. Origin of ciliated craniopharyngioma: pathological relationship between Rathke cleft cyst and ciliated craniopharyngioma. Noshuyo Byori 1995;12:97–103.

141. Adamson TE, Wiestler OD, Kleihues P, et al. Correlation of clinical and pathological features in surgically treated craniopharyngiomas. J Neurosurg 1990;73:12–17.

142. Crotty TB, Scheithauer BW, Young WF Jr, et al. Papillary craniopharyngioma: a clinicopathological study of 48 cases. J Neurosurg 1995;83:206–214.

143. Barrow DL, Spector RH, Takei Y, et al. Symptomatic Rathke's cleft cysts located entirely in the suprasellar region: review of diagnosis, management, and pathogenesis. Neurosurgery 1985;16:766–772.

144. Itoh J, Usui K. An entirely suprasellar symptomatic Rathke's cleft cyst: case report. Neurosurgery 1992;30:581–585.

145. Nishio S, Fujiwara S, Morioka T, et al. Rathke's cleft cysts within a growth hormone producing pituitary adenoma. Br J Neurosurg 1995;9:51–55.

146. Ikeda H, Yoshimoto T, Katakura R. A case of Rathke's cleft cyst within a pituitary adenoma presenting with acromegaly: do "transitional cell tumors of the pituitary gland" really exist? Acta Neuropathol (Berl) 1992;83:211–215.

147. Kepes JJ. Transitional cell tumor of the pituitary gland developing from a Rathke's cleft cyst. Cancer 1978;41:337–343.

148. Grisoli F, Vincentelli F, Raubaud C, et al. Intrasellar meningioma. Surg Neurol 1983;20:36–41.

149. Kudo H, Takaishi Y, Minami H, et al. Intrasellar meningioma mimicking pituitary apoplexy: case report. Surg Neurol 1997;48:374–381.

150. Talacchi A, Benvenuto F, Lombardo C, et al. Endosellar meningiomas: report of 2 cases and review of the literature. Clin Neurol Neurosurg 1996;98:47–51.

151. Kinjo T, al-Mefty O, Ciric I. Diaphragma sellae meningiomas. Neurosurgery. 1995;36:1082–1092.

152. Mangiardi JR, Flamm ES, Cravioto H, et al. Hemangiopericytoma of the pituitary fossa: case report. Neurosurgery 1983;13:58–62.

153. Yokota M, Tani E, Maeda Y, et al. Acromegaly associated with suprasellar and pulmonary hemangiopericytoma: case report. J Neurosurg 1985;62:767–771.

154. Kumar PP, Good RR, Skultety FM, et al. Spinal metastases from pituitary hemangiopericytic meningioma. Am J Clin Oncol 1987;10:442–448.

155. Russell DS, Rubinstein LJ. Pathology of Tumors of the Nervous System. 5th ed. London: Edward Arnold, 1989.

156. Jennings MT, Gelman R, Hochberg T. Intracranial germ cell tumors: natural history and pathogenesis. J Neurosurg 1985;63:155–167.

157. Steimle R, Raffi A, Bonneville JF, et al. Germinome (pinealome ectopique) a double localisation: supra-sellaire et cerebelleuse sans tumeur pineale. Neurochirurgie 1979;25:129–133.

158. McLendon RE, Tien RD. Tumors and tumor-like lesions of maldevelopmental origin. In: Bigner DD, McLendon RE, Bruner JM, eds. Russell and Rubinstein's Pathology of Tumors of the Nervous System. 6th ed. London: Edward Arnold, 1998:296–370.

159. Burger PC, Scheithauer BW. Tumors of the Central Nervous System: Atlas of Tumor Pathology (3rd series, fascicle 10). Washington, DC: Armed Forces Institute of Pathology.

160. Globus J. Infundibuloma: a newly recognized tumor of neurohypophyseal derivation with a note on the saccus vasculosus. J Neuropathol Exp Neurol 1942;1:59–80.

161. Scothorne C. Glioma of the posterior lobe of the pituitary gland. J Pathol Bacteriol 1955;69:109–112.

162. Rossi ML, Bevan JS, Esiri MM, et al. Pituicytoma (pilocytic astrocytoma): case report. J Neurosurg 1987;67:768–772.

163. Hurley TR, D'Angelo CM, Clasen RA, et al. Magnetic resonance imaging and pathological analysis of a pituicytoma: case report. Neurosurgery 1994;35:314–317.

164. Mathews W, Wilson CB. Ectopic intrasellar chordoma: case report. J Neurosurg 1974;40:260–263.

165. Sherwin RP, Grassi JE, Sommers SC. Hamartomatous malformations of the posterolateral hypothalamus. Lab Invest 1962;11:89–97.

166. Albright AL, Lee PA. Neurosurgical treatment of hypothalamic hamartomas causing precocious puberty. J Neurosurg 1993;78:77–82.

167. Hamilton RL. Case of the month: July 1996: precocious puberty. Brain Pathol 1997;7:711–712.

168. Guibaud L, Rode V, Saint-Pierre G, et al. Giant hypothalamic hamartoma: an unusual neonatal tumor. Pediatr Radiol 1995;25:17–18.

169. Culler FL, James HE, Simon ML, et al. Identification of gonadotropin-releasing hormone in neurons of a hypothalamic hamartoma in a boy with precocious puberty. Neurosurgery 1985;17:408–412.

170. Kang S, Allen J, Graham JM Jr, et al. Linkage mapping and phenotypic analysis of autosomal dominant Pallister-Hall syndrome. J Med Genet 1997;34:441–446.

171. Squires LA, Constantini S, Miller DC, et al. Hypothalamic hamartoma and the Pallister-Hall syndrome. Pediatr Neurosurg 1995;22:303–308.

172. Horvath E, Kovacs K, Scheithauer BW, et al. Pituitary adenoma with neuronal choristoma (PANCH): composite lesion or lineage infidelity? Ultrastruct Pathol 1994;18:565–574.

173. Towfighi J, Salam MM, McLendon RE, et al. Ganglion cell-containing tumors of the pituitary gland. Arch Pathol Lab Med 1996;120:369–377.

174. Scheithauer BW, Kovacs K, Randall RV, et al. Hypothalamic neuronal hamartoma and adenohypophyseal neuronal choristoma: their association with growth hormone adenoma of the pituitary gland. J Neuropathol Exp Neurol 1983;42:648–663.

175. Li JY, Racadot O, Kujas M, et al. Immunocytochemistry of four mixed pituitary adenomas and intrasellar gangliocytomas associated with different clinical syndromes: acromegaly, amenorrheagalactorrhea, Cushing's disease, and isolated tumoral syndrome. Acta Neuropathologica (Berlin) 1989;77:320–328.

176. Berger SA, Edberg SC, David G. Infectious disease in the sella turcica. Rev Infect Dis 1986;8:747–755.

177. Bebzel E, Shockley W, Giyanani V, et al. Primary pituitary abscess. Surg Neurol 1986;25:571–574.

178. Nelson PB, Haverkos H, Martinez AJ, et al. Abscess formation within pituitary tumors. Neurosurgery 1983;12:331–333.

179. Ranjan A, Chandy MJ. Intrasellar tuberculoma. Br J Neurosurg 1994;8:179–185.

180. Delsedime M, Aguggia M, Cantello R, et al. Isolated hypophyseal tuberculoma: case report. Clin Neuropathol 1988;7:311–313.

181. Feigenbaum SL, Martin MC, Wilson CB, et al. Lymphocytic adenohypophysitis: a pituitary mass lesion occurring in pregnancy: proposal for medical treatment. Am J Obstet Gynecol 1991;164:1549–1555.

182. Thorner MO, Vance ML, Horvath E, et al. The anterior pituitary. In: Wilson JD, Foster DW, eds. Williams Textbook of Endocrinology. Philadelphia: WB Saunders, 1992:221–310.

183. Cosman F, Post KD, Holub DA, et al. Lymphocytic hypophysitis: report of 3 new cases and review of the literature. Medicine 1989;68:240–256.

184. Horvath E, Scheithauer BW, Kovacs K, et al. Regional neuropathology: hypothalamus and pituitary. In: Graham DI, Lantos PL. Greenfield's Neuropathology. 6th ed. London: Edward Arnold, 1997:1007–1094.

185. Scheithauer BW. The neurohypophysis. In: Kovacs K, Asa SL, eds. Functional Endocrine Pathology. Boston: Blackwell Scientific Publications, 1991:170–244.

186. Shanklin W. The origin, histology and senescence of tumorlettes in the human neurohypophysis. Acta Anatomica 1953;18:1–20.

187. Liss l, Kahn E. Pituicytoma: tumor of the sella turcica: a clinicopathologic study. J Neurosurg 1958;15:481–488.

188. Friede RL, Yasargil MG. Suprasellar neoplasm with a granular cell component. J Neuropathol Exp Neurol 1977;36:769–782.

189. Teears RJ, Silverman EM. Clinicopathologic review of 88 cases of carcinoma metastatic to the pituitary gland. Cancer 1975;36: 216–220.

190. Post KD, McCormick PC, Hays AP, et al. Metastatic carcinoma in pituitary adenoma: report of two cases. Surg Neurol 1988;30: 286–292.

191. Lieberman PH, Jones CR, Dargeon HW, et al. A reappraisal of eosinophilic granuloma of bone, Hand-Schuller-Christian syndrome and letterer-Siwe syndrome. Medicine 1969;48:375–400.

192. Kepes JJ, Kepes M. Predominantly cerebral forms of histiocytosis X: a reappraisal of 'Gagel's hypothalamic granuloma,' 'granuloma infiltrans of the hypothalamus' and 'Ayala's disease' with a report of four cases. Acta Neuropathologica 1969;14:77–98.

193. Scholtz M, Firsching R, Feiden W, et al. Gagel's granuloma (localized Langerhans cell histiocytosis) in the pituitary stalk. Clin Neurol Neurosurg 1995;97:164–166.

194. Mierau GW, Favara BE, Brenman JM. Electron microscopy in histiocytosis X. Ultrastruct Pathol 1982;3:137–142.

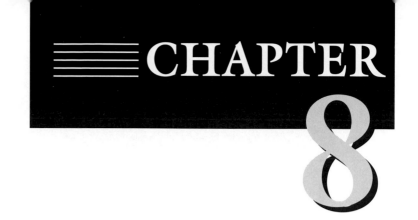

CHAPTER 8

Radiology

Neuroradiologic Evaluation of Pituitary Disorders

Edgardo J.C. Angtuaco

INTRODUCTION

The pituitary gland is a relatively small organ measuring between 12 and 15 mm in diameter and approximately 3 to 7 mm in height and is located within the central skull base. The pituitary gland maintains a complex network of relationships with surrounding neural and vascular structures to maintain its function. Despite its size, it plays a vital role in the maintenance of the internal milieu of the body, accomplishing this by the secretion of hormones that control the function of other vital glands. Dysfunction of the pituitary gland by disease involving the gland or its surroundings causes significant clinical problems. The advent of new laboratory assays and modern neuroimaging techniques has changed the medical approach to lesions in this area. The soft tissue and bone detail afforded by high-resolution magnetic resonance imaging (MRI) and computed tomographic (CT) studies has allowed for more precise evaluation and management of lesions in the sellar and parasellar area (1–7).

NORMAL ANATOMY OF THE PITUITARY

The pituitary gland is housed within the confines of the bony sella. The bony sella, otherwise referred to as the sella turcica, is a cup-shaped depression in the basisphenoid bone. Its anterior boundary is the tuberculum sella, and its posterior boundary is the dorsum sella. Anterior to the tuberculum sella is the chiasmatic sulcus. The chiasmatic sulcus continues laterally to end in the optic canal. The sella is bordered superolaterally by the anterior clinoid process, which arises medially from the lesser wing of the sphenoid. The sellar floor consists of a thin layer of cortical bone separating the pituitary fossa from the inferior sphenoid sinus. The variable degree of pneumatization of the sphenoid sinuses in humans account for the difference in the thickness of the sellar floor and the asymmetric location of the sphenoid septum. Posteriorly, the sellar floor continues in a superior direction to form the dorsum sella. Along the supero-

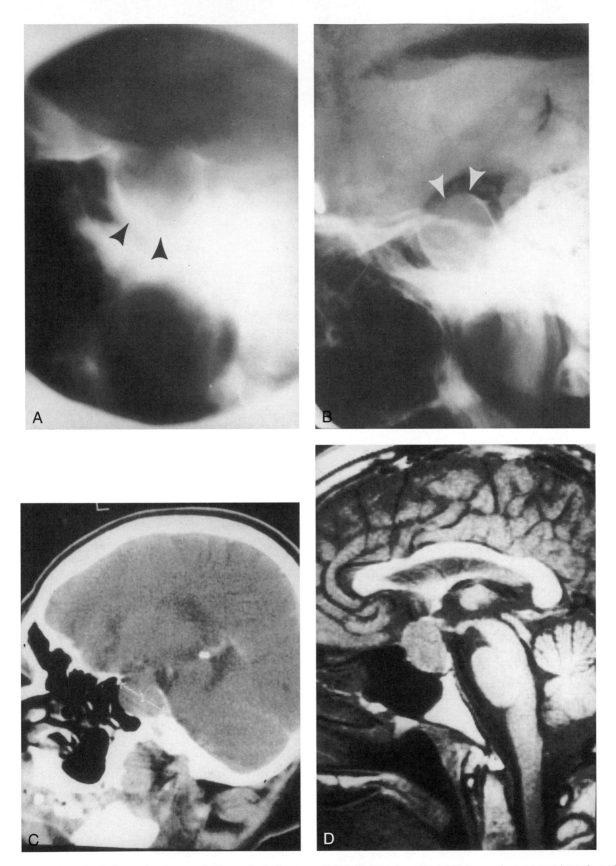

Figure 8.1. Various techniques in demonstration of pituitary macroadenoma. **A.** Sellar tomogram shows enlargement of the sella with downward extension of the sellar floor (*arrowheads*) into the sphenoid sinus. **B.** Lateral skull film of a pneumoencephalogram demonstrates air outlining the upwardly displaced diaphragma sella (*arrowheads*). Note the sellar enlargement with downward extension of the sellar floor into the sphenoid sinus.

C. Sagittal postcontrast CT image shows an enhancing pituitary mass (*arrows*) with extension superiorly into the suprasellar cistern and anteroinferiorly into the sphenoid sinus. **D.** Midsagittal postcontrast T-1 weighted image shows a homogeneously enhancing pituitary mass with superior extension into the suprasellar cistern and compression of the optic chiasm (*arrowhead*).

lateral aspects of the dorsum sella are the paired posterior clinoid processes. The basisphenoid and the basiocciput form the clivus. The junction between the basisphenoid and the basiocciput is the spheno-occipital synchondrosis, an anatomic structure readily visible as an oblique radiolucency on lateral skull radiographs in children.

The superior and lateral aspects of the pituitary gland are covered by dura. Superiorly, the anterior extent of the tentorium covers the pituitary fossa and attaches anteriorly to the anterior clinoid process and the tuberculum sella. Its posterior attachment is to the posterior clinoid processes and the dorsum sella. The dural covering of the sella is the diaphragma sella, which has a central opening containing the pituitary stalk. Laterally, the pituitary gland is enveloped by the dura of the cavernous sinus, with its two layers containing the multiseptated venous sinus. The right and left cavernous sinus has extensive interconnections located superiorly and posteriorly. The cavernous sinus receives venous blood anteriorly from the superior and inferior ophthalmic veins, laterally from the sylvian veins through the sphenoparietal sinus, and inferiorly from the veins of the pterygoid plexus. The cavernous sinus then drains posteriorly through the superior and inferior petrosal sinus to eventually end in the internal jugular vein. The cavernous sinus contains the internal carotid artery (ICA), which travel mostly in a posterior to anterior direction within the sinus. At the level of the anterior clinoid process, the ICA makes a sharp turn superiorly to exit the dura of the cavernous sinus medial to the anterior clinoid process. The ophthalmic artery is a useful angiographic landmark that separates the inferior cavernous segment of the ICA from its superior supraclinoid cisternal segment. Within the cavernous sinus lies the abducens nerve, and along its outer lateral dural layers in a superior to inferior location are the oculomotor, trochlear, and trigeminal nerves.

The pituitary gland is composed of two distinct lobes that have separate and distinct embryologic origins. The anterior lobe of the pituitary gland is thought to arise from the primitive oral cavity, the stomodeum, and the posterior lobe arises from the caudal invagination of the diencephalic neuroectoderm. The anterior pituitary gland or the adenohypophysis has three parts: the pars intermedia, which is small; the pars tuberalis, which forms most of the anterior pituitary lobe; and the pars distalis, which comprises a portion of the pituitary infundibulum and the median eminence of the hypothalamus. The neurohypophysis consists of the posterior lobe, most of the pituitary infundibulum, and the nuclei of the hypothalamus. Located around the pituitary stalk is the hypophyseal portal system, which is the major blood supply to the adenohypophysis. The neurohypophysis derives its blood supply from the hypophyseal arteries and perforating branches of the anterior and middle cerebral arteries. The pituitary gland and the infundibulum do not have a blood-brain barrier and hence readily enhance on contrast studies. The adenohypophysis secretes various stimulating hormones, such as follicle-stimulating hormone, adrenocorticotropic hormone, thyroid-stimulat-

ing hormone, prolactin, growth hormone, and luteinizing hormone, and the neurohypophysis is responsible for vasopressin and oxytocin.

Above the diaphragma sella is the suprasellar cistern, which contains cerebrospinal fluid. The anterior margin of the suprasellar cistern is bordered by the base of the frontal lobes and by the paired cisternal ICA and anterior and middle cerebral arteries. The mesial temporal lobes form its lateral boundaries, and the floor of the third ventricle forms its superior limits. From an anterior to posterior direction, the optic chiasm, the infundibular recess, the tuber cinereum, and mamillary bodies are distinctly shown on midsagittal MRIs as forming the anatomic structures of the floor of the third ventricle. The midbrain and the interpeduncular cistern form its posterior boundaries together with the tip of the basilar artery and the posterior cerebral arteries.

The small size of the pituitary gland and the smaller size of lesions that produce clinical symptoms present a considerable diagnostic challenge. Prior to the advent of modern neuroimaging techniques of CT and MRI, the use of sellar tomography was advocated to detect pituitary masses by looking for sellar enlargement or erosions of the lamina dura of the sellar floor to detect pituitary microadenomas (8). Adjunctive techniques of pneumoencephalography and contrast cisternography outlined the bulge of the suprasellar component of sellar masses (Fig. 8.1A, B). Cerebral angiography showed the displacement of the cavernous and supraclinoid ICA in sellar and parasellar lesions and detected the presence of parasellar aneurysms. These diagnostic techniques, however, presented only indirect proof of the presence of large sellar masses. The advent of CT provided a direct look at the pituitary gland. Subsequent improvement of the technology, with faster scanners capable of performing high-resolution, thin-section studies with dynamic techniques, established its importance in neurodiagnostic evaluation. The development of high-resolution MRI techniques further emphasized the vital role of these studies in establishing the presence of suspected sellar and parasellar lesions and the determination of its location and extent (1, 3, 6, 9) (Fig. 8.1C, D).

MRI AND CT TECHNIQUES

MRI is the preferred neurodiagnostic study in evaluating the pituitary gland. The MRI evaluation of the pituitary gland requires specially directed, detailed examination of the pituitary gland. Our MRI studies of the pituitary gland are done on a 1.5-T magnet, and the protocol primarily consists of high-resolution T1-weighted sagittal and coronal images of the pituitary gland performed before and after the administration of gadolinium-chelated compounds. A T2-weighted coronal study of the sella is also obtained. The T1- and T2-weighted images are done with thin sections (3-mm slice thickness) with a 10% gap, a small field of view (15 to 18 cm), a 256×160 matrix, and multiple averages (4). The coronal postgadolinium studies are performed immediately after contrast administration. In cases in which a parasellar abnormality is suspected, a brain MRI protocol is used. This usually consists of sagittal T1-weighted images (20- to 22-cm field of view), axial or coronal proton-density and T2-weighted images (fast spin-echo technique), and appropriate axial and coronal pregadolinium and postgadolinium studies. Depending on the clinical suspicion and the MRI findings, magnetic resonance angiography with three-dimensional time of flight technique with magnetization transfer technique without the use of contrast material is performed.

In select clinical instances, CT of the pituitary is obtained. Precontrast and postcontrast examinations are performed with the patient in a prone position with the head tilted up in the head holder. Coronal slices are prescribed perpendicular to the canthomeatal line, and the slice angle and sections are chosen to encompass the sella and to avoid dental artifacts. Thin slices (1.5 mm) with appropriate parameters to increase signal to noise are chosen. The contrast studies are done immediately after rapid bolus administration of 75 to 100 cc of nonionic iodinated contrast. Appropriate window and level settings for visualizing the pituitary gland are obtained. With modern CT scanners, this study is performed quickly, resulting in high-quality images of the pituitary gland with little discomfort to the patient. Helical CT of the skull base is done when bony anatomy and detection of the presence of calcification is required for diagnostic evaluation and for surgical planning. These examinations are performed without contrast administration, and helical, 1.0-mm slices are obtained usually from the basion to 1.0 to 2.0 cm above the sella. Review of the axial images as well as the coronal and sagittal reformations are done. Three-dimensional reformations are occasionally required.

Contrast dynamic studies of the pituitary gland improve visualization of microadenomas of the pituitary gland. Bonneville et al. (10, 11) report that dynamic CT studies of the sella show the microadenoma by showing displacement of the vascular tuft seen on the superior aspect of the pituitary. Dynamic MRI studies have also been done with techniques based on modification of regular spin-echo, fast spin-echo, and gradient-echo sequences (12–14). In general, gradient-echo sequences are not preferred because of the magnetic susceptibility artifacts induced by the adjacent sphenoid sinus. Elster (1) suggests a coronal fast spin-echo sequence, available on most commercial MRI scanners, of 3-mm thick sections without gaps and TR of 500 msec, eff TE of 14 msec echo train length of 8, 192 × 256 imaging matrix, 1 NEX, 18-cm field of view, with receiver bandwidth of 32 kHz. Three contiguous images are obtained every 13 seconds with intravenous contrast, and this technique is effective in demonstrating the hypointensity of the pituitary microadenoma in relation to the enhancing pituitary gland. Demonstration on MRI of the transit of contrast through the pituitary gland was accomplished using gradient-echo studies with faster temporal resolution (15). A differential enhancement of the anterior and posterior pituitary lobes was seen with early enhancement of the posterior lobe owing to its arterial blood supply and later

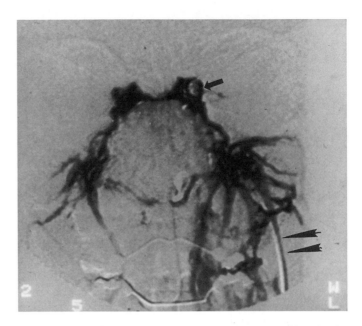

Figure 8.2. Left inferior petrosal sinus venogram. Digital subtraction angiography in the frontal projection shows a catheter (*arrowheads*) at the distal end of the inferior petrosal sinus. The multiple channels of the left inferior petrosal sinus connect to the left cavernous sinus (*arrow*), which intercommunicates with the right cavernous sinus through the circular sinus. The right cavernous sinus then drains inferiorly through the right inferior petrosal sinus to the right jugular vein. The radiolucency in the left cavernous sinus is the anatomic position of the left cavernous ICA.

enhancement of the anterior lobe owing to its venous blood supply. In patients with known microadenoma, the adenoma enhanced at the same time as the posterior lobe. Dynamic MRI studies are performed if the initial imaging studies with high-resolution T1-weighted contrast and noncontrast studies are negative in the face of hormonal abnormalities of a suspected pituitary microadenoma.

In the patient with Cushing's disease, Miller and Doppman describe the technique of inferior petrosal sinus sampling as extremely valuable in lateralizing the functional microadenoma in the pituitary gland (16–18) (Fig. 8.2). In their earlier publications, they describe the performance of this procedure and its relative safety and accuracy. Miller and Strack emphasize the effect of corticotropin-releasing factor stimulation on pituitary secretion as valuable in helping localize the site of the adenoma. Neurologic complications from this procedure are rare (17).

NORMAL MRI ANATOMY OF THE PITUITARY GLAND

On the mid-sagittal image of the head, the pituitary gland is identified as the soft tissue mass located within the sella turcica. On T1-weighted images, the anterior lobe of the pituitary gland is seen as an isointense mass occupying most of the sella. The posterior lobe of the pituitary gland located just anterior to the dorsum sella is identified as a small area of hyperintensity anterior to the dorsum sella (Fig. 8.3A). This hyperintensity is attributed to the phospholipid mem-

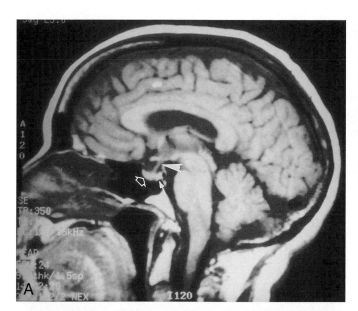

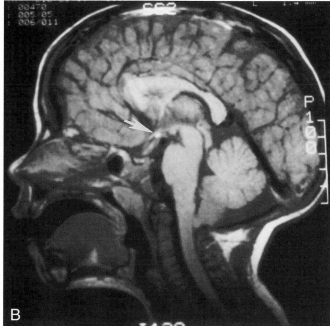

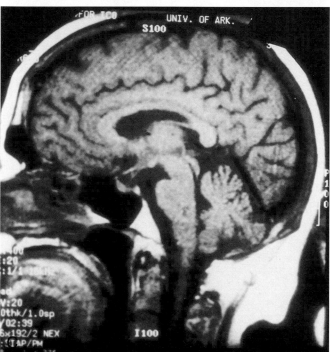

Figure 8.3. Normal midsagittal anatomy of the pituitary region. **A.** Midsagittal unenhanced MRI of the head shows the anatomic relationship of the pituitary fossa. The anterior lobe of the pituitary (*open arrowhead*) is seen as an isointense mass in the pituitary fossa. Posteriorly, the posterior lobe of the pituitary gland (*arrow*) is seen as a small area of hyperintensity. The pituitary stalk (*solid arrowhead*) extends from the pituitary gland to the floor of the third ventricle. The floor of the third ventricle from anterior to posterior is composed of the optic chiasm, the infundibular recess, the tuber cinereum, and the mamillary bodies. **B.** Pituitary dwarfism. An area of hyperintensity (*arrowhead*) is seen in the floor of the third ventricle. The associated findings of a small sella and lack of connection with the pituitary gland confirmed the diagnosis of pituitary dwarfism. **C.** Diabetes insipidus. Absence of the posterior pituitary bright spot is noted in this patient with known diabetes insipidus.

brane, to which the hormones of vasopressin and oxytocin are attached after being produced in the hypothalamus and stored in the posterior pituitary (19–23). Occasionally, this hyperintense signal is located at the hypothalamic end of the pituitary infundibulum and represents an ectopic location of the posterior pituitary hormones (24, 25) (Fig. 8.3*B*). This may be found in normal asymptomatic individuals, although this ectopic location has been described in the rare cases of trauma in which there has been transection of the pituitary stalk. Absence of the hyperintense signal is found in patients with diabetes insipidus (Fig. 8.3*C*). The pituitary

infundibulum extends in the suprasellar cistern from the superior pituitary gland to the hypothalamus at the tuber cinereum. On fluid-attenuated inversion recovery sequence, the pituitary infundibulum is normally seen as a hyperintense linear structure (23). From anterior to posterior, the anatomic structures in the floor of the third ventricle are the optic chiasm, infundibular recess, tuber cinereum, and mamillary bodies. Inferior to the pituitary gland are the air sinuses of the sphenoid sinus.

In the coronal plane, the dural borders of the pituitary gland are identified (Fig. 8.4*A*). Lateral to the pituitary

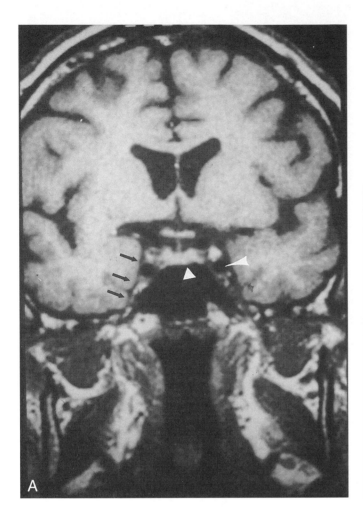

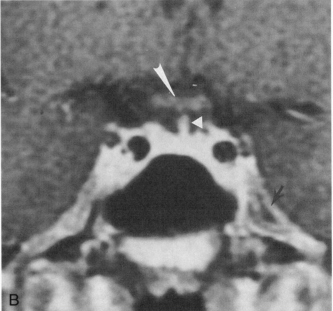

Figure 8.4.   Normal coronal MRI anatomy of the pituitary gland.
A. Coronal T1-weighted image shows the isointense anterior lobe
of the pituitary gland (*triangle*). The pituitary gland is bordered
laterally by the cavernous sinuses, and the medial dural border
it maintains with the cavernous sinus is difficult to see. The lateral
border of the cavernous sinus (*black arrows*) is identified as a
hypointense linear area separating it from the medial aspect of
the temporal lobe. Within the cavernous sinus, the hypointense
area represents the flow void (*arrowhead*) of the cavernous ICA.
B. Coronal postcontrast T-1 weighted image demonstrates intense
enhancement of the pituitary gland. The enhancing pituitary stalk
(*triangle*) extends superiorly to the floor of the third ventricle, and
the rectangular soft tissue mass is the optic chiasm (*arrowhead*).
The hypointense triangular area within the cavernous sinus (*black
arrow*) represents Meckel's cave. The cavernous ICAs abut the
lateral borders of the pituitary gland. Note similar enhancement
of the pituitary gland, cavernous sinus, and infundibulum. **C.** Midsagittal MRI image of the head in a pregnant woman shows an
enlarged pituitary gland with convex superior borders. Note the
hyperintensity of the entire pituitary gland, a normal finding in
pregnant women.

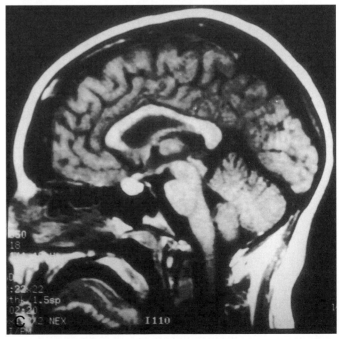

gland is the thin dura of the cavernous sinus, and the flow void of the cavernous ICA is seen within the cavernous sinus. Within the cavernous sinus and not visible on MRI is the abducens nerve. Along the outer layer of dura of the cavernous sinus, from superior to inferior, are the oculomotor, trochlear, and V1 and V2 branches of the trigeminal nerve. In the suprasellar cistern located above the pituitary gland is the midline optic chiasm and the laterally paired supraclinoid ICAs. On a more posterior section, the pituitary infundibulum is seen as the midline linear structure extending from the floor of the third ventricle to the superior border of the pituitary gland. Following contrast material, the pituitary gland and the infundibulum strongly enhance, much like the adjacent cavernous sinus (Fig. 8.4B). The pituitary gland on noncontrast studies is usually isointense and homogeneous in signal intensity. Following contrast material, there is homogeneous enhancement of the pituitary gland. The normal height of the pituitary gland ranges from 3 to 7 mm, and the upper border of the gland is usually flat to concave. In women, the height of the pituitary gland usually measures between 5 and 7 mm, and in men it measures about 3 to 5 mm. There is physiologic hypertrophy of the pituitary gland during adolescence; in women during menstruation, pregnancy, and lactation; and in patients with hypothyroidism (26–31). During pregnancy, on T1-weighted images, the enlarged pituitary gland may have hyperintense signal (Fig. 8.4C). The normal size of the enhancing pituitary stalk is 3.5 mm near the median eminence, 2.8 mm at its midpoint, and about 2 mm at its attachment to the pituitary gland.

THE ABNORMAL PITUITARY GLAND

The most common tumor in the sellar and parasellar region is a pituitary adenoma, constituting about 54% of such lesions. These are benign tumors that originate from the anterior pituitary lobe and are classified as functional or nonfunctional tumors. Radiologic size–based differentiation is made with adenomas less than 10 mm in diameter "microadenomas" and greater than 10 mm in diameter (macroadenomas).

Pituitary Microadenoma

Pituitary microadenoma is the most common sellar mass in adults. Most microadenomas produce prolactin and cause amenorrhea and galactorrhea in women. In most patients, the treatment for hyperprolactinemia produced by a microadenoma is medical treatment with bromocriptine. Indications for surgical treatment vary depending on the patient's wishes, the desire to become pregnant, and failure or inability to tolerate medical therapy (32, 33). In patients with Cushing's disease and acromegaly, surgical resection of the microadenoma is imperative to effect cure of the hormonal problem. On unenhanced CT or MRI studies, microadenomas are relatively hypodense or hypointense

relative to the normal pituitary gland (Fig. 8.5A) They are usually located along the lateral aspect of the pituitary gland. On T2-weighted sequences, the microadenomas have variable signal intensity. Following contrast studies, the microadenomas are seen as hypodense or hypointense mass relative to the strongly enhancing normal pituitary tissue and cavernous sinus (34–37) (Fig.8. 5B, C). It is important to perform the postcontrast studies immediately after a rapid bolus administration of contrast material because delay in timing may make the microadenoma isodense in relation to the normal pituitary gland. The contrast difference between the microadenoma and the normal pituitary gland may be slight, and careful attention to the images have to be done with review of the images in the diagnostic console or photography with narrow windows. Findings on high-resolution MRI studies are highly sensitive, with a 60 to 70% sensitivity on unenhanced studies and increasing by 10% on postcontrast studies (32–36). In patients with Cushing's disease, the same sensitivity is not present because of the smaller size of the tumor at presentation; in these patients, additional studies with dynamic MRI and inferior petrosal sinus sampling may help determine the location and laterality of the lesion (18, 19, 38–40). The high sensitivity of MRI to locate areas of abnormality in the pituitary gland must be tempered in light of the reduced specificity of this examination. Results of multiple studies indicate the presence of hypointense asymptomatic lesions in the pituitary gland, such as pars intermedia cyst, Rathke's cleft cyst, and nonfunctioning pituitary microadenomas. Teramoto et al. (41) reported a 6% incidence of pituitary abnormalities in 1000 unselected autopsy specimens. A prospective study by Chong et al. showed that in 20 of 52 asymptomatic volunteers and in all 14 patients with microadenomas, a focal area of hypointensity was seen in the pituitary gland (42, 43). Medical treatment with bromocriptine may reduce the size of lesions in patients with prolactinomas. Occasionally, bromocriptine therapy may cause the tumors to hemorrhage (Fig. 8.6A–C).

Pituitary Macroadenoma

Most patients with pituitary macroadenomas present because of the mass effect of the large tumor extending in the suprasellar cistern, compressing the optic chiasm, and causing symptoms of bitemporal hemianopia. The patients may also present with hypopituitarism. Most cases were recently shown to be gonadotroph adenomas. On imaging studies, macroadenomas are usually isointense with brain on T1-weighted images and intensely enhance on the contrast study (Fig. 8.7A, B). Because of their course through the diaphragma sella, a figure eight appearance can be seen (Fig. 8.7C). The tumor may show heterogeneity in its enhancement. On T-2 weighted sequences, variable signal intensity is noted. There may be extension of the tumor into the sphenoid sinus with erosion of the sellar floor. The tumor can likewise spread into the parasellar area and

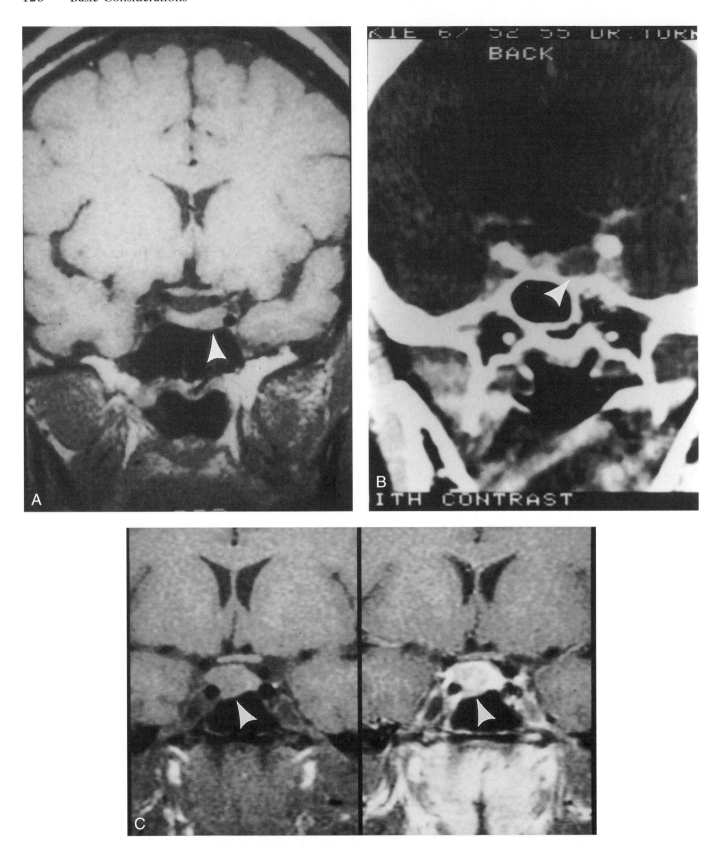

Figure 8.5.   Pituitary microadenoma. **A.** Unenhanced coronal image of the pituitary gland shows a hypointense mass (*arrowhead*) in the left lateral aspect of the pituitary gland. **B.** Enhanced CT of the pituitary gland photographed with narrow windows shows a nonenhancing hypodense mass (*arrowhead*) in the left lateral pituitary gland. **C.** Precontrast and postcontrast MRI of the pituitary gland shows similar findings of a hypointense mass in the pituitary gland (*arrowheads*). Note minimal indentation of the sellar floor.

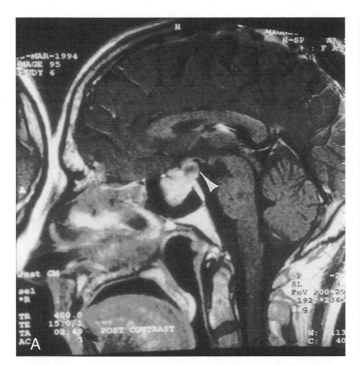

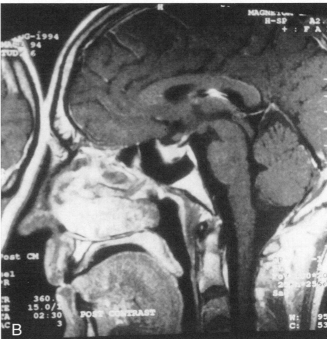

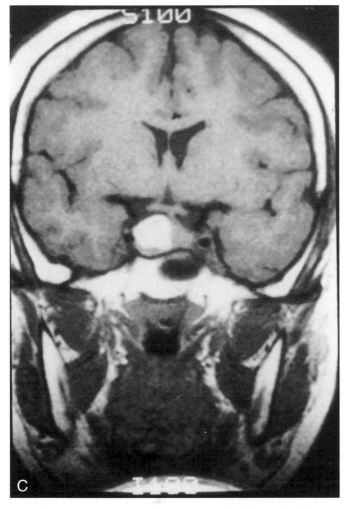

Figure 8.6. Effects of bromocriptine therapy. Sagittal T-1 weighted image **(A)** shows an enlarged enhancing pituitary gland with a superior cystic mass (arrowhead). Following bromocriptine therapy **(B)**, follow-up study shows a decrease in the size of the mass and disappearance of the cystic mass. **C.** Coronal MRI study of the pituitary gland of a known pituitary microadenoma (prolactinoma) following bromocriptine therapy shows a hyperintense area (subacute hemorrhage) in the known site of adenoma.

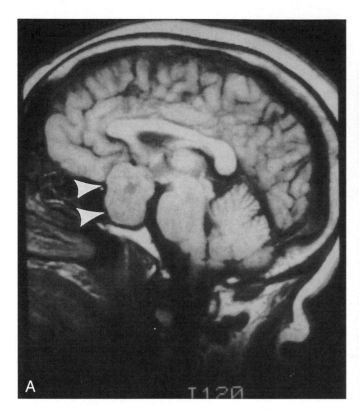

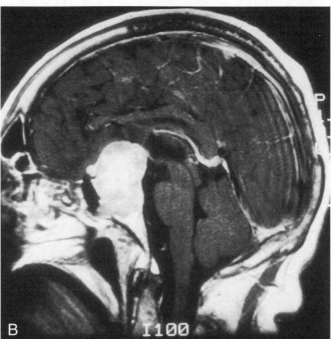

Figure 8.7. Pituitary macroadenoma. Midsagittal T1-weighted unenhanced image **(A)** shows a mostly isointense mass (*arrowheads*) in the pituitary fossa extending into the suprasellar cistern and compressing optic chiasm superoposteriorly. Enhanced MRI of the same area **(B)** shows homogeneous enhancement of the enlarged pituitary gland. **C.** Coronal T1-weighted enhanced image shows figure eight appearance of enhancing pituitary mass as mass passes through the opening of the diaphragma sella to extend into the suprasellar cistern. Notice the bulging of the pituitary mass in the right cavernous sinus, displacing the cavernous carotid artery laterally and bowing the lateral borders of the cavernous sinus.

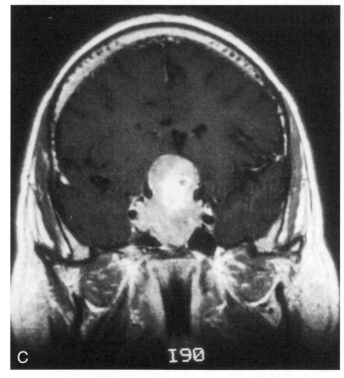

invade the cavernous sinus (44–48). Functionally active tumors like prolactinomas and growth hormone–secreting tumors are more apt to invade the cavernous sinus than are null-cell adenomas. Imaging criteria to suspect invasion of the cavernous sinus include bulging of the cavernous sinus wall, displacement of the cavernous carotid artery, and abnormal signal of the mass in the cavernous sinus.

These findings are not specific, and the only true positive finding is complete encasement by the mass of the cavernous carotid artery (Fig. 8.8). This is because of the difficulty in identifying the medial wall of the dura of the cavernous sinus, and differentiation between invasion and displacement may not be possible. Occasionally, macroadenomas may hemorrhage, and MRI findings will indicate the pres-

OTHER SELLAR/PARASELLAR MASSES

Other masses may involve the sellar and parasellar regions. The list of these abnormalities is large, and in this chapter we discuss the radiologic findings of some of the more common masses in this region.

Empty Sella Syndrome

Empty sella syndrome is the most common incidental finding on imaging studies and is usually not associated with clinical symptoms. The imaging findings are related to the increased amount of subarachnoid fluid found within the sella owing to herniation of the subarachnoid space through a widely open diaphragma sella (Fig. 8.12*A, B*). The pituitary gland appears flattened against the floor of the sella, and the sella is widened. The pituitary infundibulum maintains a midline position. Occasionally, the optic chiasm may herniate into the sella, causing visual difficulties.

Pituitary Cysts

Intrasellar cysts in the pituitary fossa are found incidentally in 20% of autopsy specimens. They are derived from arachnoid or epithelial remnants along Rathke's pouch and include pars intermedia, colloid, Rathke's pouch, arachnoid, epidermoid, and dermoid cysts. Their radiologic appearance accounts for the high incidence of pituitary abnormalities discovered in asymptomatic patients, and they are grouped together under "incidentalomas" (41–43). On CT or MRI studies, the signal characteristics of these cysts vary depending on the content of the cyst, but they are usually hypodense or hypointense lesions. On contrast studies, they do not enhance and are seen as low-density masses within the enhancing pituitary gland. The cyst size will vary, and increased accumulation of fluid is produced by the secretory cells in the cyst wall. Pituitary cysts are located anterior to the pituitary stalk.

Dermoid and epidermoid cysts occur in the suprasellar cistern, although an intrasellar location has been reported. Dermoid cysts contain dermal appendages and fat, whereas epidermoid cysts have desquamated keratin products. On MRI, dermoid cysts are hyperintense on both T1- and T2-weighted images. They do not enhance on postcontrast studies and may manifest clinically as meningitis when there is rupture of the cyst in the subarachnoid space. Epidermoid cysts have similar imaging characteristics as arachnoid cysts. They follow cerebrospinal fluid signal, but close inspection of the images may allow differentiation by the observation of slightly higher signal intensity on T1-weighted images. Diffusion imaging may help differentiate epidermoid cysts. Arachnoid cysts may also occur in the suprasellar location, and in children they have to be differentiated from an enlarged third ventricle herniating into

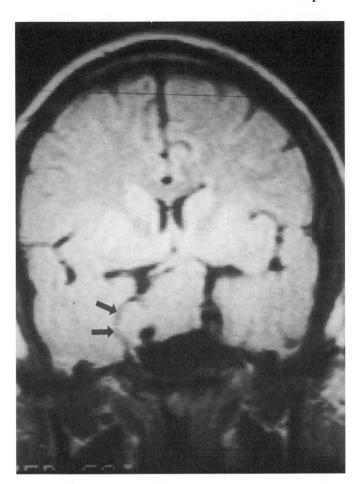

Figure 8.8. Cavernous sinus invasion. Coronal T1-weighted unenhanced image of the pituitary gland shows an enlarged pituitary gland with extension laterally into the cavernous sinus with tumor completely surrounding the carotid artery. Note the significant convexity of the lateral borders of the cavernous sinus (*arrows*).

ence and age of the hemorrhage (Fig. 8.9*A–C*). Pituitary apoplexy is known to occur in the postpartum period. Hemorrhage, however, has been found to occur in microadenomas and may be clinically occult. Cystic pituitary adenomas may also be seen (Fig. 8.10). Invasive prolactinomas with lytic involvement of the clivus or sphenoid sinus may present with a sellar mass and skull base involvement and has to be differentiated from squamous cell carcinoma of the nasopharynx or sphenoid sinus, plasmacytoma of the sphenoid sinus, and clival chordomas (Fig. 8.11*A, B*).

Postoperatively, radiologic assessment with CT or MRI is difficult because of the presence of postoperative changes of granulation tissue, fibrosis, graft, and postoperative fluid. The pituitary gland height following surgery slowly diminishes over time, and the best marker for establishing the true postoperative height of the pituitary gland after surgery is a study 8 weeks after surgical removal of the tumor. Growth in size of the tumor or recurrence of symptoms are useful criteria for the presence of tumor recurrence.

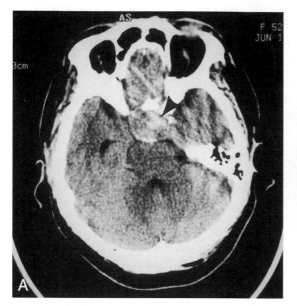

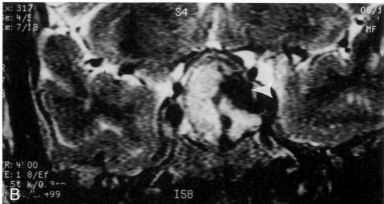

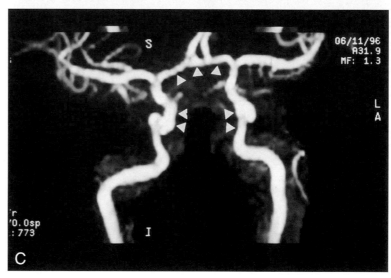

Figure 8.9. Pituitary apoplexy with hemorrhage. A. Noncontrast CT of the head shows scattered areas of hyperdensity (*arrowhead*) in a suprasellar mass. B. Coronal T2-weighted image of the pituitary gland shows an area of significant hypointensity (*arrowhead*) in the large pituitary mass, which bulges into the suprasellar cistern. These findings confirm the diagnosis of hemorrhage occurring in a pituitary macroadenoma. C. Magnetic resonance angiogram of the head using three-dimensional time of flight technique shows displacement of the parasellar carotid artery and its anterior cerebral artery branches (*triangles*) by the large sellar mass, which extended into the suprasellar cistern.

the pituitary fossa. Anterior displacement of the pituitary stalk is a helpful sign to determine the mass effect of the arachnoid cyst as it bows the membrane of Lillequist (49–51) (Fig. 8.13).

Rathke's Cleft Cyst

Rathke's pouch embryologically develops from the primitive oral cavity and grows cranially to form the adenohypophysis. Its cranial elongation forms the craniopharyngeal duct, and its distal part forms the anterior pituitary lobe. Failure to close this pouch creates a cyst that lies between the anterior and intermediate lobe of the pituitary gland (52–56). The contents of the cyst are mixed, ranging from mucoid to serous to cellular, and account for its varied appearance on MRI (Fig. 8.14A–C). The cyst is usually intrasellar, small, and typically asymptomatic. Ross et al. (52) describe the MRI appearance as related to its protein content, with low protein content appearing as low signal

on T1-weighted images and as high signal on T2-weighted images, medium protein content as high signal on both T1- and T2-weighted images, and high protein content as high signal on T1-weighted images and low signal on T2-weighted images. Occasionally, primary suprasellar location has been described. The differentiation from a craniopharyngioma that is derived from the same embryologic remnant may be made by presence of calcification in the lesion or around the cyst wall with craniopharyngioma.

Craniopharyngioma

Craniopharyngiomas are epithelial tumors that arise primarily in the sellar and suprasellar location. There is a bimodal age distribution, with tumors more commonly occurring in the young, in the first three decades of life, but also occurring in the fifth to seventh decades of life. In a recent article, Sartoretti-Schefer et al. (57) describe MRI correlation of craniopharyngiomas with the pathologic classification of adamantinous and squamous papillary types. The adamantinous type are the tumors of childhood and young adults and are characterized by the presence of large, lobulated cysts in the sellar/suprasellar location. On MRI, the cysts are hyperintense on T1-weighted images and pathologically correlate with the high protein content and free methemoglobin within the cysts (Fig. 8.15A–C). Variable amounts of cholesterol and triglycerides are present, but their concentrations do not appear to change the signal intensity of the cyst. Calcification and encasement of the arterial subarachnoid vessels are frequently found. Solid enhancing lesions are likewise noted, and the associated finding of hypointense cyst on T1-weighted images are also seen. The squamous papillary subtype is found in adults, and the tumors are frequently solid and enhance intensely. The associated cysts are hypointense on T1-weighted images and hyperintense on T2-weighted images, reflecting its watery/keratin content (Fig. 8.15D). Calcification may be present, but not as frequently as in the adamantinous type. Embryologically, craniopharyngiomas arise from remnants of Rathke's pouch that are derived from the stomodeum of the primitive oral cavity. As Rathke's pouch separates from the oral cavity, the craniopharyngeal duct that connects Rathke's pouch to the stomodeum regresses (58). The cranial end of Rathke's pouch as it meets its counterpart from the caudal evagination of the diencephalon undergoes proliferation and rotation. This embryologic development explains the occurrence of craniopharyngiomas in the sellar and suprasellar region as well as in the nasopharynx and the sphenoid sinus and along the migration route of the craniopharyngeal duct (59–63). Com-

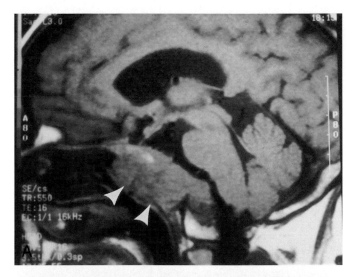

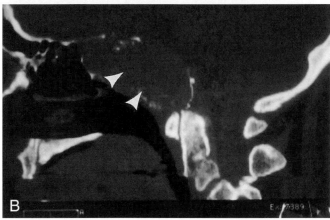

Figure 8.11. Invasive pituitary adenoma. **A.** Sagittal unenhanced T1-weighted image shows a large mass extending along the clivus (*arrowheads*). This extends inferiorly into the occipital condyle. **B.** Sagittal reconstructed CT from a helical CT of the head shows lytic mass destroying the bony outline of the sella and clivus (*arrowheads*). The patient clinically had significantly elevated levels of prolactin.

plete resection of craniopharyngiomas may not be possible in some clinical instances, and recurrence of tumor are more common in the adamantinous type of tumor. This is caused by the tight adherence of these tumors to the adjacent normal brain. Pseudoaneurysms of the adjacent ICA can occur following surgery, and an enhancing mass in the operative site should raise the suspicion of its possible presence and not be solely attributed to tumor recurrence (64).

Pituitary Metastases

Metastatic involvement to the pituitary gland and hypothalamic structures occurs from systemic or local spread. At autopsy, metastases in the pituitary gland are seen in 10% of cases. Of sellar/suprasellar masses, they make up about 1% of all cases. Lung and breast cancer are the most common primary tumors to involve the pituitary gland, and other cancers known to involve the area include prostate,

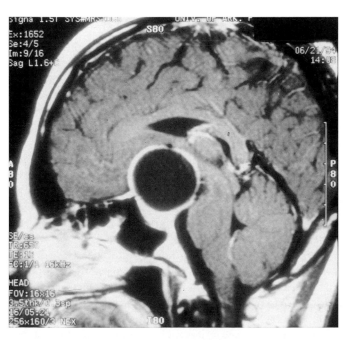

Figure 8.10. Cystic pituitary adenoma. Midsagittal enhanced T1-weighted image shows a large pituitary mass with extension of a large cystic component into the suprasellar cistern, with posterior displacement of the floor of the third ventricle.

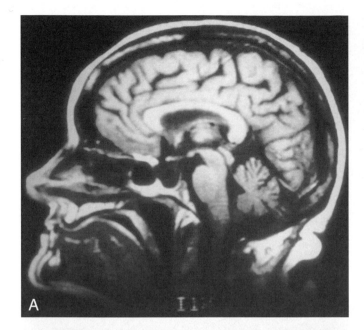

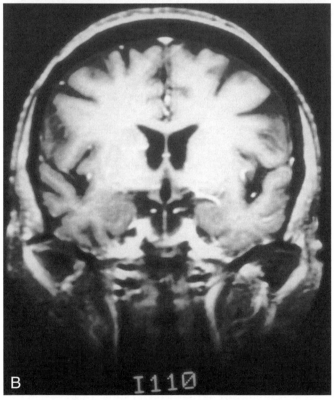

Figure 8.12. Empty sella. **A.** Sagittal T1-weighted image shows a hypointense area in the pituitary fossa with an elongated pituitary stalk. **B.** Postcontrast T1-weighted MRI of the head shows an area of hypointensity in the suprasellar cistern that extends into the pituitary fossa and inferiorly displaces the enhancing pituitary gland.

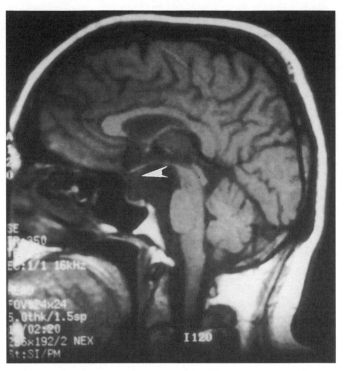

Figure 8.13. Arachnoid cyst. Midsagittal unenhanced T1-weighted image shows a hypointense mass in the posterior suprasellar cistern displacing the floor of the third ventricle superiorly and the midbrain posteriorly. Notice the anterior displacement of the infundibular stalk (*arrowhead*).

stomach, kidney, malignant melanoma, bladder, uterus, pancreas, and lymphoma/leukemia (65). Local spread of tumor to the pituitary gland may develop from primary ear, nose, throat tumors of the skull base involving the sphenoid sinus or nasopharynx. Plasmacytomas of the sphenoid sinus are not uncommon.

Most patients with systemic metastases to the pituitary gland are clinically asymptomatic. In 15% of patients, their clinical presentation is marked by acute and rapid progression, and symptoms of panhypopituitarism, diabetes insipidus, or cranial nerve palsy are present. MRI characteristics show a sellar or suprasellar mass, isointense on T1-weighted images and isointense to hyperintense mass on T2-weighted images. Strong enhancement usually follows contrast administration. Involvement of the adjacent cavernous sinus and pituitary infundibulum may be seen, which may make these indistinguishable from pituitary adenomas. A helpful differentiating point is the presence of other brain lesions.

With local spread of tumor from a nearby primary source, usually a squamous cell carcinoma of the nasopharynx or the subjacent sphenoid sinus, destruction of the midskull base is seen in association with the primary mass. This process is best shown on coronal imaging (Fig. 8.16A). An expansile lesion such as a mucocele of the sphenoid sinus may cause compression of the sellar and parasellar structures. Expansion of the bony walls of the sinus is usually present, and the contents of the mucocele is usually

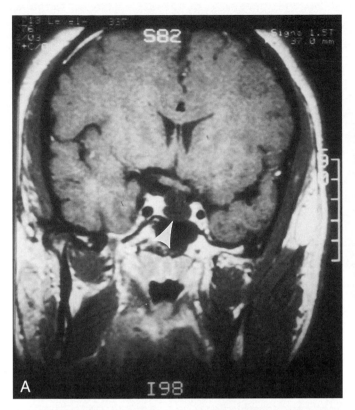

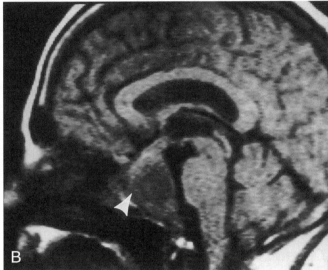

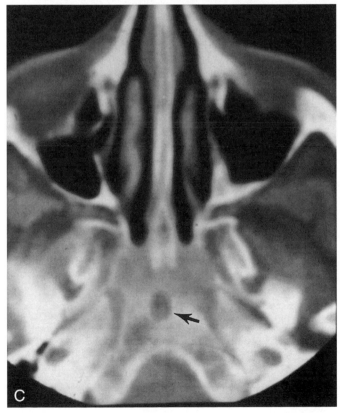

Figure 8.14. Rathke's cleft cyst. **A.** Coronal enhanced T1-weighted image shows a hypointense mass (*arrowhead*) in the sella with minimal extension in the suprasellar cistern. **B.** Sagittal unenhanced T1-weighted image shows a hypointense mass in the sellar-suprasellar area (*arrowhead*) with signal intensity higher than the adjacent cerebrospinal fluid. Mass extends in the suprasellar cistern. **C.** Cranial CT of the skull base shows a foramen (*arrow*) at the base of the clivus representing the primitive craniopharyngeal duct.

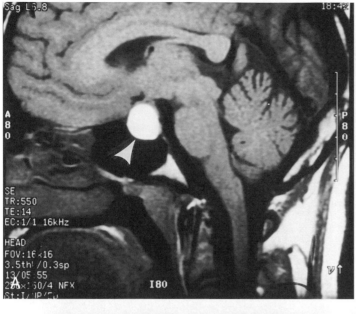

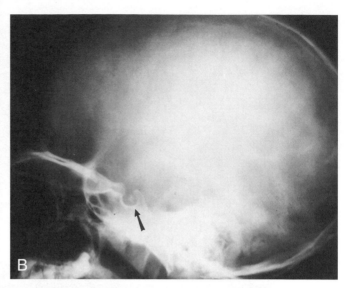

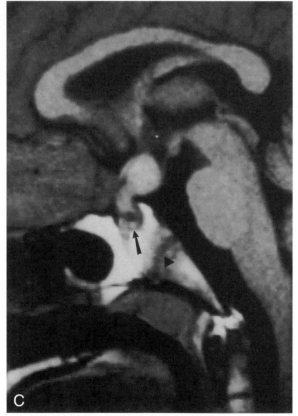

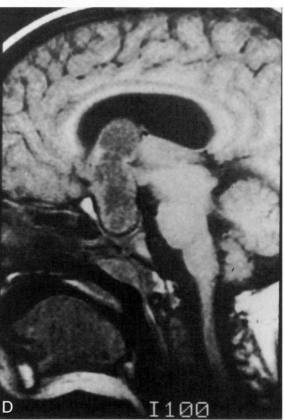

Figure 8.15. Craniopharyngioma. **A.** Sagittal unenhanced T1-weighted image shows a primary intrasellar hyperintense mass (*arrowhead*) in the pituitary fossa extending superiorly in the suprasellar cistern. This finding in a 30-year-old female is difficult to differentiate from a Rathke's cleft cyst, a primary intrasellar dermoid cyst, or a purely cystic pituitary adenoma. **B.** Lateral skull film shows a discrete focal calcified mass (*arrow*) in the pituitary fossa. **C.** Sagittal unenhanced T1-weighted image of the same case in Fig. 8.15*B* shows the calcification to be hypointense (*arrow*), and there is an associated hyperintense linear

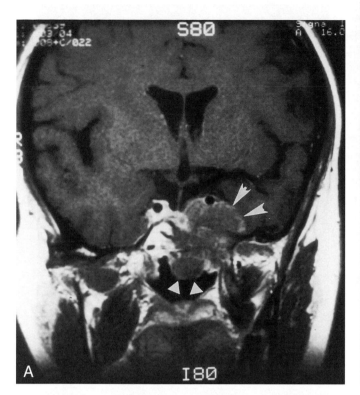

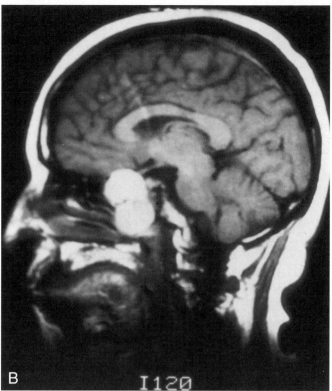

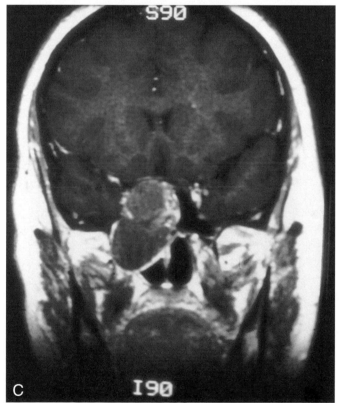

Figure 8.16.   A. Nasopharyngeal carcinoma. Coronal postcontrast T1-weighted image shows a large soft tissue mass extending from the nasopharynx (*triangles*) through the sphenoid sinus to invade the pituitary fossa and adjacent cavernous sinus (*arrowheads*). Sphenoid sinus mucocele. **B.** Midsagittal unenhanced T1-weighted image shows a hyperintense mass in the region of the sphenoid sinus. The mass displaces the pituitary fossa posteriorly and invades the planum sphenoidale. **C.** Coronal postcontrast T1-weighted image shows a hypointense mass with surrounding mucosal enhancement in the sphenoid sinus, which expands inferiorly into the nasal cavity and superiorly into the planum sphenoidale.

Figure 8.15. *(continued)* mass (*triangle*) extending in the area of the pituitary infundibulum with a hyperintense rounded mass in the suprasellar cistern displacing the chiasm anteriorly and elevating the floor of the third ventricle. The combination of these findings with calcification and hyperintense mass points to the diagnosis of craniopharyngioma. **D.** Midsagittal

T1-weighted MRI shows a hypointense mass extending from the sellar area to the suprasellar region extending superiorly and compressing the foramen of Monro. There is resultant hydrocephalus. Hypointense cysts are associated with craniopharyngiomas and are more likely to be found in the papillary squamous type.

hyperintense on T1-weighted sequences because of their high protein content and show no enhancement on the contrast studies (Fig. 8.16B, C). Thick wall enhancement occurs when there is concomitant infection (pyocele) of the involved sinus. The MRI appearance of lymphoma metastatic to the brain structures affects the basal meninges in a focal or diffuse fashion and commonly causes diffuse infiltration of the cranial nerves.

Lymphocytic Hypophysitis

Lymphocytic hypophysitis is a rare inflammatory disorder of the pituitary gland involving the adenohypophysis (66–68). Pathologic confirmation of this disease is made by the finding of lymphocytic infiltration of the anterior lobe. Clinical presentation is varied but usually occurs in women late during pregnancy or in the immediate postpartum period. Patients complain of headache and visual problems and have hypopituitarism. Imaging characteristics are that of a sellar/suprasellar mass, which is isointense on T1-weighted images and homogeneously or heterogeneously enhanced on postcontrast studies and simulate a macroadenoma. Ahmadi et al. (66) notes common associated findings of enhancement of the pituitary infundibulum, adjacent dura, and sphenoid sinus together with the pituitary enlargement.

Aneurysm

Giant aneurysms of the cavernous and supraclinoid ICA present as large masses in the sellar and parasellar region. Depending on location and size, these aneurysms may compress the contents of the cavernous sinus or optic chiasm and clinically present with cranial nerve palsy, visual field defects or symptoms secondary to their mass effect. CT scans may show erosion of the adjacent bony wall around the cavernous sinus, with circumferential or lamellar calcification within the wall of the aneurysm. In a nonthrombosed giant aneurysm on CT, the mass intensely enhances following contrast administration, and this represents the true lumen of the aneurysm (Fig. 8.17A, B) This may simulate the appearance of other masses in the sellar/suprasellar location. On MRI, the aneurysm shows a circumscribed area of flow void, with associated phase artifacts corresponding to the disturbed flow within the lumen. With partially thrombosed aneurysm, crescentic areas of intermediate to high signal intensity are seen in the wall of the aneurysm on MRI and represents methemoglobin in the wall of aneurysm. Angiography reveals the patent lumen of the aneurysm, which may be significantly smaller than the total size of the aneurysm (69, 70).

Meningioma

Meningiomas comprise the most common benign tumor of the intracranial cavity, making up 20% of all intracranial tumors. Ten percent of all meningiomas occur in the parasel-

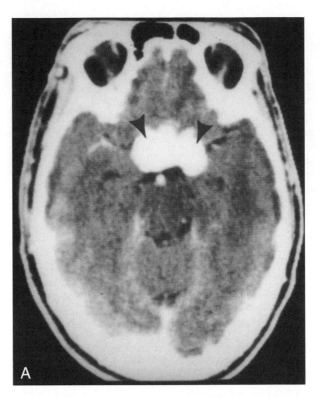

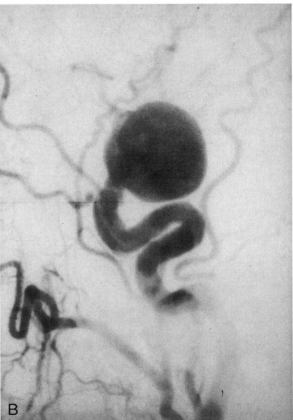

Figure 8.17. Bilateral carotid aneurysms. **A.** Postcontrast axial CT of the head shows a large enhancing mass (*arrowheads*) in the suprasellar cistern. **B.** Right common carotid arteriogram in the lateral projection shows a nonthrombosed giant aneurysm of the left supraclinoid ICA. A similar nonthrombosed aneurysm of the right supraclinoid ICA was also shown on the opposite side injection (not shown).

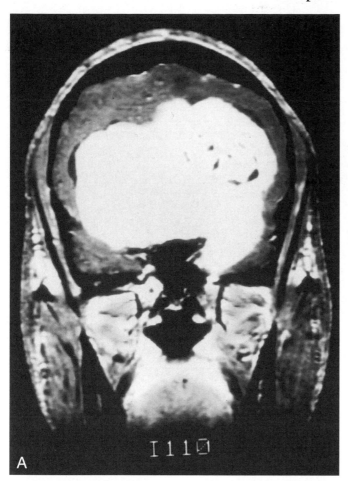

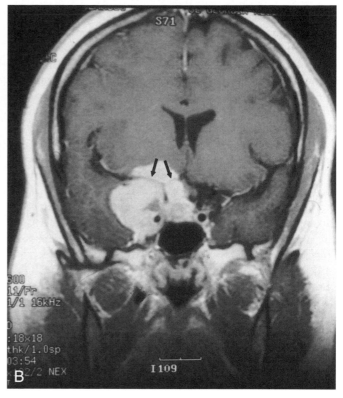

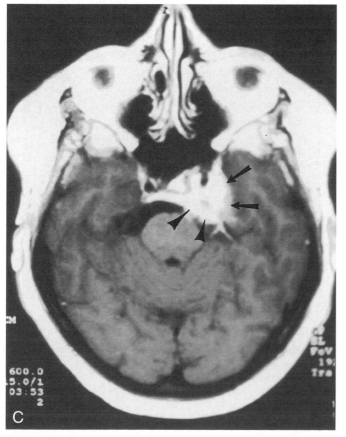

Figure 8.18.   Meningiomas (multiple sites). **A.** Coronal postcontrast T1-weighted image shows a large enhancing mass superior to the planum sphenoidale occupying most of the anterior cranial fossa and laterally into the middle cranial fossa. **B.** Postcontrast coronal T1-weighted image shows an enhancing mass that started from the anterior clinoid process and extends posteriorly in the suprasellar cistern to invade the right cavernous sinus and encompass the right supraclinoid ICA and the anterior and middle cerebral arteries (*arrows*). **C.** Postcontrast axial T1-weighted image demonstrates an enhancing mass in the posterior cavernous sinus (*arrows*) with mild extension into the posterior cranial fossa (*arrowhead*).

lar area (71–75). These may arise from the diaphragma sella, tuberculum sella, anterior or posterior clinoid processes, planum sphenoidale, walls of the cavernous sinus, or medial sphenoid wing and can involve all compartments of the cranial fossa, especially with the large sphenopetroclival type (Fig. 8.18A–C). Cranial nerve palsy, visual symptoms, and headaches are associated symptoms. Meningiomas are characterized by their broad-based dural attachment with a soft tissue mass that has clumpy, psammomatous, or ringlike calcification. MRIs show an isointense mass on all imaging sequences that homogeneously and intensely enhances on postcontrast studies. Enhancement of the associated dura is seen with a dural tail sign. Associated hyperostosis of the involved bone is seen with increased signal intensity in the marrow of the hyperostotic bone. On CT, hyperostosis is noted in about 43% of cases, with associated calcification within the mass in 20% of cases. The mass is isointense with brain on noncontrast studies and homogeneously enhances. On angiography, the mass shows a hypervascular blush usually supplied by dural vessels, but with cavernous sinus involvement, multiple branches from the cavernous internal carotid supply may be the dominant blood supply. Diaphragma sella meningiomas may be difficult to differentiate from a homogeneously enhancing mass of a pituitary macroadenoma, and differentiation may be obtained by careful search for the diaphragma sella and the differential enhancement of the tumor in relation to the normal pituitary gland.

Optic/Hypothalamic Glioma

Gliomas of the visual pathway constitute about 5% of primary brain tumors in childhood and 2% in adults. In children, about 20 to 50% are associated with neurofibromatoses type 1. Histologically, the childhood tumors are low-grade tumors of the juvenile pilocytic variety (76, 77). They may involve the intraorbital or intracranial segments of the optic pathways in a focal or diffuse fashion. Optic gliomas spread along the optic pathways and may invade the hypothalamus. CT scans may show an enlarged optic canal with a focal isodense mass of the optic nerve that variably enhances after contrast administration. MRIs show the enlarged optic nerve or chiasm, which is hypointense to isointense on T1-weighted images and hyperintense on T2-weighted images. Optic gliomas may enhance on the postcontrast MRI studies, and extended enhancement along the optic pathways to the optic tract as well as hyperintensity on T2-weighted images along that pathway may distinguish optic pathway gliomas.

Hypothalamic gliomas have similar imaging characteristics as optic pathway gliomas. Growth of these tumors occurs inferiorly and anteriorly to involve the optic chiasm and may make differentiation of primary source of tumor difficult. The principal clinical presentation of hypothalamic dysfunction indicates a hypothalamic primary origin. Optic pathway gliomas are suggested with growth along the optic tracts or findings of hyperintense signal in unassociated cerebral white matter tracts, which may indicate the presence of neurofibromatoses (Fig. 8.19).

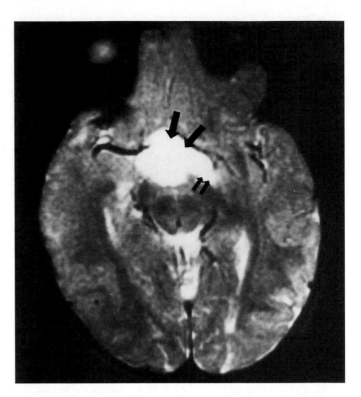

Figure 8.19. Optic glioma. Axial T2-weighted image shows a hyperintense mass (*large arrows*) in the area of the optic chiasm. There is extension of this mass along the optic pathway of the left optic tract (*small arrows*). This is indicative of an optic chiasm glioma.

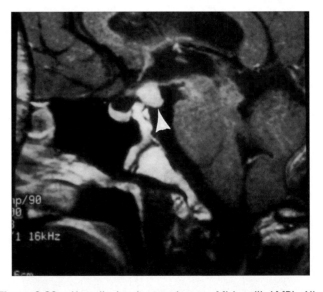

Figure 8.20. Hypothalamic germinoma. Midsagittal MRI of the head shows an enhancing pedunculated mass (*arrowhead*) in the floor of the third ventricle posterior to the pituitary infundibulum. The finding of a midline mass in either the pineal region or the hypothalamic region in a young patient should indicate its possible presence.

Germinoma

Germinomas are rare tumors of germ cell origin usually in the first three decades of life. They occur in the midline, in either the pineal gland or the hypothalamic region. Suprasellar germinomas are more common in women, and the pineal location is more common in men (78). They are usually the least malignant of the germ cell tumors but have the capacity to metastasize along the subarachnoid passageways. Patients with suprasellar germinomas clinically present with diabetes insipidus or visual disturbance or have panhypopituitarism. A suprasellar mass is usually seen on imaging studies and is isointense on T1-weighted images and hyperintense on T2-weighted images. Contrast studies usually show significant enhancement of the mass which is usually located posterior to the pituitary infundibulum at the hypothalamic end (Fig. 8.20). The mass may invade the sellar region. Germinomas may shed cells into the subarachnoid space, and contrast MRI may show the leptomeningeal spread of tumor.

Histiocytosis X

Langerhans' cell histiocytosis or histocytosis X may result in pituitary stalk thickening (79, 80). Clinically, they present with central diabetes insipidus. The MRI findings of this entity show a thickened pituitary infundibulum that enhances intensely following contrast administration. Focal

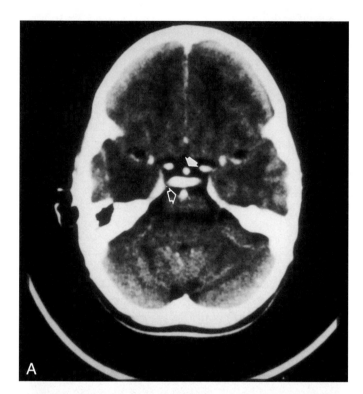
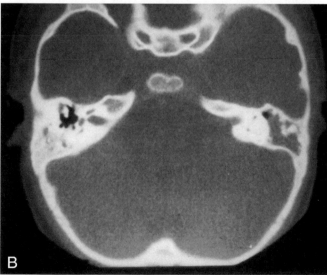

Figure 8.21. Histiocytosis X. **A.** Postcontrast axial CT scan shows the pituitary infundibulum (*solid arrowhead*) to be as large as the more posterior basilar artery (*open arrowhead*). **B.** Axial CT scan through the temporal bone shows a soft tissue mass in the left temporal bone. The combination of findings in a young patient with diabetes insipidus with an enlarged infundibular stalk and a lytic lesion of bone usually in the temporal bone indicate the diagnosis of histiocytosis X.

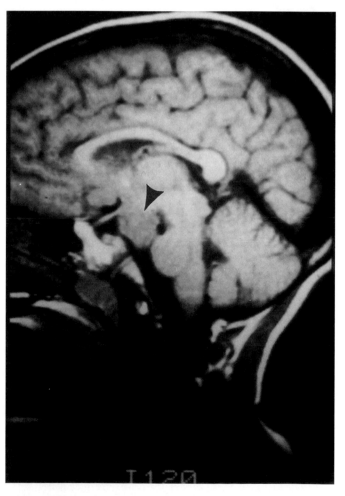

Figure 8.22. Hamartoma of tuber cinereum. Sagittal T1-weighted MRI image shows an isointense pedunculated mass (*arrowhead*) in the floor of the third ventricle centered around the tuber cinereum. In this 6-year-old male with precocious puberty, the diagnosis of hamartoma of the tuber cinereum is the most likely possibility.

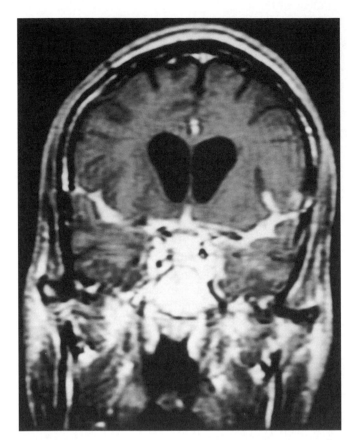

Figure 8.23. Cryptococcal meningitis. Coronal postcontrast image shows diffuse enhancement along the basilar meninges with enhancement extending into the interhemispheric fissure and both sylvian cisterns. Involvement of the meninges can be focal or diffuse, and postcontrast MRI images are the most efficacious neuroimaging tool to diagnose its presence and extent.

enhancement in the hypothalamus may be seen. The normal hyperintensity of the posterior pituitary bright spot is usually absent. On axial CT, the pituitary infundibulum is normally smaller than the basilar artery. The finding of similar or enlarged size of the infundibulum should make one suspicious of an enlarged pituitary stalk (Fig. 8.21*A*, *B*). The combination of findings of a young child with diabetes insipidus and the imaging findings of an enlarged pituitary stalk should make one suspicious of the diagnosis of Langerhans' cell histiocytosis. This diagnosis is made when there are associated masses, and a search is best done with chest radiograph, temporal bone CT, or bone scans. Other causes for infundibular stalk thickening include an infundibuloma (glioma), choristoma (granular cell tumor, myoblastoma), sarcoidosis, and metastasis.

Hamartoma of Tuber Cinereum

These are congenital nonneoplastic heterotopias found in the floor of the third ventricle and occur in children who present with precocious puberty. The tumors lie between the infundibular recess and the mamillary bodies and present as large masses in the suprasellar cistern. On MRI, the pedunculated masses are usually isointense on all imaging sequences, although cystic regions within the mass showing as hyperintense signal within the mass on T2-weighted se-

quences may be shown (Fig. 8.22). They do not enhance following contrast administration.

Sarcoidosis and Other Inflammatory Lesions

Sarcoidosis can involve the intracranial cavity as a focal infundibular mass or focal suprasellar or diffuse basal meningitis. On contrast MRI imaging studies, a focal mass in the pituitary stalk or enhancement of the basilar meninges in a focal or diffuse fashion can be seen (Fig. 8.23). Infiltration of the base of the brain via involvement of the Virchow-Robin spaces can also be found. These MRI findings are nonspecific and may be noted with subarachnoid spread with infection or tumor. Other infectious processes associated with diffuse basilar meningitis include tuberculosis, cryptococcus, blastomycosis, and other chronic infections.

Chordoma and Chondrosarcomas

Chordomas are tumors of primitive notochordal remnants that occur most frequently in the sacrum and clivus. Clival chordomas make up about 30% of all known chordomas (81). They occur typically in a midline location close to the spheno-occipital synchondroses. The tumor starts in the bony clivus but typically breaks through the cortex to present as an intracranial mass in the posterior fossa. The soft tissue mass may extend in the pituitary fossa, the sphenoid sinus, or the nasopharynx (Fig. 8.24). They can be found in an off-midline position in the cavernous sinus. Chordomas are destructive lesions, and frequent calcification of the associated soft tissue mass is seen. Noncontrast CT shows lytic

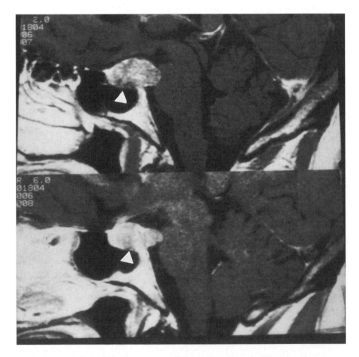

Figure 8.24. Clival chordoma. Sagittal postcontrast T1-weighted images show an enhancing mass (*triangles*) in the posterior portion of the pituitary fossa centered around the dorsum sella. There is extent anteriorly into the pituitary fossa with displacement of the infundibular stalk and posteriorly into the prepontine cistern.

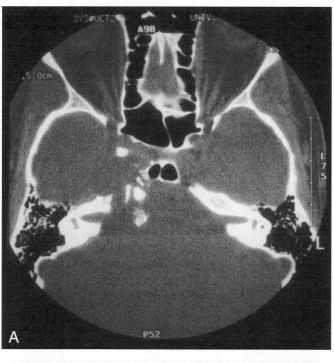

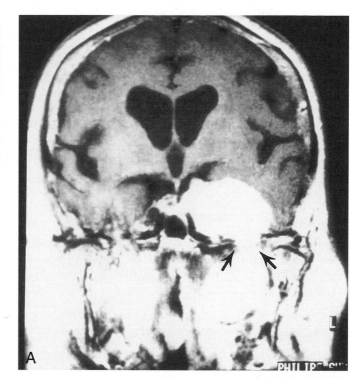

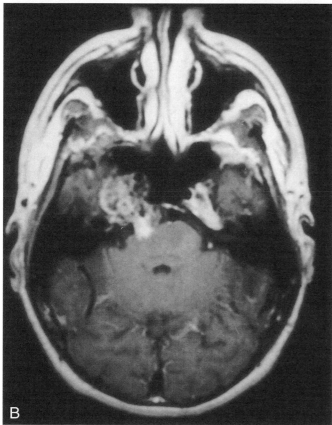

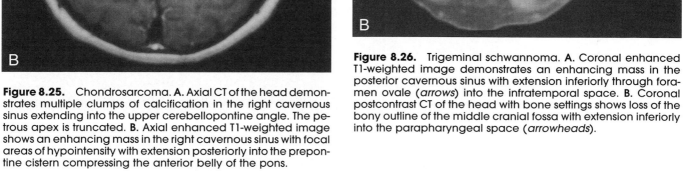

Figure 8.25. Chondrosarcoma. **A.** Axial CT of the head demonstrates multiple clumps of calcification in the right cavernous sinus extending into the upper cerebellopontine angle. The petrous apex is truncated. **B.** Axial enhanced T1-weighted image shows an enhancing mass in the right cavernous sinus with focal areas of hypointensity with extension posteriorly into the prepontine cistern compressing the anterior belly of the pons.

Figure 8.26. Trigeminal schwannoma. **A.** Coronal enhanced T1-weighted image demonstrates an enhancing mass in the posterior cavernous sinus with extension inferiorly through foramen ovale (*arrows*) into the infratemporal space. **B.** Coronal postcontrast CT of the head with bone settings shows loss of the bony outline of the middle cranial fossa with extension inferiorly into the parapharyngeal space (*arrowheads*).

involvement of the clivus with associated soft tissue calcification. On MRI, they are hypointense on T1-weighted images in relation to the adjacent hyperintense normal marrow. On T2-weighted images, they are usually hyperintense and enhance variably on the postcontrast studies. Chondrosarcomas are rare tumors that occur in the same area as chordomas. They have similar imaging characteristics and may be indistinguishable (82). The finding of a chondroid calcification on CT aids in the differential diagnosis of these masses, and the off-midline position of chondrosarcomas may help in differentiating this tumor (Fig. 8.25A, B).

Neurinomas

Schwannomas or neurofibromas may affect the cisternal or cavernous portion of cranial nerves III to VI. The tri-

geminal nerve is the most commonly involved nerve. Involvement may be focal or diffuse, involving the various divisions of the trigeminal nerve in patients with neurofibromatoses. The lesion tends to be locally expansile, causes remodeling and enlargement of the adjacent bone and skull base foramina. They are solid lesions and enhance homogeneously after contrast administration (Fig. 8.26A, B). Cystic degeneration with tumoral necrosis can occur, and the lesions may shown heterogeneity on imaging studies (83, 84). Cavernous hemangiomas are a form of vascular malformation that is usually found within the brain parenchyma. A rare location is in the cavernous sinus, and MRI characteristics that may suggest its presence include the finding of significantly hyperintense signal on T2-weighted images and strong enhancement after contrast administration (Fig. 8.27A, B).

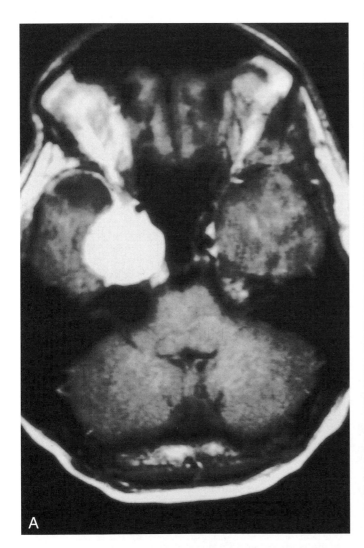
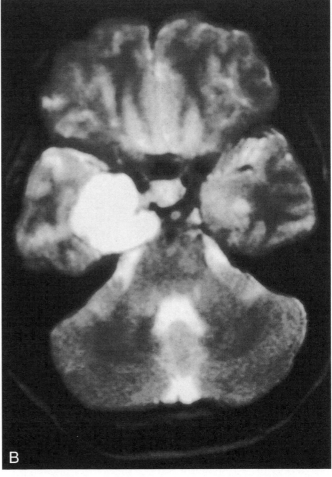

Figure 8.27. Cavernous hemangioma. **A.** Axial postcontrast T1-weighted image shows a significantly enhancing mass in the cavernous sinus with bulging of the cavernous sinus walls. **B.** Axial T2-weighted image demonstrates the mass to be hyperintense and extending posteriorly into the upper cerebellopontine angle. The MRI appearance of the mass is nonspecific but the combination of findings of a hyperintense homogenous mass on T2-weighted images and marked enhancement may lead one to suspect its presence.

REFERENCES

1. Elster A. Modern imaging of the pituitary. Radiology 1993;187:1–14.
2. Wolpert S. The radiology of pituitary adenomas. Endocrinol Metab Clin North Am 1987;16(3):553–583.
3. Montanera W, Kucharczyk W. Imaging of sellar and parasellar lesions. In: Wilkins R, Regenchary S, eds. Neurosurgery. New York: McGraw-Hill, 1996;1:1253–1272.
4. Post K, McCormick P, Bello J. Differential diagnosis of pituitary tumors. Endocrinol Metab Clin North Am 1987;16(3):609–629.
5. Felsberg G, Tien R. Sellar and parasellar lesions involving the skull base. Neuroimaging Clin N Am 1994;4(3):543–560.
6. Johnsen D, Woodruff W, Allen I, et al. MR imaging of the sellar and juxtasellar regions. Radiographics 1991;11:727–758.
7. Aron D, Tyrrell J, Wilson C. Pituitary tumors: current concepts in diagnosis and management. West J Med 1995;162:340–352.
8. Geehr R, Allen W, Rothman S, et al. Pluridirectional tomography in the evaluation of pituitary tumors. Am J Roentgenol 1978;130:105–109.
9. Karnaze M, Sartor K, Winthrop J, et al. Suprasellar lesions: evaluation with MR imaging. Radiology 1986;161:77–82.
10. Bonneville J, Catlin F, Moussa-Bacha K, et al. Dynamic computed tomography of the pituitary gland: the "Tuft Sign." Radiology 1983;149:145–148.
11. Bonneville J, Catlin F, Dietermannn J. Computed tomography of the pituitary gland. Berlin: Springer-Verlag, 1986;33–46.
12. Finnelli D, Kaufman B. Varied microcirculation of pituitary adenomas at rapid, contrast enhanced MR imaging. Radiology 1993;189:205–210.
13. Tien R. Sequence of enhancement of various portions of the pituitary gland in gadolinium-enhanced MR images: correlation with regional blood supply. Am J Roentgenol 1992;158:651–654.
14. Kucharcyzk W, Bishop J, Plewes D, et al. Detection of pituitary microadenomas: comparison of dynamic keyhole fast SE, unenhanced and conventional contrast-enhanced MR imaging. Am J Roentgenol 1994;163:671–679.
15. Yuh W, Fisher D, Nguyen H, et al. Sequential MR enhancement in normal pituitary gland and in pituitary adenoma. AJNR 1994;15:101–108.
16. Miller D, Doppman J. Petrosal sinus sampling: technique and rationale Radiology 1991;178:37–47.
17. Miller D, Doppman J, Peterman S, et al. Neurologic complications of petrosal sinus sampling. Radiology 1992;185:143–147.
18. Strack T, Schild H, Bohl J, et al. Selective bilateral blood sampling from the inferior petrosal sinus in Cushing's disease: effects of corticotropin-releasing factor and thyrotropin-releasing hormone on pituitary secretion. Cardiovasc Intervent Radiol 1993;16:287–292.
19. Fujisawa I, Asato, N, Togashi K, et al. Anterior and posterior lobes of the pituitary gland: assessment by 1.5 T MR imaging. J Comput Assist Tomogr 1987;11(2):214–220.
20. Miki Y, Matsuo M, Nishigawa S. Pituitary adenomas and normal pituitary tissue: enhancement patterns on gadopentate-enhance MR imaging. Radiology 1990;177:35–38.
21. Kucharczyk J, Kucharczyk W, Berry I. Histochemical characterization and functional significance of the hyperintense signal on MR images of the posterior pituitary. AJNR 1986; 9:1079–1083.
22. Colombo N, Berry I, Kucharczyk J. Posterior pituitary gland: appearance on MR images in normal and pathologic states. Radiology 1987;165:481–485.
23. Araki Y, Ashikaga R, Takahashi S, et al. High signal intensity of the infundibular stak on fluid-attenuated inversion recovery MR. AJNR 1997;18:89–93.
24. Benshoff E, Katz B. Ectopia of the posterior pituitary gland as a normal variant: assessment with MR imaging. AJNR 1990;11:709–712.
25. El Gammal T, Brooks B, Hoffman W. MR imaging of the ectopic bright signal of posterior pituitary regeneration. AJNR 1989;10:323–328.
26. Elster A, Sanders T, Vines F, et al. Size and shape of the pituitary gland during pregnancy and postpartum: measurement with MR imaging. Radiology 1991;181:531–535.
27. Elster A, Chen M, Williams D, et al. Pituitary gland: MR imaging of physiologic hypertrophy in adolescence. Radiology 1990;174:681–685.
28. Hinshaw D, Hasso A, Thompson J, et al. High resolution computed tomography of the postpartum pituitary gland. Neuroradiology 1984;26:299–301.
29. Swartz J, Russel K, Basile B, et al. High resolution CT appearance of the intrasellar contents in women of childbearing age. Radiology 1983;147;115–117.
30. Cox T, Elster A. Normal pituitary gland: changes in shape, size and signal intensity during the first year of life at MR imaging. Radiology 1991;179:721–724.
31. Hutchins W, Crues J, Mirza P, et al. MR demonstration of pituitary hyperplasia and regression after therapy for hypothyroidism. AJNR 1990;11:410.
32. Kulkarni M, Lee K, McArdle C. 1.5 T MR imaging of pituitary microadenomas: technical considerations and CT correlation. AJNR 1988;9:5–11.
33. Pojunas K, Daniels D, Williams A, et al. MR imaging of prolactin-secreting microadenomas. AJNR 1986;7:209–213.
34. Davis P, Hoffman J, Spencer T, et al. MR imaging of pituitary adenoma: CT, clinical and surgical correlation. Am J Roentgenol 1987;148:797–802.
35. Nichols D, Laws E, Houser O, et al. Comparison of magnetic resonance imaging and CT in preoperative evaluation of pituitary adenomas. Neurosurgery 1988;22:380–385.
36. Newton D, Dillon W, Norman D, et al. Gd-DTPA enhanced MR imaging of pituitary adenomas. AJNR 1989;10:949–958.
37. Syvertsen A, Haughton V, Williams A, et al. The CT appearance of the normal pituitary gland and pituitary microadenomas. Radiology 1979;133:385–391.
38. Dwyer A, Frank J, Doppman J. Pituitary adenomas in patients with Cushing's disease: initial experience with Gd-DTPA enhanced MR imaging. Radiology 1987;163:421–425.
39. Oldfield EH, Doppman JL, Nieman EK. Petrosal sinus sampling with and without corticotropin-releasing hormone for the differential diagnosis of Cushing's syndrome. J Virol 1992;3:149.
40. Buchfelder M, Nistor R, Fahlbusch R, et al. The accuracy of CT and MR evaluation of the sella turcica for detection of adrenocorticotropic hormone-secreting adenomas in Cushing disease. AJNR 1993;14:1183–1190.
41. Teramoto A, Hirakawa K, Sanno N, et al. Incidental pituitary lesions in unselected 1000 autopsy specimens. Radiology 1994;193:161–164.
42. Chong BW, Kucharzyk W, Singer W, et al. Pituitary gland MR: a comparative study of healthy volunteers and patients with microadenomas. AJNR 1994;15:675–679.
43. Molitch M. Incidental pituitary adenomas. Am J Med Sci 1993;306(4):262–264.
44. Kucharzyk W, Davis D, Kelly W, et al. Pituitary adenomas: high-resolution MR imaging at 1.5 T. Radiology 1986;161:761–765.
45. Bilaniuk L, Zimmerman R, Wehrli F. MRI of pituitary lesions using 1.0–1.5 T field strength. Radiology 1984;153:415–418.
46. Young S, Grossman R, Goldberg H, et al. MR of vascular encasement in parasellar masses: comparison with angiography and CT. AJNR 1988;9:35–38.
47. Sakamoto Y, Rakahashi M, Korogi Y, et al. Normaland abnormal gadopentate dimeglumine-enhanced MR imaging. Radiology 1991;178:441–445.
48. Stadnik T, Stevenaert A, Berckers A, et al. Pituitary microadenoma diagnosis with two- and three-dimensional MR imaging at 1.5T before and after injection of gadolinium. Radiology 1990;176:419–428.
49. Fox JR, AlMefty O. Suprasellar arachnoid cysts: an extension of the membrane of Lillequist. Neurosurgery 1980;7:615.
50. Rutka JT, Hoffman HJ, Dranke JM. Suprasellar and sellar tumors in childhood and adolescence. Neurosurg Clin N Am 1992;3:803.
51. Weiner SN, Pearlstein AE, Eiber A. MR imaging of intracranial arachnoid cysts. J Comput Assist Tomogr 1987;11:236.
52. Ross D, Norman D, Wilson C. Radiologic characteristics and results of surgical management of Rathke's cysts in 43 patients. Neurosurgery 1992;30:173–179.

53. Asari S, Ito T, Tsuchida S, et al. MR appearance and cyst content of Rathke cleft cysts. J Comput Assist Tomogr 1990;14(4):532–535.

54. Kucharczyk W, Peck W, Kelly W, et al. Rathke cleft cysts: CT, MR imaging, and pathologic features. Radiology 1987;165:491–495.

55. Sumida M, Uozumi T, Mukada K, et al. Rathke cleft cysts: correlation of enhanced MR and surgical findings. AJNR 1994;15:525–532.

56. Naylor MF, Scheithauer B, Forbes F, et al. Rathke cleft cyst: CT, MR, and pathology of 23 cases. J Comput Assist Tomogr 1995;19(6):853–859.

57. Sartoretti-Schefer S, Wichmann W, Aguzzi A, et al. MR differentiation of adamantinous and squamous-papillary craniopharyngiomas. AJNR 1997;18:77–88.

58. Benitez W, Sartor K, Angtuaco E. Craniopharyngiomas presenting as a nasopharyngeal mass: CT and MR findings: case report. J Comput Assist Tomogr 1988;12:1066–1072.

59. Harwood-Nash DC. Neuroimaging of childhood craniopharyngiomas. Pediatr Neurosurg 1994;21(suppl):2–10.

60. Crotty T, Scheithauer B, Young W. Papillary craniopharyngioma: a clinicopathological study of 48 cases J Neurosurg 1995;83:206–214.

61. Pusey E, Kortman K, Flannigan B, et al. MR of craniopharyngiomas: tumor delineation and characterization. AJNR 1987;8:439–444.

62. Hillman T, Peyster R, Hoover E, et al. Intrasellar craniopharyngioma: CT and MR studies. J Comput Assist Tomogr 1988;12:702–704.

63. Hald J, Eldevik O, Skalpe I. Craniopharyngioma identification by CT and MR imaging at 1.5T. Acta Radiologica 1994;36:142–147.

64. Lakhanpal S, Glasier C, James C, et al. MR and CT diagnosis of carotid pseudoaneurysm in children following surgical resection of craniopharyngioma. Pediatr Radiol 1995;25:249–251.

65. Mayr N, Yuh W, Muhonen M, et al. Pituitary metastases: MR findings. J Comput Assist Tomogr 1993;17(3):433–437.

66. Ahmadi J, Meyers G, Segall H, et al. Lymphocytic adenohypophysitis: contrast-enhanced MR imaging in five cases. Radiology 1995;195:30–34.

67. Levine S, Benzel E, Fowles M, et al. Lymphocytic adenohypophysitis: clinical, radiological and magnetic resonance imaging characterization. Neurosurgery 1988;22:937–941.

68. Quencer R. Lymphocytic adenohypophysitis: autoimmune disorder of the pituitary gland. AJNR 1980;1:343–345.

69. Atlas S, Grossman R, Goldberg H, et al. Partially thrombosed giant intracranial aneurysm: correlation of MR and pathology findings. Radiology 1987;162:111–117.

70. Hahn F, Ong E, McComb R, et al. Peripheral signal void ring in giant vertebral aneurysm: MR and pathology findings. J Comput Assist Tomogr 1992;10:1036–1040.

71. Goldsher D, Litt A, Pinto R, et al. Dural "tail" associated with meningiomas on Gd-DTPA-enhanced MR images: characteristics, differential diagnostic value and possible implications for treatment. Radiology 1990;176:447–450.

72. Breger R, Papke R, Pojunas K, et al. Benign extra-axial tumors: contrast enhancement with Gd-DTPA. Radiology 1987;163:427–429.

73. Chakeres D, Curtin A, Ford G. Magnetic resonance imaging of pituitary and parasellar abnormalities. Radiol Clin North Am 1989;27:265–281.

74. Taylor S, Barakos J, Harsh G, et al. Magnetic resonance imaging of tuberculum sellae meningiomas: preventing preoperative misdiagnosis as pituitary macroadenoma. Neurosurgery 1992;31:621–627.

75. Andrews B, Wilson C. Suprasellar meningiomas: the effect of tumor location on postoperative visual outcome. J Neurosurg 1988;69:523–528.

76. Jafar J, Crowell R. Parasellar and optic nerve lesions: the neurosurgeon's perspective. Radiol Clin North Am 1987;25:877–885.

77. Rutka J, Hoffman H, Drake J. Suprasellar and sellar tumors in childhood and adolescence. Neurosurg Clin N Am 1992;3:103–115.

78. Fujisawa I, Asato R, Okumura R. Magnetic resonance imaging of neurohypophyseal germinomas. Cancer 1991;68:1009–1015.

79. Tien R, Newton T, McDermott M, et al. Thickened pituitary stalk on MR images in patients with diabetes insipidus and Langerhans cell histiocytosis. AJNR 1990;11:703–706.

80. Graif M, Pennock J. MR imaging of histiocytosis X in the central nervous system. AJNR 1986;7:21–23.

81. Weber A, Liebsch N, Sanchez R, et al. Chordomas of the skull base. Neuroimaging Clin N Am 1994;4(3):515–527.

82. Brown E, Hug E, Weber A. Chondrosarcoma of the skull base. Neuroimaging Clin N Am 1994;4(3):529–541.

83. Yuh W, Wright D, Barloon T. MR imaging of primary tumors of trigeminal nerve and Meckel's cave. Am J Roentgenol 1988;151:577–580.

84. Yasui T, Hakuba A, Kim S. Trigeminal neuromas: operative approach in eight cases. J Neurosurg 1989;71:506–514.

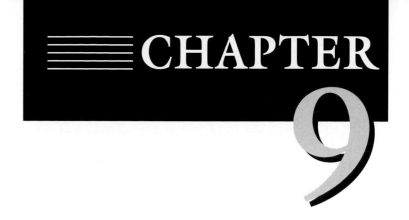

CHAPTER 9

Clinical Aspects

Clinical Presentation of Pituitary Tumors

Lewis S. Blevins, David Shore, Jonathon Weinstein, and Scott Isaacs

INTRODUCTION

Pituitary adenomas are benign monoclonal neoplasms that arise from the cells composing the anterior pituitary gland. They account for approximately 15% of all intracranial tumors (1). Pituitary adenomas can result in a variety of symptoms, signs, and disorders. Detection of microadenomas (< 1 cm) in as many as 27% of pituitaries in an unselected autopsy series suggests that most remain asymptomatic throughout life (2). Occasionally, these are incidentally detected during neuroradiologic examinations of the head for unrelated complaints (i.e., head trauma, "migraine" headaches, sinusitis, etc.) Macroadenomas (> 1 cm) usually become clinically apparent but are sometimes also incidentally detected. Careful clinical and biochemical evaluation discloses evidence of hormone overproduction or underproduction in more than one-quarter of patients with these pituitary "incidentalomas" (3). Pituitary tumors most often first become clinically apparent when patients present with recognizable features attributed to compressive mass effects, varying degrees of hypopituitarism, and

syndromes of hormone hypersecretion. The protean and insidious manifestations of many of the syndromes of hormone hypersecretion often lead to significant delays in diagnosis and management. In contrast, occasional patients present with acute life-threatening neurologic, hormonal, and metabolic abnormalities that require immediate attention.

FEATURES ATTRIBUTED TO COMPRESSIVE MASS EFFECTS

Headaches are perhaps the most common complaint of patients with pituitary adenomas (4). The discomfort is nonspecific and often described as vague, dull, or pressure-like and may be localized to the vertex, temples, or the fronto-orbital areas (5, 6). Many patients relate a progressive worsening of the intensity and frequency of their headaches. In some patients the discomfort is truly disabling, whereas in others the headaches are simply an occasional nuisance. Headaches have been ascribed to stretching or tearing of the diaphragma sellae, to invasion of the cavernous sinuses or other surrounding bony structures, and, rarely, to increased intracranial pressure (7, 8). Tumor expansion and rupture through the diaphragma sellae may result in a sudden resolution of chronic headaches and onset of visual abnormalities (9). An abrupt onset of a severe headache is usually the result of rapid tumor expansion caused by intratumoral hemorrhage or infarction. A syndrome of facial pain and numbness in the distributions of the first and second divisions of the trigeminal nerves may result from tumor invasion of the cavernous sinuses.

Visual abnormalities often provoke patients with large pituitary tumors to seek medical attention (10). Common complaints include blurred vision, decreased visual acuity, decreased night vision, tunneling of vision, and, rarely, diplopia. Occasional patients suspect they have visual problems only after minor traffic violations or accidents prompt them to question their ability to safely operate an automobile. A detailed account of the neuro-ophthalmologic manifestations is given in Chapter 10, but in addition to the classic bitemporal hemianopia, involvement of an optic tract can result in a homonymous hemianopia (11). Papilledema is unusual and, when present, may be caused by either hydrocephalus or anterior extension of the tumor. Invasion of the cavernous sinuses with compression of the oculomotor, trochlear, or abducens nerves may result in diplopia and characteristic abnormalities of the eye movements (12). Involvement of the oculomotor nerve is often accompanied by ipsilateral ptosis.

Other less common symptoms and signs depend on the extent and direction of pituitary tumor growth. For example, headaches, nausea, vomiting, urinary incontinence, ataxia, cognitive abnormalities, thermoregulatory disturbances, hyperphagia, and dementia may develop in patients with marked suprasellar extension and compression of the hypothalamus and the third ventricle (8). Frontal lobe involvement may result in personality changes, anosmia, and generalized seizures (8). Extension into the middle cranial fossa can result in compression of the cerebral peduncles, with hemiparesis, partial-complex (uncinate) seizures, and visual field deficits. Tumors that compress the hippocampus can precipitate disagreeable olfactory and gustatory auras (8). Patients with erosion of the floor of the sella and tumor extension into the sphenoid sinus may present with a cerebrospinal fluid leak, epistaxis, nasal stuffiness, and even a presumed nasopharyngeal or sinus mucosal tumor (8, 13).

The classical syndrome of pituitary apoplexy is rare despite the occurrence of intratumoral hemorrhage in as many as 17% of patients with pituitary tumors (14, 15). Numerous precipitating factors, including head trauma, anticoagulation, irradiation, surgical manipulation, treatment with bromocriptine, administration of hypothalamic peptides, and diabetic ketoacidosis, have been described. Patients with the full-blown syndrome report the abrupt onset of severe headache, nausea, and vomiting, which are often accompanied by visual field deficits, ocular paresis, meningeal signs, and an altered sensorium. Hypopituitarism is often present and probably contributes to the mortality of this disorder.

FEATURES ATTRIBUTED TO HYPOPITUITARISM

Pituitary tumors and therapeutic modalities directed against them account for more than two-thirds of all causes of hypopituitarism in adults (16). The occurrence of hypopituitarism in patients with pituitary tumors, especially macroadenomas, is common. Nelson et al. found deficiencies of one or more anterior pituitary hormones in nearly half of the de novo macroadenoma patients (17).

Several pathophysiologic mechanisms have been advanced to account for the hypopituitarism in affected patients. Tumor-induced increases in intrasellar pressure may compromise the flow of arterial blood to the residual normal pituitary and result in ischemia or infarction (18). Increased intrasellar pressure and direct mechanical compression of the infundibulum can impair the delivery of hypothalamic-releasing and hypothalamic-inhibiting factors to the adenohypophysis and result in a "stalk syndrome" characterized by hypopituitarism and mild to moderate hyperprolactinemia (18, 19). In these patients, a successful tumor resection is often accompanied by resumption of normal anterior pituitary function, presumably because of reversal of the stalk syndrome. For example, Arafah et al. demonstrated immediate recovery of adrenocorticotropic hormone (ACTH) deficiency following surgery in 17 (65%) of 26 patients with macroadenoma who also had preoperative hyperprolactinemia (19). Prolactin (PRL) levels were higher in patients who had recovery of their pituitary function than in those who did not. In another series, Nelson et al. demonstrated postoperative improvement in anterior pituitary function in only one-third of their macroadenoma patients with partial hypopituitarism (17). Half of the remaining two-thirds of hypopituitary patients developed new anterior pituitary hormone deficits following surgery, and the remainder were unchanged compared with their preoperative hormonal status. One-fifth of their patients with normal preoperative function had varying degrees of hypopituitarism following surgery. In a series reported by Faria and Tindall, a similar proportion (23%) of women with PRL-secreting pituitary adenomas and otherwise normal anterior pituitary function developed hormone deficiencies following transsphenoidal microsurgery (20). Approximately half of pituitary tumor patients treated with conventional radiotherapy develop hypopituitarism within 4 years of treatment; as many as two-thirds will ultimately develop hypopituitarism that is believed to be caused by radiation-induced hypothalamic dysfunction (21).

In the absence of pituitary apoplexy, the course of hypopituitarism in patients with pituitary tumors is insidiously progressive. Affected patients may develop partial or complete deficiencies of one or more anterior pituitary hormones. The clinical presentation of hypopituitarism varies depending on the extent, severity, and course of development of the pituitary and the resulting target gland hormone deficiencies, as well as the age and overall health of the patient and the presence or absence of clinical syndromes of hormone hypersecretion. In the remainder of this section, we will review the syndromes resulting from deficiencies of the anterior pituitary hormones.

ACTH Deficiency

ACTH deficiency results in impaired adrenocortical synthesis and secretion of cortisol, other glucocorticoid hormones, and weak adrenal androgens.

The clinical features of hypocortisolemia are relatively nonspecific. Affected patients may be asymptomatic or have malaise, fatigue, anorexia, nausea, weight loss, arthralgias, and myalgias. Unlike patients with primary adrenal insufficiency, patients with "central adrenocortical insufficiency" do not become hyperpigmented because ACTH levels are unable to increase in response to the prevailing cortisol deficiency. Adrenal androgen deficiency often results in decreased or absent axillary and pubic hair, especially when hypogonadism is also present. Acute illnesses, severe physical and psychological stressors, and medications that accelerate the metabolism of cortisol (L-thyroxine, phenytoin, rifampin, phenobarbital) may unmask partial ACTH deficiency and result in dramatic worsening of symptoms accompanied by nausea, vomiting, and orthostatic hypotension. Rare patients, especially those unable to eat, are prone to develop hypoglycemia because impaired glucose counterregulation is often seen in patients with cortisol deficiency and coexisting growth hormone (GH) deficiency. Occasionally, patients develop hyponatremia because cortisol deficiency and nausea enhance the secretion of arginine vasopressin, which results in impaired renal free water excretion (22–24). Since mineralocorticoid production remains normal under the regulatory influences of the renin-angiotensin system, affected patients do not develop hyperkalemia.

Controversy exists regarding the best screening test(s) for central adrenocortical insufficiency (25). Some advocate measurement of the morning serum cortisol level or performance of a standard ACTH stimulation test (26). Both of these provide only an indirect assessment of the integrity of the hypothalamic–pituitary–adrenal axis. In patients with diseases of the hypothalamic–pituitary unit, morning serum cortisol levels less than 90 to 140 nmol/L (< 3 to 5 µg/dL) suggest ACTH deficiency, and levels greater than 390 to 500 nmol/L (> 14 to 18 µg/dL) usually indicate normal function of the hypothalamic–pituitary–adrenal axis (27; LS Blevins Jr, unpublished data, 1996). ACTH-stimulated cortisol levels greater than 550 nmol/L (> 20 µg/dL) usually indicate a normal axis, but rare patients meeting this criterion have impaired cortisol responses to physical stressors (28). Use of the ACTH stim-

ulation test is not recommended in the evaluation of patients with presumed acute ACTH deficiency (apoplexy, immediate postoperative period) because in these patients the adrenal glands maintain normal responsiveness to exogenous ACTH for several weeks before becoming atrophic. Dynamic tests of the hypothalamic–pituitary–adrenal axis, including the insulin-induced hypoglycemia and the metyrapone tests, are often required to firmly establish a diagnosis of central adrenocortical insufficiency (29).

Thyroid-Stimulating Hormone (TSH) Deficiency

TSH deficiency results in impaired thyroidal synthesis and secretion of L-thyroxine (T4) and L-triiodothyronine (T3) (30). The resulting constellation of clinical and laboratory features is often referred to as "central hypothyroidism."

The clinical manifestations of central hypothyroidism depend on many factors, including the degree of T4 deficiency. Affected patients generally have mild to moderate symptoms compared with patients with primary hypothyroidism. Common complaints include fatigue, weakness, an increased need for sleep, weight gain, cold intolerance, impaired mentation, and constipation. Results of physical examination may reveal bradycardia, diastolic hypertension, poverty of speech and movement, and slight prolongation of the relaxation phase of the deep tendon reflexes (31). Myxedema is rarely present. Many patients with hypothyroidism fulfill the diagnostic criteria for major depression (32).

Patients with central hypothyroidism typically have low or "low normal" free T4 concentrations and free T4 indices (product of the total T4 and the T3 resin uptake). Most patients with central hypothyroidism have inappropriately "normal" serum TSH concentrations (30, 33). In these patients, TSH is immunoreactive, and thus measurable, but biologically inactive, and thus unable to maintain normal thyroid function. Altered diurnal variability (absence of the normal nocturnal surge) in the serum TSH concentration may also explain the impaired thyroidal response to normal levels of TSH (33). In contrast, in patients with primary hypothyroidism, the serum TSH concentrations are elevated, the biologic activity of the TSH is increased relative to normal TSH, and the diurnal pattern of TSH secretion is preserved. The thyrotropin-releasing hormone (TRH) stimulation test is rarely necessary in the evaluation of patients with suspected central hypothyroidism (29).

Gonadotropin Deficiency

Gonadotropin [luteinizing hormone (LH) and follicle-stimulating hormone (FSH)] deficiencies result in impaired gonadal synthesis and secretion of the sex steroid hormones and disordered production and maturation of the gametes. Thus, symptoms and signs of "central hypogonadism" are related to deficiencies of the principal sex steroid hormones (estradiol in women, testosterone in men) and infertility.

Gonadotropin deficiencies in preadolescent patients result in delayed puberty, and deficiencies before completion of sexual maturation result in arrested puberty. These patients are usually diagnosed during adolescence and early adulthood with either sexual infantilism or incomplete sexual maturation. Many patients have eunuchoidal body proportions as a result of delayed closure of the epiphyses of the appendicular skeleton. Premenopausal women have a spectrum of menstrual disorders ranging from oligomenorrhea with anovulatory menses to amenorrhea. Cyclical monthly menses almost always exclude gonadotropin deficiencies. Rarely, however, infertility is the only complaint prompting the patient to seek medical attention. Other symptoms and signs related to estrogen deficiency include hot flashes, irritability, mood swings, vaginal dryness, dyspareunia, diminished libido, and atrophy of the breasts. Postpubertal men with testosterone deficiency often admit to weakness, fatigue, a diminished libido, erectile dysfunction of varying degrees, and a decreased ejaculate volume. Irritability, mood swings, hot flashes, and infertility are frequent. Results of physical examination may reveal decreased beard and body hair growth; softened testes; and a small, flattened prostate gland. Patients of either sex often have pallor and fine wrinkling of the skin over the lateral aspects of the orbits and at the angles of the mouth.

Men and premenopausal women with central hypogonadism typically have low or normal levels of LH and FSH and low or low normal levels of the sex steroid hormones. Low or inappropriately normal FSH concentrations in postmenopausal women indicate gonadotropin deficiency (22). Anovulation may be predicted by the occurrence of menstrual flow in an amenorrheic patient within 7 to 10 days following a course of medroxyprogesterone, 10 mg orally for 10 days. Failure of the basal body temperature to rise by more than 0.5°F approximately 14 days before the onset of menses and low levels of serum progesterone on day 21 following the onset of spontaneous menses are also indicators of anovulation. Papanicolaou smears often reveal an impaired maturational index of the superficial cells of the vaginal mucosa in women with estrogen deficiency. Semen analysis may reveal morphologic and quantitative abnormalities of the sperm in hypogonadal men. The gonadotropin-releasing hormone stimulation test is rarely indicated in the evaluation of patients with obvious diseases of the hypothalamic–pituitary unit (29).

GH (or Somatotropin) Deficiency

GH has complex effects on growth and intermediary metabolism that are mediated by insulinlike growth factor-1 (IGF-1 or somatomedin-C), which is produced in cartilage and also secreted by the liver. In children and adolescents, acquired GH deficiency results in impaired linear growth and short stature. Affected children are often more than 3 standard deviations below the mean height for age-

and sex-matched controls, and their linear growth velocity is usually less than 4 cm per year. Standardized bone age radiograph results of the nondominant wrist and hand often reveal delayed skeletal maturation. Affected children usually have normal body proportions and are often overweight.

In adults, symptoms of acquired GH deficiency are nonspecific and are often difficult to distinguish from symptoms caused by deficiencies of other anterior pituitary hormones. Symptoms attributed to GH deficiency include easy fatigability, decreased exercise tolerance, muscle weakness, weight gain, and impaired psychosocial skills. Physical findings and assessments may include an increased waist:hip ratio, increased body fat content, muscle weakness, decreased work capacity, depression, poor self-image, hyperlipidemia, and osteopenia (34).

Provocative tests of GH reserve are necessary to establish and confirm a diagnosis of GH deficiency. Simple and reliable tests that usually suffice (especially in adults) include the insulin-induced hypoglycemia test and the levodopa, arginine, and clonidine stimulation tests (29).

PRL Deficiency

PRL is only one of several hormones necessary for postpartum lactation. Failure of appropriate lactation is the only known manifestation of PRL deficiency (35). In contrast to controls, who have 3- to 10-fold elevations in early postpartum serum PRL concentrations, affected patients have low or inappropriately normal PRL levels (35). In most patients with hypopituitarism, PRL deficiency is masked by the infertility caused by the associated gonadotropin deficiency. PRL deficiency will almost certainly be recognized with increasing frequency now that assisted reproductive technologies have made it possible for hypopituitary women to conceive and to have normal pregnancies.

Diabetes Insipidus (DI)

Neurogenic DI results from a heterogeneous group of disorders that impair either the hypothalamic synthesis, transport, or secretion of arginine vasopressin from the posterior pituitary gland (36). Pituitary adenomas are unusual causes of DI. Other types of intrasellar or stalk neoplasms and disease processes (craniopharyngioma, metastasis, sarcoidosis, etc.) should be suspected in patients with sellar masses and DI.

Vasopressin deficiency results in impaired renal free water conservation and subsequent polyuria. The polyuria is characterized by a 24-hour urine volume greater than 30 mL/kg body weight and either a urine osmolality less than 300 mmol/kg H_2O (< 300 mOsm/kg H_2O) or a urine specific gravity less than 1.010 (37). Daily urine volumes may range from 2.5 to more than 20 L. Plasma osmolality and serum sodium levels are typically increased because of the renal losses of free water. Thirst-induced polydipsia ensues as a natural defense against further dehydration. Denial of access to free water (i.e., unconsciousness, neurologic deficits, physical restraint, endotracheal intubation, etc.) can result in severe hypertonic dehydration characterized by hypernatremia, neuromuscular irritability, psychomotor agitation, lethargy, seizures, coma, and even death (38).

DI occurs in as many as 25% of patients following transsphenoidal pituitary surgery (36). Fortunately, DI is permanent in only 2% of these patients (39). DI is more common following surgery for macroadenomas with suprasellar extension (9.5 to 17%) than following surgery for lesions confined to the sella (1%) (40). DI usually has an abrupt onset within the first 3 postoperative days. In most patients, DI is transient and lasts for 3 to 5 days or, rarely, for several weeks (41). Although DI persisting for more than 6 months after the inciting event is usually permanent, some patients may enjoy improvement and even resolution of the disorder over several years (36). Attempts at resection of large suprasellar tumors can result in a classic triphasic response to pituitary stalk injury (41). The initial phase is characterized by an abrupt cessation of vasopressin release followed by polyuria lasting 4 to 8 days. An interphase, characterized by inappropriate vasopressin secretion resulting in concentration of the urine and plasma hypo-osmolality and hyponatremia, may last 5 to 6 days. Profound hyponatremia and related complications may develop if there is a delay in the recognition of this phase. The final phase is heralded by the return of DI, which usually persists but may ultimately improve or resolve (36, 41, 42).

Patients with severe DI often present with a plasma osmolality greater than 295 mmol/kg H_2O (> 295 mOsm/kg H_2O), a urine osmolality less than the plasma osmolality, and a serum sodium concentration greater than 145 mmol/L (> 145 mEq/L) (43). In these patients, one can proceed with a determination of the effect of exogenous vasopressin on the urine osmolality and polyuria. A classical water deprivation test may be necessary to establish a diagnosis in patients with mild to moderate neurogenic DI (36).

FEATURES ATTRIBUTED TO SPECIFIC TYPES OF PITUITARY ADENOMAS
Hyperprolactinemia

PRL-secreting pituitary adenomas represent the most common causes of hyperprolactinemia (44) (Table 9.1). These tumors arise from the lactotroph cells of the anterior pituitary gland. Although most prolactinomas are less than 10 mm in size, these tumors can become large and locally invasive. Giant macroprolactinomas associated with severe hyperprolactinemia have a predilection for young adult males and probably represent a distinct pathologic entity (45).

Hyperprolactinemia disrupts normal reproductive function by altering pulsatile gonadotropin secretion, interfer-

Table 9.1. Causes of Hyperprolactinemia

Intracranial disorders
  Prolactinoma
  Mixed GH-cell and prolactin-cell adenoma
  Mammosomatotroph adenoma
  Acidophil stem cell adenoma
  Hypothalamic tumor
  Granulomatous disorders (sarcoidosis, Langerhans' cell histiocytosis, tuberculosis)
  Metastasis (breast, lung, lymphoma)
  Traumatic stalk section (basal skull fracture, penetrating wounds, surgery)
  Pseudoprolactinoma

Pharmacologic agents
  Monoamine synthesis inhibitors (α-methyldopa)
  Monoamine depletors (reserpine)
  Dopamine receptor antagonists (phenothiazines, butyrophenones, thioxanthenes)
  Monoamine uptake inhibitors (tricyclic antidepressants)
  Oral contraceptives (estrogen)
  Narcotics (morphine, heroin)
  Metoclopramide
  Cimetidine
  Verapamil

Neurogenic disorders
  Spinal cord tumors
  Chest wall disease/injury (burns, herpes zoster)

Physiologic causes
  Pregnancy
  Nursing
  Nipple stimulation
  Exercise
  Sleep
  Stress

Others
  Hypothyroidism
  Cirrhosis
  Chronic renal failure
  Polycystic ovarian disease
  Idiopathic disease

ing with sex steroid feedback at the level of the hypothalamus, and inhibiting gonadal steroidogenesis (46). Menstrual disturbances (oligomenorrhea, amenorrhea) are present in 93% of premenopausal women with prolactinomas (47). Occasionally, patients have "regular" menses and infertility (46–49). Many of these patients have luteal phase defects owing to abnormal function of the corpus luteum. Their menstrual cycles are often of variable lengths (i.e., 21 to 40 days). Symptoms related to estrogen deficiency include hot flashes, decreased libido, vaginal dryness, and dyspareunia. Galactorrhea, which may be present in 5 to 10% of normal women, is present in approximately 83% of women with prolactinomas (46, 47, 50). The galactorrhea may be spontaneous or noted only following manipulation of the nipples of the breasts. The expressed nipple secretions may vary in appearance from milky to clear and oily. Men typically present with impotence or other forms of erectile dysfunction, diminished libido, fatigue, infertility, galactorrhea (12%), and, because 90% have macroadenomas, tumor mass effects (47, 51, 52). Hyperprolactinemia in children and adolescents can result in primary amenorrhea and varying degrees of pubertal arrest.

Laboratory abnormalities in hyperprolactinemic patients reflect central hypogonadism. Some women have increases in serum dehydroepiandrosterone sulfate and free testosterone levels because PRL stimulates the synthesis and secretion of adrenal androgens (53, 54). Semen analysis reveals oligospermia in some but not all men (52). Young women with hyperprolactinemic amenorrhea have reduced bone mineral density compared with age-matched controls (55–57). Progressive osteopenia in untreated patients may lead to devastating complications associated with osteoporosis. Men with hypogonadism as a result of hyperprolactinemia also have osteopenia and are at increased risk for spinal compression fractures (58).

PRL levels in patients with prolactinomas may vary from the upper limit of normal (15 to 20 μg/L [15 to 20 ng/mL]) to values greater than 10,000 μg/L (> 10,000 ng/mL) (45, 59). Microprolactinomas usually cause only modest elevations in the serum PRL concentration. PRL levels typically exceed 200 μg/L (200 ng/mL) in patients with macroprolactinomas; invasive tumors are often associated with extremely high PRL levels (45).

Large, nonsecreting pituitary tumors can distort the infundibulum and interfere with the transport of dopamine to normal lactotroph cells in the anterior pituitary, resulting in hyperprolactinemia; PRL levels are usually less than 200 μg/L (< 200 ng/mL). Clinically, these "pseudoprolactinomas" can be distinguished from true prolactinomas in that reduction in tumor size often can be achieved in the latter following the administration of dopamine agonists for 3 months (46, 60, 61). Primary and metastatic tumors and infiltrative disorders of the hypothalamus, infundibulum, and posterior pituitary gland can present in a similar fashion. Histologic examination of resected tissue is occasionally necessary to firmly establish a diagnosis in some hyperprolactinemic patients with sellar and parasellar tumors.

Severe primary hypothyroidism may be accompanied by thyrotroph hyperplasia caused by increased hypothalamic synthesis and secretion of TRH. Serum TSH levels are always elevated. Hypersecretion of TRH also results in lactotroph hyperplasia and subsequent hyperprolactinemia (62). PRL levels are usually less than 100 μg/L (< 100 ng/mL). Affected patients are often suspected of having pituitary disease because they present with clinical and biochemical features of hypothyroidism, hypogonadism, and hyperprolactinemia. Magnetic resonance imaging of the sella can be a trap for the unwary because marked thyrotroph and lactotroph hyperplasia can result in pituitary enlargement and mimic a pituitary tumor.

Other causes of hyperprolactinemia should be entertained in patients with normal imaging studies of the hypothalamic–pituitary unit (Table 9.1). PRL levels increase 10- to 15-fold throughout normal pregnancy (63). Associated lactotroph hyperplasia results in a doubling of the size of the pituitary gland (64). Thus, pregnancy should be excluded in amenorrheic hyperprolactinemic women before definitive therapy for presumed prolactinomas.

Acromegaly

The constellation of clinical features resulting from chronic pathologic hypersecretion of GH and IGF-1 is known as "acromegaly" (Fig. 9.1). GH-secreting pituitary adenomas cause more than 95% of cases of acromegaly. These tumors arise from the somatotroph cells of the anterior pituitary gland. Macroadenomas with suprasellar extension were present in 40% of 500 patients enrolled in a clinical study to assess the therapeutic efficacy of octreotide (65). Acromegaly is diagnosed most often in the fourth decade of life and occurs with equal frequency in men and women. Mortality in acromegalic patients compared with the general population is increased twofold to fourfold. Deaths are largely attributable to cardiovascular, respiratory, and malignant diseases (66–68).

The term acromegaly, derived from the Greek akron (extremity) and megale (great), describes only a few of several common manifestations of GH excess, namely, disproportionate enlargement of the distal regions of the skeleton (65) (Fig. 9.2). GH-induced swelling of the soft tissues is the result of increased deposition of glycosaminoglycan in the dermis and GH-induced sodium and water retention by the kidneys (69, 70). Enlargement of the bones and swelling of the soft tissues of the hands and feet results in increased breadth, which usually is manifest as increased ring, glove, and shoe size. The hands are often described as "spadelike." The skin of the distal extremities is thickened and doughy. The heel pad is thickened, and the calcaneus is often not ballottable (69).

Overgrowth of the skull and facial bones produces several characteristic features of acromegaly (Fig. 9.3). Enlargement of the frontal sinuses results in frontal bossing often described as a thickened brow. Increased breadth of the zygomas results in prominence of the upper cheeks. Growth of the mandible results in prognathism accompanied by malocclusion, temporomandibular joint dysfunction, and interdental spacing (Fig. 9.4). Dentists are often the first to notice these specific changes. Cartilaginous enlargement and soft tissue swelling results in increased prominence of the nose, lips, ears, and nasolabial folds. Some patients develop deep furrows in the scalp and forehead (cutis verticis gyrata). Macroglossia is common, and the lateral aspects of the tongue are often scalloped.

Arthralgias may be attributed to involvement of the bony, cartilaginous, ligamentous, and tendinous structures of joints. Classical osteoarthritis may affect the knees, hips, and shoulders. Joint crepitus is a common physical finding, but effusions and other signs of acute inflammation are infrequent. Roentgenographic findings include osteophytosis, angular joint deformities, articular space calcifica-

ACROMEGALY

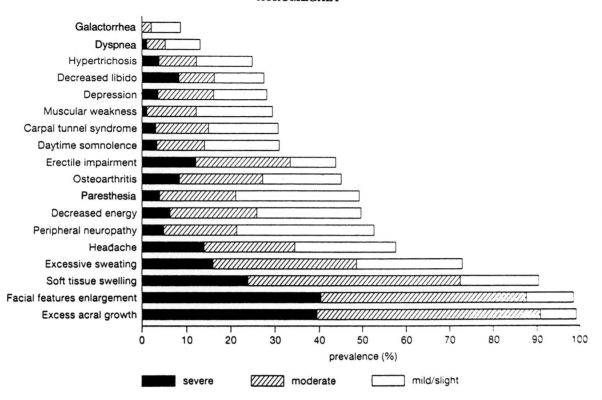

Figure 9.1. Prevalence of various symptoms and signs in 500 patients with acromegaly. (Reprinted with permission from Ezzat S, Forester MJ, Berchtold P, Redelmeier DA, Boerlin V, Harris A. Acromegaly: clinical and biochemical features in 500 patients. Medicine 1994;73:233–240.)

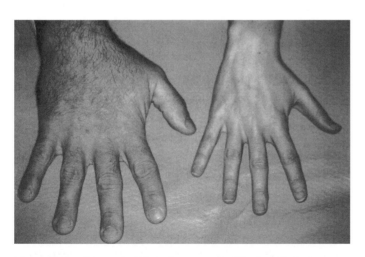

Figure 9.2. Characteristic enlargement of the hand of an acromegalic patient. Note the increased breadth of the digits and wrist compared with the hand of a normal examiner.

tion, joint space narrowing, and periarticular subchondral cyst formation (71). Tendons and ligaments may become lax, resulting in joint destabilization and misalignment. Altered biomechanics can result in secondary degenerative changes in other large, weightbearing joints. Vertebral body enlargement and growth and calcification of the cos-

tal cartilages results in dorsal kyphosis and the typical barreled chest. Laxity of the spinal ligaments contributes to back fatigue.

Many patients complain of hyperhidrosis, excessive body odor, and acne. These manifestations are related to overactivity of the eccrine and apocrine sweat glands and the sebaceous glands (72, 73). Other dermatologic features include acanthosis nigricans, hypertrichosis, generalized hyperpigmentation, suppurative hidradenitis, and thickening and hardening of the nails (72). Skin tags are commonly found in the axillae and groins and on the truncal regions.

Fatigue, decreased energy, and weakness are common complaints despite generalized muscle fiber hypertrophy and increased muscle mass. Peripheral neuropathies are not uncommon and may be enhanced by uncontrolled diabetes mellitus. Affected patients may have abnormal reflexes and impaired temperature, light touch, superficial pain, and vibration sensations. Paresthesias in the lower extremities are common. Progressive neuropathy may ultimately lead to charcot joints, neuropathic ulcers, and significant disability. Carpal tunnel syndrome is occasionally the initial manifestation of acromegaly. Compression of the median nerve in the carpal tunnel by soft tissue overgrowth can result in wasting of the thenar eminence, decreased thumb abduction, decreased handgrip strength, paresthesias, and disa-

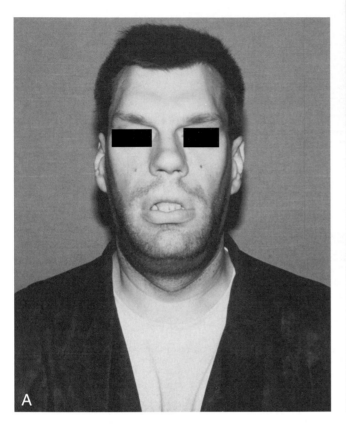

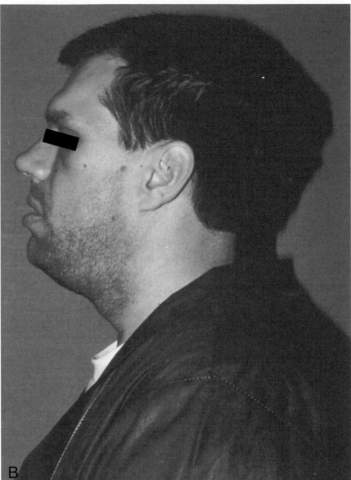

Figure 9.3.   Frontal **(A)** and lateral **(B)** views of an acromegalic patient. Note the coarsened facies, prominent brow, thickening of the mandible, and prognathism.

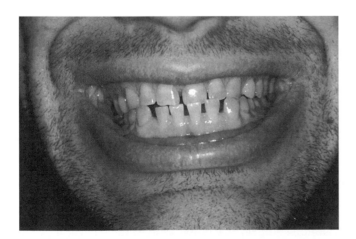

Figure 9.4.   Interdental spacing and malocclusion are common findings in acromegalic patients.

bility. Spinal changes can result in nerve root compression and spinal stenosis, problems that contribute to the back discomfort often seen in acromegalic patients.

Systemic arterial hypertension is found in approximately half of the patients (65, 73). The pathogenesis of hypertension in acromegalic patients is partly explained by direct actions of GH on the renal sodium pump resulting in retention of sodium and water and consequent volume expansion (71). Left ventricular hypertrophy may lead to impaired diastolic filling and decreased exercise performance. Congestive heart failure may ensue. Some patients have a distinct cardiomyopathy thought to be related to direct effects of GH on the myocardium (74). Ventricular arrhythmias may result from interstitial fibrosis of the myocardial conduction system. Hypertension, diabetes mellitus, and hyperlipidemia increase the likelihood of atherosclerotic vascular disease. Coronary artery disease is present in 4 to 11% of patients (65, 73).

Thickening of the vocal cords and expansion of the paranasal sinuses results in deepening of the voice with enhanced resonance. Sleep apnea may be caused by upper airway obstruction, central mechanisms, or a combination of these (75). Airway obstruction is usually a result of tongue, pharyngeal, and upper airway soft tissue growth. Central mechanisms of sleep apnea in acromegalic patients are poorly understood but may be related to altered control of the respiratory centers. GH and IGF-1 levels are higher in patients with central sleep apnea than in patients with obstructive sleep apnea. Sleep apnea is associated with the presence of systemic arterial hypertension and is more common in patients older than 50 years of age. Clinical manifestations include nighttime restlessness, daytime somnolence, fatigue, irritability, restless legs, headaches, and impaired concentration. Affected patients are at increased risk for myocardial infarction, stroke, and motor vehicle accidents.

Impaired glucose tolerance and overt diabetes mellitus are seen in 36% and 30% of acromegalic patients, respectively (65). GH is a glucose counterregulatory hormone that increases hepatic glucose output and decreases glucose use by peripheral tissues. Hyperglycemia results when pancreatic β-cell insulin production fails to reverse and correct these metabolic abnormalities. Hypertriglyceridemia may accompany glucose intolerance and is caused, in part, by abnormalities in hepatic triglyceride lipase and lipoprotein lipase. Hypercalciuria, hypercalcemia, and nephrolithiasis are not uncommon and may even precede the diagnosis of acromegaly. These problems are most likely related to GH-induced increases in bone turnover and enhanced vitamin D action resulting in increased fractional absorption of dietary calcium from the gastrointestinal tract (76).

Organomegaly (cardiomegaly, hepatomegaly, goiter, etc.) is often noted during examination of acromegalic patients. Acromegaly is associated with an increased risk of adenomatous colon polyps and other gastrointestinal tract neoplasms (77–80). Risk factors for colon carcinoma in acromegalic patients include age older than 50 years, more than three skin tags, a history of colon polyps, and a family history of colon cancer (81). GH and IGF-1 may promote neoplastic growth via direct stimulatory effects on epithelial cell proliferation, or they may act as mitogens via induction of c-*myc* proto-oncogene expression (79). Other malignancies (thyroid, breast, gastric, and esophageal carcinomas, meningiomas) have been reported with increased frequency in patients with acromegaly (69). Acromegaly is occasionally one of the phenotypic expressions of multiple endocrine neoplasia type 1 (82). This rare autosomal-dominant disorder is characterized by pituitary tumors, parathyroid hyperplasia, and pancreatic islet-cell neoplasms.

Acromegaloidism and insulin resistance share many of the clinical features of acromegaly (83) (Fig. 9.5). Thus, demonstration of pathologic GH hypersecretion is required to firmly establish a diagnosis of acromegaly. Numerous diagnostic criteria have been proposed (84). GH levels are usually elevated and do not suppress below 88 pmol/L (2 ng/mL) within 2 hours of oral administration of glucose (100 g). IGF-1 and IGFBP-3 levels are usually

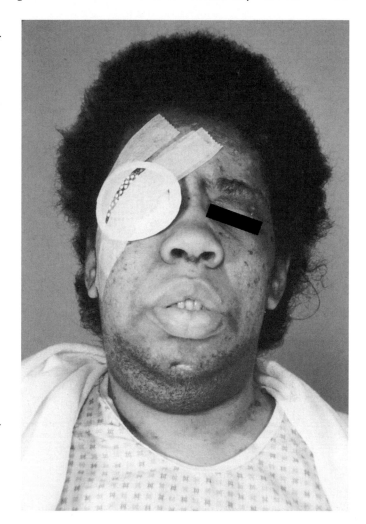

Figure 9.5. Acromegaloidism in a patient with insulin resistance.

elevated. Patients with somatotroph hyperplasia owing to ectopic GHRH-secreting neuroendocrine tumors often have elevated GHRH levels.

Cushing's Syndrome

Cushing's syndrome, first described by Harvey Cushing in 1912, is a constellation of clinical features resulting from pathologic hypercortisolism (85) (Table 9.2). Depending on the pathophysiology of the hypercortisolism, this disorder may be classified as ACTH dependent or ACTH independent. In the ACTH-dependent forms (Table 9.3), chronic ACTH hypersecretion promotes adrenocortical growth and increased synthesis and secretion of glucocorticoids, androgens, and intermediate steroids that possess mineralocorticoid activity. The clinical features of the disorder are a direct result of the effects of supraphysiologic levels of these hormones on various tissues and metabolic processes.

ACTH-secreting pituitary tumors (Cushing's disease) account for more than two-thirds of cases of spontaneous

Table 9.2. *Clinical Features of Cushing's Syndrome*

Clinical Features	%
Obesity	97
Weight gain	91
Plethora	94
Moon facies	88
Menstrual irregularity	84
Hirsutism in women	81
Hypertension	74
Bruising	62
Lethargy/depression	62
Striae	56
Muscle weakness	56
Buffalo hump	54
Ankle edema	50
Osteoporosis	50
Headache	47
Backache	43
Impaired glucose tolerance	37
Muscle weakness	29
Dyspnea	26
Recurrent infections	25
Abdominal pain	21
Acne	21
Fractures	19
Urolithiasis	15
Alopecia	13
Diabetes mellitus	13
Hyperpigmentation	4

Modified from Ross EJ, Linch DC. Cushing's syndrome-killing disease: discriminatory value of signs and symptoms aiding early diagnosis. Lancet 1982;2:646–649.

Table 9.3. *Differential Diagnosis of ACTH-Dependent Cushing's Syndrome*

Pituitary dependent
ACTH-producing pituitary adenoma
  Microadenoma
  Macroadenoma
Corticotroph hyperplasia
  Primary (idiopathic)
  CRH-producing gangliocytoma
  CRH-producing neuroendocrine tumor

Pituitary independent (ectopic)
Bronchial carcinoid
Thymic carcinoid
Small cell bronchogenic carcinoma
Medullary thyroid carcinoma
Pheochromocytoma
Pancreatic islet cell carcinoma
Metastatic colon carcinoma
Ovarian carcinoma

Cushing's syndrome (86). These tumors are derived from the corticotroph cells of the anterior pituitary gland. Approximately three-quarters of patients have microadenomas (87). These tumors are small (mean diameter, 5 mm) and are often not visualized with the aid of conventional neuroradiologic imaging procedures. Nearly 20% of patients harbor macroadenomas, and half of them present with frankly invasive tumors (87). Clinical and biochemical features of corticotroph hyperplasia, present in 4% of patients with presumed Cushing's disease in a recent series, can mimic a pituitary adenoma (87).

Most patients have an ill-defined onset and insidious progression of symptoms and signs of hypercortisolism. A review of the clinical history and old photographs of affected patients may reveal that hypercortisolism has been present for many years (Fig. 9.6). Several clinical features of hypercortisolism (obesity, hypertension, glucose intolerance) are fairly common in the general population and thus do not reliably identify affected patients. Central obesity, proximal myopathy, ecchymoses, widened purplish striae, and osteopenia are more specific for hypercortisolism (88, 89). Most patients are diagnosed in the third to fifth decades of life. There is a definite female preponderance of Cushing's disease (86, 87).

Obesity is one of the first manifestations of hypercortisolism. Some patients may literally double their body weight, whereas others report only minimal increases in weight but are aware of a central redistribution of body fat. Characteristic physical features are a result of visceral, retroperitoneal, mediastinal, and subcutaneous fat accumulation. The abdomen is often protuberant. The supraclavicular, infraclavicular, and cervicodorsal ("buffalo hump") fat pads are rounded and puffy. Widened and rectangular or "moon" facies develop because of fat deposition in the preauricular areas, temporal fossae, and cheeks (Fig. 9.7). Effects of glucocorticoids, catecholamines, and insulin on fat metabolism and regional variations in the density of glucocorticoid receptors in adipose tissues have been implicated in the pathophysiology of fat redistribution in patients with hypercortisolism (86, 90).

Atrophy of the skin is more prominent over the distal aspects of the upper and lower extremities. Fragility of the connective tissues of the dermis predispose to ecchymoses that can occur following minimal trauma. Widened (> 1 cm) violaceous striae may develop across the flanks, buttocks, inner aspects of the thighs, axillary folds, breasts, and upper arms (Fig. 9.8). Occasionally, patients have thinned reddish striae similar to those seen after rapid weight gain and in pregnant patients. Facial plethora, hypertrichosis, hirsutism, male pattern hair loss, steroid acne, tinea versicolor, acanthosis nigricans, and poor wound healing with a propensity for wound dehiscence and infection are other common cutaneous manifestations of chronic hypercortisolism (86, 88–90). Hyperpigmentation is unusual in patients with ACTH-secreting pituitary adenomas, and its presence should alert the treating physician to the possibility of an ectopic ACTH-secreting neuroendocrine tumor.

Muscle atrophy can result in fatigue, proximal myopathy, decreased strength, and thinning of the extremities, which accentuates the other changes in body habitus. Proximal myopathy and weakness are characterized by disability related to dysfunction of the muscles about the shoulder and hip girdles. Affected patients often report difficulty climbing stairs, arising from a sitting position, combing

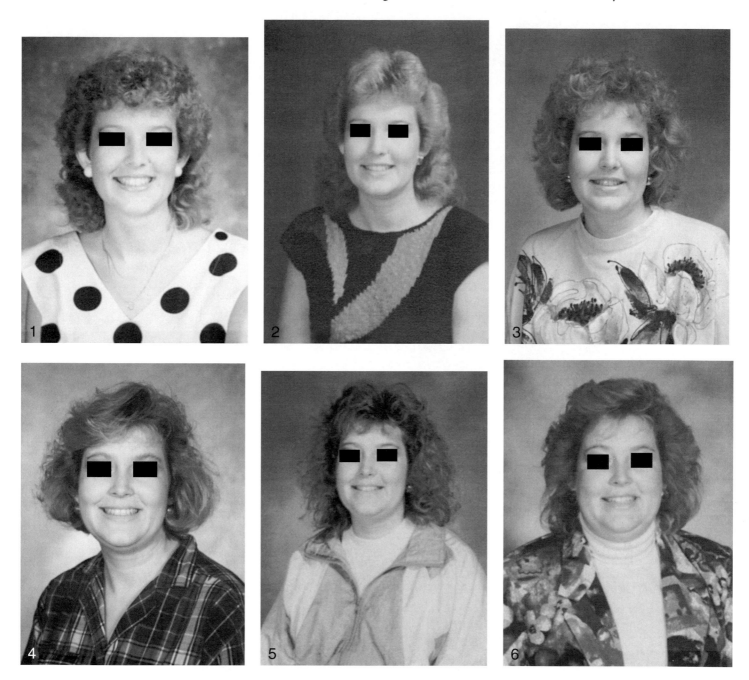

Figure 9.6. Serial photographs at 2-year intervals for 10 years illustrating the onset and insidious progression of facial features of Cushing's syndrome caused by an ACTH-secreting pituitary macroadenoma.

their hair, and performing repetitive work-related tasks involving use of the upper extremities.

Glucocorticoids inhibit intestinal calcium absorption and promote renal calcium wasting. These actions lead to secondary hyperparathyroidism and increased bone resorption. Glucocorticoids directly inhibit new bone formation by suppressing osteoblastic function and decreasing replication and differentiation of osteoblast precursors (91). Most patients with active Cushing's syndrome have marked osteopenia in the lumbar spine and femoral neck (92, 93). Patients with severe disease may experience compression fractures with resulting back pain, loss in height, and ky-

phosis. Spontaneous fractures of the ribs and pelvis are not uncommon. Hypercalciuria may lead to nephrolithiasis, which, when complicated by urinary tract obstruction and infection, can be life threatening.

Impaired glucose tolerance is seen in three-quarters of affected patients. Overt diabetes mellitus is present in only 10 to 15% of patients (89, 94). Increased hepatic glucose output, muscle glycogenolysis, and insulin resistance related to accretion of body fat can result in glucose intolerance when endogenous insulin secretory capacity fails to reverse and correct these metabolic abnormalities. Hypercortisolism has complex effects on lipid metabolism, result-

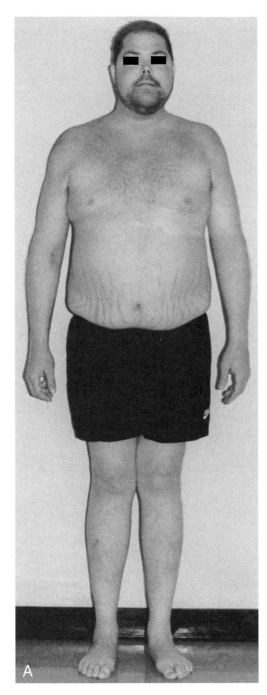

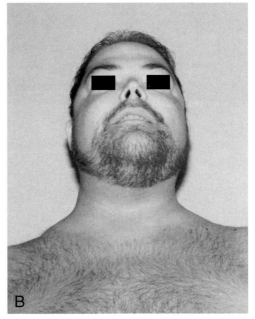

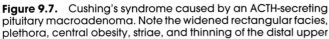

Figure 9.7. Cushing's syndrome caused by an ACTH-secreting pituitary macroadenoma. Note the widened rectangular facies, plethora, central obesity, striae, and thinning of the distal upper and lower extremities caused by muscle atrophy **(A)** and the convex fullness of the supraclavicular fossae **(B)**.

ing in increased circulating levels of all lipid fractions (total cholesterol, HDL, LDL, VLDL, triglycerides) (95).

Hypertension is an early manifestation of glucocorticoid excess and occurs in nearly three-quarters of affected patients. The pathogenesis of hypertension in Cushing's syndrome is complex and reflects the interplay of numerous systems regulating plasma volume, vascular resistance, and cardiac output (96, 97). The hypertension is usually mild but can be severe and may result in left ventricular hypertro-

phy followed by diastolic dysfunction and congestive heart failure (97). Hypokalemia, unusual in patients with ACTH-secreting pituitary adenomas, may result from the mineralocorticoid effect of high intrarenal levels of cortisol, secretion of steroid intermediates that possess mineralocorticoid activity, or activation of the renin-angiotensin system. Hypertension, diabetes mellitus, insulin resistance, and hypercholesterolemia are risk factors for the development of atherosclerotic vascular disease. An increased inci-

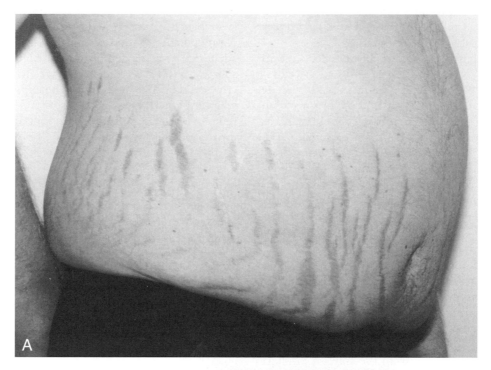

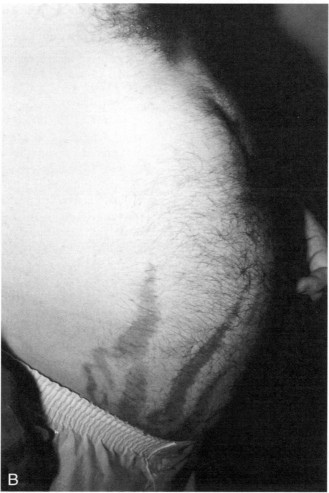

Figure 9.8. Variations in the appearance of striae in two patients with Cushing's syndrome.

dence of perioperative thromboembolic events in patients with Cushing's syndrome has been attributed to a documented hypercoagulable state (98–100).

Glucocorticoids have complex inhibitory effects on inflammatory and cellular immune responses to infectious agents. As a result, patients with Cushing's syndrome are prone to develop common bacterial and opportunistic infections (101). Skin and skin structure infections (cellulitis, perirectal abscess, wound) with common bacterial pathogens are common. Mucocutaneous candidiasis and tinea versicolor are common, whereas disseminated opportunistic fungal infections (cryptococcosis, histoplasmosis, aspergillosis, Pneumocystis carinii pneumonia) are uncommon. Disseminated strongyloidiasis and listeriosis are unusual but must be considered in the differential diagnosis of patients with systemic infections. Hypercortisolism may alter the clinical manifestations of infection, resulting in absence of fever, pain, and other cardinal signs of inflammation. In many cases, infectious processes are life threatening by the time they are recognized.

Hypercortisolism results in functional suppression of hypothalamic gonadotropin-releasing hormone and disruption of LH and FSH secretion from the anterior pituitary gland. These abnormalities result in varying degrees of reversible hypogonadism in more than three-quarters of affected patients (87–89).

Clinically important psychological disturbances are common. Self-reported perceptions of the effects of hypercortisolism on mental functioning include mood swings, irritability, depression, memory lapses, unclear thinking, impaired concentration, and disruption of sleep (102). More than half of adult patients have a major affective disorder (90). Predominant features of Cushing's syndrome in children include weight gain, growth retardation, and premature sexual development (93, 103, 104). Children often have generalized obesity rather than central obesity. Myopathy and thinning of the extremities are uncommon.

The syndrome of ectopic ACTH hypersecretion must be considered in the differential diagnosis of all patients with ACTH-dependent Cushing's syndrome (105, 106) (Table 9.3). The clinical presentations of many of these patients, especially those with bronchial carcinoid tumors, mimic the presentation of Cushing's disease (107, 108). Further, the classic syndrome of ectopic ACTH hypersecretion, characterized by an explosive onset of rapid weight loss, edema, myopathy, carbohydrate intolerance, and hypokalemic alkalosis, may be seen in rare patients with Cushing's disease and significant hypersecretion of ACTH and cortisol.

Patients suspected of having ACTH-secreting pituitary adenomas must be studied in a stepwise fashion to avoid potentially catastrophic diagnostic and therapeutic errors. Demonstration of clinical and biochemical features of pathologic hypersecretion of cortisol are required to establish a diagnosis of Cushing's syndrome (109, 110). The ACTH-dependent nature of the Cushing's syndrome is confirmed by the presence of normal or overtly elevated levels of plasma ACTH in hypercortisolemic patients (111). A preoperative diagnosis of an ACTH-secreting pituitary adenoma rests on demonstration of the pituitary as the source of ACTH as evidenced by results of dynamic endocrine studies, neuroradiologic imaging procedures, and, when indicated, measurements of ACTH levels in blood samples obtained from the inferior petrosal sinuses following the administration of ovine corticotropin-releasing hormone (112–115).

Hyperthyroidism

Hyperthyroidism caused by a TSH-secreting pituitary adenoma was first described in 1970 (116). This rare disorder is now recognized with increasing frequency because serum TSH measurements are routine in the evaluation of patients with hyperthyroidism (117, 118). TSH-secreting pituitary adenomas are derived from the thyrotroph cells of the anterior pituitary gland. They are usually diagnosed in the third to sixth decades of life and are more common in women than in men (119).

Macroadenomas are found in 93% of patients with TSH-secreting pituitary adenomas (117, 120–123). Many of these patients have clinical features attributed to large, invasive tumors. Nearly all patients have hyperthyroidism and diffuse goiters (117, 120, 123). Unfortunately, the usual delay between diagnosis of hyperthyroidism and recognition of a TSH-secreting pituitary adenoma is about 6 years (117, 119). Failure to recognize the TSH-dependent nature of the hyperthyroidism often leads to inappropriate therapy directed against the thyroid gland with I-131, antithyroid drugs, and surgery. Many patients have refractory or recurrent hyperthyroidism despite attempts to eradicate the thyroid gland because persistent TSH secretion results in hypertrophy and hyperfunction of remnant thyroid tissue. Therapy directed against the thyroid gland to decrease circulating levels of thyroid hormones may promote aggressive pituitary tumor growth and invasiveness, a situation analogous to Nelson's syndrome after adrenalectomy in patients with ACTH-secreting pituitary adenomas (117).

Symptoms of hyperthyroidism include nervousness, sweating, heat intolerance, palpitations, fatigue, weakness, increased appetite, and hyperdefecation. Common physical findings include tachycardia, hyperkinesis, warm velvety skin, widened palpebral fissures, stare, lid lag, a fine tremor of the outstretched hands, and hyperreflexia with a rapid relaxation phase of the deep tendon reflexes. Unilateral exophthalmos has been described and attributed to tumoral invasion of the orbit. Otherwise, features specific for Graves' disease, including thyroid orbitopathy, acropachy, and pretibial myxedema, are absent in patients with TSH-secreting pituitary adenomas.

Serum total and free thyroid hormone levels are elevated in nearly all patients but may be normal or even low in patients successfully treated with I-131 and thyroidectomy (119–121, 123). Serum TSH levels are always inappropriately normal or frankly elevated. TSH levels as low as 1.1 μIU/L (1.1 μIU/mL) and as high as 568 μIU/L (568 μIU/mL) have been reported (117, 121). Basal TSH levels do not correlate with tumor size or invasiveness (117).

Two observations may explain the occurrence of hyperthyroidism in patients with TSH-secreting pituitary adenomas who have normal circulating TSH levels. First, these patients seem to secrete TSH molecules that are more biologically active than "normal" TSH (117). Second, tumoral secretion of TSH is variable and erratic, resulting in loss of the normal diurnal variation in TSH concentration (117). As a result, TSH secretion for a 24-h period may be elevated despite normal random serum TSH levels. α-Subunit levels are usually elevated and the α-subunit-to-TSH molar ratio exceeds 1.0 in nearly all patients (117, 123). The molar ratio is calculated by dividing the α-subunit concentration, in nanomoles per liter, by the serum TSH concentration, in micro international units per liter, and multiplying the result by 10. Dynamic testing of the serum TSH responses to various agents has not yielded consistent results in patients with TSH-secreting pituitary tumors. The lack of a rise in serum TSH levels following TRH administration may, however, be helpful in distinguishing patients with TSH-secreting microadenomas from patients with selective pituitary resistance to thyroid hormone (120, 123).

Nonfunctional Pituitary Adenomas

Patients with sellar masses and no obvious clinical features of a syndrome of anterior pituitary hormone hypersecretion are often said to have "nonfunctioning" or "nonsecreting" pituitary tumors. In fact, these patients may have any one of several subtypes of pituitary adenomas or other disorders mimicking pituitary tumors (Table 9.4). Thorough preoperative clinical, biochemical, and radiologic investigations and routine postoperative histologic and immunohistochemical examinations of resected tissue are necessary to correctly diagnose and classify these patients.

Approximately one-quarter of patients with documented pituitary tumors harbor clinically nonfunctioning adenomas (124, 125). A few of these are truly nonfunctioning oncocytomas. Results of immunohistochemical, dispersed cell culture, and advanced molecular studies have proved that most of them are, in fact, gonadotropin-producing adenomas (126–130). These tumors are derived from a single neoplastic clone of a gonadotropin-producing anterior pituitary cell. They occur with an equal frequency in men and women and are most commonly diagnosed in middle-aged patients. The gonadotropins (FSH, LH) and their subunits (β-FSH, β-LH, and α-subunit) are inefficiently produced, and, as a result, less than half of affected patients have elevated gonadotropin levels (130, 131). Paradoxically, most patients with these tumors do not have clinical features related to gonadotropin excess but instead present with mass effects and central hypogonadism (130, 131) (Table 9.5). Clinical scenarios suggesting the pres-

Table 9.4. Differential Diagnosis of Nonfunctioning Pituitary Adenomas

Null-cell adenoma
Oncocytoma
Gonadotropin-secreting adenoma
Clinically silent hormone-producing adenoma
  ACTH
  PRl
  GH
  TSH
  α-Subunit
  Plurihormonal
Hormone-secreting tumor with subtle features of hormone excess
Other intrasellar or parasellar processes
  Cyst
  Meningioma
  Craniopharyngioma
  Chordoma
  Granular cell myoblastoma
  Lymphoma
  Metastatic carcinoma
  Sarcoidosis
  Lymphocytic hypophysitis
  Granulomatous hypophysitis
  Aneurysm

Table 9.5. Clinical Presentation of Gonadotropin-Producing Pituitary Adenomas

Symptoms/Signs	Percent
Symptoms	
Visual complaints	43
Hypopituitarism	22
Headache	8
Multiple features	10
Incidental (asymptomatic)	17
Signs	
Visual field deficits	68
Hypopituitarism	77
Hyperprolactinemia	33
Elevated FSH	42
FSH > 2× upper limit of normal	9
Elevated LH	36
LH > 2× upper limit of normal	19
Elevated α-subunit	3

Adapted from Young WF Jr, Scheithauer BW, Kovacs KT, Horvath E, Davis DH, Randall RV. Gonadotroph adenoma of the pituitary gland: a clinicopathologic analysis of 100 cases. Mayo Clin Proc 1996;71:649–656.

ence of gonadotropin-secreting tumors in patients harboring apparent nonfunctioning tumors include (a) an elevated serum FSH concentration in a man with hypogonadism; (b) elevated LH and total testosterone concentrations in a man with normal gonadal function, especially in the setting of partial hypopituitarism; (c) an elevated serum FSH concentration in an amenorrheic premenopausal woman; (d) an elevated serum FSH concentration in a postmenopausal woman with documented hypopituitarism; and (e) isosexual precocious puberty in a boy (130, 132–134). In many of these patients, gonadotropin-secreting adenomas can be confirmed preoperatively by the gonadotropin response following the administration of TRH (130, 132). Serum concentrations of FSH and β-LH increase in some affected patients but do not rise at all in patients with normal (nonneoplastic) gonadotrophs and other types of pituitary adenomas.

Clinically silent nonsecreting or nonfunctioning tumors can also arise from other anterior pituitary cell types (135). In patients harboring these tumors, the absence of clinical evidence of hormone hypersecretion may reflect impaired synthesis, secretion, or biologic activity of the final hormone product (124). ACTH-producing pituitary tumors are perhaps the most well characterized of these clinically silent tumors. Horvath et al. found 17 silent ACTH-producing adenomas in a study of 300 unselected pituitary tumors (136). Immunohistochemical detection of ACTH 1–39, ACTH 19–39, β-lipotropin, and β-endorphin was taken as evidence of tumoral ACTH production. These tumors, which are usually large, invasive, and aggressive, have a tendency to recur following primary therapy (135, 137). Recurrences may be heralded by the onset and progression of typical clinical and biochemical features of hypercortisolism in patients whose tumors have acquired the ability to synthesize and secrete ACTH (137). Silent GH-producing tumors have also been described (138–140). Clinical features of acromegaly are characteristically absent despite moderate elevations in GH and IGF-1 levels. These patients usually have large, invasive, and aggressive tumors.

Occasionally, patients are misdiagnosed as having nonfunctioning tumors when the subtle and protean clinical manifestations of anterior pituitary hormone hypersecretion are overlooked. These patients are often correctly diagnosed on review of their clinical presentation in light of immunohistochemical findings or as clinical features evolve during follow-up in patients with residual and recurrent tumors.

Plurihormonal Adenomas

Plurihormonal pituitary adenomas synthesize and/or secrete more than one anterior pituitary hormone. These adenomas, more commonly recognized by immunocytochemical analysis of resected tumor tissue than by standard clinical evaluation, probably account for 10 to 15% of all anterior pituitary neoplasms. Plurihormonal adenomas may be composed of one cell type (monomorphous) that secretes several hormones or of several cell types (plurimorphous) that each secrete one hormone (141–143).

Thirty to fifty percent of patients with acromegaly harbor tumors that also secrete PRL. In many acromegalic patients, the coexisting hyperprolactinemia is erroneously attributed to stalk syndrome. These tumors may be one of three well-recognized subtypes: mixed GH-cell and PRL-cell adenomas, mammosomatotroph (GH-predominant) adenomas, or acidophil stem cell (PRL-predominant) adenomas (144–148). Successful tumor resection usually restores the serum PRL concentration to normal. Acromegalic patients with persistently elevated postoperative serum PRL concentrations should be assessed to determine whether they have residual tumor requiring adjunctive therapy. Interestingly, acromegalic patients with these plurihormonal adenomas are more likely to respond to treatment with dopamine agonists than are patients with pure GH-secreting adenomas (149).

GH-secreting adenomas that also secrete one of the anterior pituitary glycoprotein hormones (LH, FSH, TSH) and the α-subunit of the glycoprotein hormones have been described (150–153). ACTH- and PRL-secreting plurimorphous adenomas and ACTH- and α-subunit–secreting tumors also have been reported (154–157). Half of TSH-secreting pituitary adenomas are histologically plurihormonal (119). Acromegaly and hyperprolactinemia have been described in patients harboring these tumors (119, 120).

Occasionally, patients thought to harbor plurihormonal tumors may actually have several pituitary adenomas (158). Blevins et al. described a patient with acromegaly and Cushing's syndrome who had synchronous GH- and ACTH-secreting adenomas (159). Tolis et al. reported a patient with acromegaly and hyperprolactinemia resulting from two discrete adenomas, one secreting GH and the other secreting PRL (160). Silent microadenomas have been found during histologic examination of normal pituitary resected at surgery for nonsecreting pituitary adenomas.

REFERENCES

1. Kovacs K, Scheithauer B, Horvath E, et al. The World Health Organization classification of adenohypophysial neoplasms. Cancer 1996;78:502–510.
2. Burrow GN, Wortzman G, Rewcastle NB, et al. Microadenomas of the pituitary and abnormal sellar tomograms in an unselected autopsy series. N Engl J Med 1981;304:156–158.
3. Molitch ME, Russell EJ. The pituitary incidentaloma. Ann Intern Med 1990;112:925–931.
4. Ontjes DA, Nay RL. Pituitary tumors. Cancer J Clin 1976;26:330–350.
5. Bakay L. The results of 300 pituitary adenoma operations. J Neurosurg 1950;7:240–255.
6. Caplan B, Day AL, Quisling R, et al. Hemorrhage into pituitary adenomas. Surg Neurol 1983;20:280–287.
7. Banna M. Pathology and clinical manifestations. In: Hankinson J, Banna M, eds. Pituitary and Parapituitary Tumors. Philadelphia: WB Saunders, 1976.
8. Robinson F, Goodrich I. Neurological manifestations of extrasellar expanding pituitary adenomas. In: Goodrich I, Lee KJ, eds. The Pituitary: Clinical Aspects of Normal and Abnormal Function. New York: Elsevier Science Publishers, 1987.
9. Bailey P. Hypophyseal Adenomas: Intracranial Tumors. Springfield: Charles C Thomas, 1983.
10. Stefanis GS, Cavanaugh HD, Tindall GT. Ophthalmological aspects of pituitary tumors. In: Tindall GT, Collins WF, eds. Clinical Management of Pituitary Disorders. New York: Raven Press, 1979.
11. Lesser R. Neuroophthalmic aspects of pituitary disease. In: Goodrich I, Lee KJ, eds. The Pituitary: Clinical Aspects of Normal and Abnormal Function. New York: Elsevier Science Publishers, 1987.

12. Robert CM Jr, Feigenbaum JA, Stern WE. Ocular palsy occurring with pituitary tumors. J Neurosurg 1973;38:17–19.
13. Rothrock JF, Laguna JF, Reynolds AF. CSF rhinorrhea from untreated pituitary adenoma. Arch Neurol 1982;39:442–443.
14. Bills DC, Meyer FB, Laws ER, et al. A retrospective analysis of pituitary apoplexy. Neurosurgery 1993;33:602–609.
15. Cardoso ER, Peterson EW. Pituitary apoplexy: a review. Neurosurgery 1984;14:363–373.
16. Rosén T, Bengtsson BC. Epidemiology of adult onset hypopituitarism in Göteborg, Sweden during 1956–1993. 10th International Congress of Endocrinology, 1996.
17. Nelson AT Jr, Tucker HstG, Becker DP. Residual anterior pituitary function following transsphenoidal resection of pituitary macroadenomas. J Neurosurg 1984;61:577–580.
18. Lees PD, Pickard JD. Hyperprolactinemia, intrasellar pituitary tissue pressure, and the pituitary stalk compression syndrome. J Neurosurg 1987;67:192–196.
19. Arafah BM, Kailani SH, Nekl KE, et al. Immediate recovery of pituitary function after transsphenoidal resection of pituitary macroadenomas. J Clin Endocrinol Metab 1994;79:348–354.
20. Faria MA Jr, Tindall GT. Transsphenoidal microsurgery for prolactin-secreting pituitary adenomas: results in 100 women with the amenorrhea-galactorrhea syndrome. J Neurosurg 1982;56:33–43.
21. Snyder PJ, Fowble BF, Schatz NJ, et al. Hypopituitarism following radiation therapy of pituitary adenomas. Am J Med 1986;81:457–462.
22. Krishna AY, Blevins LS. Case report: reversible gastroparesis in patients with hypopituitary disease. Am J Med Sci 1996;312:43–45.
23. Oelkers W. Hyponatremia and inappropriate secretion of vasopressin (antidiuretic hormone) in patients with hypopituitarism. N Engl J Med 1989;321:492–496.
24. Kamoi K, Tamura T, Tanake K, et al. Hyponatremia and osmoregulation of thirst in vasopressin secretion in patients with adrenal insufficiency. J Clin Endocrinol Metab 1993;77:1584–1588.
25. Blevins LS. Serum cortisol is not an accurate predictor of the integrity of the hypothalamic-pituitary-adrenocortical axis. Clin Endocrinol 1995;42:101–104.
26. Watts NB, Tindall GT. Rapid assessment of corticotropin reserve after pituitary surgery. JAMA 1988;259:708–711.
27. Jones Sl, Trainer PJ, Perry L, et al. An audit of the insulin tolerance test in adult subjects in an acute investigational unit over one year. Clin Endocrinol 1992;37:387–397.
28. Streeten DHP, Anderson GH Jr, Bonaventura MN. The potential for serious consequences from misinterpreting normal responses to the rapid adrenocorticotropin test. J Clin Endocrinol Metab 1996;81:285–290.
29. Blevins LS. Dynamic tests of pituitary function. In: Hurst JW, ed. Medicine for the Practicing Physician. 4th ed. Stamford: Appleton and Lange, 1996.
30. Pinchera A, Martino E, Faglia G. Central hypothyroidism. In: Braverman LE, Utiger RD, eds. The Thyroid. 6th ed. Philadelphia: Lippincott, 1991.
31. Hall R, Scanlon MF. Hypothyroidism: clinical features and complications. J Clin Endocrinol Metab 1979;8:29–38.
32. Joffe RT, Sokolv STH. Thyroid hormones, the brain and affective disorders. Clin Rev Neurobiol 1994;8:45–63.
33. Samuels MH, Ridgway EC. Central hypothyroidism. Endocrinol Metab Clin North Am 1992;21:903–919.
34. Cuneo RC, Salomon F, McGauley GA, et al. The growth hormone deficiency syndrome in adults. Clin Endocrinol 1992;37:387–397.
35. Shamanesh M, Ali Z, Pourmand M, et al. Pituitary function tests in Sheehan's syndrome. Clin Endocrinol 1980;12:303–311.
36. Blevins LS, Wand GS. Diabetes insipidus. Crit Care Med 1992;20:69–79.
37. Robertson GL. Differential diagnosis of polyuria. Annu Rev Med 1988;39:425–442.
38. Geheb MA. Clinical approach to the hyperosmolar patient. Crit Care Clin 1987;5:797–815.
39. Black P, Cervas NT, Candia GL. Incidence and management of complications of transsphenoidal operation for pituitary adenomas. Neurosurgery 1987;20:920–923.
40. Cohen AR, Cooper PR, Kupersmith MJ, et al. Visual recovery after transsphenoidal removal of pituitary adenomas. Neurosurgery 1985;17:446–452.
41. Verbalis JG, Robinson AG, Moses AM. Postoperative and post-traumatic diabetes insipidus. In: Czernichow P, Robinson AG, eds. Diabetes Insipidus in Man: Frontiers of Hormone Research. Vol 13. Basel: S. Karger, 1985.
42. Moses AM. Long-standing post-traumatic diabetes insipidus. Medical Grand Rounds 1983;2:117–128.
43. Vokes TJ, Robertson GL. Disorders of antidiuretic hormone. Endocrinol Metab Clin North Am 1988;17:281–299.
44. Arguello C, Blevins LS. Prolactinomas: diagnosis and management. Contemp Neurosurg 1995;17:13.
45. Loh K-C, Shlossberg AH, Ritmaster RS, et al. Giant prolactinomas: a retrospective review. The Endocrinologist 1996;6:257–263.
46. Molitch ME. Prolactin. In: Melmed S, ed. The Pituitary. Ann Arbor: Blackwell Science, 1995.
47. Molitch ME. Prolactinoma. In: Melmed S, ed. The Pituitary. Ann Arbor: Blackwell Science, 1995.
48. Kredentser JV, Hoskins CF, Scott JZ. Hyperprolactinemia: a significant factor in female infertility. Am J Obstet Gynecol 1981;139:264–267.
49. Huang K-E, Bonfiglio TA, Muschler EK. Transient hyperprolactinemia in infertile women with luteal phase deficiency. Obstet Gynecol 1991;78:651–655.
50. Jacobs HS, Frank S, Murray MAF, et al. Clinical and endocrine features of hyperprolactinemic amenorrhea. Clin Endocrinol 1976;5:439.
51. Carter JN, Tyson JE, Tolis G, et al. Prolactin-secreting tumors and hypogonadism in 22 men. N Engl J Med 1978;229:847.
52. Segal LS, Polishuk WZ, Ben-David M. Hyperprolactinemic male infertility. Fertil Steril 1976;26:1425.
53. Carter JN, Tyson JE, Warne GL, et al. Adrenocortical function in hyperprolactinemic women. J Clin Endocrinol Metab 1977;45:973.
54. Glickman SP, Rosenfield RL, Bergenstal RM, et al. Multiple androgenic abnormalities, including free testosterone, in hyperprolactinemic women. J Clin Endocrinol Metab 1982;55:251.
55. Klibanski A, Neer RM, Beitens IZ, et al. Decreased bone density in hyperprolactinemic women. N Engl J Med 1980;303:1511.
56. Schlechte JM, Sherman B, Martin R. Bone density in amenorrheic women with and without hyperprolactinemia. J Clin Endocrinol Metab 1983;56:1120.
57. Klibanski A, Greenspan SL. Increase in bone mass after treatment of hyperprolactinemic amenorrhea. N Engl J Med 1986;315:542–546.
58. Greenspan SL, Near RM, Ridgway EC, et al. Osteoporosis in men with hyperprolactinemic hypogonadism. Ann Intern Med 1986;104:777–782.
59. Feingenbaum SL, Downey DE, Wilson CB, et al. Transsphenoidal pituitary resection for preoperative diagnosis of prolactin-secreting pituitary adenoma in women: long-term follow-up. J Clin Endocrinol Metab 1996;81:1711–1719.
60. Molitch ME, Elton RL, Blackwell RE, et al. Bromocriptine as primary therapy for prolactin-secreting macroadenomas: results of a prospective multi-center study. J Clin Endocrinol Metab 1985;60:698–705.
61. Bevan JS, Webster J, Burke CW, et al. Dopamine agonists and pituitary tumor shrinkage. Endocrinol Rev 1992;13:220–240.
62. Chan AW, MacFarlane IA, Fox PM, et al. Pituitary enlargement and hyperprolactinemia due to primary hypothyroidism: errors and delays in diagnosis. Br J Neurosurg 1990;4:107–112.
63. Tyson JE, Hwang P, Guyda H, et al. Studies of prolactin secretion in human pregnancy. Am J Obstet Gynecol 1972;113:14–20.
64. Gonzalez JG, Elizondo G, Saldivar D, et al. Pituitary gland growth during normal pregnancy: an in vivo study using magnetic resonance imaging. Am J Med 1988;85:217–220.
65. Ezzat S, Forester MJ, Berchtold P, et al. Acromegaly: clinical and biochemical features in 500 patients. Medicine 1994;73:233–240.
66. Rajasoorya C, Holdaway IM, Wrightson P, et al. Determinants of clinical outcome and survival in acromegaly. Clin Endocrinol 1994;41:95–102.
67. Bates AS, Van't Hoff W, Jones JM, et al. Does treatment of acromegaly affect life expectancy? Metabolism 1995;44(suppl 1):1–5.
68. Bengtsson B-A, Eden S, Ernest E, Odén A, Sjögren B. Epidemiology and long-term survival in acromegaly. Acta Med Scand 1988;223:327–335.
69. Hennessey JV, Jackson IM. Clinical features and differential diag-

nosis of pituitary tumours with emphasis on acromegaly. Ballière's Clin Endocrinol Metab 1995;9:271–314.

70. Snow MH, Piercy DA, Robson V, et al. An investigation into the pathogenesis of hypertension in acromegaly. Clin Sci Mol Med 1977;53:87–91.

71. Layton MW, Fudman EJ, Barkan A, et al. Acromegalic arthropathy. Arthritis Rheum 1988;31:1022–1027.

72. Thiboutot DM. Dermatological manifestations of endocrine disorders. J Clin Endocrinol Metab 1995;80:3082–3087.

73. Nabarro JDN. Acromegaly. Clin Endocrinol 1987;26:481–512.

74. Klein I, Ojamaa K. Cardiovascular manifestations of endocrine disease. J Clin Endocrinol Metab 1992;72:2:339–342.

75. Grunstein RR, Ho KY, Sullivan CE. Sleep apnea in acromegaly. Ann Intern Med 1991;115:527–532.

76. Takamoto S, Tsuchiya H, Onishi T, et al. Changes in calcium homeostasis in acromegaly treated by pituitary adenomectomy. J Clin Endocrinol Metab 1985;61:7–11.

77. Barzilay J, Heatley GJ, Cushing GW. Benign and malignant tumors in patients with acromegaly. Arch Intern Med 1991;151:1629–1632.

78. Terzolo M, Tappero G, Borretta G, et al. High prevalence of colonic polyps in patients with acromegaly. Arch Intern Med 1994;154:1272–1276.

79. Cats A, Dullaart RPF, Kleibeuker JH, et al. Increased epithelial cell proliferation in the colon of patients with acromegaly. Cancer Res 1996;56:523–526.

80. Delhougne B, Deneux C, Abs R, et al. The prevalence of colonic polyps in acromegaly: a colonoscopic and pathological study in 103 patients. J Clin Endocrinol Metab 1995;80:3223–3226.

81. Melmed S. Acromegaly. In: Melmed S, ed. The Pituitary. Ann Arbor: Blackwell Science, 1995.

82. Burgess JR, Shepherd JJ, Parameswanan V, et al. Somatotrophinomas in multiple endocrine neoplasia type 1: a review of clinical phenotype and insulin-like growth factor-1 levels in a large multiple endocrine neoplasia type 1 kindred. Am J Med 1996;100:544–547.

83. Melmed S. Acromegaly. N Engl J Med 1990;322:966–977.

84. Chang-DeMoranville BM, Jackson IMD. Diagnosis and endocrine testing in acromegaly. Endocrinol Metab Clin North Am 1992;21:649–668.

85. Cushing H. The basophil adenomas of the pituitary body and their clinical manifestations. In: The Pituitary Body and Its Disorders: Clinical States Produced by Disorders of the Hypophysis Cerebri. Philadelphia: JB Lippincott, 1912.

86. Bertagna X, Raux-Demay M-C, Guilhaume B, et al. Cushing's Disease. In: Melmed S, ed. The Pituitary. Ann Arbor: Blackwell Science, 1995.

87. Tindall GT, Khajavi M, Christy JH, et al. Natural history of treated Cushing's disease due to pituitary macroadenomas. In: von Werder K, Fahlbusch R, eds. Pituitary Adenomas: From Basic Research to Diagnosis and Therapy. Amsterdam BV: Elsevier Science, 1996:183–187.

88. Nugent CA, Warner HR, Dunn JT, et al. Probability, theory and the diagnosis of Cushing's syndrome. J Clin Endocrinol Metab 1964;24:621–627.

89. Ross EJ, Linch DC. Cushing's syndrome-killing disease: discriminatory value of signs and symptoms aiding early diagnosis. Lancet 1982;2:646–649.

90. Yanovski JA, Cutler GB Jr. Glucocorticoid action in the clinical features of Cushing's syndrome. Endocrinol Metab Clin North Am 1994;23:487–509.

91. Canalis E. Mechanisms of glucocorticoid action in bone: implications to glucocorticoid-induced osteoporosis. J Clin Endocrinol Metab 1996;81:3441–3447.

92. Hermus AR, Smals AG, Swinkels LM, et al. Bone mineral density and bone turn over before and after surgical cure of Cushing's syndrome. J Clin Endocrinol Metab 1995;80:2859–2865.

93. Leong GM, Mercado-Asis LB, Reynolds JC, et al. The effect of Cushing's disease on bone mineral density, body composition, growth and puberty: a report of an identical adolescent twin pair. J Clin Endocrinol Metab 1996;81:1905–1911.

94. Ganda OP. Prevalence and incidence of secondary and other types of diabetes. In: Diabetes in America. 2nd ed. Bethesda: NIH NIDDK. Publication 95–1468.

95. Duell PB. Hypertriglyceridemia: pathophysiology, diagnosis and treatment. The Endocrinologist 1992;2:321–331.

96. Danese RD, Aron DC. Cushing's syndrome in hypertension. Endocrinol Metab Clin North Am 1994;23:299–324.

97. Boscaro M, Sonino N, Fallo F, et al. Hypertension and Cushing's syndrome. In: Lüdecke DK, Chrousos GP, Tolis G, eds. ACTH, Cushing's Syndrome, and Other Hypercortisolemic States. New York: Raven Press, 1990:203–210.

98. Sjöberg HE, Blombäck M, Granberg PO. Thromboembolic complications, heparin treatment and the increase in coagulation factors in Cushing's syndrome. Acta Med Scand 1976;199:95–98.

99. Dal-Bo-Zanon R, Fornaserio L, Boscaro M, et al. Clotting changes in Cushing's syndrome: elevated factor VII activity. Folia Hematol 1983;110:268–277.

100. Jackson JA, Trowbridge A, Smigiel M. Fatal thromboembolism after successful transsphenoidal hypophysectomy for Cushing's disease. South Med J 1990;883:960–962.

101. Aucott JN. Glucocorticoids and infection. Endocrinol Metab Clin North Am 1994;23:655–670.

102. Gotch PM. Cushing's syndrome from the patient's perspective. Endocrinol Metab Clin North Am 1994;23:607–617.

103. Besser GM, Savage MO. Cushing's disease in childhood. Trends Endocrinol Metab 1996;7:213–216.

104. Magiakou MA, Mastorakos G, Oldfield EH, et al. Cushing's syndrome in children and adults. N Engl J Med 1994;331:629–636.

105. Doppman JL. The search for occult ectopic ACTH-producing tumors. The Endocrinologist 1992;2:41–46.

106. Doppman JL, Neiman L, Miller DL, et al. Ectopic adrenocorticotropic hormone syndrome: localization studies in 28 patients. Radiology 1989;172:115–124.

107. Limper AH, Carpenter PC, Scheithauer B, et al. The Cushing's syndrome induced by bronchial carcinoid tumors. Ann Intern Med 1992;117:209–214.

108. Leinung MC, Young WF Jr, Whitaker MD, et al. Diagnosis of corticotropin-producing bronchial carcinoid tumors causing Cushing's syndrome. Mayo Clin Proc 1990;65:1314–1321.

109. Yanovski JA. The dexamethasone-suppressed corticotropin releasing hormone test and the differential diagnosis of hypercortisolism. The Endocrinologist 1995;5:169–175.

110. Kaye TB, Crapo L. The Cushing's syndrome: an update on diagnostic tests. Ann Intern Med 1990;112:434–444.

111. Findling JW, Engeland WC, Raff H. The use of immunoradiometric assay for the measurement of ACTH in human plasma. Trends Endocrinol Metab 1990;1:283–287.

112. Avgerinos PC, Yanovski JA, Oldefield EH, et al. The metyrapone and dexamethasone suppression tests for the differential diagnosis of the adrenocorticotropin-dependent Cushing's syndrome: a comparison. Ann Intern Med 1994;121:318–327.

113. Flack MR, Oldfield EH, Cutler GB Jr, et al. Urine-free cortisol in the high-dose dexamethasone suppression test with a differential diagnosis of Cushing's syndrome. Ann Intern Med 1992;116:211–217.

114. Dichek HL, Nieman LK, Oldfield EH, et al. A comparison of the standard high dose dexamethasone suppression test and the overnight 8 mg dexamethasone suppression test for the differential diagnosis of adrenocorticotropin-dependent Cushing's syndrome. J Clin Endocrinol Metab 1994;78:418–422.

115. Oldfield EH, Doppman JL, Nieman LK, et al. Petrosal sinus sampling with and without corticotropin-releasing hormone for the differential diagnosis of Cushing's syndrome. N Engl J Med 1991;325:897–905.

116. Hamilton CR Jr, Adams LC, Maloof F. Hyperthyroidism due to thyrotropin-producing pituitary chromophobe adenoma. N Engl J Med 1970;283:1077–1080.

117. Gesundheit N, Petrick PA, Nissim M, et al. Thyrotropin-secreting pituitary adenomas: clinical and biochemical heterogeneity. Ann Intern Med 1989;111:827–835.

118. Losa M, Giovanelli M, Persani L, et al. Criteria of cure and follow-up of central hyperthyroidism due to thyrotropin-secreting pituitary adenomas. J Clin Endocrinol Metab 1996;81:3084–3090.

119. Mindermann T, Wilson CB. Thyrotropin-producing pituitary adenomas. J Neurosurg 1993;79:521–527.

120. Smallridge RC, Smith CE. Hyperthyroidism due to thyrotropin-secreting pituitary tumors. Arch Intern Med 1983;143:503–507.

121. Beckers A, Abs R, Mahler C, et al. Thyrotropin-secreting pituitary adenomas: report of seven cases. J Clin Endocrinol Metab 1991;72:477–483.

122. Wynne AG, Gharib H, Scheithauer BW, et al. Hyperthyroidism

due to inappropriate secretion of thyrotropin in 10 patients. Am J Med 1992;92:15–24.

123. Smallridge RC. Thyrotropin-secreting pituitary tumors. Endocrinol Metab Clin North Am 1987;16:765–792.

124. Klibanski A. Nonsecreting pituitary tumors. Endocrinol Metab Clin North Am 1987;16:793–804.

125. Katznelson L, Alexander JM, Klibanski A. Clinically nonfunctioning pituitary adenomas. J Clin Endocrinol Metab 1993;76:1089–1094.

126. Jameson JL, Klibanski A, Black PMcL, et al. Glycoprotein hormone genes are expressed in clinically nonfunctioning pituitary adenomas. J Clin Invest 1987;80:1472–1478.

127. Klibanski A, Alexander JM, Bikkal HA, et al. Somatostatin regulation of glycoprotein hormone and free subunit secretion in clinically nonfunctioning and somatotroph adenomas in vitro. J Clin Endocrinol Metab 1991;73:1248–1255.

128. Asa SL, Gerrie BM, Singer W, et al. Gonadotropin-secretion in vitro by human pituitary null cell adenomas and oncocytomas. J Clin Endocrinol Metab 1986;62:1011–1019.

129. Black PM, Hsu DW, Klibanski A, et al. Hormone production in clinically nonfunctioning pituitary adenomas. J Neurosurg 1987;66:244–250.

130. Synder PJ. Gonadotroph adenomas. In: Melmed S, ed. The Pituitary. Cambridge: Blackwell Science, 1995:559–575.

131. Young WF Jr, Scheithauer BW, Kovacs KT, et al. Gonadotroph adenoma of the pituitary gland: a clinicopathologic analysis of 100 cases. Mayo Clin Proc 1996;71:649–656.

132. Daneshdoost L, Gennarelli TA, Bashey HM, et al. Recognition of gonadotroph adenomas in women. N Engl J Med 1991;324:589–594.

133. Ambrosi B, Basstti M, Ferrario R, et al. Precocious puberty in a boy with a PRL-LH- and FSH-secreting pituitary tumour: hormonal and immunocytochemical studies. Acta Endocrinol 1990;122:569–576.

134. Faggiano M, Criscuolo T, Perrone I, et al. Sexual precocity in a boy due to hypersecretion of LH and prolactin by a pituitary adenoma. Acta Endocrinol 1983;102:167–172.

135. Horvath E, Kovacs K. The adenohypophysis. In: Kovacs K, Asa SL, eds. Functional Endocrine Pathology. Boston: Blackwell Scientific Publications, 1991:245–281.

136. Horvath E, Kovacs K, Killinger DW, et al. Silent corticotrophic adenomas of the human pituitary gland: a histologic, immunocytologic, and ultrastructural study. Am J Pathol 1980;98:617–638.

137. Bates AS, Buckley N, Boggild MD, et al. Clinical and genetic changes in a case of Cushing's carcinoma. Clin Endocrinol 1995;42:663–670.

138. Kovacs K, Lloyd R, Horvath E, et al. Silent somatotroph adenomas of the human pituitary. Am J Pathol 1989;134:345–353.

139. Tourniaire J, Trouillas J, Chalendar D, et al. Somatotropic adenoma manifested by galactorrhea without acromegaly. J Clin Endocrinol Metab 1985;61:451–453.

140. Klibanski A, Zervas NT, Kovacs K, et al. Clinically silent hypersecretion of growth hormone in patients with pituitary tumors. J Neurosurg 1987;66:806–811.

141. Heitz PU. Multihormonal pituitary adenomas. Horm Res 1979;10:1–13.

142. Scheithaur BW, Horvath E, Kovacs K, et al. Plurihormonal pituitary adenomas. Semin Diagn Pathol 1986;3:69–82.

143. Horvath E, Kovacs K. Pituitary gland. Pathol Res Pract 1988;183:129–142.

144. Lloyd RV, Cano M, Chandler WF, et al. Human growth hormone and prolactin secreting pituitary adenoma analyzed by *in situ* hybridization. Am J Pathol 1989;134:605–613.

145. Horvath E, Kovacs K, Killinger DW, et al. Mammosomatotroph cell adenoma of the human pituitary: a morphological entity. Virchows Arch A Pathol Anat Histopathol 1983;398:277–289.

146. Horvath E, Kovacs K, Singer W, et al. Acidophil stem cell adenoma of the human pituitary. Arch Pathol Lab Med 1977;101:594–599.

147. Horvath E, Kovacs K, Singer W, et al. Acidophil stem cell adenoma of the human pituitary. Cancer 1981;47:761–771.

148. Nyquist P, Laws ER, Elliott E. Novel features of tumors that secrete both growth hormone and prolactin in acromegaly. Neurosurgery 1994;35:179–183.

149. Lamberts SW, Liuzzi A, Chiodini PG, et al. The value of plasma prolactin levels in the prediction of the responsiveness of growth hormone secretion to bromocriptine and TRH in acromegaly. Eur J Clin Invest 1982;12:151–155.

150. Kovacs K, Horvath E, Ezrin C, et al. Adenoma of the human pituitary producing growth hormone and thyrotropin: a histologic immunocytologic and fine-structural study. Virchows Arch A Pathol Anat Histopathol 1982;395:59–68.

151. Beck-Peccoz P, Piscitelli G, Amr S, et al. Endocrine, biochemical, and morphological studies of a pituitary adenoma secreting growth hormone, thyrotropin and alpha-subunit: evidence for secretion of TSH with increased bioactivity. J Clin Endocrinol Metab 1986;62:704–711.

152. Horvath E, Kovacs K, Scheithauer BW, et al. Pituitary adenomas producing growth hormone, prolactin and one or more glycoprotein hormones: a histologic, immunohistochemical, and ultrastructural study of four surgically removed tumors. Ultrastruct Pathol 1983;5:171–183.

153. Oppenheim DS, Kana AR, Sangha JS, et al. Prevalence of alpha-subunit hypersecretion in patients with pituitary tumors: clinically nonfunctioning in somatotroph adenomas. J Clin Endocrinol Metab 1990;70:859–864.

154. Sherry SH, Guay AT, Lee AY, et al. Concurrent production of adrenocorticotropin and prolactin from two distinct cell lines in a single pituitary adenoma: a detailed immunohistochemical analysis. J Clin Endocrinol Metab 1982;55:947–955.

155. Gyama JIT, Ishibashi M, Teramoto A, et al. Prolactin secretion by mixed ACTH-prolactin pituitary adenoma cells in culture. Acta Endocrinol 1985;108:456–463.

156. Berg KY, Scheithauer BW, Felix I, et al. Pituitary adenomas that produce adrenocorticotropic hormone and alpha-subunit: clinicopathological, immunohistochemical, ultrastructural, and immunoelectron microscopic studies in 9 cases. Neurosurgery 1990;26:397–403.

157. Mahler C, Verhelst J, Klaes R, et al. Cushing's disease in hyperprolactinemia due to a mixed ACTH- and prolactin-secreting pituitary macroadenoma. Pathol Res Pract 1991;187:598–602.

158. Kontogeorgos G, Kovacs K, Horvath E, et al. Multiple adenomas of the human pituitary. J Neurosurg 1991;74:243–247.

159. Blevins LS Jr, Hall GS, Madoff DH, et al. Case report: acromegaly and Cushing's disease in a patient with synchronous pituitary adenomas. Am J Med Sci 1992;304:294–297.

160. Tolis G, Bertrand G, Carpenter S, et al. Acromegaly and galactorrhea-amenorrhea with two pituitary adenomas secreting growth hormone or prolactin. Ann Intern Med 1978;89:345–348.

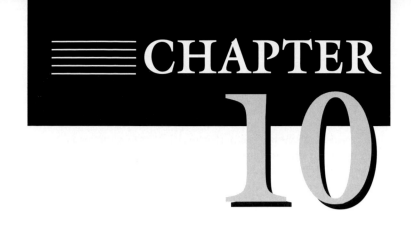

CHAPTER 10

Neuro-Ophthalmology of Pituitary Tumors

Cargill H. Alleyne Jr. and Nancy J. Newman

HISTORICAL HIGHLIGHTS

Anatomy and Physiology

Perhaps the earliest description of the optic chiasm was made by Rufus of Ephesus, who lived during the Galenic period (1). Although he realized that the structure was involved in vision, it was not until 1870 that Gudden conclusively demonstrated that removal of the eye in newborn rabbits led to atrophy of the optic nerve and chiasm (2). Sir Isaac Newton first postulated that the optic nerves partially decussate in the chiasm (3).

The word "pituitary" is derived from the Latin "pituita," which means phlegm. The concept of the pituitary gland as a structure that excretes waste products or phlegm through the nose and pharynx was initiated by Aristotle (384 to 322 BC) and perpetuated by Galen (130 to 200 AD) (4). With the emergence of the Renaissance anatomists, not the least of whom was Vesalius (1514 to 1564), a crude form of the anatomy of the pituitary gland was described (4). Benda, in 1900, and Erdheim, in 1903, described the gland's microanatomy (4). Although observations on the function of the pituitary began in the 1800s when Mohr described a patient with obesity and a pituitary tumor and Marie showed the relationship between the pituitary and acromegaly, it was not until 1909, with the publication of

Cushing's work entitled "Is the Pituitary Gland Essential to the Maintenance of Life?" that the modern study of neuroendocrinology was born (4).

Diagnosis

According to Heublein (5), Oppenheim, in 1898, was the first to diagnose a pituitary tumor by x-ray. Foix is credited with first identifying oculomotor nerve palsy as an early sign of a pituitary adenoma (6), and Weinberger et al. (6), in 1940, reported 6 cases of pituitary adenomas presenting with ocular palsies in a series of 169 patients. Jefferson also wrote extensively on ocular motor palsies in pituitary tumors (7–9). The first report of pituitary apoplexy was made by Bailey in 1898 (10). Another early report of pituitary apoplexy was provided by Bleibtreu in 1905 (11).

Treatment

Horsely first removed the pituitary gland of a human in 1889 via a subtemporal approach (12) and subsequently performed nine such procedures for tumor removal. Krause (13), in 1900, recommended a subfrontal approach to the pituitary. The birth of the transsphenoidal approach to pituitary tumors began with publications by Scholffer and by von Eiselsberg in 1907, and later by Hochenegg and Kosher (4). These radical transnasal procedures were later refined by Kanavel, Hirsch, and others (4). By 1914, Cushing had performed 74 transsphenoidal procedures in 68 patients, and by 1939 he had performed 171 transsphenoidal operations for chromophobe adenomas (4). Cushing and Walker, in 1915, analyzed 81 cases of chiasmal compression and showed that surgical decompression could lead to restoration of vision (14).

Treatment of pituitary adenomas by radiotherapy was first reported in 1909 by Beclere (15) and Gramegna (16).

TOPOGRAPHIC DIAGNOSIS OF LESIONS IN THE REGION OF THE PITUITARY

An understanding of the mechanisms involved in the neuro-ophthalmologic manifestations of pituitary tumors is facilitated by a thorough knowledge of the anatomy of the optic nerves, chiasm, tract, and other structures in the parasellar area. Knowledge of both normal variants and anomalies is essential for an accurate diagnosis. This section provides a review of the anatomic basis of the neuro-ophthalmologic deficits seen in pituitary tumors.

Afferent System

Optic Nerves

The optic nerves enter the cranium via the optic canals located in the superomedial aspect of the sphenoid bone. Renn and Rhoton (17) investigated the microsurgical anatomy of the sellar region in 50 cadavers and found that the average length of the optic nerve from the optic canal to the anterior chiasm was 12 mm, with a range of 8 to 19 mm. The cross-sectional configuration of the optic nerves just proximal to the canal was consistently oblong, with a mean width of 5 mm and a mean height of 3 mm. The distance between the medial aspect of the nerves at the optic canal averaged 14 mm, with a range of 9 to 24 mm. The angle between the nerves ranged from 50° to 80°. The approach of the optic nerves to the chiasm is inclined 45° from the horizontal (18) (Fig. 10.1).

Preferential optic nerve involvement in pituitary tumors is more likely if the tumor exhibits extensive anterior growth or if the chiasm is postfixed (see below). A fragility of the anastomotic blood supply to the posterior portion of the optic nerve may also contribute to its involvement. The resultant field defect can thus be monocular and is usually a superior temporal defect. Arcuate, central, or cecocentral defects also may result (Fig. 10.2). Bilateral nasal field defects may occur rarely if growth of a tumor between the optic nerves compresses them laterally against the supraclinoid internal carotid arteries or the A1 segment of the anterior cerebral arteries, thus injuring the temporal fibers of each optic nerve. Compression of the posterior optic nerve

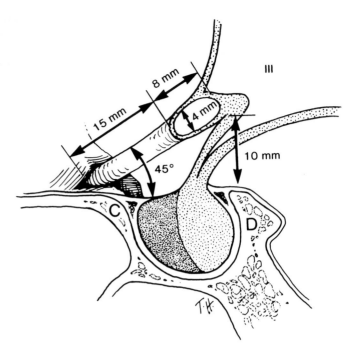

Figure 10.1. Relationships of the optic nerves and optic chiasm to the sellar structures and third ventricle (III). *C*, anterior clinoid; *D*, dorsum sellae. (Reprinted with permission from Miller NR. Walsh and Hoyt's Clinical Neuro-Ophthalmology. 4th ed. Baltimore: Williams & Wilkins, 1982;1:63.)

against the overlying anterior cerebral artery, the roof of the optic canal, or the falciform ligament (the dural band connecting the anterior clinoid processes) may cause an inferior altitudinal defect. Involvement of the junction of the posterior optic nerve and anterior chiasm, where crossed ventral fibers loop anteriorly (Wilbrand's knee), can result in a hemianopic or central scotoma in the ipsilateral eye and a superior temporal defect in the contralateral eye—the so-called "junctional scotoma" (19).

Optic Chiasm

The relationship of the optic chiasm to the tuberculum sella was investigated by Bergland et al. (20). Usually the optic chiasm is situated over the diaphragma sella, which is a rectangular or circular fold of dura mater averaging 11 mm by 8 mm that forms the roof of the sella turcica (17). Occasionally, the optic chiasm can overlie the tuberculum sella (said to be prefixed) or the dorsum sellae (said to be postfixed). Bergland et al. (20) found a normal chiasm in 80%, a prefixed chiasm in 9%, and a postfixed chiasm in 11% of specimens (Fig. 10.3). In the study by Renn and Rhoton (17), a normal chiasm was seen in 75%, a prefixed chiasm in 10%, and a postfixed chiasm in 15% of specimens. These relationships are not merely of academic importance but have a direct bearing on the configuration of the visual field defect resulting from an encroaching pituitary tumor. The chiasm is in direct contact with the third ventricle posteriorly and superiorly and the chiasmatic cistern anteriorly and inferiorly (Fig. 10.1).

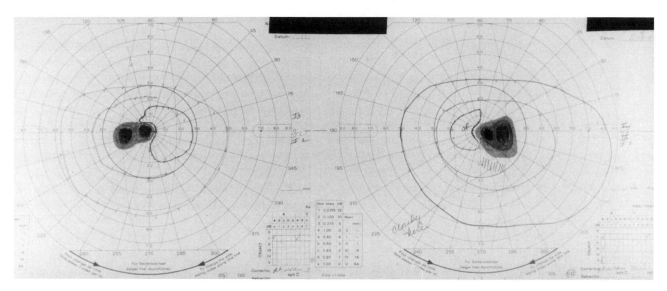

Figure 10.2. The patient is a 25-year-old woman who presented with headaches and blurred vision mostly in the temporal field of the right eye. She was found to have a high prolactin level. Her visual acuity was 20/20, and there was slight temporal pallor noted bilaterally (right slightly worse than left).

Goldmann visual fields showed cecocentral defects bilaterally (larger on the right than the left). A computed tomographic scan revealed a pituitary tumor compressing the posterior optic nerves bilaterally, consistent with a postfixed chiasm.

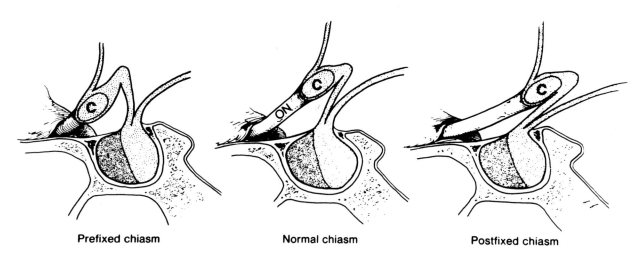

Prefixed chiasm   **Normal chiasm**   **Postfixed chiasm**

Figure 10.3. Schematic drawing of three sagittal sections of the optic chiasm and sellar region showing the positions of a prefixed chiasm above the tuberculum sellae (*left*), a normal chiasm above the diaphragma sellae (*center*), and a postfixed chiasm above the dorsum sellae (*right*). *C*, chiasm; *ON*, optic nerve. (Reprinted with permission from Miller NR. Walsh and Hoyt's Clinical Neuro-Ophthalmology. 4th ed. Baltimore: Williams & Wilkins, 1982;1:62.)

Some of the seminal studies of the retinotopic fiber anatomy were done by Ronne (21), Polyak (22), Hoyt and Luis (23), and Wilbrand (24), among others. About 53% of the axons in both optic nerves decussate in the chiasm (25). These decussating fibers originate from the nasal retina, which subserves the temporal hemifield. The crossed fibers that lie ventrally loop anteriorly into the distal portion of the contralateral optic nerve (Wilbrand's knee) before continuing through the optic chiasm and then the contralateral optic tract. Although there is some new pathologic evidence that the "knee" described by Wilbrand may only occur grossly when there is long-standing ipsilateral optic nerve atrophy (J Horton, personal communication, March 1997), the clinical–anatomic correlates still hold. As these fibers make the transition from chiasm to tract, their position changes from ventral (in the chiasm) to ventrolateral (in the tract). The fibers destined to cross that lay dorsal in the optic nerve traverse the chiasm posteriorly and directly enter the dorsomedial optic tract. Most fibers in the chiasm are projections from the macular region. The crossing macular fibers mainly occupy the central and posterior portions of the chiasm.

A pattern of bitemporal hemianopia produced by a single lesion uniquely localizes that lesion to the optic chiasm (Fig. 10.4). Early involvement of the crossing macular fibers can produce a bitemporal hemianopic sco-

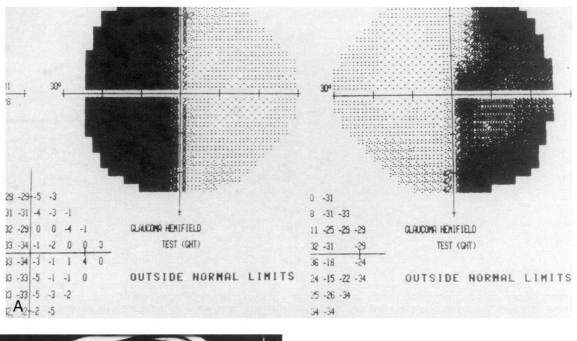

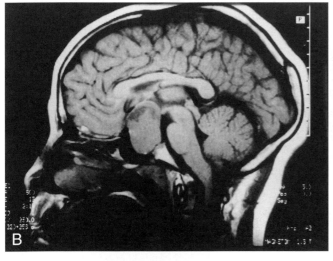

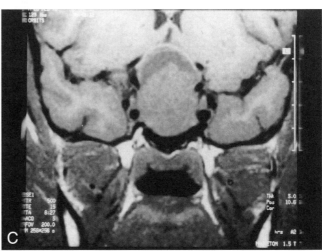

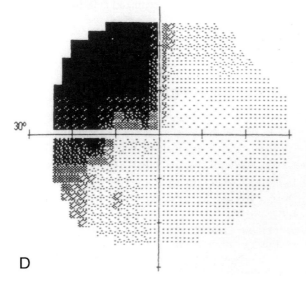

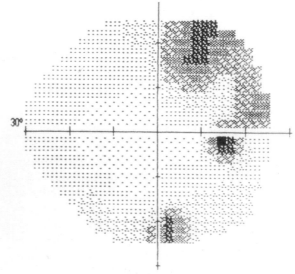

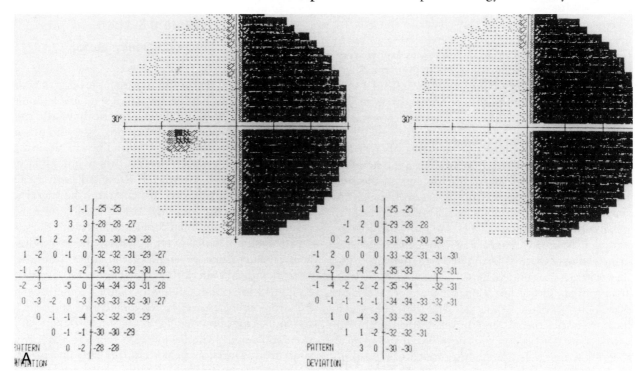

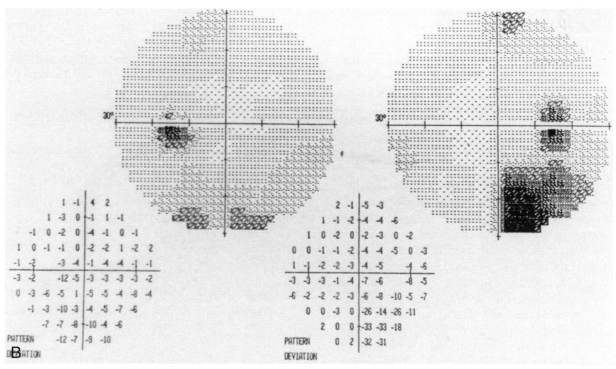

Figure 10.5. The patient is a 62-year-old man with a 1-month history of loss of vision in the right visual field of both eyes. His visual acuity was 20/20 OD and 20/40 OS, and Humphrey visual fields revealed a dense right homonymous hemianopia **(A)**.

MRIs showed a pituitary adenoma compressing the left optic tract, consistent with a prefixed chiasm. Postoperatively, his visual fields improved considerably **(B)**.

Figure 10.4. The patient is a 15-year-old boy with occasional complaints of blurred vision and headaches and a 1-year history of galactorrhea. He had no facial, axillary, or pubic hair, and had small genitalia. His visual acuity was 20/20 OD and 20/40 OS. With attempts to refract, he read only the nasal halves of each eye chart. His PRL level was more than 4,000 µg/L (> 4,000 ng/mL), and he had panhypopituitarism. After 2 weeks of bro-

mocriptine therapy, he underwent a transsphenoidal adenomectomy. Illustrated are his preoperative Humphrey automated visual fields showing a complete bitemporal defect **(A)**. Sagittal **(B)** and coronal **(C)** views of a T1-weighted MRI showing a large pituitary adenoma with suprasellar extension. A postoperative improvement in visual fields is noted **(D)**.

toma. The exact mechanism of this characteristic pattern of visual loss in pituitary tumors is somewhat controversial. If compression of the optic chiasm from below were the only pathologic mechanism involved, then the fibers subserving the upper visual field would be affected and a superior altitudinal defect would result. In fact, the superonasal field is generally the last quadrant to manifest a defect.

Bergland et al. (20) found that the median bar of the chiasm was supplied by a plexus of vessels from the superior hypophyseal arteries. They invoked early compression of this inferior plexus by pituitary tumors to explain the bitemporal field defects observed with chiasmal compression. Compression of the draining venules and intrinsic capillaries resulting in stagnant anoxia and conduction block is another mechanism that has been cited by Hoyt (26). Another hypothesis, expounded by O'Connell (27), is that the crossing fibers in the optic chiasm are more resistant to displacement by virtue of the fact that they interweave with fibers from the contralateral nerves. When the chiasm is displaced, a greater tension thus develops in the crossed fibers than in the uncrossed, laterally located fibers. In addition, Hedges (28) found that the inflation of a balloon in the sella of cadavers caused selective stretching of the superior fibers in the median bar of the chiasm.

In addition to bitemporal hemianopia, chiasmal compression occasionally causes a monocular temporal arcuate defect extending from the blind spot to the vertical meridian. This may be explained by the fact that the axons from the retina remain associated until they reach the chiasm.

Optic Tract

The optic tracts begin at the optic chiasm and diverge anterior to the interpeduncular space, between the tuber cinereum and the anterior perforated substance anteriorly. They pass posteriorly around the cerebral peduncle and above the posterior cerebral arteries to synapse in the lateral geniculate body. The crossed and uncrossed fibers of the optic chiasm converge as they enter each optic tract. The macular fibers lie dorsolaterally, and the fibers from the upper retinas and lower retinas are situated dorsomedially and ventrolaterally, respectively. Some of the fibers in the optic tract give rise to branches that ascend to the pretectal regions of the midbrain prior to the lateral geniculate. These fibers subserve the pupillary light reflex.

The optic tracts are more likely to be injured with a pituitary tumor growing posterosuperiorly or with a prefixed optic chiasm. If the optic tract on one side is involved, an homonymous visual field defect results (Fig. 10.5). These defects are typically incomplete and incongruous (29–31). A relative afferent pupillary defect may be seen contralateral to the involved tract. This occurs because the tract contains more crossed than uncrossed fibers.

Efferent System

The Cavernous Sinus and Ocular Motor Cranial Nerves

The paired cavernous sinuses, rich plexuses of veins that surround the internal carotid arteries, lie just lateral to the pituitary fossa. They are bound anteriorly by the tuberculum sella and the anterior clinoid processes and posteriorly by the posterior clinoid processes. The lateral wall of the cavernous sinus has been described as two dural layers between which cranial nerves III, IV, and V_1 travel (32–34) (Fig. 10.6). Cranial nerve III penetrates the lateral wall of the cavernous sinus near the roof and slightly medial to cranial nerve IV, and then courses anteriorly to the superior orbital fissure. Cranial nerve IV enters the cavernous sinus at the posterosuperior angle of the lateral wall and runs parallel with and inferior to cranial nerve III. Cranial nerve V_1 enters inferiorly and slopes slightly superiorly to the superior orbital fissure. Exceptionally, V_2 and part of the trigeminal ganglion may lie in the inferolateral wall of the cavernous sinus. Cranial nerve VI enters the cavernous sinus from Dorello's canal, courses laterally around the proximal cavernous carotid artery, and runs parallel and medial to cranial nerve V_1. It lies free in the cavernous sinus and occasionally splits into up to five rootlets (34). Sympathetic fibers from the superior sympathetic ganglion ascend with the internal carotid artery through the foramen lacerum and then join the undersurface of cranial nerve VI

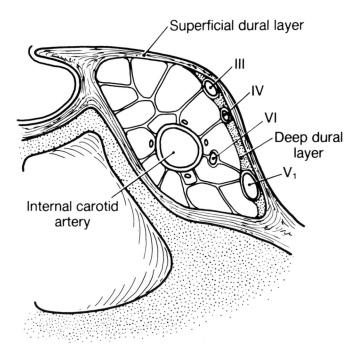

Figure 10.6. Diagram of the cavernous sinus as described by Umansky and Nathan showing that the lateral wall is composed of two layers: a superficial layer and a deep layer. The deep layer is formed by the sheaths of the oculomotor (*III*), trochlear (*IV*), and ophthalmic (*VI*) nerves, with a reticular membrane between these sheaths. V_1, abducens nerve. (Reprinted with permission from Miller NR. Walsh and Hoyt's Clinical Neuro-Ophthalmology. 4th ed. Baltimore: Williams & Wilkins, 1985;2:576.)

at the level where it crosses the internal carotid artery. The sympathetic fibers then join branches of cranial nerve V_1 after traveling with cranial nerve VI for 1 to 2 cm (32).

Any or all of the above structures in the cavernous sinus may be affected by an invasive tumor of the pituitary. Involvement of cranial nerve III causes impaired downgaze and medial gaze, diplopia, ptosis, and mydriasis. Involvement of cranial nerves IV and VI causes superior oblique and lateral rectus palsies, respectively. Injury to cranial nerve V_1 produces loss of sensation or pain in the upper face, decreased corneal sensation, and an impaired corneal reflex. Sympathetic fiber dysfunction leads to a third-order Horner's syndrome. Extraocular muscle paresis features prominently in pituitary apoplexy, which is discussed further in a later section of this chapter.

Several mechanisms have been proposed to explain the occurrence of cranial nerve III palsy with pituitary tumors. The transmission of pressure by a laterally expanding tumor to the wall of the cavernous sinus (35) and compression of cranial nerve III between the tumor and the interclinoid ligament at its point of entry into the cavernous sinus (7, 36, 37) have both been advocated. The tumor also may invade the wall of the cavernous sinus and directly compress the nerve (7) or its blood supply (38). Similar mechanisms may explain the palsies of other cranial nerves in the cavernous sinus when associated with pituitary tumors. In addition, cranial nerve VI may be affected if the sella turcica is located relatively posterior in the sphenoid bone; in this case, the nerve would be vulnerable to compressive effects of a tumor at Dorello's canal prior to its entrance into the cavernous sinus.

Invasion of the cavernous sinus by tumor may also precipitate signs of ocular venous obstruction such as proptosis (39) and mechanical restriction of eye movement similar to that seen in patients with carotid–cavernous fistulae. Expansion of a pituitary tumor posterosuperiorly into the third ventricle may result in the obstruction of cerebrospinal fluid flow. Ophthalmologic findings that may result from hydrocephalus include impairment of upgaze, pupillary light-near dissociation, convergence–retraction nystagmus, and papilledema. The injury to the ocular motor nerves by pituitary tumors may not always occur in the cavernous sinus but may occur in the subarachnoid space, or even at the level of the brainstem (7, 36).

NEURO-OPHTHALMOLOGIC MANIFESTATIONS OF PITUITARY DISEASE
Symptoms
Visual Loss

The onset and course of visual loss associated with pituitary tumors may take many forms. A large field defect may be noticed abruptly when in reality it may have been present months or years earlier. A gradual, insidious deterioration may be reported, or there may be periods of rapid visual failure interspersed with periods of retardation or cessation of visual deterioration. Genuine sudden loss of vision may rarely occur and may mimic retrobulbar neuritis, although eye pain is usually absent (40–42). Sudden loss of vision is characteristic of the acute chiasmal compression that occurs during pituitary apoplexy. Wilson and Falconer (43), in a retrospective study of 50 patients with chromophobe pituitary adenomas, found that a steady progression of visual failure was the most common presentation, seen in 50% of patients. Rapid progression was reported by 27% of patients, and intermittent progression by 12.5% of patients.

The presence of a bitemporal defect may give rise to a group of sensory complaints that consists of difficulties with depth perception. These complaints are attributed to "chiasmatic postfixational blindness" (44) (Fig. 10.7). Images in the midline past the point of fixation fall on the nasal retina, which is blind in patients with bitemporal hemianopia. Such images therefore disappear from view. Pregnant women with pituitary tumors compose a subset of patients that deserves special mention. Visual loss is a known risk of pregnancy in women with pituitary tumors. A study of 65 consecutive women with pituitary adenomas during 111 pregnancies was conducted by Kupersmith et al. (45) to assess this potential risk. Sixty patients had increased levels of serum prolactin (PRL) or growth hormone and five did not. During 103 pregnancies, none of the 57 patients with microadenomas developed visual loss, whereas 6 of 8 women with macroadenomas developed visual loss during pregnancy. Other studies describe a 5% incidence of visual loss during pregnancy in patients with microadenomas (46, 47).

Diplopia

Of 100 cases of proven pituitary tumors recorded by Lyle and Clover (48), diplopia was reported in 20 cases. No impairment of the extraocular muscles could be demonstrated in 13 of these patients. Diplopia was the presenting complaint in 7 of 1000 cases of pituitary adenoma reviewed by Hollenhorst and Younge (49) and 1 of 100 cases reviewed by Wray (50).

A group of sensory complaints that may result from a bitemporal visual field defect is intermittent diplopia in the absence of extraocular muscle paresis and is known as the "hemifield slide" phenomenon (Fig. 10.8). The visual fields of patients with complete bitemporal hemianopias represent the temporal projection from each eye. There are no corresponding retinal points to visually link the hemifields of the two eyes. This loss of physiologic linkage results in a tendency for the hemifields to overlap, or to separate vertically or horizontally if there is an underlying tendency for the eyes to be slightly misaligned, i.e., a "phoria" (44).

Pituitary Apoplexy

The term "pituitary apoplexy" has been applied both to massive infarction or hemorrhage of the pituitary occur-

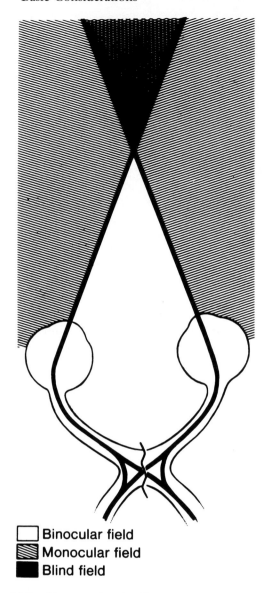

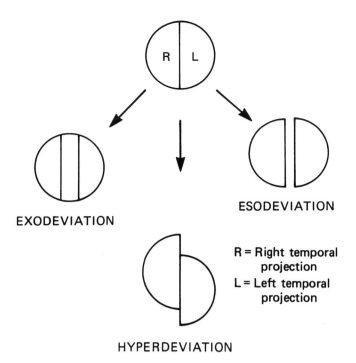

EXODEVIATION

ESODEVIATION

R = Right temporal
projection
L = Left temporal
projection

HYPERDEVIATION

Figure 10.8. Diagram showing the "hemifield slide phenomenon" experienced by patients with bitemporal hemianopias. Patients with a preexisting exophoria or intermittent exotropia will have overlapping of the intact nasal fields, whereas patients with a preexisting esophoria or intermittent esotropia will have separation of the nasal hemifields, causing a blind area in the center of the field. Patients with preexisting hyperdeviations will complain of vertical separation of images crossing the vertical meridian. (Reprinted with permission from Miller NR. Walsh and Hoyt's Clinical Neuro-Ophthalmology. 4th ed. Baltimore: Williams & Wilkins, 1982;1:124.)

☐ Binocular field
▨ Monocular field
■ Blind field

Figure 10.7. Diagram showing the formation of a blind, triangular area of visual field that occurs just beyond fixation in patients with complete, bitemporal hemianopias. Such patients have intact binocular vision in the triangular area up to fixation and uniocular vision temporal and anterior to the triangular blind region. (Reprinted with permission from Miller NR. Walsh and Hoyt's Clinical Neuro-Ophthalmology. 4th ed. Baltimore: Williams & Wilkins, 1982;1:124.)

ring in association with acute necrotic changes in preexisting pituitary tumors and to infarction or hemorrhagic necrosis of a nontumorous pituitary gland (51, 52). The occurrence of symptomatic hemorrhagic infarction of the pituitary has been reported at a rate of up to 10% in a large series (53). Mohr and Hardy (54) reported clinical pituitary apoplexy in 0.6% of 663 cases of pituitary adenomas but found significant hemorrhage and necrotic changes in 9.5% of the cases. The sudden expansion of a pituitary tumor with necrosis is associated with a constellation of findings, both neuro-ophthalmologic and non–neuro-ophthalmologic. The latter findings include headache, altered con-

sciousness, nausea and vomiting, stiff neck, photophobia, endocrine dysfunction, facial paresthesias, seizures, focal hemispheric symptoms, and cerebellar symptoms. A detailed account of the non–neuro-ophthalmologic findings in pituitary apoplexy can be found in chapter 8.

The neuro-ophthalmologic manifestations of pituitary apoplexy are diverse. The visual apparatus may suffer the sudden compressive or irritative effect of a pituitary tumor undergoing spontaneous infarction with expansion. This may result in visual blurring, visual field defects, and binocular or monocular visual loss (54–58). Diplopia and ophthalmoplegia are prominent features of pituitary apoplexy (36, 51, 55, 56, 59) (Fig. 10.9). They are not a result of direct tumor involvement but rather the sudden increase in size of the tumor results in increase in pressure on the lateral wall of the cavernous sinus and (presumably) deformation of the course of the cranial nerves. Ischemic injury or a combination of compressive and ischemic causes is also possible. The oculomotor nerve is usually most frequently involved, followed by the abducens and trochlear nerves. Other rare ophthalmologic manifestations of pituitary apoplexy include elements of the dorsal midbrain syndrome, such as pupillary light-near dissociation (60) and convergence–retraction nystagmus (61). The leakage of blood into the subarachnoid space may precipitate symptoms of meningeal irritation, including photophobia.

Other Unusual Symptoms

Shults et al. (62) reported a series of six patients with ocular neuromyotonia characterized by periods of sustained involuntary contraction of one or more of the extraocular muscles caused by spontaneous excitation of the ex-

traocular cranial nerves. Four of the six patients had a history of invasive pituitary adenoma treated with radiotherapy. They suggested that compressed irradiated axons are susceptible to spontaneous discharge.

Exophthalmos is an extremely rare presentation of pituitary adenomas (63–67). This can result from invasion of the tumor into the orbit or into the cavernous sinus, the latter with resultant venous stasis and proptosis.

Recurrent blepharoptosis has been reported as the presenting symptom of a pituitary tumor in an 11-year-old

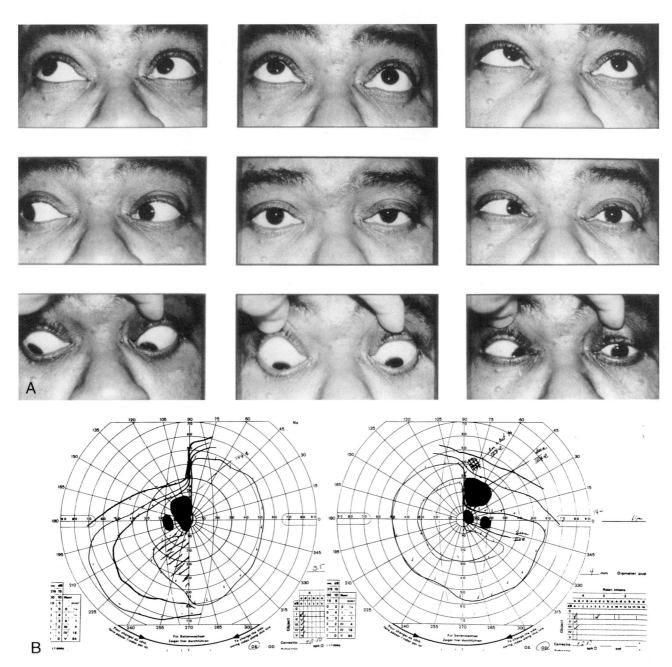

Figure 10.9. The patient is a 53-year-old man with a known pituitary tumor who presented with a 2-day history of sudden onset of headache, lethargy, decreased vision in the left eye, and double vision with left lateral gaze. His visual acuity was 20/25 OD and 20/100 OS. He had ptosis on the left and palsies of the left sixth nerve and superior division of the third nerve **(A)**. Goldmann visual field testing revealed bitemporal superior quadrantanopias with macular involvement on the left **(B)**.

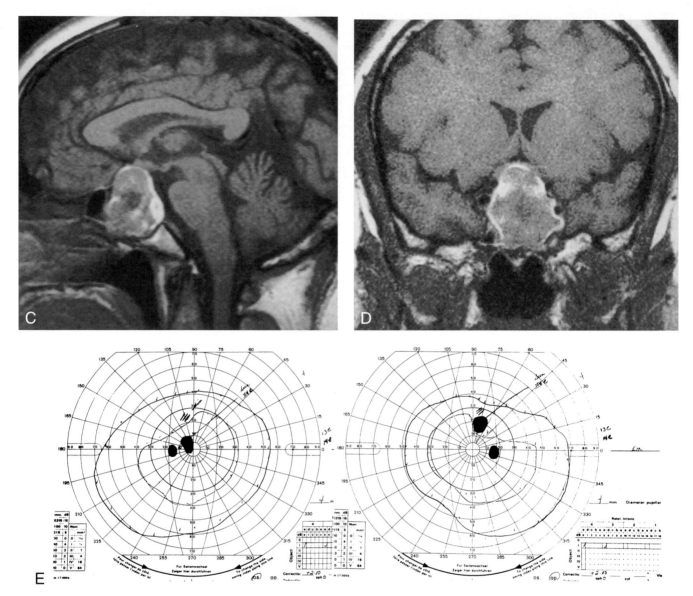

Figure 10.9. *(continued)* A T1-weighted MRI (**C**, sagittal view; **D**, coronal view) revealed a large pituitary adenoma with suprasellar extension and heterogenous signal intensity consistent with intratumoral hemorrhage. A transsphenoidal adenomectomy was performed, and postoperatively his visual defects improved considerably (**E**).

child (68). The suggested mechanism was displacement of the dura through which the oculomotor nerve passes with secondary stretch of the nerve. It was presumed that fibers innervating the levator palpebrae superioris muscle were more sensitive to stretch.

Visual hallucinations, both formed (69–71) and unformed (69), have been associated with pituitary adenomas. Brief images of unformed shapes and lights probably result from direct pressure on the optic apparatus by the tumor. More complex, formed hallucinations are best characterized as release phenomena resulting from sensory deprivation from visual loss. When concurrent symptoms suggestive of seizures are described with the hallucinations, cortical irritation has been suggested as the mechanism (69, 70).

Signs

Afferent System

Visual Field Defects

As noted in five large studies dating from before 1955 to 1981, the prevalence of visual signs (and symptoms) in patients with pituitary tumors has progressively declined during the past four or five decades (49, 50, 72–74) (Table 10.1). In 1955, Chamblin et al. (72) reviewed 156 patients with pituitary adenomas or craniopharyngiomas and found a prevalence of visual field defects of 86%. Of these patients with visual field defects, 32% had decreased central vision in at least one eye. Hollenhorst and Younge (49) reviewed 1000 patients with pituitary tumors, most of whom had been diagnosed between 1940 and 1962. Seventy percent

Table 10.1. Signs and Symptoms in Patients with Pituitary Tumors in Five Studies Covering Different Periods of Time

Signs and Symptoms	Chamblin et al.[72] (156 Patients, Before 1955)	Hollenhorst and Younge[49] (1,000 Patients, 1940-1962)	Klauber et al.[73] (51 Patients, 1967-1974)	Wray[50] (100 Patients, 1974-1976)	Anderson et al.[74] (200 Patients, 1976-1981)
Amenorrhea/impotence, %	—	5	—	21	70
Headache, %	—	14	45	24	46
Visual, %	86	70	69	31	9
Optic atrophy, %	50	34	47	19	2
Extraocular muscle palsy, %	5	6	—	4	1

Modified from Anderson D, Faber P, Marcovitz S, et al. Pituitary tumors and the ophthalmologist. Ophthalmology 1983;90:1268.

of these patients had visual field defects, but this sign was the presenting complaint in only 42% and the main presenting complaint in only 35% of patients. In a study by Klauber et al. (73) in which 51 patients with pituitary tumors were studied between 1967 and 1974, 69% of patients had visual field defects. Wray (50) examined 100 patients with pituitary tumors between 1974 and 1976 and found that 31% had visual field defects, although in only 17% was this a presenting complaint. By contrast, visual field defects were seen in only 9% of 200 patients seen between 1976 and 1981 in a study by Anderson et al. (74). A comparison of these five studies reveals not only that the incidence of ophthalmologic findings is decreasing in patients with pituitary tumors, but also that the incidence of neuroendocrine findings is increasing (Table 10.1). Reasons cited for this change include the development of hormone assays, improved radiographic detection methods, and earlier treatment by selective transsphenoidal adenomectomy (74). Because pituitary adenomas can now be removed selectively without damage to surrounding normal gland, this surgery is now performed earlier to correct hormonal excess rather than as a last resort to save vision. Increased patient awareness of symptoms and increased accessibility to health care may also play a role.

In the study by Hollenhorst and Younge of 1000 patients with pituitary tumors presenting at the Mayo Clinic (49), the most common types of visual field defects encountered were bitemporal hemianopia (30.0%), superior bitemporal defects (10.1%), blindness in one eye and a temporal defect in the other (8.1%), and junctional patterns (5.6%) (56). Less common defects noted were homonymous hemianopia (4.2%), superior temporal defects in one eye (3.3%), central or temporal scotoma in both eyes (2.7%), and temporal scotoma in one eye (1.2%). Defects seen in less than 1% of patients were a central scotoma in one eye (0.8%), inferior temporal defect in one eye (0.4%), arcuate scotoma in one eye (0.4%), inferior temporal defect in both eyes (0.4%), and arcuate scotoma in one eye and temporal defect in the other (0.3%). "Miscellaneous defects" that could not be assigned to one of the above groups were seen in 2.7% of patients.

Funduscopic Examination

Chiasmal compression may cause early changes in the peripapillary nerve fiber bundle layer as a result of drop out of axons (75, 76). These changes, known as "guttering" or "rake defects," can best be seen with red-free light and photography (77). Prolonged compression can cause temporal pallor, or, if only decussating fibers are lost, "band" or "bow-tie" atrophy (78). The latter pattern is seen because the decussating fibers originate in the nasal retina and enter the disc nasally and temporally (Fig. 10.10).

The prevalence of optic pallor observed in the Mayo Clinic study was 34% (676 of 1995 eyes), about half the prevalence of visual field defects (49). In contrast, only 2% of patients in the study by Anderson et al. (74) were described as having optic atrophy. Poon et al. (79) noted that optic disc pallor was a relatively insensitive sign in identifying patients with visual pathway compression (behind visual field loss, color loss, and acuity loss). In addition, the identification of optic pallor is somewhat subject to observer variability. Wilson and Falconer (43) noted unequivocal pallor of one or both optic discs in 28 (56%) of 50 patients with chromophobe pituitary adenomas. They noted that optic atrophy may present even when the subjective duration of visual failure is short. They also noted that in all patients with chiasmal compression (regardless of the type of visual field defect), optic atrophy always occurred within 2 years of onset of visual symptoms. There was no relationship between the presence of optic atrophy and the progression of visual failure.

Papilledema is a rare finding in patients with pituitary adenomas. In the Mayo Clinic study it was seen in only 3 of 1000 patients (49). All of these patients harbored large tumors. Suprasellar pituitary tumors (e.g., craniopharyngiomas) are more likely to obstruct cerebrospinal fluid pathways and hence cause papilledema.

Efferent System

Ocular Dysmotility

The prevalence of ocular dysmotility in patients with pituitary tumors has also decreased in recent times and ranges from 1 to 6% (49, 50, 73–79) (Table 10.1). Fifty-

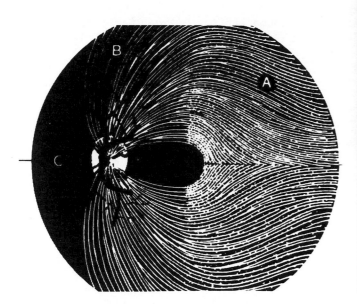

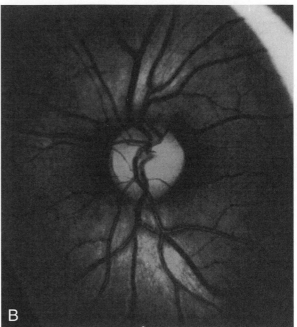

Figure 10.10. Diagram of "band" or "bow-tie" atrophy in patients with temporal hemianopia from chiasmal compression. **A.** A diagram of the left fundus. The nasal retinal fibers, subserving the temporal hemifield of vision, enter the disc in the pattern shown. Because the nasal retinal fibers are defined by those fibers nasal to the fovea, nasal retinal fibers will include those originating nasal to the disc and those originating temporal to the disc but nasal to the fovea. Regions marked *A, B,* and *C* in the diagram denote areas of nerve fiber layer preservation, partial loss, and complete loss, respectively. **B.** The appearance of the optic nerve in the left eye. With long-standing chiasmal compression, the nasal retinal fibers become atrophic, and pallor may be seen in a pattern corresponding to the location of these fibers on the disc, so-called "bow-tie" atrophy. (Reprinted with permission from Miller NR. Walsh and Hoyt's Clinical Neuro-Ophthalmology. 4th ed. Baltimore: Williams & Wilkins, 1982;1:125.)

nine of one thousand patients with pituitary tumors presented with cranial nerve palsies in a series collected prior to 1973 (49). Of these, 12 patients had multiple palsies of cranial nerves III and IV, or III and VI, 2 had bilateral paralysis of cranial nerve III, and 32 had either cranial nerve III or VI palsies. In addition, 13 patients developed palsy of cranial nerve III, IV, or VI after surgery and 8 developed palsy at the time of tumor recurrence.

Cranial nerve III is the most frequently involved ocular motor nerve in pituitary tumors (50, 80), and the levator palpebral superioris is most commonly affected. A third nerve palsy is occasionally the presenting sign or the only neurologic sign observed (38, 81–83). Although cranial nerve VI is thought to be relatively protected from involvement by pituitary tumors by virtue of its anatomic location in the cavernous sinus, there are several reports of isolated cranial nerve VI involvement (50, 80, 84). Ocular motor nerve palsy can also rarely be the presenting symptom of lymphocytic hypophysitis and tumors metastatic to the pituitary (85, 86).

Nystagmus

Pituitary tumors and other parasellar lesions may also lead to the rare phenomenon of see-saw nystagmus, in which elevation and intorsion of one eye alternates with depression and extorsion of the other eye. The mechanism causing see-saw nystagmus is uncertain. The association with bitemporal hemianopia in some patients has prompted speculation that an underlying sensory release phenomenon, perhaps related to the hemifield slide, may be at play (87). See-saw nystagmus also has been associated with vascular disease of the upper brainstem in patients without bitemporal hemianopia (88). This phenomenon is not specific for lesions in and around the parasellar area and has been reported with diencephalic, medullary, and pontine lesions and with obstructive hydrocephalus (88–91). Convergence–retraction nystagmus is a manifestation of the dorsal midbrain syndrome and usually results from lesions directly involving the mesencephalic tegmentum. It has been described in association with pituitary apoplexy when the lesions are large or hydrocephalus is apparent (61).

Pupillary Abnormalities

Of the 100 cases of proven pituitary tumors recorded by Lyle and Clover (48), abnormalities in pupillary reaction were recorded in 20 cases. They attributed these changes in 18 patients to the visual defect, presumably relative afferent pupillary defects from asymmetrical involvement of the anterior visual pathways. Pupillary abnormalities, especially anisocoria with ipsilateral mydriasis, is a common sign in pituitary apoplexy from cranial nerve III involvement (60).

VISUAL OUTCOME

Prognosis of Visual Outcome

The goals of pituitary tumor therapy should include (*a*) control of tumor growth, (*b*) normalization of pituitary function, and (*c*) preservation or restoration of visual function. The therapeutic options available to the clinician include surgery, medical therapy, radiotherapy, or expectant observation without intervention. Multimodal therapy is frequently used.

Several studies have been aimed at identifying preoperative factors that are predictive of outcome after surgery for pituitary adenomas. Cohen et al. (92) retrospectively reviewed 100 consecutive patients with pituitary adenomas who underwent decompression of the optic nerves and chiasm by the transsphenoidal approach. They found that preoperative visual acuity was highly predictive of outcome. Only 62% of eyes with visual acuity equal to or worse than 20/100 preoperatively showed improvement, whereas 89% of eyes with visual acuity better than 20/100 were normal or improved postoperatively. The duration of preoperative visual complaints correlated inversely with outcome for both visual acuity and visual fields. Improvement in visual acuity and fields was less likely to occur in patients who had undergone a previous operation. In this study, age was also a significant factor (independent of the preoperative status) in predicting both postoperative visual acuity and visual fields, with younger patients achieving a better outcome. The authors found that except for cases of frank atrophy, where an improvement in vision was never seen, the color of the optic disc had no bearing on visual outcome.

Although many studies corroborate the predictive value of preoperative visual acuity and duration of preoperative visual symptoms (93–95), and some also show a correlation between tumor size and visual recovery (73, 93), others failed to find a correlation between visual recovery and preoperative visual acuity (96), visual fields (96), age of the patient (97), and size of the tumor (97, 98). The sentiments expressed by Trobe et al. (94), however, ring true: "Although the correlation of duration of symptoms, preoperative acuity, and tumor size with outcome may not always be firm, it is sufficient to underscore the importance of early diagnosis and treatment of these potentially curable lesions." Although some studies have not found a correlation between either the time from onset of apoplexy to treatment or the severity of visual deficits and the outcome (99), Bills et al. (100) reported a significantly better outcome in visual acuity in those patients decompressed within the first week and found a similar trend with regards to visual field defects, which did not reach significance. They noted "good recovery" of vision in a patient decompressed 14 days after apoplexy and emphasized that although patients with unilateral or bilateral blindness should undergo decompression as soon as possible, patients presenting late after pituitary apoplexy may also benefit from surgery.

Rush et al. (101), in a study of the effect of radiation therapy alone for pituitary adenomas causing visual impairment, documented the determinants of visual field and visual acuity outcome. Visual field improvement occurred in patients whose pretreatment visual field defects were less than a dense homonymous hemianopia (grades 1 through 3), in patients without diffuse optic atrophy, and in patients who were younger than the median age of 69 years. Visual acuity improvement occurred in patients with only minor visual acuity impairment, in patients without diffuse optic atrophy, and in patients with only mild visual loss prior to radiation therapy. Normal color vision and the absence of an afferent pupillary defect were also predictive of improvement. Hughes et al. (102) analyzed the outcome of 268 patients receiving radiation therapy alone and those receiving postoperative radiotherapy. In the latter group, visual field defects and/or visual failure was noted at presentation in 128 of 160 patients. The patients with pretreatment visual dysfunction had a 10-year progression-free survival rate of 80%, which was not significantly different than the 32 patients who had no visual disturbance.

Outcome After Medical Therapy

PRL-secreting tumors are the most common type of pituitary adenomas, accounting for 40 to 50% of all pituitary tumors. The ergot derivative bromocriptine (Parlodel) binds to dopamine receptors with 5 to 10 times greater affinity than does dopamine (103). There are now numerous reports of improvement in visual function in patients with prolactinomas treated with this drug (Fig. 10.11). Moster et al. (104) described 10 patients with prolactinomas and visual dysfunction who were treated primarily with bromocriptine. Nine patients had improved visual fields or acuity associated with decreased tumor size and serum PRL level, usually within a few days of initiating bromocriptine therapy. Molitch et al. (105) also reported improvement in 9 of 10 patients with pretreatment visual field defects in a series of 27 patients harboring PRL-secreting macroadenomas. Lesser et al. (106) noted an improvement in vision in eight patients with PRL-secreting macroadenomas treated with bromocriptine (106). Follow-up ranged from 18 to 56 months. Landholt et al. (107) described improvement in a patient with third and fourth nerve paresis associated with a recurrent pituitary adenoma that was treated with bromocriptine (107). King et al. (108) noted resolution of bitemporal visual field defects and dysfunction of cranial nerves V and VI during 6 months in a patient with an invasive prolactinoma. The improvement in visual function with bromocriptine therapy is often rapid and usually occurs within 24 to 72 hours of initiation of therapy (109–113). The long-acting and repeatable form of bromocriptine (Parlodel-LAK) has also shown some benefit, with improvement in 3 of 8 patients with visual defects in a series of 29 patients with macroprolactinomas (114).

Several other relatively new agents have been evaluated for the medical treatment of pituitary tumors. CV

205–502, or quinagolide (octahydrobenzo [g] quinolone), is a nonergot long-acting PRL inhibitor and a pure D_2 agonist. Grochowicki et al. (115) evaluated the visual function of 13 patients with macroprolactinomas treated with this agent. Mean follow-up was 30 months. No change was seen in nine patients (six had normal visual fields and three had previous visual field defects after surgery). In four patients, visual function dramatically improved (one patient experienced regression of a third nerve palsy and three patients noted disappearance of a chiasmal syndrome between 4 and 8 weeks after therapy). Resolution of ophthalmoplegia has also been noted with this agent (116, 117). Other dopamine agonists, lisuride and mesulergine, are being studied (118).

Medical therapy of growth hormone–secreting and thy-rotropic adenomas has also been effective in improving visual function. Warnet et al. (119) administered the long-acting somatostatin analog octreotide (SMS 201–995) to eight patients with pituitary macroadenomas of varying types. An improvement in both visual fields and visual acuity occurred in six patients (within 4 to 6 hours of treatment in two of these patients). In two patients, gonadotropic adenomas were unresponsive. Maximal improvement occurred within 6 to 45 days and was sustained during the 1- to 12-month follow-up period. Tumor shrinkage was demonstrated in only one patient. The adenomas secreting growth hormone and thyroid-stimulating hormone and the silent corticotropin-secreting adenomas responded, as did the nonfunctioning adenomas. The authors concluded that therapy with SMS 201–995 can rapidly improve the

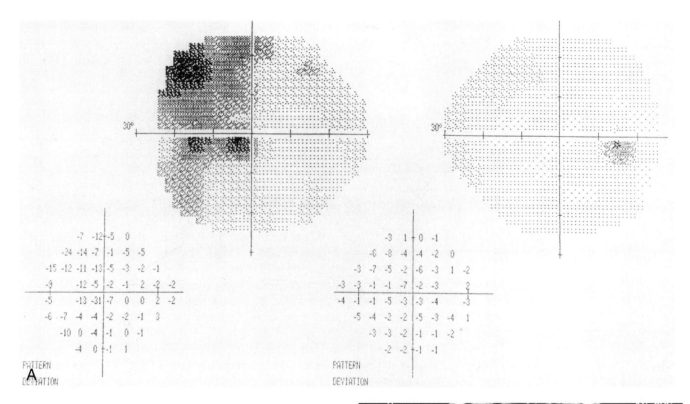

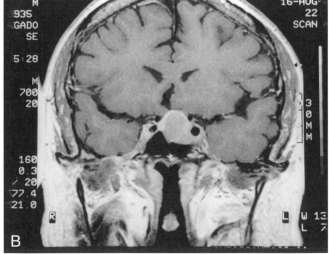

Figure 10.11. The patient is a 59-year-old man with a 2-year history of mild problems with left eye vision and impotence. His PRL level was elevated. His visual acuity was 20/15 OD and 20/20 OS. A left temporal field defect was seen on Humphrey visual fields **(A)**. A T1-weighted MRI with gadolinium revealed a large pituitary tumor causing compression of the optic pathways **(B,** coronal view). Treatment with bromocriptine resulted in symptomatic improvement within 3 days. At 4-month follow-up, his visual fields were normal **(C)**, and the pituitary tumor had regressed on the MRI **(D,** coronal view).

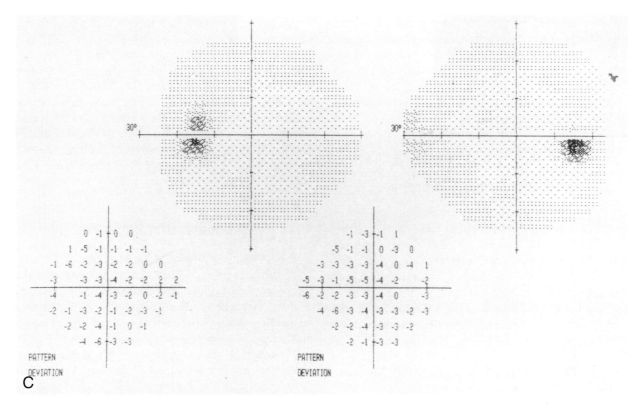

```
        0  -1 +0   0                          -1  -3 +-1   1
     1  -5 -1 |-1  -1  -1                  -5 -1  -1 | 0  -3   0
  -1 -6 -2 -3 |-2  -2   0   0          -3  -3  -3 -3 |-4   0  -4   1
  -3    -3 -3 |-4  -2  -2   2   2    -5 -3  -1 -5 -5 |-4  -2      -2
  -4    -1 -4 |-3  -2   0  -2  -1    -6 -2  -2 -3 -3 |-4   0      -3
 -2 -1 -3 -2 |-1  -2  -3  -1         -4 -6 -3  -4 |-3  -3  -2  -3
   -2 -2 -4 |-1   0  -1                -2 -2 -4 |-3  -3  -2
      -4 -6 +-3  -3                       -2 -1 +-3  -3

PATTERN                               PATTERN
DEVIATION                             DEVIATION
C
```

Figure 10.11. *(continued)*

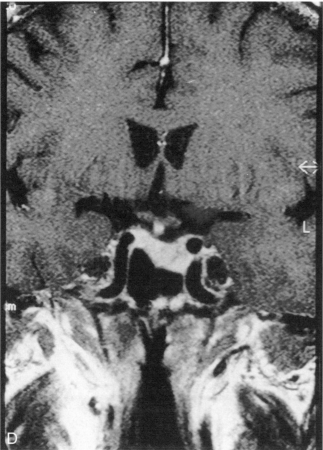

chiasmal syndrome caused by pituitary macroadenomas and that this effect may be independent of a reduction in tumor volume and independent of the type of adenoma. Vance and Harris (120), in a multicenter study of 189 patients with acromegaly treated with octreotide, noted an improvement in three of eight patients with visual field defects; five patients were unchanged.

As a better understanding of the genesis and endocrinology of the various types of pituitary tumors is achieved, we can expect an improvement in the medical arsenal available in the treatment of these tumors.

Outcome After Surgical Therapy

In a study of visual recovery after transsphenoidal adenomectomy by Cohen et al. (92), visual acuity was normal or improved in 79% of the eyes and visual fields were normal or improved in 74% of the eyes. Preoperatively, all patients had objective signs of visual acuity or field defects. Blaauw et al. (93), in a study of the effect of transsphenoidal adenomectomy on 60 patients, found an improvement in visual acuity and visual fields in 63% and 70% of eyes, respectively. An improvement in visual acuity and/or visual fields was noted in 78% of eyes.

In the Mayo Clinic series, 714 patients with pituitary adenomas underwent visual testing before and after transsphenoidal adenomectomy (31). Preoperatively, visual acuity was decreased in 115 patients. Postoperatively, visual acuity was normal or improved in 53 patients (46.5%), unchanged in 60 patients (52.2%), and worse in 2 patients (1.7%). Visual fields, which were abnormal in 230 patients, were normal or improved in 168 patients (73%), unchanged in 52 patients (22.6%), and worse in 10 patients (4.3%). There were five patients whose vision was normal preoperatively but not postoperatively; thus, the total number of patients who experienced worsened vision after surgery was 17 (2.3%).

Ciric et al. (98), in their study of 108 patients with pituitary macroadenomas who underwent 117 transsphenoidal procedures and 5 craniotomies, documented a preoperative visual deficit in 59 patients. Postoperatively, the visual acuity and visual fields had recovered or improved in 90% of patients, and no worsening of vision occurred. Other studies have documented similar rates of visual recovery (121–123). Significant improvement in visual function usually occurs within 24 hours of surgical decompression (124–126).

In patients surgically treated for pituitary apoplexy, an improvement in the visual acuity, visual fields, and ocular motility is generally seen. In a retrospective analysis of 37 patients with pituitary apoplexy, Bills et al. (100) found an improvement in visual acuity deficits, visual field deficits, and ocular paresis in 88%, 95%, and 100% of patients, respectively. Several other authors have reported, to varying degrees, recovery of blindness from apoplexy with surgical decompression (127–129) but more than any other ophthalmologic deficit, ocular paresis is most likely to resolve (123, 127–129). Resolution of ocular paresis with conservative management has also been noted (130).

A comparison was made between the transfrontal and transsphenoidal approaches by Sullivan and O'Day (96). Improvement in visual acuity was noted in 63% of eyes in patients operated on through the transfrontal route and in 50% of eyes in patients undergoing transsphenoidal adenomectomy. When eyes with normal preoperative acuity were excluded from analysis, however, no statistically significant difference was noted. With respect to visual fields, the improvement rates for the transfrontal and the transsphenoidal approaches were 56% and 81%, respectively, when the eyes with normal preoperative fields were excluded.

Outcome After Radiotherapy

Radiotherapy has historically been reserved for patients with residual and recurrent tumors after surgical therapy, for patients medically unfit for surgery, or for patients with tumors refractive to medical therapy. As such, there are relatively few large studies that evaluate the efficacy of radiotherapy alone on pituitary tumors.

Movsas et al. (131) retrospectively reviewed the records of 86 patients treated with radiotherapy for pituitary tumors to analyze the long-term effects of this therapy on visual fields and acuity. Twenty-one patients had preoperative and postoperative visual field testing. All patients but one (who had an inoperable invasive macroadenoma) were irradiated after one or more transsphenoidal resections or a craniotomy. The mean radiation dose was 50 Gy, and the median follow-up was 48 months. Of the 38 sighted eyes, 27 had normal vision before and after radiation, 7 showed improvement, and 4 had a stable defect. No radiation-induced deterioration occurred in visual fields or acuity.

Rush et al. (132) studied the effect of radiation therapy alone on 25 pituitary macroadenomas causing visual impairment. Radiation doses of 4000 to 5000 cGy were administered for 4 to 5 weeks, and median follow-up was 36 months. Eighteen (78%) of 23 patients evaluated noted improvement. Visual field deterioration occurred in four patients as a result of tumor recurrence, tumor hemorrhage, possible radiation necrosis, and optic chiasm prolapse.

Good ophthalmologic results have been obtained in the treatment of acromegaly by radiotherapy. Of 25 patients treated by Dowsett et al. (133), visual fields remained normal and visual acuity stable in 21 patients without pretreatment visual deficits. Four patients with prior visual field deficits improved. There were no complications of therapy.

The reversal of bilateral blindness caused by a recurrent hemangiopericytoma of the pituitary fossa by treatment with transsphenoidal implantation of a single high-activity iodine-125 seed has been reported (134). Stereotactic radiosurgery has also been used for the treatment of recurrent pituitary lesions, but the data are scant (135).

NEURO-OPHTHALMOLOGIC COMPLICATIONS OF THERAPY

Complications After Medical Therapy

Bromocriptine, an ergot derivative that functions as a dopamine receptor agonist, is widely used to shrink PRL-secreting macroadenomas (136). Neuro-ophthalmologic complications of bromocriptine therapy are extremely rare. Neuropsychiatric symptoms, including visual hallucinations, may occur in 1 to 2% of patients (137). This results especially if the lysergic acid diethylamide fragment of the bromocriptine molecule undergoes hydrolysis (138).

The rapid shrinkage of a large invasive prolactinoma induced by treatment with oral bromocriptine has been reported in association with a sixth nerve palsy that resolved over 6 weeks (139). The authors admitted the possibility of coincident diseases but thought that the sixth nerve injury was probably related to rapid tumor shrinkage and resultant deformation of the nerve.

If bromocriptine therapy is initiated and subsequently stopped in a patient with a pituitary adenoma, the initial tumor shrinkage is not maintained. Tumor reexpansion, sometimes associated with rapid deterioration in vision, has been reported within 7 to 14 days of ceasing therapy (140, 141).

Reenlargement of macroprolactinomas during bromocriptine therapy (142, 143) and pituitary apoplexy occurring in a patient after the initiation of bromocriptine therapy (144) also have been reported sporadically.

There is a recent report of chiasmal herniation complicating bromocriptine therapy (145). New bilateral visual field defects developed 8 months after therapy for a macroprolactinoma, and a magnetic resonance image (MRI) revealed chiasmal prolapse. After reduction of the bromocriptine dose, the visual field abnormality resolved during the ensuing 4 months.

Complications After Surgical Therapy

Following the surgical removal of a pituitary tumor, the suprasellar cistern may extend into the pituitary fossa, a phenomenon known as the "secondary empty sella syndrome." Progressive visual impairment may develop as the optic nerves and chiasm prolapse into the empty sella (146, 147). Suggested mechanisms for the visual deficit include vascular injury (148, 149) and scarring and traction (146, 148). Improvement in vision has been documented after chiasmapexy (147).

In an attempt to decrease the occurrence of the aforementioned complication of pituitary surgery, the sella and sphenoid sinus are usually packed with fat or muscle. Excessive packing of the sella has resulted in chiasmal compression and incomplete visual recovery (150). Improvement of visual function was noted with removal of the fat.

Worsening of visual acuity and visual fields after transsphenoidal surgery has been noted in 0 to 11% and 0 to 4% of patients, respectively, in large series (31, 92, 96, 121,

123). Barrow and Tindall (151) reported 11 patients who suffered significant visual loss after transsphenoidal surgery from a series of more than 1100 operations. The mechanisms of visual loss included direct injury or devascularization of the optic apparatus, fracture of the orbit, postoperative hematoma, cerebral vasospasm, and prolapse into an empty sella. Risk factors for visual complications of surgery included the presence of a pituitary macroadenoma, previous visual impairment, a "bottleneck" or dumbbell-shaped tumor, previous surgery and/or radiation therapy, and, possibly, use of a lumbar subarachnoid catheter during operation.

Complications After Radiotherapy

The empty sella syndrome, discussed in the previous section, may also result after radiation therapy.

Radiation optic neuropathy and chiasmopathy are a subset of the more extensive delayed radionecrosis of the central nervous system, which occurs with an incidence of 0.25 to 25% after radiotherapy (152–155). In a review of the literature from 1961 to 1985, Kline et al. (156) documented 22 cases of radiation optic neuropathy following radiotherapy for pituitary tumors, and added 4 cases of their own. Radiation optic neuropathy usually occurs within 3 years of completion of radiotherapy, with a peak incidence at 12 to 18 months. The presentation is usually an acute, unilateral loss of vision, but the other eye can also lose vision weeks or months later. Although the pattern of visual loss is usually a central scotoma and arcuate defects consistent with optic nerve involvement, a bitemporal hemianopia may also occur. Results of funduscopic examination reveal a normal or, eventually, a pale optic nerve.

The gross pathologic findings in patients with cerebral radionecrosis are loss of the gray-white distinction with edema and foci of hemorrhage. Microscopically, the hallmark of radiation damage is thickened, hyalinized blood vessels with fibrinoid necrosis. Endothelial proliferation and areas of reactive gliosis abound. Examination of the optic apparatus reveals demyelination, fibrinoid necrosis, astrocytic proliferation and endothelial hyperplasia. MRIs often reveal enlargement and focal gadolinium enhancement of the optic chiasm and tract (157–159) and can help exclude the diagnosis of tumor recurrence (Fig. 10.12).

The theories on the mechanism of delayed radiation injury to the central nervous system include direct injury to the brain parenchyma (160) and primary vascular injury with secondary neural damage (152). An older theory invoked alteration of the antigenic structure of the brain, resulting in an autoimmune vasculitis (161).

A retrospective study by Harris and Levene (162) revealed 5 patients with radiation optic neuropathy from a group of 55 patients with pituitary adenomas or craniopharyngiomas treated with irradiation. No patient who received less than 250 rad/day fractions showed visual loss, and the researchers recommended that the fraction size should not exceed 200 rad/day.

In a study by Aristizabal et al. (163) of 12 patients with pituitary adenomas treated by external irradiation, 1 patient

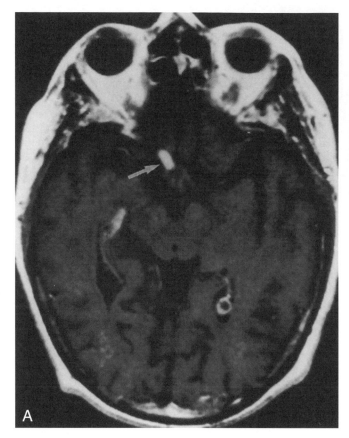

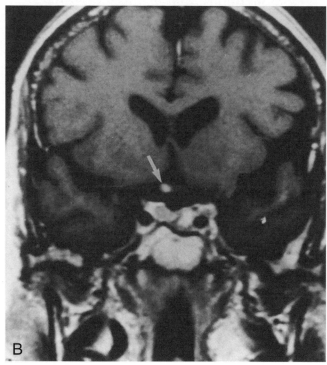

Figure 10.12. The patient is a 72-year-old woman who presented with diplopia and a left partial third nerve palsy. Her PRL level at presentation was 300 μg/L (300 ng/mL), and an MRI revealed a large sellar mass with suprasellar extension and invasion of the left cavernous sinus. She underwent a transsphenoidal procedure with subtotal resection of a pituitary adenoma. She received postoperative radiation therapy to the pituitary fossa, and her third nerve palsy and diplopia resolved. Thirty-five months later the patient developed headaches and visual loss, referable to the right optic nerve, occurring during a several-day period. An MRI with gadolinium revealed no recurrent tumor. Although unenhanced T1- and T2-weighted images through the orbits and optic nerves were normal, axial **(A)** and coronal **(B)** enhanced T1-weighted images revealed enhancement of the right optic nerve immediately in the prechiasmic portion (*arrow*). The nerve was slightly enlarged compared with the normal left side. A presumptive diagnosis of radiation optic neuropathy was made. Her visual loss did not resolve. (Reprinted with permission from Hudgins PA, Newman NJ, Dillon WP, Hoffman JC Jr. Radiation-induced optic neuropathy. AJNR 1992;13: 235–236.)

developed brain necrosis and 4 developed blindness. The authors found that the risk of complications increases from 0 to 25% as the dose exceeds a time-dose fractionation of 80 (5000 rad). Because cases of radiation optic neuropathy have been reported in patients receiving less than 5000 cGy or a fraction size less than 200 cGy (156, 163), inherent susceptibility to radiation therapy undoubtedly plays a role in the occurrence of radiation optic neuropathy.

Other potential risk factors for radiation optic neuropathy and chiasmopathy cited include the combination with chemotherapeutic agents, which may potentiate the effect of radiation, preexisting vasculopathy (including acromegaly, carotid atherosclerosis, and, possibly, diabetes mellitus), and childhood, when the relatively immature nervous system may be especially predisposed to radiation injury (164, 165).

REFERENCES

1. Sachs E. The History and Development of Neurological Surgery. New York: Paul B. Hoeber, 1952:29.
2. Meyer A. Historical Aspects of Cerebral Anatomy. New York: Oxford University Press, 1971:47.
3. Rucker CW. The concept of a semidecussation of the optic nerves. Arch Ophthalmol 1958;59:159–171.
4. Davey LM. Early historical aspects of the pituitary gland. In: Goodrich I, Lee KJ, eds. The Pituitary. Amsterdam: Elsevier Science Publishers, 1987.
5. Heublein GW. Some observations concerning the hypophysial fossa. Am J Roentgenol Rad Therapy 1946;46:299–319.
6. Weinberger LM, Adler FH, Grant FC. Primary pituitary adenoma and the syndrome of the cavernous sinus. Arch Ophthalmol 1940; 24:1197–1236.
7. Jefferson G. Extrasellar extensions of pituitary adenomas. Proc R Soc Med 1940;33:433–458.
8. Jefferson G. Concerning injuries, aneurysms and tumours involving the cavernous sinus. Trans Ophthalmol Soc UK 1953;73: 117–152.
9. Jefferson G. The Invasive Adenomas of the Anterior Pituitary. Liverpool: University Press, 1955.
10. Bailey P. Pathological report of a case of akromegaly with special

reference to the lesions in the hypophysis cerebri and in the thyroid gland; and of a case of hemorrhage into the pituitary. Philadelphia Med J 1898;1:789–792.

11. Bleibtreu L. Ein Fall von akromegalie (Zerstorung der Hypophysis durch Blutung). Munch Med Wochenschr 1905;52:2079–2080.

12. Horsely V. On the technique of operations on the central nervous system. Br Med J 1906;2:411–423.

13. Krause F. Surgery of the Brain and Spinal Cord. Vol 1, translated by Haubold HA. New York: Rebman, 1912:117–120; Vol 2, translated by Thorek M, pp 792–802.

14. Cushing H, Walker CB. Distortion of the visual fields in cases of brain tumor, IV: chiasmal lesions with special reference to bitemporal hemianopsia. Brain 1915;37:341–400.

15. Beclere A. The radiotherapeutic treatment of tumors of the hypophysis, giantism and acromegaly. Arch Roentgenol Radiol 1909;14:147–150.

16. Gramegna A. Un cas d'acromegalie traite par la radiotherapie. Revue Neurolog Fr 1909;17:15–17.

17. Renn WH, Rhoton AL. Microsurgical anatomy of the sellar region. J Neurosurg 1975;43:288–298.

18. Miller NR. Anatomy and physiology of the optic chiasm. In: Walsh and Hoyt's Clinical Neuro-Ophthalmology. 4th ed. Baltimore: Williams & Wilkins, 1982;1:60–68.

19. Traquir HM. An Introduction to Clinical Perimetry. 4th ed. St. Louis: CV Mosby, 1944.

20. Bergland RM, Ray BS, Torack M. Anatomical variations in the pituitary gland and adjacent structures in 225 human autopsy cases. Neurosurgery 1968;28:93–99.

21. Ronne H. Ueber doppelseitige hemianopsie mit erhaltener makula. Klin Monatsbl Augenheilkd 1914;53:470–487.

22. Polyak SL. Projection of the retina upon the cerebral cortex, based upon experiments with monkeys. In: Proceedings of the Association for Research in Nervous and Mental Disease. Baltimore: Williams & Wilkins, 1934;13:535–537.

23. Hoyt WF, Luis O. The primate chiasm: details of visual fiber organization studied by silver impregnation techniques. Arch Ophthalmol 1963;70:69–85.

24. Wilbrand HL. Schema des verlaufs der sehnervenfasern durch das chiasm. Z Augenheilk 1926;59:135–144.

25. Kupfer C, Chumbley, Downer J deC. Quantitative histology of optic nerve, optic tract and lateral geniculate nucleus of man. J Anat 1967;101:393–401.

26. Hoyt WF. Correlative functional anatomy of the optic chiasm-1969. Clin Neurosurg 1970;17:189–208.

27. O'Connell JEA. The anatomy of the optic chiasm and heteronymous hemianopia. J Neurol Neurosurg Psychiatry 1973;36:710–723.

28. Hedges TR. Preservation of the upper nasal field in the chiasmal syndrome: an anatomic explanation. Trans Am Ophthalmol Soc 1969;67:131–141.

29. Bynke H. Pituitary tumors with ocular manifestations: incidence of cases and clinical findings 1946–1984. Neuro-ophthalmol 1986;6:303–311.

30. Anderson DF, Faber P, Marcovitz S, et al. Pituitary tumors and the ophthalmologist. Ophthalmology 1983;90:1265–1270.

31. Trautmann JC, Laws ER Jr. Visual status after transsphenoidal surgery at the Mayo Clinic. Am J Ophthalmol 1983;96:200–208.

32. Johnston J, Parkinson D. Intracranial sympathetic pathways associated with the sixth nerve. J Neurosurg 1974;40:236–243.

33. Umansky F, Nathan H. The lateral wall of the cavernous sinus with special reference to the nerves related to it. J Neurosurg 1982;56:228–234.

34. Harris FS, Rhoton AL. Anatomy of the cavernous sinus: a microsurgical study. J Neurosurg 1976;45:169–180.

35. Walsh FB. Bilateral total ophthalmoplegia with adenoma of the pituitary gland: report of two cases; an anatomic study. Arch Ophthalmol 1949;42:646–654.

36. Symonds CP. Ocular palsy as the presenting symptom of pituitary adenoma. Bull Johns Hopkins Hosp 1962;111:72–82.

37. Cairns HWB. Peripheral ocular palsies from the neurosurgical point of view. Trans Ophthalmol Soc UK 1938;58:464–482.

38. Saul RF, Hilliker JK. Third nerve palsy: the presenting sign of a pituitary adenoma in five patients and the only neurological sign in four patients. J Clin Neuro-ophthalmol 1985;5:185–193.

39. Trumble HC. Observations on large tumours which have spread widely beyond the confines of the sella turcica. Br J Surg 1951;39:7–24.

40. Scott TV, Schatz NJ, Lee KF. Malignant pituitary adenoma: a cause of sphenoid hyperostosis and monocular blindness. Arch Ophthalmol 1974;91:123–125.

41. Huber A; Blodi FC, ed and trans. Eye Signs and Symptoms in Brain Tumors. 3rd ed. St. Louis: CV Mosby, 1976:202–228.

42. Milas RW, Sugar O, Dobben G. Benign pituitary adenoma associated with hyperostosis of the sphenoid bone and monocular blindness: case report. J Neurosurg 1977;46:107–110.

43. Wilson P, Falconer MA. Patterns of visual failure with pituitary tumors: clinical and radiological correlations. Br J Ophthalmol 1968;52:94–110.

44. Kirkham TH. The ocular symptomatology of pituitary tumors. Proc R Soc Med 1972;65:517–518.

45. Kupersmith MJ, Rosenberg C, Kleinberg D. Visual loss in pregnant women with pituitary adenomas. Ann Intern Med 1994;121:473–477.

46. Gemzell C, Wang CF. Outcome of pregnancy in women with pituitary adenoma. Fertil Steril 1979;31:363–372.

47. Thorner MO, Edwards CR, Charlesworth M, et al. Pregnancy in patients presenting with hyperprolactinaemia. Br Med J 1979;2:771–774.

48. Lyle TK, Clover P. Ocular symptoms and signs in pituitary tumours. Proc R Soc Med 1961;54:611–619.

49. Hollenhorst RW, Younge BR. Ocular manifestations produced by adenomas of the pituitary gland: analysis of 1000 cases. In: Kohler PO, Ross GT, eds. Diagnosis and Treatment of Pituitary Tumors. Amsterdam: Excerpta Medica, 1973:53–68.

50. Wray SH. Neuro-ophthalmological manifestations of pituitary and parasellar lesions. Clin Neurosurg 1976;24:86–117.

51. Rovit RL, Fein JM. Pituitary apoplexy: a review and reappraisal. J Neurosurg 1972;37:280–288.

52. Lopez IA. Pituitary apoplexy. J Oslo City Hosp 1970;20;17–27.

53. Wakai S, Fukushima T, Teramoto A, et al. Pituitary apoplexy: its incidence and clinical significance. J Neurosurg 1981;55:187–193.

54. Mohr G, Hardy J. Hemorrhage, necrosis, and apoplexy in pituitary adenomas. Surg Neurol 1982;18:181–189.

55. Conomy JP Ferguson JH, Brodkey JS, et al. Spontaneous infarction in pituitary tumors: neurologic and therapeutic aspects. Neurology 1975;25:580–587.

56. Reid RL, Quigley ME, Yen SSC. Pituitary apoplexy: a review. Arch Neurol 1985;42:712–719.

57. Peterson P, Christiansen KH, Lindholm J. Acute monocular disturbances mimicking optic neuritis in pituitary apoplexy. Acta Neurol Scand 1988;78:101–103.

58. Robinson JL. Sudden blindness with pituitary tumours: report of three cases. J Neurosurg 1972;36:83–85.

59. Silvestrini M, Matteis M, Cupini LM, et al. Ophthalmoplegic migraine-like syndrome due to pituitary apoplexy. Headache 1994;34:484–486.

60. Nichols BD, Romanchuk KG. Pituitary apoplexy presenting with light-near dissociation of the pupils. J Clin Neuro-ophthalmol 1987;7:139–143.

61. Poisson M, Van Effentere R, Mashaly R. Pituitary apoplexy with retraction nystagmus. Ann Neurol 1980;7:286.

62. Shults WT, Hoyt WF, Behrens M, et al. Ocular neuromyotonia: a clinical description of six patients. Arch Ophthalmol 1986;104:1028–1034.

63. Ortiz JM, Stein SC, Nelson P, et al. Pituitary adenoma presenting as unilateral proptosis. Arch Ophthalmol 1992;110:283.

64. Jackson H. Orbital tumors. J Neurosurg 1962;19:551–567.

65. De Divitis E, Cerillo A. Adenome hypophaysaire a developpement intraorbitaire. Neurochirurgie 1973;19:561–566.

66. Sammartino A, Bonavolonta G, Pettinato G, et al. Exophthalmos caused by an invasive pituitary adenoma in a child. Ophthalmologica 1979;179:83–89.

67. Daita G, Yonemasu Y, Hashizume A. Unilateral exophthalmos caused by an invasive pituitary adenoma. Neurosurgery 1987;21:716–718.

68. Small KW, Buckley EG. Recurrent blepharoptosis secondary to a pituitary tumor. Am J Ophthalmol 1988;106:760–761.

69. Ram Z, Findler G, Gutman I, et al. Visual hallucinations associated with pituitary adenoma. Neurosurgery 1987;20:292–296.

70. Dawson DJ, Enoch BA, Shepherd DI. Formed visual hallucinations with pituitary adenomas. Br Med J 1984;289:414.

71. Weinberger EA, Grant FC. Visual hallucinations and their neuro-optical correlates. Arch Ophthalmol 1940;23:166–199.

72. Chamblin M, Davidoff LM, Feiring EH. Ophthalmological changes produced by pituitary tumors. Am J Ophthalmol 1955; 40:353–368.

73. Klauber A, Rasmussen P, Lindholm J. Pituitary adenoma and visual function: the prognostic value of clinical, ophthalmological and neuroradiologic findings in 51 patients subjected to operation. Acta Ophthalmol 1978;56:252–263.

74. Anderson D, Faber P, Marcovitz J, et al. Pituitary tumors and the ophthalmologist. Ophthalmology 1983;90:1265–1270.

75. Frisen L, Hoyt WF. Insidious atrophy of retinal nerve fibers in multiple sclerosis: Funduscopic identification in patients with and without visual complaints. Arch Ophthalmol 1974;92:91–97.

76. Lundstrom M, Frisen L. Atrophy of the nerve fibers in compression of the chiasm: degree and distribution of ophthalmoscopic changes. Acta Ophthalmol 1976;54:623–640.

77. Newman NM. Ophthalmoscopic observation of the retinal nerve fiber layer. Trans Am Acad Ophthalmol Otolaryngol 1977;83: 786–796.

78. Hoyt WF, Rios-Montenegro EN, Behrens MM, et al. Homonymous hemioptic hypoplasia. Br J Ophthalmol 1972;56:537–545.

79. Poon A, McNeill P, Harper A, et al. Patterns of visual loss associated with pituitary macroadenomas. Aust N Z J Ophthalmol 1995; 23:107–115.

80. Robert CM, Feigenbaum JA, Stern WE. Ocular palsy occurring with pituitary tumors. J Neurosurg 1973;38:17–19.

81. Yen MY, Liu JH, Jaw SJ. Ptosis as the early manifestation of pituitary tumours. Br J Ophthalmol 1990;74:188–191.

82. Hsu TH. Sudden onset of unilateral third nerve paresis in a patient with Cushing syndrome. Arch Neurol 1977;34:196–198.

83. Wykes WN. Prolactinoma presenting with intermittent third nerve palsy. Br J Ophthalmol 1986;70:706–707.

84. Lopez R, David NJ, Gargano F, et al. Bilateral sixth nerve palsies in a patient with massive pituitary adenoma. Neurology 1981;31: 1137–1138.

85. Supler ML, Mickle JP. Lymphocytic hypophysitis: report of a case in a man with cavernous sinus involvement. Surg Neurol 1992; 37:472–476.

86. Cullom ME, Savino PJ. Adenocarcinoma of the prostate presenting as a third nerve palsy. Neurology 1993;43:2146–2147.

87. Gittinger JW Jr. Ophthalmological evaluation of pituitary adenomas. In: Jackson IMD, Reichlin S, eds. The Pituitary Adenoma. New York: Plenum Press, 1980:276–277.

88. Daroff RB. See-saw nystagmus. Neurology 1965;15:874–877.

89. Fein JM, Williams RDB. See-saw nystagmus. J Neurol Neurosurg Psychiatry 1969;32:202–207.

90. Kinder RSL, Howard GM. See-saw nystagmus. Am J Dis Child 1963;106:331–332.

91. Williams IM, Dickinson P, Ramsay RJ, et al. See-saw nystagmus. Aust J Ophthalmol 1982;10:19–25.

92. Cohen AR, Cooper PR, Kupersmith MJ, et al. Visual recovery after transsphenoidal removal of pituitary adenomas. Neurosurgery 1985;17:446–452.

93. Blaauw G, Braakman R, Cuhadar M, et al. Influence of transsphenoidal hypophysectomy on visual deficit due to a pituitary tumour. Acta Neurochir (Wien) 1986;83:79–82.

94. Trobe JD, Tao AH, Schuster JJ. Perichiasmal tumors: diagnostic and prognostic features. Neurosurgery 1984;15:391–399.

95. Symon L, Jakubowski J. Transcranial management of pituitary tumours with suprasellar extension. J Neurol Neurosurg Psychiatry 1979;42:973–982.

96. Sullivan LJ, O'Day J. Visual outcomes of pituitary adenoma surgery: St. Vincent's Hospital 1968–1987. J Clin Neuro-ophthalmol 1991;11:262–267.

97. Lennerstrand G. Visual recovery after treatment for pituitary adenoma. Acta Ophthalmol 1983;61:1104–1117.

98. Ciric I, Mikhael M, Stafford T, et al. Transsphenoidal microsurgery of pituitary macroadenomas with long-term follow-up results. J Neurosurg 1983;59:395–401.

99. McFadzean RM, Doyle D, Rampling R, et al. Pituitary apoplexy and its effect on vision. Neurosurgery 1991;29:669–675.

100. Bills DC, Meyer FB, Laws ER Jr, et al. A retrospective analysis of pituitary apoplexy. Neurosurgery 1993;33:602–609.

101. Rush SC, Kupersmith MJ, Lerch I, et al. Neuro-ophthalmological assessment of vision before and after radiation therapy alone for pituitary macroadenomas. J Neurosurg 1990;72:594–599.

102. Hughes MN, Llamas KJ, Yelland ME, et al. Pituitary adenomas: long-term results for radiotherapy alone and post-operative radiotherapy. Int J Radiat Oncol Biol Phys 1993;27:1035–1043.

103. Borowski D, Rose LI. Bromocriptine update. Clin Pharmacol 1984;30:1984.

104. Moster ML, Savino PJ, Schatz NJ, et al. Visual function in prolactinoma patients with bromocriptine. Ophthalmology 1985;92: 1332–1341.

105. Molitch ME, Elton RL, Blackwell RE, et al. Bromocriptine as primary therapy for prolactin-secreting macroadenomas: results of a prospective multi-center study. J Clin Endocrinol Metab 1985;60: 698–705.

106. Lesser RL, Zheutlin JD, Boghen D, et al. Visual function improvement in patients with macroprolactinomas treated with bromocriptine. Am J Ophthalmol 1990;109:535–543.

107. Landholt AM, Wuthrich R, Fellmann H. Regression of pituitary prolactinoma after treatment with bromocriptine. Lancet 1979;1: 1082–1083.

108. King LW, Molitch ME, Gittinger JW, et al. Cavernous sinus syndrome due to prolactinoma: resolution with bromocriptine. Surg Neurol 1983;19:280–284.

109. Clayton RN, Webb J, Heath JA, et al. Dramatic and rapid shrinkage of a massive invasive prolactinoma with bromocriptine: a case report. Clin Endocrinol 1985;22:573–581.

110. Grimson BS, Bowman ZL. Rapid decompression of anterior intracranial visual pathways with bromocriptine. Arch Ophthalmol 1983;101:604–606.

111. Kahn SE, Miller JL. Rapid resolution of visual field defects and reduction in macroprolactinoma size with bromocriptine therapy: a case report. S Afr Med J 1982;62:696–699.

112. Vaidya RA, Aloorkar SD, Rege NR, et al. Normalization of visual fields following bromocriptine treatment in hyperprolactinemic patients with visual field constriction. Fertil Steril 1978;19: 632–636.

113. Brisman MH, Katz G, Post KD. Symptoms of pituitary apoplexy rapidly reversed with bromocriptine: case report. J Neurosurg 1996;85:1153–1155.

114. Beckers A, Petrossians P, Abs R, et al. Treatment of macroprolactinomas with the long-acting and repeatable form of bromocriptine: a report on 29 cases. J Clin Endocrinol Metab 1992;75:272–280.

115. Grochowicki M, Khalfallah Y, Vighetto A, et al. Ophthalmic results in patients with macroprolactinomas treated with a new prolactin inhibitor CV 205–502. Br J Ophthalmol 1993;77:785–788.

116. Vance ML, Lipper M, Klibanski A, et al. Treatment of prolactin-secreting pituitary macroadenomas with the long-acting non-ergot dopamine agonist CV 205–502. Ann Intern Med 1990;112: 668–673.

117. Kvistborg A, Halse J, Bakke S, et al. Long-term treatment of macroprolactinomas with CV 205–502. Acta Endocrinol 1993;128: 301–307.

118. Wen PY, Loeffler JS. Advances in the diagnosis and management of pituitary tumors. Curr Opin Oncol 1995;7:56–62.

119. Warnet A, Timsit J, Chanson P, et al. The effect of somatostatin analogue on chiasmal dysfunction from pituitary macroadenomas. J Neurosurg 1989;71:687–690.

120. Vance ML, Harris AG. Long-term treatment of 189 acromegalic patients with the somatostatin analog octreotide: results of the International Multicenter Acromegaly Study Group. Arch Intern Med 1991;151:1573–1578.

121. Harris PE, Afshar F, Coates P, et al. The effects of transsphenoidal surgery on endocrine function and visual fields in patients with functionless pituitary tumours. QJM 1989;71:417–427.

122. Findlay G, McFadzean RM, Teasdale G. Recovery of vision following treatment of pituitary tumours: application of a new system of visual assessment. Trans Ophthalmol Soc UK 1983;103:212–216.

123. Ebersold MJ, Quast LM, Laws ER Jr, et al. Long-term results of nonfunctioning pituitary adenomas. J Neurosurg 1986;64: 713–719.

124. Kayan A, Earl CJ. Compressive lesions of the optic nerves and chiasm: pattern of recovery of vision following surgical treatment. Brain 1975;98:13–28.

125. Wilson CB, Dempsey LC. Transsphenoidal microsurgical removal of 250 pituitary adenomas. J Neurosurg 1978;48:13–22.

126. Miller NR, Calvert PC, Zinreich JS, et al. Quantitative analysis of visual results following transsphenoidal surgery for pituitary adenomas. Neuro-ophthalmol Jpn 1986;3:431.

127. Kaplan B, Day AL, Quisling R, et al. Hemorrhage into pituitary adenomas. Surg Neurol 1983;20:280–287.
128. Symon L, Mohanty S. Haemorrhage in pituitary tumours. Acta Neurochir (Wien) 1982;65:41–49.
129. Onesti ST, Wisiniewski T, Post KD. Clinical versus subclinical pituitary apoplexy: presentation, surgical management, and outcome in 21 patients. Neurosurgery 1990;26:980–986.
130. David NJ, Gargano FP, Glaser JS. Pituitary apoplexy in clinical perspective. In: Glaser JS, Smith JL, eds. Neuro-ophthalmology 1975: Symposium at the University of Miami and the Bascom Palmer Eye Institute. St. Louis: CV Mosby, 1975:140–165.
131. Movsas B, Movsas TZ, Steinberg SM, et al. Long-term visual changes following pituitary irradiation. Int J Radiat Oncol Biol Phys 1995;33:599–605.
132. Rush SC, Kupersmith MJ, Lerch I, et al. Neuro-ophthalmological assessment of vision before and after radiation therapy alone for pituitary macroadenomas. J Neurosurg 1990;72:594–599.
133. Dowsett RJ, Fowble B, Sergott RC, et al. Results of radiotherapy in the treatment of acromegaly: lack of ophthalmologic complications. Int J Radiat Oncol Biol Phys 1990;19:453–459.
134. Kumar PP, Good RR, Cox TA, et al. Reversal of visual impairment after interstitial irradiation of pituitary tumor. Neurosurgery 1986; 18:82–84.
135. Degerblad M, Rahn T, Bergstrand G, et al. Long-term results of stereotactic radiosurgery to the pituitary gland in Cushing's disease. Acta Endocrinol 1986;112:310–314.
136. McGregor AM, Scanlon MF, Hall K, et al. Reduction in size of a pituitary tumor by bromocriptine therapy. N Engl J Med 1979; 300:291–293.
137. Fossati P, Dewailly D, Thomas-Desrousseaux P, et al. Medical treatment of hyperprolactinemia. Horm Res 19485;22:228–238.
138. Parkes D. Bromocriptine. N Engl J Med 1979;301:873–878.
139. Dunne JW, Stewart-Wynne EG, Pullan PT. Abducent palsy after rapid shrinkage of a prolactinoma. J Neurol Neurosurg 1987;50: 496–498.
140. Barrow DL, Tindall GT, Kovacs K, et al. Clinical and pathological effects of bromocriptine on prolactin-secreting and other pituitary tumors. J Neurosurg 1984;60:1–7.
141. Clark JDA, Wheatley T, Edwards OM. Rapid enlargement of non-functioning pituitary tumour following withdrawal of bromocriptine. J Neurol Neurosurg Psychiatry 1985;48:287.
142. Breidal HD, Topliss DJ, Pike JW. Failure of bromocriptine to maintain reduction in size of a macroprolactinoma. Br Med J 1983; 287:451–452.
143. Dallabonzana D, Spelta B, Oppizzi G, et al. Reenlargement of macroprolactinomas during bromocriptine treatment: report of two cases. J Endocrinol Invest 1983;6:47–50.
144. Alhajje A, Lambert M, Crabbe J. Pituitary apoplexy in an acromegalic patient during bromocriptine therapy: case report. J Neurosurg 1985;63:288–292.
145. Taxel P, Waitzman DM, Harrington JF Jr, et al. Chiasmal herniation as a complication of bromocriptine therapy. J Neuro-ophthalmol 1996;16:252–257.
146. Lee WM, Adams JE. The empty sella syndrome. J Neurosurg 1968; 28:351–356.
147. Welch K, Stears JC. Chiasmapexy for the correction of traction on the optic nerves and chiasm associated with their descent into an empty sella turcica: case report. J Neurosurg 1971;35:760–764.
148. Morello G, Frera C. Visual damage after removal of hypophysial adenomas: possible importance of vascular disturbances of the optic nerves and chiasma. Acta Neurochir (Wien) 1966;15:1–10.
149. Poppen JL. Discussion: symposium on pituitary tumors-IV. J Neurosurg 1962;19:25.
150. Slavin ML, Lam BL, Decker RE, et al. Chiasmal compression from fat packing after transsphenoidal resection of intrasellar tumor in two patients. Am J Ophthalmol 1993;115:368–371.
151. Barrow DL, Tindall GT. Loss of vision after transsphenoidal surgery. Neurosurgery 1990;27:60–68.
152. Pennybacker J, Russell DS. Necrosis of the brain due to radiation therapy: clinical and pathological observations. J Neurol Neurosurg Psychiatry 1948;11:183–198.
153. Boden G. Radiation myelitis of the brain-stem. J Fac Radiol 1950; 2:79–84.
154. Sato O, Tamura A, Teraoka A, et al. Results of treatment for pituitary adenomas. Brain Nerve (Tokyo) 1973;25:285–294.
155. Takeuchi J, Hanakita J, Abe M, et al. Brain necrosis after repeated radiotherapy. Surg Neurol 1976;5:89–93.
156. Kline LB, Kim JY, Ceballos R. Radiation optic neuropathy. Ophthalmology 1985;92:1118–1126.
157. Tachibana O, Yamaguchi N, Yamashima T, et al. Radiation necrosis of the optic chiasm, optic tract, hypothalamus, and upper pons after radiotherapy for pituitary adenoma, detected by gadolinium-enhanced, T1-weighted magnetic resonance imaging: case report. Neurosurgery 1990;27:640–643.
158. Zimmerman CF, Schatz NJ, Glaser JS. Magnetic resonance imaging of radiation optic neuropathy. Am J Ophthalmol 1990;110: 389–394.
159. Hudgins PA, Newman NJ, Dillon WP, et al. Radiation-induced optic neuropathy: characteristic appearance on gadolinium-enhanced MR. AJNR 1992;13:235–238.
160. Arnold A, Bailey P, Harvey RA. Intolerance of the primate brain-stem and hypothalamus to conventional and high energy radiations. Neurology 1954;4:575–585.
161. Crompton MR, Layton DD. Delayed radionecrosis of the brain following therapeutic x-radiation of the pituitary. Brain 1961;84: 85–101.
162. Harris JR, Levene MB. Visual complications following irradiation for pituitary adenomas and craniopharyngiomas. Radiology 1976; 120:167–171.
163. Aristizabal S, Caldwell WL, Avila J. The relationship of time-dose fractionation factors to complications in the treatment of pituitary tumors by irradiation. Int J Radiat Oncol Biol Phys 1977;2: 667–673.
164. Schatz NJ. Discussion, in Kline LB, et al. Radiation optic neuropathy. Ophthalmology 1985;92:1126.
165. Atkinson AB, Allen IV, Gordon DS, et al. Progressive visual failure in acromegaly following external pituitary irradiation. Clin Endocrinol 1979;10:469–479.

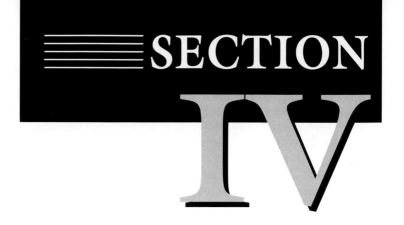

SECTION IV

*Management of
Pituitary Tumors*

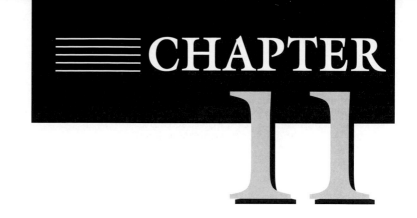

CHAPTER 11

Hyperprolactinemia: Physiology and Clinical Approach

Laurence Katznelson and Anne Klibanski

PROLACTIN PHYSIOLOGY AND PATHOPHYSIOLOGY

Prolactin (PRL) is a peptide hormone synthesized and secreted by the pituitary lactotroph cell. The physiologic role of PRL is to initiate and maintain lactation, and levels rise progressively during pregnancy and peak at term (100 to 300 µg/L [100 to 300 ng/mL]) (1). Lactation begins when estradiol levels fall at delivery. The nursing stimulus promotes acute PRL release via afferent spinal neural pathways; within 20 to 30 minutes of nursing, PRL levels increase 60-fold (2). With established nursing, nipple stimulation elicits progressively less PRL release, and, in the weeks following initiation of lactation, both basal and nursing-stimulated PRL pulses decrease (2). Within 4 to 6 months postpartum, basal PRL levels should return to normal, and a nursing-induced rise does not occur despite continued lactation.

PRL is secreted in a pulsatile fashion with 4 to 14 pulses per day (3). The PRL pulse amplitude is highly variable between individuals, with peak levels as well as peak frequency occurring during the late hours of sleep (4). However, changes in PRL pulse characteristics are not associated with a specific sleep stage. Rises in serum PRL concentration occur within an hour of eating in normal individuals but not in individuals with prolactinomas. The protein component of meals seems to be the main stimulus to PRL secretion (5). PRL levels rise in normal individuals during stress, including acute physical exertion, surgery, sexual intercourse, insulin-induced hypoglycemia, and seizures. The biologic significance of these increases in PRL concentration during stress is not known.

Results of several studies suggest that PRL secretion varies during the menstrual cycle, with PRL levels significantly higher during the ovulatory and luteal phases, particularly at midcycle (6). This increase is likely attributable to increased circulating estradiol levels during these phases of the cycle. In addition, PRL levels are slightly higher in premenopausal women than in men. This is probably the result of a direct effect of estrogen on pituitary PRL secretion because postmenopausal women have lower circulating PRL levels that are comparable with those of normal men (7). Therefore, a serum PRL level should be evaluated in the context of a careful review of the clinical situation in which the sample was drawn, such as the proximity to a meal, time of day, timing of a recent breast examination, and phase of the menstrual cycle.

189

Figure 11.1. Regulation of PRL secretion. PRL release is under tonic inhibition by dopamine, the most important PRL-inhibiting factor. PRL release is stimulated by several factors, including vasoactive intestinal peptide (*VIP*) and thyroid-releasing hormone (*TRH*). Estrogens and pregnancy stimulate PRL release.

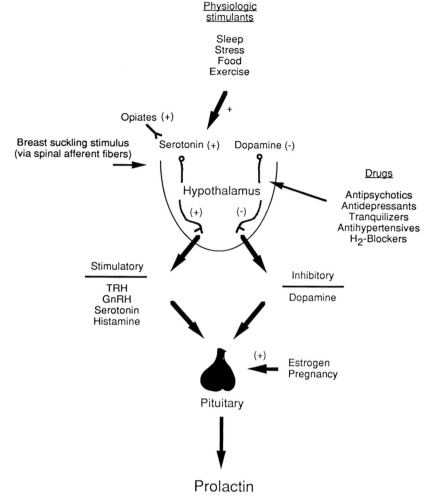

Normal PRL secretion is controlled by both inhibitory and stimulatory factors (Fig. 11.1). However, in contrast to the regulation of other pituitary hormones, PRL secretion is predominantly under tonic inhibitory control. Dopamine, the main physiologic inhibitor of PRL secretion, is transported from the hypothalamus to the pituitary gland via the hypophyseal stalk circulation to inhibit PRL biosynthesis and secretion directly from lactotroph cells (8, 9). Damage to the hypothalamus or the hypophyseal stalk, e.g., tumor compression (both pituitary and nonpituitary lesions), infiltrative disorders, trauma, surgery, or radiation scarring, can interfere with normal dopaminergic inhibitory control, resulting in hyperprolactinemia.

Pharmacologic causes of hyperprolactinemia are often mediated through alterations of dopaminergic tone (Table 11.1). Use of antihypertensive drugs, such as reserpine and methyldopa, can result in hyperprolactinemia by causing dopamine depletion in the tuberoinfundibular neurons. Use of calcium channel blocker agents such as verapamil may increase PRL levels, although the underlying mechanism is largely unknown. PRL level elevations have been seen in patients undergoing therapy with angiotensin-converting enzyme inhibitors such as enalapril. Chronic opiate

use, cocaine abuse, and therapy with H_2-antagonists such as cimetidine have been associated with hyperprolactinemia. Use of psychotropic agents is a frequent cause of hyperprolactinemia (10). Treatment with phenothiazines and haloperidol may cause PRL release act by blockade of dopamine receptors. Tricyclic antidepressant use may cause modest hyperprolactinemia in up to one-fourth of patients. Use of psychotropic agents that affect the serotonergic axis, such as fluoxetine hydrochloride (Prozac), may also cause hyperprolactinemia.

Estrogens are important physiologic stimulators of PRL release and cause increased PRL levels during pregnancy (11). Chronic exposure to estrogens results in an increase in lactotroph number and size (i.e., "pregnancy cells"), and pituitary volume normally increases during pregnancy because of lactotroph hyperplasia (12). Although pharmacologic estrogen administration can raise serum PRL levels, the estrogen concentrations in typical oral contraceptives (i.e., 35 mcg ethinyl estradiol) and postmenopausal estrogen replacement do not cause hyperprolactinemia. In a recent study, cyclic conjugated estrogen (Premarin) and medroxyprogesterone acetate (Provera) were administered to 29 premenopausal hyperprolactinemic women at replace-

Table 11.1. *Pathologic and Pharmacologic Causes of Hyperprolactinemia*

Pituitary disease
　Prolactin-secreting tumors
　Acromegaly
　Cushing's disease
　Empty sella syndrome
Pituitary stalk section
　Clinically nonfunctioning pituitary tumors
　Trauma
Hypothalamic infiltrative or degenerative disease
　Craniopharyngiomas
　Meningiomas
　Dysgerminomas
　Gliomas
　Lymphoma
　Metastatic disease
　Tuberculosis
　Sarcoidosis
　Eosinophilic granuloma
　Irradiation
Neurogenic
　Chest wall trauma
　Chest wall lesions
　Herpes zoster
　Breast stimulation
Medications
　Phenothiazines
　Tricyclic antidepressants
　Metoclopramide
　Cimetidine
　Methyldopa
　Reserpine
　Calcium channel blockers
　Fluoxetine hydrochloride (Prozac)
Other
　Renal failure
　Liver disease
　Primary hypothyroidism
　Ectopic hormone production
　Seizures

Adapted with permission from Molitch ME. Pathologic hyperprolactinemia. Endocrinol Metab Clin North Am 1992;21:877-901.

ment doses for a mean of 4 years (13). Serum PRL levels did not change significantly in these women, and, in the 15 patients with microprolactinomas, tumor size did not increase as assessed by computed tomography. Therefore, it is unlikely that routine contraceptive or replacement estrogen doses result in significant tumor progression.

Thyrotropin-releasing hormone also stimulates PRL secretion, although the physiologic role of thyrotropin-releasing hormone in modulating PRL secretion is not established (14). PRL levels may be elevated in patients with primary hypothyroidism presumably because of thyrotropin-releasing hormone stimulation and/or hypothyroid-induced changes in dopaminergic tone. Although luteinizing hormone release is synchronous with PRL secretion, the role of gonadotropin-releasing hormone (GnRH) in the normal physiologic control of PRL secretion is unknown.

Other causes of hyperprolactinemia include chronic renal disease, probably because of altered metabolism or clearance of PRL or decreases in dopaminergic tone (15). Hemodialysis usually does not reverse the hyperprolactinemia, and therapy with dopamine agonists may lower PRL without improving gonadal function. Nipple stimulation, chest wall trauma or surgery, and herpes zoster infection of the breast may result in increased PRL levels (16).

PRL-secreting pituitary adenomas are a frequent cause of pathologic hyperprolactinemia. Prolactinomas are the most common type of pituitary tumor and may account for as many as 40 to 50% of all pituitary tumors (17). Hyperprolactinemia may be detected in as many as 20% of patients with acromegaly and has been reported in patients with Cushing's disease. Hyperprolactinemia in patients with acromegaly may be caused by a mixed somatotroph–lactotroph tumor or may be secondary to stalk compression in patients with macroadenomas. Although elevated serum PRL levels are found in only a few patients with acromegaly, immunohistochemical analysis demonstrates that most somatotroph tumors have positive staining for both growth hormone and PRL. The presence of acromegaly and Cushing's disease should be evaluated in hyperprolactinemic patients with suggestive clinical manifestations. This is particularly true in young women with acromegaly who have not had the disease for a sufficient duration to develop acral changes and whose first clinical manifestation of acromegaly may be PRL-associated reproductive disease.

CLINICAL MANIFESTATIONS OF HYPERPROLACTINEMIA

The clinical signs and symptoms of hyperprolactinemia are the result of both the biochemical effects of hyperprolactinemia and, in the case of macroadenomas, complications secondary to tumor mass (Table 11.2).

Hyperprolactinemia is a common cause of amenorrhea, and approximately 20% of women with secondary amenor-

Table 11.2. *Symptoms Associated with Hyperprolactinemia*

Hypogonadism
　Amenorrhea
　Oligomenorrhea
　Infertility
　Impotence
　Decreased libido
Galactorrhea
Hirsutism, acne
Headaches
Mass effect (if macroprolactinoma)
　Visual loss
　Cranial neuropathies
　Hypopituitarism
　Temporal lobe seizures

rhea have elevated PRL levels (18). Women with hyperprolactinemia may have more subtle abnormalities in gonadal function, including oligomenorrhea or luteal phase insufficiency. A subset of infertile women have been described with mild hyperprolactinemia in whom fertility was restored with bromocriptine therapy. In some cases, hyperprolactinemia causing infertility has been intermittent and may only be detected in the periovulatory phase of the menstrual cycle. Galactorrhea is present in up to 25% of parous women with regular menses and normal serum PRL levels. However, patients with "idiopathic" galactorrhea may also demonstrate intermittent hyperprolactinemia. In a recent study, eight of nine normoprolactinemic women with galactorrhea had elevated levels of PRL during sleep (19). In addition, several studies have shown that infertile, normoprolactinemic women with luteal phase defects may show improved luteal function and/or fertility following administration of dopamine agonist therapy (19). A single PRL value determined during the day may not rule out the presence of a pathologic hyperprolactinemic state, and multiple determinations, particularly in the periovulatory phase of the menstrual cycle, may be necessary to make this diagnosis.

Hypogonadism is a common sequelae of hyperprolactinemia. In women, hypogonadism is accompanied by several symptoms, including menstrual dysfunction, dry vaginal mucosa and dyspareunia, and diminished libido. Decreased androgen secretion in men may present with decreased libido, impotence, infertility owing to oligospermia, and gynecomastia. Galactorrhea is rare in hyperprolactinemic men as well as postmenopausal women, and this is likely because of the lack of estrogen priming of the breast. There are multiple potential mechanisms underlying the hypogonadism caused by hyperprolactinemia. Evidence suggests that the hypogonadism is central because of impaired pulsatile GnRH secretion. Hypogonadism is typically associated with decreased or inappropriately normal luteinizing hormone and follicle-stimulating hormone levels relative to the state of estrogen or androgen deficiency, consistent with central hypogonadism. PRL, probably via alterations in dopamine inhibitory tone, decreases hypothalamic GnRH secretion, with a resultant disruption of normal pulsatile luteinizing hormone secretion (20). The restoration of ovulatory menstrual periods in hyperprolactinemic women during pulsatile exogenous GnRH administration is consistent with the hypothesis that suppression of endogenous GnRH is the key mechanism underlying hypogonadism in women (21). This study both clarified the mechanisms of hyperprolactinemic hypogonadotropic hypogonadism and demonstrated a potential therapy to induce ovulation in hyperprolactinemic women. Therefore, infertile patients with prolactinomas who are unresponsive or unable to tolerate dopamine agonist therapy and who are not surgical candidates may undergo ovulation induction with pulsatile GnRH. PRL may also stimulate androgen secretion, particularly at the level of the adrenal gland, resulting in increased serum levels of dehydroepiandrosterone sulfate and testosterone (22). Elevated androgen levels may be accompanied by clinical sequelae of androgen excess, such as hirsutism.

If the hyperprolactinemia is caused by a pituitary macroadenoma or a large nonpituitary mass, the lesion could cause compression of the normal, adjacent pituitary gland, thereby compromising normal gonadotroph function. Mass effects from the tumor could also lead to visual symptoms resulting from compression of the optic chiasm, cranial nerve palsies via extension laterally into the cavernous sinus, headaches, and, rarely, seizures.

Patients with hyperprolactinemia often describe headaches, which seem to be out of proportion to the size of the underlying tumor. Hyperprolactinemic patients without demonstrable tumors on scan may also suffer from headaches that may diminish or subside completely following institution of therapy.

METABOLIC CONSEQUENCES OF HYPERPROLACTINEMIA

Hyperprolactinemia in women is accompanied by an absolute or relative estrogen deficiency state. Mean serum estradiol levels in premenopausal amenorrheic women with hyperprolactinemia are comparable with those seen in normal women in the early follicular phase of the menstrual cycle. Therefore, estradiol levels are fixed at a relatively low level, and exposure to the higher serum estradiol levels found in the late follicular and luteal phases of the menstrual cycle does not occur. A subset of hyperprolactinemic women may have undetectable serum estradiol levels compared with those seen in postmenopausal women. This estrogen deficiency results in both trabecular and cortical bone loss. Hyperprolactinemic women have been demonstrated to have trabecular osteopenia, with spinal bone density up to 25% below normal (23, 24). The cause of this decrease in bone density seems to be hypogonadism and not PRL itself because bone density is normal in eumenorrheic hyperprolactinemic women (23). Figure 11.2 shows the progressive decline in spinal bone mineral density associated with untreated hyperprolactinemia (25). Group 1 refers to 12 women with amenorrhea throughout the study, group 2 refers to 9 women with normalization of menses after study entry, and group 3 refers to 8 women with normal menses before and during the study. Resumption of menses following therapy was associated with an increase in spinal bone mineral density during a mean of 1.8 years. However, bone density typically still remained lower than that of normal control subjects. Therefore, prolonged amenorrhea in such patients may result in a permanent increase in fracture risk throughout life. An important and as yet unanswered question is the natural history of hyperprolactinemia in postmenopausal women and the relative risks and benefits of estrogen replacement in such women.

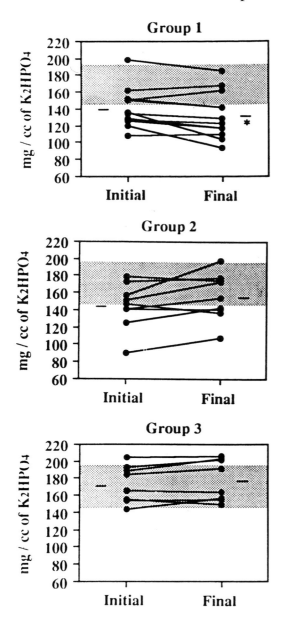

Figure 11.2. Initial and final trabecular bone mineral density in women with hyperprolactinemia. *Group 1* refers to women who were amenorrheic throughout the study, *group 2* refers to women with resumption of menses with treatment after study entry, and *group 3* refers to women with hyperprolactinemia and normal menses. The *shaded area* represents the mean ± SD of bone density in 41 normal women. *, *P* = .04 compared with initial mean bone density. (Reprinted with permission from Biller BM, Baum HB, Rosenthal DI, et al. Progressive trabecular osteopenia in women with hyperprolactinemic amenorrhea (see comments). J Clin Endocrinol Metab 1992;75:692–697.)

DIAGNOSTIC EVALUATION OF HYPERPROLACTINEMIA

After excluding pregnancy as a cause of hyperprolactinemia, measurement of the PRL level should be repeated, if possible, in the morning in a nonstressed and fasting state. All causes of hyperprolactinemia should be excluded before a tumor is considered (Table 11.1). Primary hypo-

thyroidism, liver disease, and chronic renal disease should be excluded. A careful history of medications should be obtained. Substantial elevations in PRL concentration, greater than 150 µg/mL (> 150 ng/mL), in a nongravid state usually indicate the presence of a PRL-secreting pituitary tumor. In an actively secreting lactotroph tumor, radiographic estimates of tumor size and PRL levels should correlate such that significantly elevated levels of PRL are associated with larger tumors. Prolactinomas are classified as microadenomas (< 10 mm) and macroadenomas (> 10 mm). Therefore, the presence of a substantial elevation in serum PRL level in association with a pituitary lesion greater than 10 mm by radiographic imaging is consistent with the diagnosis of a macroprolactinoma. A significant discrepancy between tumor volume and the degree of hyperprolactinemia should raise the suspicion of a "clinically nonfunctioning pituitary tumor" or a sella lesion of nonpituitary origin.

Most women with hyperprolactinemia have microadenomas. This is in contrast to men, in whom most tumors are macroadenomas. This may be because women may present earlier for evaluation than men because of complaints of menstrual disturbances. However, it is unknown whether gender-based differences in basic tumor biology exist.

A continuing challenge is the diagnosis of and management of patients with psychiatric disorders who are receiving neuroleptics and are found to have an elevated PRL level. Patients receiving neuroleptics often have reproductive abnormalities both in association with and independent of hyperprolactinemia. We recommend a magnetic resonance image (MRI) scan for patients whose PRL levels are greater than 100 µg/L (> 100 ng/mL), and we assume that levels under this value are consistent with neuroleptic administration. This strategy is based on the finding that most patients receiving neuroleptics with modest PRL elevations have no evidence of a pituitary abnormality on scan. However, if patients with PRL levels less than 100 µg/L (< 100 ng/mL) have any complaints suggestive of local mass effects or of other pituitary hypersecretory or hyposecretory syndromes, then imaging studies should be performed.

When an elevated serum PRL level is not associated with a clear secondary cause, an MRI scan should be performed. If the scan shows normal sellar and extrasellar contents, and there is no clear secondary cause of the hyperprolactinemia, then the diagnosis of idiopathic hyperprolactinemia is made. These cases may represent occult microprolactinomas with an anatomic lesion beyond the sensitivity of the scanning technique.

MANAGEMENT OF HYPERPROLACTINEMIA

The overall therapeutic goals in the management of hyperprolactinemia are to suppress excessive PRL secretion, to reduce or stabilize tumor size, and to preserve or restore normal physiologic anterior pituitary function. For patients with microadenomas, there are three available options: no therapy, with close clinical biochemical and radiologic observation; medical therapy with a dopamine agonist; and, rarely, surgery. All patients with macroprolactinomas require therapy. Dopamine agonist administration is the primary therapy of choice, and, rarely, surgery or radiation may be used. Determination of the appropriate treatment option for a patient is an individual one that takes into account the presence of mass effects, biochemical consequences of the hyperprolactinemia, desire for fertility, and tolerance of dopamine agonist therapy.

An important therapeutic consideration is the size of the prolactinoma. Patients are categorized into those who have macroprolactinomas (> 10 mm) and those who have microprolactinomas (< 10 mm). Microprolactinomas are typically intrasellar and are not associated with evidence of local mass effects. Other anterior pituitary hormone functions, such as thyrotroph, corticotroph, and somatotroph function, are typically normal. In addition, studies investigating the natural history of microprolactinomas have shown that in most cases, PRL levels usually remain stable and, in some cases, spontaneously normalize. The degree of serum PRL elevation and menstrual function at the time of presentation are prognostic factors predicting the likelihood of spontaneous resolution. In a study of 41 patients with idiopathic hyperprolactinemia who were followed up for a mean of 5.5 years, 67% of patients whose initial PRL values were less than 57 µg/L (< 57 ng/mL) had normalization of PRL (26). In contrast, none of the patients with initial PRL values greater than 60 µg/L (> 60 ng/mL) normalized. In the study by Sisam et al. (27) of 38 patients with untreated microprolactinomas who were followed up for an average of 50.5 months, 36.6% had an increase, 55.3% had a spontaneous decrease, and 13.1% had no change in PRL levels. A prospective study by Schlechte et al. (28) of untreated hyperprolactinemic women showed that patients who were eumenorrheic at the time of diagnosis were more likely to have normalization of PRL values over time, whereas patients with oligomenorrhea or amenorrhea were more likely to have no change or increases in PRL values. Therefore, basal menstrual function is an important variable in predicting the natural history of this disease.

An important consideration in the treatment of microprolactinomas is that most such tumors do not increase in size. In one study of 43 patients with presumed microadenomas with a mean follow-up of 5.4 years, only 2 patients showed evidence of tumor progression (29). In the prospective study by Schlechte et al. (28), 27 women were followed up for an average of 5.2 years. Radiologic evidence of tumor growth occurred in up to 22% of cases; however, it was rarely accompanied by clinical symptoms. Patients with untreated microprolactinomas who demonstrate an increase in tumor size on follow-up MRI scans should be seriously considered for medical therapy.

Abnormal gonadal function owing to hyperprolactinemia is a second important therapeutic consideration. Hyperprolactinemia may lead to ovulatory disorders ranging from amenorrhea to luteal phase defects resulting in infertility (19). If an elevated PRL level is found in a woman desiring fertility, then therapy should be instituted. Amenorrhea and oligomenorrhea are associated with an increased risk of osteoporosis and a significantly increased risk of fracture (23, 24). Because the risk of osteoporosis associated with hyperprolactinemia is significant and may be, at least in part, reversible with therapy, hypogonadism in the presence of hyperprolactinemia is a clear indication for therapy.

Hyperandrogenism secondary to hyperprolactinemia may result in hirsutism, oily skin, and an acneform rash. In some hyperprolactinemic women, the presence of androgen excess symptoms may be an additional indication for therapy. Men with hyperprolactinemia often describe decreased libido and erectile dysfunction. Hypogonadal symptoms are reversible with therapy in most cases if there has not been permanent damage to the gonadotroph axis because of large tumor size. Long-standing androgen deficiency in men with prolactinomas also leads to both cortical and trabecular bone loss, and normalization of androgens may lead to improvement in bone density (30).

Galactorrhea affects as many as 30% of women with hyperprolactinemia. Although galactorrhea in itself is not an absolute indication for therapy, if the degree of galactorrhea is significantly bothersome to the patient, dopamine agonist therapy is recommended.

Headaches are frequently a result of the expanding tumor mass, and, therefore, therapy resulting in a decrease in tumor size should lead to improvement in the headaches. Many patients with hyperprolactinemia without a large mass describe headaches that are out of proportion to the tumor size. Although such headaches may be caused by migraine or other causes, a trial of therapy to normalize PRL levels may be tried successfully in some patients.

MEDICAL THERAPY

Almost all patients with hyperprolactinemia can be effectively treated medically with a dopamine agonist. Bromocriptine (Parlodel), the most frequently used dopamine agonist, lowers serum PRL levels in patients with pituitary tumors and all other causes of hyperprolactinemia. Bromocriptine has been the primary medical therapy for patients with hyperprolactinemic disorders for approximately two decades. Bromocriptine therapy normalizes PRL levels and leads to resumption of ovulatory function and menses in 80 to 90% of patients (31). In some patients, ovulatory function is restored, although PRL levels are decreased but not normalized. This suggests that in some patients, reduction but not normalization of PRL levels may be sufficient for return of gonadal function. However, if fertility is a goal, normalization of PRL levels should be achieved because of the concern of ongoing ovulatory defects. Bromocriptine is also useful in treating patients with normoprolactinemic galactorrhea because such patients often have intermittent or nocturnal hyperprolactinemia (19).

The effects of bromocriptine therapy are rapid in onset (1 to 2 hours), but normalization of serum PRL levels may take weeks or longer. Discontinuation of the drug is typically followed by a return of hyperprolactinemia to basal values. Side effects of bromocriptine therapy, including nausea, headache, dizziness, nasal congestion, and constipation, may occur and may be dose limiting. Side effects may be minimized by starting with a low dose at night, e.g., 1.25 mg (half a tablet), with a snack, and increasing by 1.25 mg during 4- to 5-day intervals as tolerated. This is continued until a dose that normalizes PRL levels is reached. The rate of dose escalation is dictated by the clinical situation, such as the presence of mass effects and medication tolerance. Side effects, particularly gastrointestinal, usually improve with either continuing the medication at the same dose or by temporarily reducing the dose. If patients stop taking the medication for a few days, therapy should be re-instituted at a lower dose because side effects are likely to return. Chronic therapy may result in side effects including painless cold-sensitive digital vasospasm, alcohol intolerance, and dyskinesia. Psychiatric and affective reactions include fatigue, depression, insomnia, and anxiety as well as the precipitation of acute psychosis. Therefore, caution must be taken in the consideration of bromocriptine administration in patients with prolactinomas and a tendency toward psychosis. To reduce the gastrointestinal tract side effects, bromocriptine has recently been administered intravaginally. Reductions in PRL levels similar to those attained with oral bromocriptine have been achieved with the intravaginal route (32, 33). However, long-term patient compliance has not been demonstrated.

Bromocriptine therapy results in significant tumor shrinkage in up to 75% of patients with macroadenomas and is the initial option for patients with macroprolactinomas. Tumor size reduction may occur early, in days, weeks, or over many months. This is frequently accompanied by improvement in visual field abnormalities and pituitary function. Visual field deficits have been reported to improve within hours of institution of medical therapy. Of 27 patients with macroadenomas treated with bromocriptine, 64% had a reduction in tumor size by at least 50% (34). The fall in PRL level does not always correlate with reduction in tumor size. Therefore, it is critical to monitor visual fields carefully in patients presenting with neuro-ophthalmologic symptoms as well as serial MRI scans.

Most men with diagnosed prolactinomas have macroadenomas. In men with hyperprolactinemia-induced hypogonadism and normal residual pituitary function, it may take 3 to 6 months for testosterone levels to increase and normal sexual function to be restored after PRL levels normalize.

Pergolide (Permax) is a dopamine agonist approved by the US Food and Drug Administration for the treatment of Parkinson's disease. Although not approved for use in the management of hyperprolactinemia, pergolide may be efficacious in reducing PRL levels in patients with hyperprolactinemia (35).

There are other dopamine agonists under investigation, including the long-acting preparations parlodel LAR and cabergoline. Cabergoline is an ergoline derivative with selective, potent, and long-lasting dopaminergic properties and has been shown to be highly effective in the management of hyperprolactinemia. Its two advantages are long half-life (dosing once or twice a week) and its improved side effect profile compared with bromocriptine. Administration of cabergoline to patients with microprolactinomas results in normalization of PRL levels in 95% of cases (36). In a recent study, the administration of cabergoline to 15 patients with macroprolactinomas resulted in a decrease in tumor size in 73%, a decrease in PRL levels in 94%, and normalization of PRL levels in 73% of patients (37). The efficacy of cabergoline therapy in reducing serum PRL levels in patients with macroadenomas is demonstrated in Figure 11.3. In addition, as shown in Figure 11.4, Webster et al. (38) demonstrated in a double-blind study that cabergoline was more effective and better tolerated than bromocriptine in the management of hyperprolactinemia. Cabergoline therapy will likely be an important advance in the management of patients with hyperprolactinemia.

Although medical therapy is a primary mode of management for virtually all patients with prolactinomas, surgery may be indicated in several circumstances. The presence of apoplexy is an important indication for immediate surgery because of the necessity to evacuate the hemorrhage, and such patients are not first managed with dopamine agonists. Surgery may also be indicated in patients who have

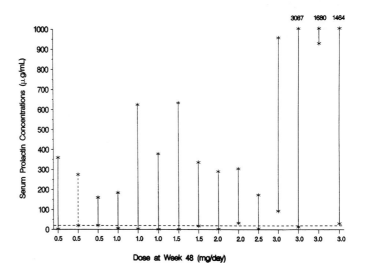

Figure 11.3. Serum PRL levels at baseline and after 48 weeks of cabergoline administration in 15 patients with macroprolactinomas. The *dotted horizontal line* indicates normal serum PRL levels (< 20 μg/L (< 20 ng/mL)). The *dotted vertical line* refers to a patient with a normalized PRL level at week 6 who did not complete 48 weeks because of a complication (pituitary hemorrhage). (Reprinted with permission from Biller BMK, Molitch ME, Vance ML, et al. Treatment of prolactin-secreting macroadenomas with the once-weekly dopamine agonist cabergoline. J Clin Endocrinol Metab 1996;81:2338–2343.)

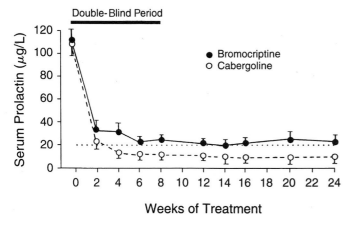

Figure 11.4. Mean serum PRL levels in 459 women with hyperprolactinemic amenorrhea treated with cabergoline or bromocriptine. Idiopathic hyperprolactinemia or a microprolactinoma was present in 446 of these women. The *dotted line* indicates the upper limit of the normal range. (Reprinted with permission from Webster J, Piscitelli G, Polli A, et al. A comparison of cabergoline and bromocriptine in the treatment of hyperprolactinemic amenorrhea: Cabergoline Comparative Study Group (see comments). N Engl J Med 1994;331:904–909.)

failed medical therapy. Surgical indications also include the presence of large tumors with visual field deficits unresponsive to bromocriptine therapy, inability to tolerate dopamine agonist therapy because of side effects, and cystic tumors that do not respond to medical therapy. A transsphenoidal approach is almost exclusively used. When performed by experienced surgeons, the major mortality rate is less than 0.27% and the major morbidity rate is less than 3% (39). In a few cases, postoperative diabetes insipidus occurs and is rarely permanent. Management is usually conservative, with fluid replacement and desmopressin acetate (DDAVP) as needed. The development of the syndrome of inappropriate antidiuretic hormone secretion in the week or more following surgery should be monitored by serial sodium levels as an outpatient. Although the risk of developing new pituitary insufficiency postoperatively is rare with experienced neurosurgeons, assessment of postoperative pituitary function is critical. Resumption of normal gonadal function should be monitored, thyroid function tests should be repeated in approximately 4 weeks, and cortisol reserve should be assessed in the immediate postoperative period to determine the need for postoperative glucocorticoid replacement.

Surgical cure is clearly a function of two factors, the size of the tumor and the experience of the neurosurgeon. Cure, defined by a normal postoperative serum PRL level, is found in approximately 71% of patients with microprolactinomas and 32% of patients with macroprolactinomas (31). Because cure rates are dependent on the size of the tumor, it was hypothesized that preoperative therapy with a dopamine agonist to decrease tumor size would improve surgical cure rates. However, studies have not demonstrated an improved cure rate with preoperative bromocriptine therapy. In addition, chronic bromocriptine therapy

may lead to tumor fibrosis, making surgical intervention more difficult.

An important concern is the significant recurrence rate following PRL surgical cure. In one series, the recurrence rates were as high as 39% and 80% in patients with microprolactinomas and macroprolactinomas, respectively, up to 5 years after surgery (40). In a more recent study of patients followed up for a mean of 9.2 years after successful surgery, the overall recurrence rate was 26% (41). As shown in Figure 11.5, an immediate postoperative serum PRL value of less than 5 μg/L (< 5 ng/mL) was associated with recurrence rates of 23% and 14% in patients with microadenomas and macroadenomas, respectively. Therefore, patients who have undergone successful surgery for prolactinomas should be serially monitored to ensure remission.

Conventional radiotherapy (4500 to 5000 rad) or proton beam therapy may be indicated in patients with larger tumors in whom definitive therapy is desired who are unable to tolerate chronic medical therapy. Given the long delay between therapy and normalization of PRL levels, medical therapy is typically required for years. In addition, radiation therapy is associated with a high likelihood of partial hypopituitarism or panhypopituitarism.

Many women with hyperprolactinemia present with infertility, and bromocriptine is typically used to normalize PRL levels and allow normal ovulation to occur. Because of estrogen-stimulated lactotroph hyperplasia, the high estrogen levels during pregnancy may lead to tumor growth

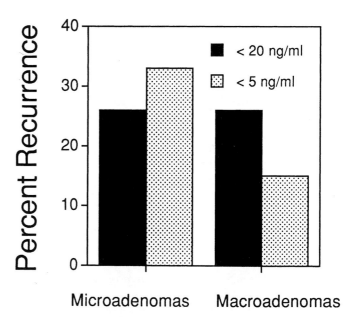

Figure 11.5. Recurrence rates in women with microprolactinomas and macroprolactinomas after initial successful surgery who were followed up for a mean of 9.2 years. *Solid columns* refer to patients with immediate postoperative serum PRL values less than 20 μg/L (< 20 ng/mL), and the *shaded columns* less than 5 μg/L (< 5 ng/mL). (Adapted from Feigenbaum S, Downey D, Wilson C, et al. Transsphenoidal pituitary resection for preoperative diagnosis of prolactin-secreting pituitary adenoma in women: long term follow-up. J Clin Endocrinol Metab 1996;81: 1711–1719.)

with resulting complications because of mass effect. Clinically significant tumor enlargement (headaches or visual deficits or both) has been described in up to 5.5% of patients with microprolactinomas (42). In patients with microprolactinomas, bromocriptine administration should be discontinued after pregnancy is established, and serial visual field monitorings should be done. In the asymptomatic patient, serial MRI scans and PRL level measurements are not indicated because therapeutic intervention is dictated by the development of symptoms of mass effect such as neuro-ophthalmologic signs or headaches rather than criteria based on absolute PRL levels or change in tumor size on scan. In contrast, 15.5 to 35.7% of patients with macroadenomas are at risk for clinically significant tumor enlargement, which can occur during any trimester (43). There is no clear evidence that surgical decompression prior to

pregnancy will prevent symptomatic tumor enlargement during pregnancy. In addition, surgery in patients desiring fertility may result in gonadotroph destruction. If there is no evidence of local mass effects after pregnancy is established, bromocriptine therapy is typically discontinued. The decision to reinstitute therapy depends on the development of clinical symptoms. If a complication caused by tumor growth does occur, it is rapidly reversible with the reinstitution of bromocriptine therapy, which is then continued through term. Based on a large international experience, there is no evidence that bromocriptine is teratogenic (44). Breast-feeding is not contraindicated in patients with microadenomas and in patients with prolactinomas, the suckling stimulus does not elicit an increase in PRL levels. However, patients with macroadenomas should continue to be followed up closely, and the decision to institute therapy is dependent on tumor size and clinical symptoms.

REFERENCES

1. Rigg LA, Lein A, Yen SS. Pattern of increase in circulating prolactin levels during human gestation. Am J Obstet Gynecol 1977;129:454–456.
2. Noel GL, Suh HK, Frantz AG. Prolactin release during nursing and breast stimulation in postpartum and nonpostpartum subjects. J Clin Endocrinol Metab 1974;38:413–423.
3. Veldhuis JD, Johnson ML. Operating characteristics of the hypothalamo-pituitary-gonadal axis in men: circadian, ultradian, and pulsatile release of prolactin and its temporal coupling with luteinizing hormone. J Clin Endocrinol Metab 1988;67:116–123.
4. Sassin JF, Frantz AG, Weitzman ED, et al. Human prolactin: 24-hour pattern with increased release during sleep. Science 1972;177:1205–1207.
5. Carlson HE. Prolactin stimulation by protein is mediated by amino acids in humans. J Clin Endocrinol Metab 1989;69:7–14.
6. Franchimont P, Dourcy C, Legros JJ, et al. Prolactin levels during the menstrual cycle. Clin Endocrinol 1976;5:643–650.
7. Vekemans M, Robyn C. Influence of age on serum prolactin levels in women and men. Br Med J 1975;4:738–739.
8. Schettini G, Cronin MJ, MacLeod RM. Adenosine 3',5'-monophosphate (cAMP) and calcium-calmodulin interrelation in the control of prolactin secretion: evidence for dopamine inhibition of cAMP accumulation and prolactin release after calcium mobilization. Endocrinology 1983;112:1801–1807.
9. Leblanc H, Lachelin GC, Abu-Fadil S, et al. Effects of dopamine infusion on pituitary hormone secretion in humans. J Clin Endocrinol Metab 1976;43:668–674.
10. Rivera JL, Lal S, Ettigi P, et al. Effect of acute and chronic neuroleptic therapy on serum prolactin levels in men and women of different age groups. Clin Endocrinol 1976;5:273–282.
11. Raymond V, Beaulieu M, Labrie F, et al. Potent antidopaminergic activity of estradiol at the pituitary level on prolactin release. Science 1978;200:1173–1175.
12. Scheithauer BW, Sano T, Kovacs KT, et al. The pituitary gland in pregnancy: a clinicopathologic and immunohistochemical study of 69 cases. Mayo Clin Proc 1990;65:461–474.
13. Corenblum B, Donovan L. The safety of physiological estrogen plus progestin replacement therapy and with oral contraceptive therapy in women with pathological hyperprolactinemia. Fertil Steril 1993;59:671–673.
14. Bowers CY, Friesen HG, Hwang P, et al. Prolactin and thyrotropin release in man by synthetic pyroglutamyl-histidyl-prolinamide. Biochem Biophys Res Commun 1971;45:1033–1041.
15. Cowden EA, Ratcliffe WA, Ratcliffe JG, et al. Hyperprolactinaemia in renal disease. Clin Endocrinol 1978;9:241–248.
16. Boyd AE, Spare S, Bower B, et al. Neurogenic galactorrhea-amenorrhea. J Clin Endocrinol Metab 1978;47:1374–1377.
17. Klibanski A, Zervas NT. Diagnosis and management of hormone-secreting pituitary adenomas. N Engl J Med 1991;324:822–831.
18. Franks S, Murray MA, Jequier AM, et al. Incidence and significance of hyperprolactinaemia in women with amenorrhea. Clin Endocrinol 1975;4:597–607.
19. Asukai K, Uemura T, Minaguchi H. Occult hyperprolactinemia in infertile women. Fertil Steril 1993;60:423–427.
20. Park SK, Keenan MW, Selmanoff M. Graded hyperprolactinemia first suppresses LH pulse frequency and then pulse amplitude in castrated male rats. Neuroendocrinology 1993;58:448–453.
21. Polson DW, Sagle M, Mason HD, et al. Ovulation and normal luteal function during LHRH treatment of women with hyperprolactinaemic amenorrhoea. Clin Endocrinol 1986;24:531–537.
22. Lobo RA, Kletzky OA, Kaptein EM, et al. Prolactin modulation of dehydroepiandrosterone sulfate secretion. Am J Obstet Gynecol 1980;138:632–636.
23. Klibanski A, Biller BM, Rosenthal DI, et al. Effects of prolactin and estrogen deficiency in amenorrheic bone loss. J Clin Endocrinol Metab 1988;67:124–130.
24. Koppelman MC, Kurtz DW, Morrish KA, et al. Vertebral body bone mineral content in hyperprolactinemic women. J Clin Endocrinol Metab 1984;59:1050–1053.
25. Biller BM, Baum HB, Rosenthal DI, et al. Progressive trabecular osteopenia in women with hyperprolactinemic amenorrhea (see comments). J Clin Endocrinol Metab 1992;75:692–697.
26. Martin TL, Kim M, Malarkey WB. The natural history of idiopathic hyperprolactinemia. J Clin Endocrinol Metab 1985;60:855–858.
27. Sisam DA, Sheehan JP, Sheeler LR. The natural history of untreated microprolactinomas. Fertil Steril 1987;48:67–71.
28. Schlechte J, Dolan K, Sherman B, et al. The natural history of untreated hyperprolactinemia: a prospective analysis. J Clin Endocrinol Metab 1989;68:412–418.
29. March CM, Kletzky OA, Davajan V, et al. Longitudinal evaluation of patients with untreated prolactin-secreting pituitary adenomas. Am J Obstet Gynecol 1981;139:835–844.
30. Greenspan SL, Neer RM, Ridgway EC, et al. Osteoporosis in men with hyperprolactinemic hypogonadism. Ann Intern Med 1986;104:777–782.
31. Molitch ME. Pathologic hyperprolactinemia. Endocrinol Metab Clin North Am 1992;21:877–901.
32. Kletzky OA, Vermesh M. Effectiveness of vaginal bromocriptine in treating women with hyperprolactinemia. Fertil Steril 1989;51:269–272.
33. Vermesh M, Fossum GT, Kletzky OA. Vaginal bromocriptine: pharmacology and effect on serum prolactin in normal women. Obstet Gynecol 1988;72:693–698.
34. Molitch ME, Elton RL, Blackwell RE, et al. Bromocriptine as primary therapy for prolactin-secreting macroadenomas: results of a

prospective multicenter study. J Clin Endocrinol Metab 1985;60: 698–705.

35. Kletzky OA, Borenstein R, Mileikowsky GN. Pergolide and bromocriptine for the treatment of patients with hyperprolactinemia. Am J Obstet Gynecol 1986;154:431–435.

36. Webster J, Piscitelli G, Polli A, et al. Dose-dependent suppression of serum prolactin by cabergoline in hyperprolactinaemia: a placebo controlled, double blind, multicentre study: European Multicentre Cabergoline Dose-finding Study Group. Clin Endocrinol 1992;37: 534–541.

37. Biller BMK, Molitch ME, Vance ML, et al. Treatment of prolactin-secreting macroadenomas with the once-weekly dopamine agonist cabergoline. J Clin Endocrinol Metab 1996;81:2338–2343.

38. Webster J, Piscitelli G, Polli A, et al. A comparison of cabergoline and bromocriptine in the treatment of hyperprolactinemic amenorrhea: Cabergoline Comparative Study Group (see comments). N Engl J Med 1994;331:904–909.

39. Zervas NT. Surgical results in pituitary adenomas: results of an international study. In: Black PM, Zervas NT, Ridgway EC, et al., eds. Secretory Tumors of the Pituitary Gland. New York: Raven Press, 1984:377–385.

40. Serri O, Rasio E, Beauregard H, et al. Recurrence of hyperprolactinemia after selective transsphenoidal adenomectomy in women with prolactinoma. N Engl J Med 1983;309:280–283.

41. Feigenbaum S, Downey D, Wilson C, et al. Transsphenoidal pituitary resection for preoperative diagnosis of prolactin-secreting pituitary adenoma in women: long term follow-up. J Clin Endocrinol Metab 1996;81:1711–1719.

42. Gemzell C, Wang CF. Outcome of pregnancy in women with pituitary adenoma. Fertil Steril 1979;31:363–372.

43. Molitch ME. Pregnancy and the hyperprolactinemic woman. N Engl J Med 1985;312:1364–1370.

44. Turkalj I, Braun P, Krupp P. Surveillance of bromocriptine in pregnancy. JAMA 1982;247:1589–1591.

Prolactinomas

Roger H. Frankel and George T. Tindall

INTRODUCTION

Prolactinomas constitute the largest group of pituitary adenomas, with approximately 30% of these tumors falling into this subset (1–3). They are pituitary tumors that autonomously secrete prolactin, a polypeptide hormone, and that occur most commonly in women of reproductive age.

This chapter covers aspects of surgical decision-making and management in the treatment of patients with prolactin-secreting pituitary adenomas. Medical and radiation therapy will be evaluated briefly regarding their role in treatment of patients with these tumors. Other chapters in this text discuss these topics in greater detail. Our discussion emphasizes the management of prolactinomas. Advances in neuroendocrinology and the introduction of sensitive neuroradiologic diagnostic techniques have made major inroads regarding how prolactinomas are diagnosed. Expansion of therapeutic options has impacted the treatment of this disease as well.

We discuss the preoperative diagnostic evaluation, operative aspects of patient care pertaining to specific problems imposed by prolactinomas, and surgical outcome as well as the place of surgical intervention. Detailed surgical technique is presented elsewhere in this book.

PHYSIOLOGY

Prolactin is produced and secreted by acidophilic cells in the anterior pituitary, under positive and negative regulation by hypothalamic releasing and inhibiting factors. Hypothalamic modulation of prolactin, unlike that of other anterior pituitary hormones, is predominantly inhibitory. Prolactin inhibitory factors are produced in the hypothalamus and released into the portal venous system and in turn prevent an unrestrained release of prolactin by the lactotroph adenohypophyseal cells. Dopamine is the most common of the naturally occurring prolactin inhibitory factors, which act at the D2 receptors in the lactotroph cell membrane (4–6); others include gonadotropin-associated peptide (7) and gamma aminobutyric acid. Pituitary stalk section and any mass lesion in the sellar region, adenomatous or other, that has mass effect on the stalk can cause prolactin hypersecretion. The vascular supply of the pituitary gland is derived from the superior hypophyseal arteries that drain into the hypothalamic–pituitary portal system. These vessels extend from the median eminence to the stalk and finally to the pituitary gland (8–10). Interruption of this source of hormonal input from the hypothalamus into the pituitary gland causes mild hypersecretion of prolactin by interrupting the flow of prolactin inhibitory factors. In the case of a mass lesion, this can result in the increase of prolactin secretion that is known as a "pseudoprolactinoma" or "stalk effect." The prolactin inhibitory mechanism is also mediated by the hypothalamic catecholamines dopamine and norepinephrine and blocked by dopaminergic blocking agents such as phenothiazines, tricyclic antidepressants, methyldopa, and reserpine. A prolactin-releasing factor, possibly regulated by serotonin, has been identified in hypothalamic extracts.

All of the physiologic effects of prolactin are not understood. Prolactin release occurs during sleep, stress, exercise, pregnancy, and nipple stimulation. Prolactin is essential for stimulation of breast tissue growth and for initiation and maintenance of lactation in humans. Breast tissue requires appropriate stimulation by the interaction of several hormones, including estrogen, progestins, corticosteroids, growth hormone, and insulin, prior to lactation occurring. Prolactin secretion increases steadily during pregnancy and peaks at parturition. The plasma level of prolactin rapidly declines to normal levels in the postpartum period. Prolactin function in males is unclear, but it seems to be necessary for normal sperm production. Hyperprolactinemia inhibits 5-alpha-reductase, which converts inactive testosterone to the biologically active dihydrotestosterone. This hormone is needed in high concentrations within the testicular tubules for spermatogenesis to occur.

Hyperprolactinemia is associated with osteoporosis, as reported by Klibanski and others (11, 12). This is because of the stimulation of postmenopausal levels of estrogen by elevated prolactin levels. These investigators described decreased bone density in 14 hyperprolactinemic women, which correlated with the relative or absolute estrogen deficiency that may accompany hyperprolactinemia. Cann et al. (13) found decreased spinal mineralization in amenorrheic women as well. In 1986, Greenspan et al. (14) found an analogous relationship between osteoporosis and hyperprolactinemic hypogonadism in males. Sartorio et al. (15) found that the concentration of osteocalcin, a specific marker of bone formation, was significantly lower in their studies of 29 patients with microprolactinomas than in the control population.

PATHOLOGY

Prolactinomas may be classified into microadenomas, which are 10 mm or less in greatest diameter, and macroadenomas, which are greater than 10 mm in greatest diameter.

Based on the staining characteristics of pituicytes with hematoxylin and eosin, subtypes of chromophobe, acidophil, basophil, and mixed adenomas were described. During the past several years, the introduction of radioimmunoassay techniques, electron microscopy, and immunocytochemistry have permitted closer study of the pathologic characteristics of pituitary adenomas, as outlined elsewhere in this text (16). This has made the traditional microscopic classification of pituitary tumors of little prognostic importance. Detailed pathologic descriptions of pituitary adenomas, including prolactinomas, using the techniques just mentioned are provided in Chapter 7 of this book.

CLINICAL PRESENTATION

Clinical manifestations of the resultant hyperprolactinemia caused by hormone hypersecretion by these adenomas differs between the sexes. In women, the principal findings consist of amenorrhea, galactorrhea, and reproductive dysfunction. Prolactinomas tend to be larger in men than in women at the time they come to medical attention. The reason for this difference is uncertain, but the sensitivity of women to the symptoms of hyperprolactinemia may result in the tumors being found earlier. This correlates with the fact that in men and postmenopausal women, the tumors are less symptomatic and usually come to medical attention when symptoms of mass effect occur.

Because of their larger tumors, the clinical picture in men is often characterized by signs and symptoms of mass effect. However, men with prolactinomas may present with decreased libido, impotence, and oligospermia. Men may also have galactorrhea; however, the incidence is rare. Prolactin-secreting tumors may present with mass effect and/or hyperprolactinemic endocrinopathy (17). Mass effect may cause compression of the adjacent hypothalamus, or normal pituitary tissue, causing hypothalamic dysfunction or hypopituitarism, respectively. Other symptoms resulting from mass effect include visual acuity and field defects that typically present as bitemporal hemianopia; headaches; rarely, third, fourth, and sixth cranial nerve palsies; and hydrocephalus. A more detailed discussion of clinical findings in patients with prolactinomas can be found in Chapter 12.

Results of a few small studies with limited follow-up suggest that the progression of untreated prolactinomas is both slow and unpredictable. In approximately 95% of patients with microprolactinomas, no increase in tumor size occurs for 4 to 6 years (18–21). This finding is supported by several studies. In a series of 38 patients with microprolactinomas followed with serial computed tomographic studies for an average of 31.7 months, Sisam et al. (22) did not demonstrate significant tumor growth in any patient. However, Weiss et al. (23), in a series of 27 similar patients followed for 6 years, noted evidence of tumor progression in 3 patients (10%). These findings are consistent with a prospective report in which 30 untreated women with hyperprolactinemia were monitored for 3 to 7 years (20). In this study, serum prolactin levels increased in 6 of the women, decreased in 10 of the women, and did not change in the remainder of the women.

The endocrinopathy associated with prolactinomas is a result of the hyperprolactinemia and is symptomatically identical to that of any other cause of elevated serum prolactin levels. Thus, an adequate medical history is necessary to rule out causes for hyperprolactinemia other than that related to a mass lesion in the sellar region. Conditions such as hypothyroidism (24), renal failure (25), cirrhosis of the liver (26), phenothiazine use, tricyclic or monoamine oxidase inhibitor antidepressant ingestion, use of butyrophenones or metoclopramide, and use of antihypertensives, including methyldopa, reserpine, and verapamil, are also associated with elevations in serum prolactin levels (27). After obtaining a detailed history, the appropriate imaging and serologic testing should be performed to identify the cause of the elevated serum prolactin value.

DIAGNOSTIC EVALUATION

Initial evaluation for a suspected prolactin-secreting tumor can be divided into two major categories: endocrinologic workup and neuroradiologic imaging, which are detailed in Chapters 11 and 8, respectively.

Endocrine Testing

Baseline studies should be performed to determine the degree of pituitary dysfunction, if any, and the level of severity of the problem. These results can then be used to monitor the efficacy of the chosen treatment regimen. Endocrine evaluation includes baseline pituitary target organ tests and two measurements of fasting serum prolactin levels. The pituitary–thyroid axis is tested with thyroid-stimulating hormone, triiodothyronine, and levothyroxine levels. The gonadal axis is evaluated with luteinizing hormone, follicle-stimulating hormone, estradiol, and testosterone studies. The pituitary–adrenal axis is tested with AM cortisol and cosyntropin stimulation if necessary. Antidiuretic hormone is assessed via electrolyte studies. Occasionally, a carefully performed water deprivation test is necessary. The pituitary target organ tests determine the presence and extent of pretreatment pituitary endocrine dysfunction and provide a measure for treatment efficacy and endocrinologic complications. Performance of a pregnancy test should be carried out to exclude this condition as a cause for prolactin elevation.

In patients with pituitary tumors who have a moderately elevated serum prolactin level (e.g., 60 to 150 μg/L [60 to 150 ng/mL]), it is difficult to identify the cause of hyperprolactinemia. These modest elevations in serum prolactin concentration may result from either stalk or hypothalamic compression or occasionally from tumor secretion. Intrasellar lesions not of pituitary origin as well as nonfunctional pituitary adenomas can cause mild hyperprolactinemia.

A fasting level of prolactin greater than 150 μg/L (> 150 ng/mL) highly suggests that the cause of the hyperprolactinemia is a pituitary adenoma. Very high serum prolactin levels of more than 1000 μg/L (> 1000 ng/mL) signify tumor invasiveness, which usually means that the lesion has extended into the cavernous sinus (28).

Neuroimaging Studies

Diagnostic imaging is important in making the diagnosis of a structural lesion and in planning an approach to it by pinpointing its location. Historically, skull x-rays, cerebral angiography, and coronal thin-section computed tomography were performed to evaluate the sellar region. The first two modalities are limited to evaluating erosive sellar enlargement or vascular malformations and tumor blush, respectively. These studies were supplanted by computed tomographic scanning because the latter could directly show the contents of the sella. The better tissue resolution and ease of multiplanar imaging has made magnetic resonance imaging (MRI) the definitive imaging modality for evaluation of pituitary adenomas. MRI studies of the sellar and parasellar region require thin slices (< 2.5 mm) and high-field–strength scanners and are routinely performed both with and without gadolinium enhancement. T1-weighted images performed with a short TE and a short TR spin echo sequence provide excellent anatomic detail of the sella, optic chiasm, and cavernous sinus. Most prolactinomas are isointense-to-hypointense to the normal gland and cerebral cortex on the T1-weighted sequence and are variable in intensity with T2 weighting. Detailed discussion of neuroimaging can be found in Chapter 8.

MANAGEMENT

Several therapeutic options are available for managing prolactinomas. We will consider the roles and timing of a conservative approach (i.e., periodic observation), medical therapy, surgery, and radiation in the treatment of these tumors. The most appropriate therapy depends on several factors, including tumor size; serum prolactin level; the patient's age, overall health, and associated surgical risk factors; tolerance or compliance with medical therapy; and whether the patient desires fertility. Some controversy exists over the optimal management of prolactinomas. This uncertainty focuses on whether medical or surgical therapy should be the primary treatment of choice for prolactinomas. Both have been shown to provide either control or cure. The precise indications, contraindications, and potential benefits of these treatment options are still incompletely defined (29).

Conservative Therapy

In certain situations, it may be appropriate not to institute any definitive therapy for prolactinomas. An example would be a young woman with a small tumor on MRI (i.e., 6 to 8 mm) associated with modest hyperprolactinemia who does not desire pregnancy. Tumor size plays a role in choosing conservative therapy as well. In approximately 95% of patients with microprolactinomas, there is no increase in tumor size for 4 to 6 years, as mentioned above (18–21). Thus, if a patient does not desire pregnancy and does not have symptoms of mass effect such as visual loss, a less aggressive treatment regimen could be instituted. Periodic clinical, MRI, and serum prolactin levels as well as bone densitometry should be obtained in following these patients (30). In all other cases, a conservative management plan is not appropriate. This is especially true of patients who have macroprolactinomas. Although the tumors may not be invasive or cause mass effect on local structures, treatment, be it surgical or medical, should be instituted because there is a smaller safety margin before irreparable injury to surrounding structures may occur.

Medical Therapy

Medical therapy at present consists of treatment with dopamine agonists. The most common is the ergot derivative bromocriptine (2-bromo-α-ergocryptine mesylate) (31). Its action is through the inhibition of prolactin mRNA transcription. Decreased protein synthesis results in decreased sizes and quantities of organelles and cellular shrinkage (32). DNA synthesis and cell multiplication is also affected (33). A small but clinically insignificant tumoricidal activity is associated with bromocriptine therapy, as reported in one study (34).

Bromocriptine is an effective agent, with studies showing 80 to 90% of patients having normoprolactinemia and/or return of menses (35, 36). As might be expected, there is a variable response to the drug. Bromocriptine binds to dopamine D2 receptors on lactotrophs, and its effectiveness has been found to correspond with the number of receptors present. A 40% decrease in receptors has been found in tumors that have minimal response to bromocriptine therapy, and a 90% decrease in receptors has been found in tumors that grow despite bromocriptine administration (37, 38). Tumor shrinkage can occur within a few days. Decrease in size can be delayed for as long as months, with incremental shrinkage noted on surveillance scans over years. This decrease in size does not correlate with the initial prolactin level.

Analysis of data from 19 series that totaled 236 patients with macroprolactinomas showed that 77% had a decrease in tumor size in an observation period ranging from 6 months to 10 years (39). Microadenoma response was similar in one report of 15 patients (40). Six tumors disappeared, five decreased by 50%, and four were unchanged in a period of 3 to 12 months.

These results have generated enthusiasm among clinicians and have led to the recommendation by some that the drug be used as the sole primary treatment for patients with prolactinomas. The implication is that surgery should be reserved only for therapeutic failures (30, 41–43). This approach is unsound for several reasons. Indications for nonmedical treatment as first-line therapy exist and are discussed below. In addition, approximately 10% of prolactinomas fail to respond to bromocriptine therapy (35, 43, 44), as described above. Another difficulty is that bromocriptine therapy is usually lifelong, and patient compliance may not always be high, making therapy less effective (44). The results of surgery, in appropriately selected patients, are comparable with those of pharmacotherapy, without the need for continued medical therapy.

Women with microprolactinomas who desire pregnancy and who have a serum prolactin level of less than 150 μg/L (< 150 ng/mL) are candidates for bromocriptine therapy. The primary goal of therapy in this situation is to reduce the level of serum prolactin so that normal ovulation occurs. Tumors with modest elevations of prolactin levels may not be prolactinomas, and the elevated prolactin may be caused by stalk effect. This form of treatment addresses the endocrine dysfunction without actually treating the tumor. The drug therapy is then discontinued after conception. Bromocriptine therapy alone is contraindicated in patients with macroprolactinomas who desire pregnancy because of risk of tumor growth during pregnancy. Patients with prolactinomas associated with serum prolactin levels greater than 1000 μg/L (> 1000 ng/mL) are better treated with bromocriptine alone because the surgical cure rate with these locally invasive tumors is poor (45).

Patients with prolactinomas can be medically treated in two ways. Bromocriptine can be a primary therapy, as described above, or can be used adjunctively to surgical treatment. Advantages and disadvantages of either approach exist. Bromocriptine as primary treatment is associated with a high positive response rate to the medication initially. However, the patient may experience side effects of drug use, including nausea, vomiting, dizziness, postural hypotension, headache, agitation, depression, mania, and others (46). Another serious complication of the drug, particularly in very large responsive tumors, is spontaneous cerebrospinal fluid (CSF) leak (47, 48).

Adjunctive use of bromocriptine is another therapeutic option. However preoperative treatment has not resulted in the significant improvement in surgical results owing to tumor shrinkage in our experience. It occasionally does make the lesions more accessible. Preoperative treatment of macroprolactinomas with bromocriptine may reduce the tumor bulk sufficiently so that later surgical management might better achieve a cure. Neal and Weiss (44) reported a series of 19 patients in whom they observed that an improved surgical cure rate was found in patients whose tumors responded well to bromocriptine therapy. Perrin et al. (49) reported a small retrospective series of 40 patients with prolactinomas in which half were treated preoperatively with bromocriptine and half were untreated. The surgical cure rate of the bromocriptine-treated group was higher than that of the control group in all tumor sizes. Microprolactinomas treated with bromocriptine had an 87.5% cure rate versus a 50% cure rate without use of the drug. Macroprolactinomas were cured 33% of the time with bromocriptine pretreatment and 17% of the time without use of the drug. Our experience with this method of therapy has not convinced us that this combined regimen is consistently effective (50, 51).

In addition, we have observed, as have other authors, that prolonged bromocriptine therapy makes the prolactinoma more fibrous and tougher in consistency. This may be caused by the perivascular fibrosis that occurs in some patients after several months of therapy (52–54). Surgical cleavage planes are obliterated, and the chances for a surgical cure are decreased. Landolt et al. (55, 56) have shown that surgical cure rates fall from 81 to 33%, whereas other studies do not show as clear a correlation (49).

Though standard bromocriptine therapy is most common in the United States, several analogs are available or in trials, including pergolide (57), cabergoline (58), quinagolide (CV205–502) (59, 60), lergotrile, mesulergine, and terguride. In addition to these drugs, two alternate dosing regimens are available for bromocriptine: intravaginal bromocriptine (61) and Parlodel LAR, an injectable depot form of bromocriptine requiring monthly dosing. The intravaginal dose minimizes gastrointestinal symptoms of bromocriptine therapy, and the injectable form allows less frequent dosing and faster elevation of serum levels of bromocriptine. Advantages of some of the other drugs include removal of the ergot derivative, thereby lessening some of the side effects. Pergolide and quinagolide were found to be no better than bromocriptine in a randomized double-blind study (62). The most promising of the drugs is cabergoline, which has a longer duration of action than bromocriptine, requiring semiweekly doses. A randomized double-blind trial found higher efficacy in allowing resumption of ovulation or pregnancy with cabergoline at 72% than bromocriptine at 52% (63). For further information on the medical therapy of prolactinomas, see Chapter 11.

Criteria For Cure

To consider a patient cured, several criteria should be met, including normalization of the serum prolactin level to less than 25 μg/L (< 25 ng/mL). This level of prolactin suggests that the prolactin-secreting tumor was successfully resected. Normoprolactinemia for at least 5 years is a good indicator of cure. However, persistent hyperprolactinemia following surgery may not necessarily be caused by residual tumor. Pituitary stalk injury of tumoral or iatrogenic origin may be the cause. If the postoperative value remains below 100 μg/L (< 100 ng/mL) without increase over time, it usually reflects stalk damage (64).

Another useful criteria suggestive of cure is cessation of galactorrhea and resumption of normal menstrual periods. These findings almost always coincide with normal serum prolactin levels. In the occasional patient, menstrual periods return and galactorrhea ceases and serum prolactin levels remain mildly elevated. The converse is also true, and patients may still experience these symptoms despite normal serum prolactin levels.

Surgical Indications

Situations in which transsphenoidal surgery should be considered include:

1. Patient does not tolerate dopaminergic therapy secondary to side effects or compliance problems;

2. Patient does not desire to take lifelong medication;

3. Patient with serum prolactin level between 150 and 500 μg/L (150 and 500 ng/mL);

4. Prolactinoma associated with large cystic components or apoplexy (a surgical emergency);

5. Prolactinoma with mass effect causing visual symptoms or pituitary insufficiency despite medical therapy (1 to 2 weeks);

6. Recurrent prolactinoma followed by medical and radiation therapy;

7. Patient has onset of CSF rhinorrhea secondary to bromocriptine therapy requiring tumor resection and surgical repair of the CSF leak;

8. Woman with prolactinoma who desires pregnancy;

9. Pregnant patient presenting with symptomatic mass effect, such as progressive visual loss; and

10. Patient has prolactinoma that does not respond to primary bromocriptine treatment.

Factors Influencing Surgical Results

Preoperative prolactin level and tumor size and extension are important factors that influence the outcome of surgical removal of prolactinomas. These factors should be carefully evaluated when making a treatment decision.

Contraindications to surgery in patients with prolactinomas is a function of preoperative prolactin level. Studies have shown that a surgical cure rate is inversely proportional to serum prolactin. Faria and Tindall (65) found postoperative normalization of prolactin level after transsphenoidal adenectomy in 76% of patients with preoperative prolactin levels less than 200 μg/L (< 200 ng/mL) and in 46% of patients with prolactin levels greater than 200 μg/L (> 200 ng/mL). Domingue et al. (66) reported therapeutic failure in 32% of their patients with prolactinomas. These patients had prolactin levels greater than 200 μg/L (> 200 ng/mL) and/or subtotal tumor resection. Bertrand et al. (67) reported a 50% control rate in patients with serum prolactin levels between 200 and 500 μg/L (200 and 500 ng/mL), a 36% control rate in patients with serum prolactin levels between 500 and 1000 μg/L, and a 22% control rate in patients with serum prolactin levels greater than 1000 μg/L (> 1000 ng/mL). Hardy (68) had similar findings with 48%, 21%, and 6% in the respective groups. Barrow et al. (28) divided preoperative serum prolactin levels into three groups. Group A ranged from 200 to 500 μg/L (200 to 500 ng/mL), group B ranged from 500 to 1000 μg/L (500 to 1000 ng/mL), and group C was greater than 1000 μg/L (> 1000 ng/mL). Surgical cure rates were 68% in group A, 30% in group B, and 14% in group C. Thus, an inverse relationship between cure rate and preoperative level of serum prolactin is documented by several reported series. These findings support the recommendation for surgery in patients with prolactin levels less than 500 μg/L (< 500 ng/mL) and medical therapy for prolactinoma patients with serum levels of prolactin greater than 1000 μg/L (> 1000 ng/mL). Besides this specific contraindication for prolactinoma resection, the more general guidelines for surgical patient selection apply.

In addition to prolactin level, several studies have shown that microadenomas achieve the best surgical results (32, 65, 66, 69, 70). Hardy et al. (70) achieved normal levels in 90% of patients with localized microadenomas following transsphenoidal surgery. Patients with adenomas limited to the sella had normal prolactin levels 53% of the time, and patients with invasive adenomas were normoprolactinemic only 43% of the time (70). Chang et al. (32) supported these results in their study in which 16 of 17 women with prolactin-secreting microadenomas and 2 of 7 women with macroadenomas had return of normal menses following surgery.

In summary, patients with microadenomas are more likely to have low preoperative prolactin levels. This group of patients achieves the best surgical results, with a cure rate of approximately 75%. Patients with macroadenomas usually have much higher preoperative prolactin levels, and the cure rate in this group falls progressively as the levels of prolactin increase.

Type Of Surgical Approach

Transsphenoidal microsurgery is associated with low morbidity and mortality rates. The complication rate from published series of transsphenoidal procedures is approximately 4% (71, 72). The most common complications are CSF leakage, hypopituitarism, and diabetes insipidus. Transsphenoidal surgery also provides tumor removal and sparing of the normal pituitary gland in most patients (73–76). It is the procedure of choice in almost all patients with prolactinoma requiring surgical intervention. Patients who benefit most from a different surgical procedure (i.e., craniotomy) fall into one of two categories. If there is significant extrasellar extension of the tumor into the anterior and/or middle fossa, a craniotomy may be the procedure of choice. In addition, a suprasellar tumor with a significant constriction at the level of the diaphragma sellae ("dumbbell configuration") is also better managed with a craniotomy or a combined approach of transsphenoidal and craniotomy. These procedures are described in Chapters 27 and 28.

Surgical Technique

Although detailed descriptions of transsphenoidal microsurgery have been reported in numerous papers (65, 66, 77–79) and will be covered in Chapter 26, certain techniques will be briefly mentioned. The sphenoid sinus aera-

tion is examined on sagittal views of the MRI. A conchal or presellar sphenoid sinus requires that the head holder be placed in an anteroposterior orientation to allow unobstructed C-arm fluoroscopy or lateral plain skull x-ray imaging to positively identify the sellar floor. We have found that almost all patients can be approached through an endonasal, as opposed to a sublabial, incision without difficulty. Regardless of whether a sublabial or an endonasal incision is used, it is important that the surgeon develop a plane along one side of the nasal septum, allowing it to be spared.

If the tumor is large with a significant amount of suprasellar extension, a lumbar drain is placed after general endotracheal anesthesia has been induced, but just prior to patient positioning. Access to the subarachnoid space gives the surgeon the option to alter CSF pressure by either withdrawing or instilling either CSF or sterile Ringer's solution and thus either forcing tumor into the operative field (by instilling fluid) or lifting the diaphragma sellae out of the sella (by withdrawing CSF) during the surgical procedure.

The last technique that we use in these cases is performed after tumor resection is completed. Instillation of absolute ethanol into the sella is performed. The alcohol is allowed to remain in place for 5 minutes to allow tumor cell lysis to occur and to remove any microscopic remnants of tumor that may not be visualized under operating microscope magnification. Alcohol is not used in the sella if there has been a tear in the diaphragma sellae.

Results Of Treatment

Surgical results published in 30 series that included prolactinomas were compiled to make the most complete assessment of surgical treatment of these tumors. Tumor size and preoperative prolactin levels as well as tumor extension influence the outcome of surgical resection of prolactinomas. Overall outcome is superior in microadenoma resection than in macroadenomas, with a greater than twofold cure rate reported (39). As mentioned earlier, preoperative prolactin levels have also been found to play a role in determining outcome. The control rate of prolactinomas was found to be inversely proportional to the preoperative prolactin level.

Results of the studies cited earlier as well as others support a cure rate of 48 to 68% in patients with preoperative prolactin levels between 200 and 500 μg/L (200 and 500 ng/mL); the cure rate is higher when patients with preoperative prolactin levels less than 200 μg/L (< 200 ng/mL) are included. These cure rates drop significantly with inclusion of patients with prolactin levels greater than 500 μg/L (> 500 ng/mL). The range of therapeutic effectiveness of surgery runs 21 to 36% in patients with preoperative prolactin levels between 500 and 1000 μg/L (500 and 1000 ng/mL) and 6 to 22% in patients with preoperative prolactin levels higher than 1000 μg/L (> 1000 ng/mL).

Radiation Treatment

At present, radiation is delivered in two forms, conventional and stereotactic radiosurgery (80–83). The response to the radiation is similar in that there is a slowly decreasing prolactin level in most patients. Rush and Newall (81) found a decrease in serum prolactin levels in all 10 patients receiving conventional radiation therapy and normalization of prolactin levels in 70% of patients. Grossman et al. (84) found decreased serum prolactin levels in 26 of 27 patients, but only 33% had normal levels. Sheline et al. (85) reported an average prolactin level decrease in 75 to 90% of patients with radiotherapy as the only treatment. In addition, the prolactin level was normalized in 30% of the treated patients. Tsagarakis et al. (83) studied the effect of external beam megavoltage radiotherapy in 36 patients with prolactinomas for 3 to 11 years. Serum prolactin level was normalized in half of the patients. In addition, 23% of patients had dysfunction of the gonadal axis, and 94% of patients had inadequate growth hormone production. Disturbances of the thyroid and adrenal axes occurred in 14% of patients.

As stereotactic radiosurgery has become more widespread, it has been added more often to the list of treatments for prolactinoma. Contraindications include very large tumor size and proximity to optic structures. Ideally, a 5-mm free margin between the optic chiasm and tumor margins is needed. Levy et al. (86) treated 20 patients with prolactinomas with stereotactic radiosurgery and had a 60% complete response rate, which falls in the range seen for conventional external beam treatments. Ganz et al. (87) treated three patients with the Gamma knife and tumor shrinkage was found in all three patients. However, only partial response was noted in normalization of prolactin levels.

Clinical benefits from radiation, either conventional or stereotactic, must be balanced with the adverse effects of brain irradiation, including hypopituitarism, optic apparatus injury, delayed brain radionecrosis, cranial nerve injury, and carcinogenesis. These are often long-lasting, irreparable injuries. Given the lower risks involved in medical and surgical therapy, use of radiation therapy should be limited to a secondary role (81–83, 88). This includes patients with recurrent tumor or incomplete tumor resection and patients in whom medical therapy has failed or is contraindicated (80). Primary radiation therapy in the absence of these factors or routine postoperative irradiation is not indicated.

Tumor Recurrence

Prolactinoma recurrence following transsphenoidal surgery has not been extensively studied. However, several large series suggest that the overall recurrence rate is 5 to 10% (65, 66, 77, 89). This rate increases in patients who are treated with craniotomy or who have irradiation as the primary therapy. In addition, macroadenomas and invasive prolactinomas are associated with an increased risk of recurrence.

All of the treatment modalities discussed above have been used to treat recurrent prolactinomas. As might be expected, clinical decision-making for choosing appropriate therapies is different than that used initially. Unresponsiveness to a particular therapy and complications associated with surgery and prior radiation should be taken into account. We have found that recurrent prolactinomas can usually be managed with bromocriptine administration. Transsphenoidal debulking may be useful in certain circumstances in combination with medical therapy. Radiation therapy is also useful in these circumstances. Stereotactic radiosurgery has not been studied as fully, but it seems to hold promise for delivering higher doses of radiation to the tumor and lower doses to surrounding normal structures in properly selected cases.

REFERENCES

1. Nasr H, Mozaffarian G, Pensky J, et al. Prolactin secreting pituitary tumors in women. J Clin Endocrinol Metab 1972;35:505–512.
2. Randall RV, Scheithauer BW, Laws ER Jr, et al. Pituitary tumors associated with hyperprolactinemia: a clinical and immunohistochemical study of 97 patients operated on transsphenoidally. Mayo Clin Proc 1985;60:753–762.
3. Riedel M, Noldus J, Saeger W, et al. Sellar lesions associated with isolated hyperprolactinemia: morphological, immunocytochemical, hormonal and clinical results. Acta Endocrinol 1986;113:196–203.
4. el Azouzi M, Hsu DW, Black PM, et al. The importance of dopamine in the pathogenesis of experimental prolactinomas. J Neurosurg 1990;72:273–281.
5. Lechan RM. Neuroendocrinology of pituitary hormone regulation. Endocrinol Metab Clin North Am 1987;16:475.
6. Maurer RA. Dopaminergic inhibition of protein synthesis and prolactin mRNA accumulation in cultured pituitary cells. J Biol Chem 1980:8092–8097.
7. Nikolics K, Mason AJ, Szonyi E. A prolactin inhibiting factor within the precursor for human gonadotropin-releasing hormone. Nature 1985;316:511.
8. Bergland RM, Page RB. Can the pituitary secrete directly into the brain? (affirmative anatomical evidence). Endocrinology 1978;102:1325.
9. Bergland RM, Page RB. Pituitary-brain vascular relations: a new paradigm. Science 1979;204:18.
10. Page RB, Bergland RM. The neurohypophyseal capillary bed, I: anatomy and arterial supply. Am J Anat 1977;148:345.
11. Howlett TA, Wass JA, Grossman A, et al. Prolactinomas presenting as primary amenorrhea and delayed or arrested puberty: response to medical therapy. Clin Endocrinol 1989;30:131–140.
12. Klibanski A, Neer RM, Beitins IZ, et al. Decreased bone density in hyperprolactinemic women. N Engl J Med 1980;303:1511–1514.
13. Cann CE, Martin MC, Genant HK, et al. Decreased spinal mineral content in amenorrheic woman. JAMA 1984;251:62–69.
14. Greenspan SL, Neer RM, Ridgeway C, et al. Osteoporosis in men with hyperprolactinemic hypogonadism. Ann Intern Med 1986;104:777–782.
15. Sartorio A, Conti A, Ambrosi B, et al. Osteocalcin levels in patients with microprolactinoma before and during medical treatment. J Endocrinol Invest 1990;13:419–422.
16. Kovacs K, Horvath E. Pathology of pituitary adenomas. Bull L A Neurol Soc 1977;42:92–110.

17. Blackwell RE. Hyperprolactinemia: evaluation and management. Endocrinol Metab Clin North Am 1992;21:105–124.
18. Koppelman MCS, Jaffe MJ, Rieth KG, et al. Hyperprolactinemia, amenorrhea, and galactorrhea. Ann Intern Med 1984;100:115.
19. March CM, Kletzky OA, Davajan V, et al. Longitudinal evaluation of patients with untreated prolactin–secreting pituitary adenomas. Am J Obstet Gynecol 1981;139:835.
20. Schlechte J, Dolan K, Sherman B, et al. The natural history of untreated hyperprolactinemia: a prospective analysis. J Clin Endocrinol Metab 1989;68:412–418.
21. Weiss MH, Yadley RR, Gott P, et al. Bromocriptine treatment of prolactin-secreting tumors: surgical implications. Neurosurgery 1983;12:640–642.
22. Sisam DA, Sheehan JP, Sheeler. The natural history of untreated microprolactinomas. Fertil Steril 1987;48:67–71.
23. Weiss MH, Teal J, Gott P, et al. Natural history of microprolactinomas: six-year follow-up. Neurosurgery 1983;12:180–183.
24. Honbo KS, Herle AJV, Kellet KA. Serum prolactin levels in untreated primary hypothyroidism. Am J Med 1978;64:782.
25. Hou SH, Grossman S, Molitch ME. Hyperprolactinemia in patients with renal insufficiency and chronic renal failure requiring hemodialysis or chronic ambulatory peritoneal dialysis. Am J Kidney Dis 1985;6:245.
26. Morgan MY, Jakobovits AW, Gore MB. Serum prolactin in liver disease and its relationship to gynecomastia. Gut 1978;19:170.
27. De Rivera JL, Lal S, Ettigi P. Effect of acute and chronic neuroleptic therapy on serum prolactin levels in men and women of different age groups. Clin Endocrinol (Oxf) 1986;5:273.
28. Barrow DL, Mizuno J, Tindall GT. Management of prolactinomas associated with very high serum prolactin levels. J Neurosurg 1988; 68:554–558.
29. Cunnah D, Besser M. Management of prolactinomas. Clin Endocrinol (Oxf) 1991;34:231–235.
30. Melton LJ, Eddy DM, Johnston CC. Screening for osteoporosis. Ann Intern Med 1990;112:516–528.
31. Molitch ME, Elton RL, Blackwell RE. Bromocriptine as primary therapy for prolactin-secreting macroadenomas: results of a prospective multicenter study. J Endocrinol Metab 1985;60:698–705.
32. Chang RJ, Keye WR Jr, Young JR, et al. Detection, evaluation, and treatment of pituitary microadenomas in patients with galactorrhea and amenorrhea. Am J Obstet Gynecol 1977;128:356–363.
33. MacLeod RM, Lehmeyer JE. Suppression of pituitary tumor growth and function by ergot alkaloids. Cancer Res 1973;33:849.
34. Mori H, Maeda T, Saitoh Y, et al. Changes in prolactinomas and somatotropinomas in humans treated with bromocriptine. Pathol Res Pract 1988;183:580–583.
35. Bevan JS, Webster J, Burke CW, et al. Dopamine agonists and pituitary tumor shrinkage. Endocr Rev 1992;13:220–240.
36. Molitch ME, Reichlin S. The amenorrhea, galactorrhea and hyperprolactinemia syndromes. In: Stollerman GD, ed. Advances in Internal Medicine. Chicago: Year Book Medical Publishers 1980;26: 37–65.
37. Molitch ME, Elton RL, Blackwell RL, et al. Bromocriptine as primary therapy for prolactin secreting macroadenomas: results of a prospective multicenter study. J Clin Endocrinol Metab 1985;60: 698.
38. Pelligrini I, Rasolonjanahary R, Gunz G, et al. Resistance to bromocriptine in prolactinomas. J Clin Endocrinol Metab 1989;69: 500–509.
39. Molitch ME. Prolactinoma. In: Melmed S, ed. The Pituitary. Cambridge: Blackwell Science, 1995:458.
40. Bonneville JF, Poulignot D, Cattin F, et al. Computed tomographic demonstration of the effects of bromocriptine on pituitary microadenoma size. Radiology 1982;143:451.
41. Alford FP, Arnott R. Medical management of pituitary tumors. Med J Aust 1992;157:57–60.
42. Molitch ME. Management of prolactinomas. Annu Rev Med 1989; 40:225–232.
43. Tan SL, Jacobs HS. Management of prolactinomas. Br J Obstet Gynaecol 1986;93:1025–1029.
44. Neal JH, Weiss MH. Management of prolactin-secreting pituitary adenomas. West J Med 1991;153:546–547.
45. Editorial: Management of prolactinoma. Lancet 1990;336:661.
46. Drug Evaluations Annual 1991. Milwaukee: American Medical Association, 1991:350, 351, 920, 946, 963, 964.
47. Hildebrandt G, Zierski J, Christophis P, et al. Rhinorrhea following dopamine agonist therapy of invasive macroprolactinoma. Acta Neurochir (Wien) 1989;96:107–113.
48. Holness RO, Shlossberg AH, Heffernan LP. Cerebrospinal fluid rhinorrhea caused by bromocriptine treatment of prolactinoma. Neurology 1984;34:111–113.
49. Perrin G, Treluyer C, Trouillas J, et al. Surgical outcome and pathological effects of bromocriptine preoperative treatment in prolactinomas. Pathol Res Pract 1991;187:587–592.
50. Barrow DL, Tindall GT, Kovacs K, et al. Clinical and pathological effects of bromocriptine on prolactin-secreting and other pituitary tumors. J Neurosurg 1984;60:1–7.
51. Tindall GT, Kovacs K, Horvath E, et al. Human prolactin-producing adenomas and bromocriptine: a histological, immunocytochemical, ultrastructural, and morphometric study. J Clin Endocrinol Metab 1982;55:1178.
52. Bevan JS, Adams CBT, Burke CW, et al. Factors in the outcome of transsphenoidal surgery for prolactinoma and nonfunctioning pituitary tumour, including preoperative bromocriptine therapy. Clin Endocrinol (Oxf) 1987;26:541–556.
53. Esiri MM, Bevan JS, Burke CW, et al. Effect of bromocriptine treatment on the fibrous tissue content of prolactin secreting and nonfunctioning macroadenomas of the pituitary gland. J Clin Endocrinol Metab 1986;63:383.
54. Faglia G, Moriondo P, Travaglini P, et al. Influence of previous bromocriptine therapy on surgery for microprolactinoma. Lancet 1983;1:133.
55. Landolt AM, Keller PJ, Froesch E, et al. Bromocriptine: does it jeopardize the result of later surgery for prolactinomas? Lancet 1982;2:657–658.
56. Landolt AM. Prolactinomas: preoperative bromocriptine treatment. Perspect Neurol Surg 1990;1(2):105–115.
57. Kleinberg DL, Boyd LAE, Wardlaw S, et al. Pergolide for the treatment of pituitary tumors secreting prolactin or growth hormone. N Engl J Med 1983;309:704–709.
58. Mattei JM, Ferrari C, Baroldi P, et al. Prolactin lowering effect of acute and once weekly repetitive oral administration of cabergoline at two dose levels in hyperprolactinemic patients. J Clin Endocrinol Metab 1988;66:193–198.
59. Serri O, Beauregard H, Lesage J, et al. Long term treatment with CV 205–502 in patients with prolactin-secreting pituitary macroadenomas. J Clin Endocrinol Metab 1990;71:682–687.
60. Vance ML, Lipper M, Klibanski A, et al. Treatment of prolactin-secreting pituitary macroadenomas with the long-acting non-ergot dopamine agonist, CV 205–502. Ann Intern Med 1990;112: 668–673.
61. Vermesh M, Fossum GT, Kletzy OA. Vaginal bromocriptine: pharmacology and effect of serum prolactin in normal women. Obstet Gynecol 1988;72:693–698.
62. Verhelst HA, Froud ALJ, Touzel R, et al. Acute and long-term effects of once daily oral bromocriptine and a new long acting non-ergot dopamine agonist, quinagolide, in the treatment of hyperprolactinaemia: a double blind study. Acta Endocrinol 1991;125:385.
63. Webster J, Piscitelli G, Polli A, et al. A comparison of cabergoline and bromocriptine in the treatment of hyperprolactinaemic amenorrhea. N Engl J Med 1994;331:904.
64. Tindall GT, Reisner A. Prolactinomas. In: Wilkins RH, Rengachary SS, eds. Neurosurgery. New York: McGraw-Hill, 1996: 1299–1307.
65. Faria MA, Tindall GT. Transsphenoidal microsurgery for prolactin-secreting pituitary adenomas: results in 100 women with the amenorrhea-galactorrhea syndrome. J Neurosurg 1982;56:33–43.
66. Domingue JN, Richmond IL, Wilson CB. Results of surgery in 114 patients with prolactin-secreting pituitary adenomas. Am J Obstet Gynecol 1980;137:102–108.
67. Bertrand G, Tolis G, Montes J. Immediate and long-term results of transsphenoidal microsurgical resection of prolactinomas in 92 patients. In: Tolis G, Stefanis C, Mountokalakis T, Labrie F, eds. Prolactin and Prolactinomas. New York: Raven Press, 1983: 441–452.
68. Hardy J. Transsphenoidal microsurgery of prolactinomas: report on 355 cases. In: Tolis G, Stefanis C, Mountokalakis T, Labrie F, eds. Prolactin and Prolactinomas. New York: Raven Press, 1983: 431–440.
69. Aubourg PR, Derome PJ, Peillon F, et al. Endocrine outcome after transsphenoidal adenomectomy for prolactinoma: prolactin levels

and tumor size as predicting factors. Surg Neurol 1980;14: 141–143.

70. Hardy J, Beauregard H, Robert F. Prolactin-secreting pituitary adenomas: transsphenoidal microsurgical treatment. In: Robyn C, Harter M, eds. Progress in Prolactin Physiology and Pathology. Amsterdam: Elsevier/North-Holland Biomedical Press, 1978: 361–370.

71. Laws ER Jr, Kern EB. Complications of transsphenoidal surgery. Clin Neurosurg 1976;23:401.

72. Tindall GT, Barrow DL. Disorders of the pituitary. St. Louis: CV Mosby, 1986:498.

73. Laws ER, Ebersol MJ, Piepgras DG, et al. The role of surgery in the management of prolactinoma. In: MacLeod RM, Thorner MO, Scapagnini U, eds. Prolactin, Basic and Clinical Correlates. New York: Springer-Verlag, 1985:849–853.

74. Laws ER, Fode NC, Redmond MJ. Transsphenoidal surgery following unsuccessful prior therapy. J Neurosurg 1985;63:823.

75. Leavens ME, McCutcheon IF, Samaan NA. Management of pituitary adenomas. Oncology 1992;6(6):69–79.

76. Wilson CB. Role of surgery in the management of pituitary tumors. Neurosurg Clin N Am 1990;1(1):139–159.

77. Laws ER Jr, Kern EB. Pituitary tumors treated by transnasal microsurgery: 7 years of clinical experience with 539 patients. In: Sano K, Takakura K, Fukushima T, eds. Functioning Pituitary Adenoma: Proceedings of the First Workshop on Pituitary Adenomas. Tokyo: 1980:25–34.

78. Post KD, Biller BJ, Adelman LS, et al. Selective transsphenoidal adenomectomy in women with galactorrhea-amenorrhea. JAMA 1979;242:158–162.

79. Tindall GT, Collins WF Jr, Kirchner JA. Unilateral septal technique for transsphenoidal microsurgical approach to the sella turcica: technical note. J Neurosurg 1978;49:138–142.

80. Moberg E, af Trampe E, Wersall J, et al. Long-term effects of radiotherapy and bromocriptine treatment in patients with previous surgery for macroprolactinomas. Neurosurgery 1991;29:200–204.

81. Rush SC, Newall J. Pituitary adenoma: the efficacy of radiotherapy as the sole treatment. Int J Radiat Oncol Biol Phys 1989;17:165–169.

82. Thoren M, Saaf M, Degerblad M, et al. Stereotactic irradiation for pituitary diseases. Horm Res 1988;30:1013.

83. Tsagarakis S, Grossman A, Plowman PN, et al. Megavoltage pituitary irradiation in the management of prolactinomas: long-term follow-up. Clin Endocrinol 1991;34:399–406.

84. Grossman A, Cohen BL, Charlesworth M, et al. Treatment of prolactinomas with megavoltage radiotherapy. BMJ 1984;288:1105.

85. Sheline GE, Grossman A, Jones AE, et al. Radiation therapy for prolactinomas. In: Black PMcL, Zervas NT, Ridgeway EC, Martin JB, eds. Secretory Tumors of the Pituitary Gland. New York: Raven Press, 1984;93–108.

86. Levy RP, Fabrikant JI, Frankel KA, et al. Heavy charged particle radiosurgery of the pituitary gland: clinical results of 840 patients. Proceedings of European Particle Accelerator Conference. Nice, France: June 14, 1990.

87. Ganz JC, Backlund EO, Thorsen FA. The effects of gamma knife surgery of pituitary adenomas on tumor growth and endocrinopathies. Stereotact Funct Neurosurg 1992;61(suppl 1):30–37.

88. Adams CB. The management of pituitary tumours and postoperative visual deterioration. Acta Neurochir (Wien) 1988; 94:103–116.

89. Pelkonen R, Grahne B, Hirvonen E, et al. Pituitary function in prolactinoma: effect of surgery and postoperative bromocriptine therapy. Clin Endocrinol 1981;14:335–348.

CHAPTER 13

Cushing's Disease

Kathryn E. Graham and Mary H. Samuels

INTRODUCTION

The diagnosis of Cushing's disease can be one of the most challenging problems faced by a physician. This stems from the fact that the clinical presentation of Cushing's syndrome can overlap that of simple obesity, essential hypertension, depression, adult-onset diabetes, or polycystic ovary disease, which are some of the most common entities seen by the primary care physician. In addition, the biochemical findings of stress-induced hypercortisolemia can be identical to those of Cushing's syndrome. Finally, distinguishing between the three most common causes of Cushing's syndrome (Cushing's disease caused by a pituitary adenoma, ectopic adrenocorticotropic hormone [ACTH] syndrome, and adrenal adenoma) can be difficult because of problems with sensitivity and specificity of both biochemical tests and imaging procedures. In this chapter, we review the normal and disordered physiologic function of the hypothalamic–pituitary–adrenal axis and the clinical manifestations of Cushing's syndrome. The differential diagnosis of Cushing's syndrome and the diagnostic evaluation are discussed. Finally, treatment options are outlined, including recommendations for preoperative and postoperative medical management of patients with Cushing's disease.

NORMAL PHYSIOLOGIC FUNCTION OF THE HYPOTHALAMIC-PITUITARY-ADRENAL AXIS

The hypothalamic–pituitary–adrenal axis responds to environmental stressors and mediates the body's "stress reaction." Neuronal input from several areas of the brain (including the suprachiasmatic nucleus, amygdala, hippocampus, locus ceruleus, and raphe nuclei of the brainstem) converge on the paraventricular nucleus of the hypothalamus (1). The integration of these signals results in release of the peptide corticotropin releasing hormone (CRH) into the hypophyseal portal system, which courses along the infundibulum to the pituitary gland. Stimulation of corticotrophs in the pituitary by CRH results in increased transcription of the gene for pro-opiomelanocortin (POMC) and stimulation of ACTH secretion. POMC is translated and processed extensively in pituitary corticotrophs to yield ACTH as well as beta-endorphin and several other small peptides. This can be clinically relevant because occasionally tumors, especially ectopic tumors, secrete poorly processed POMC molecules (2) that may not be detected in standard assays.

ACTH is secreted from the pituitary gland into the systemic circulation in discrete pulses, where it has trophic effects on the adrenal gland as well as stimulatory effects on adrenal glucocorticoid and androgen synthesis and release. Because of its trophic effects, increased ACTH secretion in patients with ACTH-dependent Cushing's syndrome results in bilateral adrenal cortical hyperplasia.

The regulation of both CRH and ACTH is by a classic negative feedback loop. Cortisol inhibits CRH synthesis and release, blocks the action of CRH (as well as other secretagogues for ACTH) on corticotrophs, and inhibits POMC transcription and ACTH release (3). Normal feedback inhibition is lost in patients with Cushing's syndrome and is the basis for several diagnostic tests (such as the peripheral ovine CRH stimulation test and dexamethasone suppression tests), which will be described in later sections.

Other known secretagogues for ACTH include vasopressin, central catecholamines, angiotensin II, serotonin, atrial natriuretic factor, cholecystokinin, and vasoactive intestinal peptide (4). The only one that is clinically significant is vasopressin, which potentiates the action of CRH on ACTH secretion (3). Because of this variety of secretagogues, several agents have been explored for use in the evaluation of Cushing's syndrome, including vasopressin (5, 6), naloxone (7, 8), and loperamide (9), but they generally lack significant clinical utility.

Secretion of ACTH, cortisol, and CRH normally demonstrates a circadian rhythm, with the highest levels beginning at about 4:00 AM and decreasing throughout the day to a nadir between midnight and 2:00 AM. This circadian rhythm is the result of higher-amplitude ACTH pulses in the morning and decreased pulse activity at night (10). In stressful situations, secretion of CRH, ACTH, and cortisol are all increased, but unless the stress is extreme, the normal circadian rhythm is preserved, albeit at higher cortisol levels. Disruption of the circadian rhythm is seen in patients with Cushing's syndrome (11, 12), as demonstrated in Figure 13.1, and may aid in the diagnosis of Cushing's syndrome (13), as discussed in subsequent sections.

PATHOPHYSIOLOGIC CHARACTERISTICS OF CUSHING'S SYNDROME

Cushing's syndrome is broadly defined as pathologic hypercortisolemia. It must be distinguished from pseudo-Cushing's syndrome, which is hypercortisolemia that results from a number of other conditions, such as depression, stress, and alcoholism (14–16). The hypercortisolemia in pseudo-Cushing's syndrome can be accompanied by the physical features of Cushing's syndrome but is not considered pathologic because the hypercortisolemia resolves with treatment of the underlying disorder (17, 18).

The variety of causes of true Cushing's syndrome are broadly classified as ACTH-dependent and ACTH-independent and are listed in Figure 13.2 (7, 19). ACTH-dependent Cushing's syndrome accounts for approximately 80% of cases and can be caused by pituitary adenoma, pituitary hyperplasia, ectopic tumor-secreting ACTH, or the rare ectopic CRH-secreting tumor. ACTH-independent causes account for approximately 20% of cases and include adrenal adenomas, carcinomas, and nodular hyperplasia. Exogenous glucocorticoid administration is also an ACTH-independent cause and is the most common overall cause of Cushing's syndrome but is almost always obvious. However, the rare patient with surreptitious use of glucocorticoids can be a diagnostic challenge.

Most patients with endogenous Cushing's syndrome have Cushing's disease, caused by oversecretion of ACTH by a pituitary corticotroph adenoma. Approximately 90% of these tumors are microadenomas (< 1 cm), and they are often so small that magnetic resonance imaging (MRI) studies are negative (20). The tumors often demonstrate basophilic staining of POMC glycoprotein by the periodic acid–Schiff reaction. They are usually single discrete tumors, but occasionally diffuse or nodular corticotroph hyperplasia can be seen (3). In some cases of corticotroph

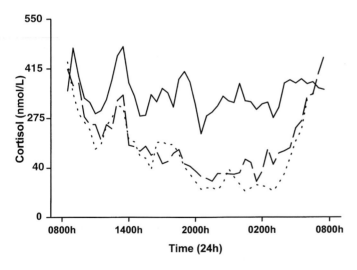

Figure 13.1. Diurnal variation in cortisol secretion in patients with surgically proven Cushing's syndrome (n = 4) (*solid line*), patients with mild hypercortisolemia and/or clinical features suggestive of Cushing's syndrome who were determined not to have Cushing's syndrome (n = 13) (*dashed line*), and healthy subjects (n = 9) (*dotted line*). Patients with Cushing's syndrome clearly have loss of the nocturnal nadir in cortisol secretion, whereas patients with pseudo-Cushing's syndrome have slightly higher cortisol levels but normal diurnal variation. (Adapted from Samuels MH, Brandon D, Isabel L, et al. Cortisol production rates in patients with suspected Cushing's syndrome. X International Congress of Endocrinology. San Francisco, June 1996.)

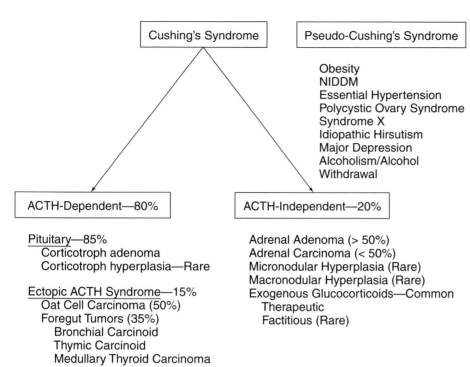

Figure 13.2. Differential diagnosis of Cushing's syndrome. *ACTH*, adrenocorticotropic hormone; *NIDDM*, non–insulin-dependent diabetes mellitus; *CRH*, corticotropin releasing hormone.

hyperplasia, pituitary stimulation by ectopic secretion of CRH has been documented (21).

The ultrastructural appearance of adenomatous cells differs from that of normal pituitary corticotrophs. Adenomatous cells are large, with large nuclei and prominent nucleoli and smaller secretory granules. Crooke's hyaline change consists of cytoplasmic accumulation of cytokeratin, a glassy, homogeneous, slightly acidophilic substance (22). However, this finding is nonspecific, seen in all types of glucocorticoid excess (23). Although their secretion is usually monohormonal, these tumors may demonstrate immunoreactivity to the other POMC-derived peptides (3). In addition, a small percentage of tumors (20%) cosecrete other pituitary hormones, most commonly prolactin (24).

In most cases of Cushing's disease, corticotroph adenomas are monoclonal and are believed to be of primary pituitary origin (25). In up to half of cases, pituitary hyperplasia alone or hyperplasia surrounding the adenoma is seen, suggesting chronic stimulation from hypothalamic CRH. However, the lack of ACTH immunoreactivity in surrounding tissue, the adrenal insufficiency after surgery, and clonality studies all strongly support a pituitary, rather than a hypothalamic, origin of the disease. Despite their monoclonal nature, no specific somatic mutations have been found consistently in corticotroph adenomas (25).

The most common ectopic ACTH-secreting tumors are malignant oat cell lung carcinomas. These are usually obvious and present with signs of the malignancy instead of signs of Cushing's syndrome. The remaining ectopic tumors are occult and often neuroendocrine in origin: carcinoids, medullary thyroid carcinoma, pancreatic islet cell tumors, and pheochromocytomas. These are usually benign, but can rarely metastasize.

A spectrum of adrenal pathologic findings can be seen in the different causes of Cushing's syndrome. Adrenal adenomas that cause Cushing's syndrome are usually single, but primary adrenal Cushing's syndrome can also consist of multiple small nodules. Adrenal carcinomas are usually large (> 5 cm) and may be metastatic at presentation. A number of patients with either ACTH-dependent or ACTH-independent Cushing's syndrome have macronodular adrenal hyperplasia, which may represent autonomy of adrenal tissue after long-standing ACTH stimulation (26). Rarely, bilateral micronodular adrenal hyperplasia (also known as "pigmented nodular adrenal dysplasia") is a cause of Cushing's syndrome. It is believed to be the result of autoimmune production of adrenal-stimulating immunoglobulins and may be associated with other entities in a syndrome referred to as the "Carney complex" (26).

CLINICAL MANIFESTATIONS

Cushing's syndrome causes profound changes in multiple organ systems. The clinical presentation is usually similar among the various causes of Cushing's syndrome, which

Table 13.1. *Clinical Signs and Symptoms of Cushing's Syndrome*

Sign/Symptom	Sensitivity (%)	Specificity (%)
Hypokalemia (K+ < 3.6)	25	96
Ecchymoses	53	94
Osteoporosis	26	94
Weakness	65	93
Diastolic blood pressure ≥ 105 mm Hg	39	83
Red or violaceous striae	46	78
Acne	52	76
Central obesity	90[a]	71
Hirsutism	50	71
Plethora	82	69
Oligomenorrhea	72	49
Generalized obesity	3[a]	38
Abnormal glucose tolerance	88	23

Signs and symptoms of Cushing's syndrome are listed in order of decreasing specificity. Note that many of the most common symptoms are not very specific and that the most discriminatory symptoms (hypokalemia, ecchymoses, osteoporosis, and weakness) are seen in only a fraction of patients (4, 28–32).
[a] The diagnoses of central obesity and generalized obesity are mutually exclusive; in this study (28), the criteria for central obesity favored this diagnosis. In other studies, generalized obesity is reported in up to 60% of patients (29–32).

supports the concept that most of the changes are secondary to glucocorticoid excess. Exceptions to this include changes secondary to elevated levels of ACTH itself, such as hyperpigmentation from the melanotropic effect of ACTH (4), and changes secondary to ACTH stimulation of adrenal androgens (e.g., hirsutism in women). In addition, some patients with ectopic ACTH syndrome have a more rapid onset of symptoms and a higher frequency of hypokalemic metabolic alkalosis (27); and if the tumor is a rapidly growing malignancy, they may have weight loss and cachexia. The spectrum of signs and symptoms observed in patients with Cushing's syndrome reflects the number of tissues that normally respond to glucocorticoids and is discussed below by body system and in Table 13.1 (4, 28–32). For unclear reasons, Cushing's disease is more common in women (8:1), and ectopic ACTH syndrome is more common in men (3:1) (29).

Body Composition

The most profound physical manifestation of glucocorticoid excess is related to changes in adipocyte function. Increased fat deposition is an early phenomenon of glucocorticoid excess and is nearly universal in patients with Cushing's syndrome (28). As opposed to generalized obesity, which is common in the general population, the fat deposition of Cushing's syndrome occurs in a truncal pattern, with sparing or even wasting of the extremities (33). Increased fat deposition is seen in the subcutaneous areas of the face and neck, mediastinum, and peritoneum. This pattern is also referred to as "centripetal obesity" and is defined by an elevated waist-to-hip ratio (> 1.0 in men and > 0.8 in women). This pattern of fat deposition results

in the classic "moon facies" and "buffalo hump" of Cushing's syndrome (30). Fat deposition in the supraclavicular fossae is a particularly specific sign for Cushing's syndrome (4).

Bone/Muscle

In contrast to the anabolic effects on adipose tissue, cortisol induces catabolism of muscle, including stimulation of muscle glycogenolysis and inhibition of muscle protein synthesis. This results in muscle weakness and atrophy, which is often most prominent in the large proximal muscles. Clinically, patients may complain of difficulty in rising from a lying or seated position or in climbing stairs. Interestingly, much of the fat deposition and muscle atrophy can be blunted in patients with Cushing's syndrome who exercise (4).

Glucocorticoids affect bone by several mechanisms, including increased resorption by osteoclasts, impaired osteoblast function, impaired calcium absorption, and secondary hyperparathyroidism leading to osteoporosis and fractures (34). Because osteoporosis is unusual in simple obesity, its presence in an obese patient should raise the possibility of Cushing's syndrome. In children, linear growth is often arrested, whereas weight continues to increase (35). Despite increased bone resorption, hypercalcemia is rare, but hypercalciuria and nephrolithiasis may be seen (4). Although avascular necrosis is common in patients with iatrogenic hypercortisolism, it is rare in those with endogenous Cushing's syndrome.

Skin/Hair

Glucocorticoids have several effects on cutaneous tissue, including atrophy of the epidermis, weakening of supporting muscle and fascia, and exposure of subcutaneous vascular tissue. This results in poor wound healing, ecchymoses, telangiectasias, purpura, and central facial erythema and plethora. Perioral dermatitis and acne can also be seen (30). Violaceous striae larger than 1 cm in diameter are highly specific for Cushing's syndrome; however, pink, reddish or thin, silver striae are commonly associated with weight gain alone (4, 30). Acanthosis nigricans may be seen in patients with Cushing's syndrome, as with any condition that causes insulin resistance (30). Soft pale villous hypertrichosis is the most common change seen in the hair of patients with Cushing's; however, hirsutism can be seen if androgens are also secreted, such as in ACTH-dependent disease and the rare adrenal carcinoma (30).

Metabolism

Hypercortisolemia results in direct simulation of hepatic gluconeogenesis. Together with the catabolic changes in muscle, this results in significant increases in hepatic glucose output. In addition, insulin resistance is often seen (36), and frank diabetes mellitus occurs in 10 to 15% of patients (4). Hyperlipidemia can be seen secondary to stimulation of very–low-density lipoprotein, low-density lipoprotein, high-density lipoprotein, and triglyceride synthesis (30). Electrolyte abnormalities are uncommon unless there is severe hypercortisolemia, in which case hypokalemic alkalosis may result from the mineralocorticoid activity of cortisol at the renal tubule (37). This is more common in patients with adrenal carcinoma or ectopic ACTH syndrome but can be seen with any cause of Cushing's syndrome.

Neuropsychiatric

A variety of neuropsychiatric disturbances occur in patients with Cushing's syndrome, ranging from fatigue, emotional lability, irritability, anxiety, insomnia, loss of memory, poor concentration, and appetite changes to depression, mania, delusions, and hallucinations. In one study (38), these symptoms were found to correlate roughly with cortisol and ACTH levels. Pseudotumor cerebri and spinal lipomatosis are two rare but potentially serious complications of Cushing's syndrome (30).

Immunologic/Hematologic

Excessive glucocorticoids have suppressive effects on multiple functions of both B and T cells and neutrophils. Thymic, splenic, and lymph node involution are seen. Immunoglobulin synthesis and phagocytic activity are reduced, and cytokine production is significantly altered (30). The overall result of these changes is an increased incidence of fungal skin infections and opportunistic infections (39). In addition, clinical signs of inflammation (such as fever, peritoneal signs, etc.) may be masked by the suppressive effects of glucocorticoids. Increased hemoglobin concentrations may be seen, and levels of some clotting factors are elevated. Although the incidence of thromboembolic events has been reported to be increased, this is disputed (30).

Cardiovascular

Hypertension is a common finding in patients with Cushing's syndrome because of increased plasma and extracellular volume, stimulation of the renin–angiotensin system, effects of cortisol and other adrenal steroid intermediates at the mineralocorticoid receptor, and increased sensitivity to catecholamine effects (37, 40). Lipid abnormalities are also common; all three of these cardiovascular risk factors (insulin resistance and diabetes mellitus, hypertension, and hyperlipidemia) contribute to the excess cardiovascular disease seen in patients with Cushing's syndrome (4).

Gastrointestinal

Gastrointestinal complications are rare in patients with endogenous Cushing's syndrome, although peptic ulceration and acute pancreatitis are seen in patients with iatrogenic hypercortisolism (30).

Endocrine

Hypercortisolemia suppresses thyroid-stimulating hormone secretion, inhibits T4 to T3 conversion, and results in mild reductions in T3, T4, and thyroid-binding globulin levels (30). Inhibition of the gonadotropin-releasing hormone pulse generator results in hypogonadism and can cause oligoamenorrhea in women, impotence in men, and decreased libido in both sexes. These changes usually resolve with treatment of hypercortisolemia (30).

LIMITATIONS IN THE CLINICAL DIAGNOSIS OF CUSHING'S SYNDROME

Although the true incidence of Cushing's syndrome is not known, it is estimated to be between one and five per million population (4, 31, 41). Obviously, Cushing's syndrome is rare compared with the incidence of the other diseases considered in the differential diagnosis (Fig. 13.2). However, although rare, Cushing's syndrome clearly causes excess morbidity and mortality, primarily because of infections and cardiovascular events, and is estimated at four times that of the general population (31, 42). It is therefore essential that the diagnosis of this curable disease be made in a timely fashion.

The physical manifestations of advanced Cushing's syndrome can be dramatic, including a combination of severe weight gain, prominent striae, diffuse ecchymoses, spontaneous fractures, and significant proximal muscle weakness. Fortunately, the disease is often suspected earlier than in previous years, before the devastating complications of the disease occur. However, because of this, patients are currently evaluated when they have more subtle clinical findings, which can be difficult to distinguish from normal variation. Furthermore, many of the signs and symptoms are nonspecific and overlap more common entities such as simple obesity, non–insulin-dependent diabetes mellitus, etc. The presence of several of these features together should increase the suspicion of Cushing's syndrome (7). Unfortunately, other syndromes that include several of these features, such as polycystic ovary syndrome (comprising hirsutism, chronic anovulation, and insulin resistance) and syndrome X (comprising hypertension, insulin resistance, and hyperlipidemia), are also much more common than Cushing's syndrome (43). Thus, even with multiple features consistent with Cushing's syndrome, the probability of a patient having Cushing's syndrome is low.

Essentially, there are no symptoms with high enough sensitivity and specificity to reliably make a clinical diagnosis of Cushing's syndrome. This point is illustrated by the data shown in Table 13.1, which lists the prevalence (equivalent to the sensitivity) of symptoms seen in patients with Cushing's syndrome in order of their specificity. Note that the symptoms that have the highest specificity for the disease (ecchymoses, muscle weakness, hypokalemia, and osteoporosis) (28) are seen in only a fraction of patients with Cushing's syndrome.

A recent onset of symptoms or a change in symptoms is more suspicious for Cushing's syndrome; however, most physicians are faced with patients who have long-standing symptoms. Essentially, the physician must have a low threshold for screening patients with these common symptoms but must recognize that most patients who are screened will be found not to have the disorder.

BIOCHEMICAL EVALUATION

The authors' recommended algorithm for evaluating patients suspected of having Cushing's syndrome is shown in Figure 13.3. The specific tests used to evaluate a patient with suspected Cushing's syndrome may differ, however,

depending on the preferences of the consulting endocrinologist or referral center. In general, the evaluation consists of three steps. The first step is diagnosing Cushing's syndrome by demonstrating pathologic hypercortisolism. The primary distinction in this step is between patients with Cushing's syndrome and those with similar physical findings from other common diseases. In addition, the physician must distinguish patients with Cushing's syndrome from those with hypercortisolemia from pseudo-Cushing's syndrome.

Once Cushing's syndrome is diagnosed, the second step is to distinguish between ACTH-dependent and ACTH-independent disease. If found to be ACTH dependent, the final step involves distinguishing Cushing's disease, caused by a pituitary adenoma, from ectopic ACTH syndrome. Each of these steps may involve multiple testing procedures, each with their own limitations. It is essential that the diagnosis be clear at each step before proceeding to subsequent steps for interpretation of test results to be valid.

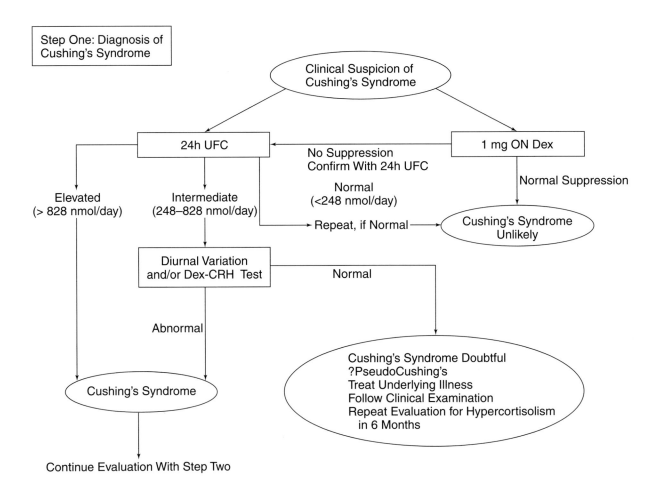

Figure 13.3. Step one: diagnosis of Cushing's syndrome. Suggested algorithm for the initial evaluation of a patient suspected of having Cushing's disease. Measurement of 24-hour urine-free cortisol (*UFC*) is the preferred method of diagnosing Cushing's syndrome, although screening with a 1 mg overnight dexamethasone suppression test (ON Dex) with confirmation by 24-hour UFC is acceptable. Intermediate levels of hypercortisolemia may require evaluation of diurnal variation or the dexamethasone-suppressed oCRH stimulation test (Dex-CRH test). *If UFC is done by radioimmunoassay, the high-performance liquid chromatography normal range will be lower.

Step One: Diagnosis of Cushing's Syndrome

After the clinical suspicion of Cushing's syndrome has been raised, the initial step in the biochemical evaluation involves demonstrating hypercortisolism. Often this step is the most difficult one in the evaluation of Cushing's syndrome because of problems with specificity of the dexamethasone suppression test and the overlap of the biochemical findings in patients with pseudo-Cushing's syndrome and Cushing's syndrome. In the past, this step has involved measurement of cortisol metabolites in 24-hour urine samples in the 2-day, low-dose dexamethasone suppression test. Unfortunately, this test lacks both sensitivity and specificity (44, 45). There are currently two accepted tests to demonstrate hypercortisolism with acceptable accuracy: (*a*) measurement of basal 24-hour urine free cortisol (UFC) excretion and (*b*) the 1 mg overnight dexamethasone suppression test.

24-Hour UFC Determination

Measurement of 24-hour UFC concentration is one of the most reliable methods for demonstrating hypercortisolism. The cortisol level determination is done either by high-performance liquid chromatography, which is very specific, with a normal range up to 1380 nmol/L (50 μg/dL), or by radioimmunoassay after solvent extraction, with a normal range up to 2480 nmol/L (90 μg/dL). Either method, when performed in a good laboratory, provides excellent reliability. Simultaneous measurement of creatinine concentration in the same sample helps ensure that the sample collection was complete. When evaluated in large numbers of patients, an elevated 24-hour UFC level has a sensitivity of 95% for diagnosing Cushing's syndrome (45) and results in only 1% false-positive results in normal patients. In non-Cushing's obese patients, the false-positive rate may be as high as 5% because nonpathologic increases in cortisol production rates and cortisol metabolism can be seen in patients with simple obesity (44). If clinical suspicion persists after obtaining a single normal 24-hour UFC value, the test should be repeated; if three of four trials of 24-hour UFC determinations are normal, the likelihood of Cushing's syndrome is low.

Rarely, a patient may manifest intermittent or cyclic hypercortisolemia, in which case, the symptoms of Cushing's syndrome often abate during periods of nonsecretion (46). Obviously, this can be confusing to diagnose, and, if suspected, the physician must ensure that the evaluation is undertaken when the patient is symptomatic. A similar caveat exists when patients are treated with medications that reduce hypercortisolemia (see the following sections).

Patient inconvenience and difficulties with completing the 24-hour collection are the main problems with the 24-hour UFC determination, which is otherwise the procedure of choice for diagnosing Cushing's syndrome.

1 mg Overnight Dexamethasone Suppression Test

A simpler test to perform is the 1 mg overnight dexamethasone suppression test. One milligram of dexamethasone is administered by mouth at 11:00 PM, and a serum cortisol level is drawn at 8:00 AM the next morning. A normal response is suppression of the cortisol level to less than 140 nmol/L (5 μg/dL). This test has excellent sensitivity for diagnosing Cushing's syndrome, resulting in less than a 1% false-negative rate. However, it suffers from poor specificity, with false-positive rates estimated by different investigators between 12 and 30% (47). Because of the extremely low prevalence of Cushing's syndrome, this false-positive rate means that a patient with a nonsuppressed cortisol level after dexamethasone administration has only a 1 in 11,000 chance of having Cushing's syndrome. Many disease processes result in false-positive test results, including stress, alcoholism, and neuropsychiatric disease, especially depression. In addition, medications such as estrogens that increase cortisol-binding globulin levels (28) and therefore increase total cortisol levels can also lead to false-positive results. False-negative test results can be caused by renal failure (47) and by use of medications that increase hepatic p450 enzyme activity and therefore dexamethasone metabolism, such as phenytoin, phenobarbital, and rifampin (48). Because of its excellent sensitivity, it is a good screening test, and normal suppression of serum cortisol levels following administration of 1 mg of dexamethasone is strong evidence that the patient does not have Cushing's syndrome. However, lack of suppression is nonspecific and requires further evaluation and confirmation of hypercortisolism by a 24-hour UFC determination.

Salivary Cortisol Level Determination

Cortisol can be detected in the salivary ultrafiltrate with levels that closely approximate serum free cortisol levels (49). Because of the simple and noninvasive method of collection, determination of salivary cortisol concentration throughout the day and after dexamethasone suppression has been proposed as an alternative to 24-hour urine collections and serum cortisol level determinations (50). Unfortunately, this has been validated in only small numbers of patients, and currently the reliability of salivary cortisol level determinations is not consistent, precluding widespread application of this method.

Mild Hypercortisolism and Pseudo-Cushing's Syndrome

If the patient demonstrates clear hypercortisolism by a 24-hour UFC collection (e.g., > 830 nmol [> 300 μg] free cortisol per day in a patient who is not acutely ill or severely depressed), the diagnosis of Cushing's syndrome is clear. However, lesser degrees of hypercortisolism often require further investigation to distinguish mild Cushing's syndrome from pseudo-Cushing's syndrome. Pseudo-Cushing's syndrome results in hypercortisolism and, at times, physical features identical to those of Cushing's disease. Although the cause is unclear, it is believed to involve excessive hypothalamic CRH secretion (4). The hypercortisolemia is clearly secondary to the underlying disease process and resolves with treatment of the underlying disease. The initial examination of a patient suspected of having Cushing's syndrome should always include evaluation for alcohol use, depression, and other psychiatric disorders as well as underlying illnesses.

Two biochemical features have emerged as promising to distinguish Cushing's syndrome from pseudo-Cushing's syndrome. The first is the observation that patients with most causes of pseudo-Cushing's syndrome retain the normal circadian variation in ACTH and cortisol secretion, albeit, with higher amplitude pulses, as shown in Figure 13.1 (11–13, 15, 51). Thus, some measure of diurnal variation, e.g., hourly 24-hour cortisol sampling or a single sleeping midnight cortisol level that reaches an appropriate nadir (< 210 nmol/L [< 7.5 μg/dL]) suggests pseudo-Cushing's syndrome (13). This normal diurnal variation seems to be retained in mild to moderate depression, but results of a recent report suggest that patients with severe depression (requiring inpatient treatment) may not reach this level of cortisol nadir despite retention of some diurnal variation (51). In addition, some patients with alcoholic pseudo-Cushing's syndrome have abnormal diurnal cortisol variation, so measurement of nocturnal cortisol levels may be misleading in this patient group (52).

The second potential biochemical test to distinguish pseudo-Cushing's syndrome from true Cushing's syndrome is the dexamethasone-suppressed CRH stimulation test. The basis of this test is the additive differences in the responses to dexamethasone and CRH between normal pituitary corticotrophs in pseudo-Cushing's syndrome and ACTH-secreting cells of a pituitary or ectopic tumor causing Cushing's syndrome. In patients with pseudo-Cushing's syndrome, normal corticotrophs are suppressed by dexamethasone use, and this suppression cannot be overcome by CRH. In contrast, the abnormal ACTH secretion from pituitary adenomas and ectopic tumors is relatively resistant to dexamethasone suppression and hyperresponsive to CRH. (Adrenal adenomas are autonomous and secrete cortisol independent of both hormones and therefore will be detected correctly with this test.) Combining both medications improves the accuracy of the test. To perform the test, the patient is treated with dexamethasone, 0.5 mg by mouth every 6 hours for 2 days. At 8:00 AM on the third day, 2 hours after the last dexamethasone dose, ovine CRH (oCRH), 1 μg/kg or 100 μg, is administered by intravenous bolus. Cortisol and ACTH levels are drawn at baseline and 15 and 30 minutes after the oCRH. A 15-minute cortisol level greater than 40 nmol/L (> 1.4 μg/dL) has been shown to distinguish even mild Cushing's syndrome from pseudo-Cushing's syndrome with 100% sensitivity and specificity (53).

Although both measurement of diurnal variation and the dexamethasone-suppressed CRH test look promising, the number of patients evaluated with each of these techniques is still small, and further evaluation of both of these tests is necessary before their clinical utility can be stated confidently. If a reliable diagnosis of Cushing's syndrome cannot be established using these tests, the physician should reevaluate the patient at regular intervals. A patient who has an underlying disease causing pseudo-Cushing's syndrome requires treatment of the underlying disorder and follow-up to demonstrate resolution of the hypercortisolism and a lack of progression of features of Cushing's syndrome. In contrast, a patient with early or mild Cushing's syndrome will usually evidence gradual progression of symptoms.

Step Two: Distinguish ACTH-Dependent from ACTH-Independent Cushing's Syndrome

Once a patient has been definitively shown to have Cushing's syndrome by the above tests, the physician must distinguish ACTH-independent causes (usually adrenal adenomas or exogenous glucocorticoids, but rarely adrenal carcinomas or micronodular hyperplasia) from ACTH-dependent causes (pituitary adenomas and ectopic ACTH syndrome), as outlined in Figure 13.4. This step in the evaluation begins with measurement of a random plasma ACTH level, usually by a two-site immunochemiluminescent or immunoradiometric assay. Analysis by the older radioimmunoassay technique suffers from both poor sensitivity and poor specificity (44). If the ACTH is nonsuppressed, either "normal" or elevated (e.g., ACTH level > 2 pmol/L [> 10 pg/mL]), the patient clearly has ACTH-dependent Cushing's syndrome and the physician can proceed to step 3 of the evaluation, detailed in the following section and in Figure 13.5. However, if the ACTH level is low, the patient may still have ACTH-dependent disease because ACTH secretion from both pituitary adenomas and ectopic tumors has been shown to be pulsatile and even episodic. Further, some tumors secrete poorly processed POMC molecules, referred to as "big ACTH," that are not detected by standard assays. Therefore, a low random ACTH level does not exclude ACTH-dependent disease.

The peripheral oCRH test is used to distinguish ACTH-dependent disease from ACTH-independent disease in Cushing's patients with low random ACTH levels. The basis of this test stems from the observation that ACTH-secreting tumors (pituitary or ectopic) usually respond to CRH, in contrast to the suppressed pituitary corticotrophs in ACTH-independent disease. In this test, basal ACTH levels are drawn, then oCRH (1 μg/kg or 100 μg) is given and plasma ACTH levels are determined 15 and 30 minutes later.

A peak ACTH level less than 2 pmol/L (< 10 pg/mL) indicates ACTH-independent disease. The primary differential causes are exogenous glucocorticoid administration and primary adrenal disease. Patients who are prescribed

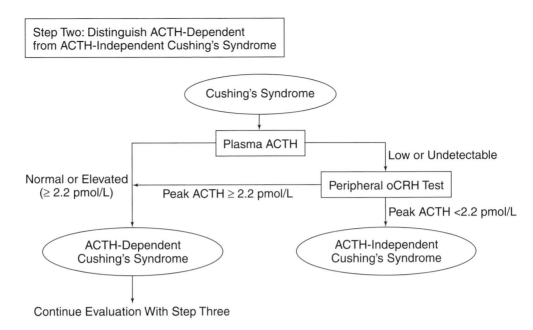

Figure 13.4. Step two: distinguish ACTH-dependent from ACTH-independent disease. Measurement of a random plasma ACTH level can demonstrate ACTH-dependent Cushing's syndrome if the level is 2 pmol/L (10 pg/mL) or higher. If low, performance of the peripheral oCRH test will exclude ACTH-independent disease if the peak plasma ACTH level remains below 2 pmol/L (< 10 pg/mL).

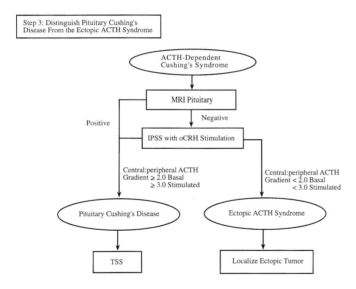

Figure 13.5. Step three: distinguish pituitary Cushing's disease from ectopic ACTH syndrome. The final step is to localize the ACTH source. The only test that accomplishes this with 100% accuracy is inferior petrosal sinus sampling (*IPSS*). The specificity of MRI is sufficient, however, that if MRI demonstrates a lesion, one reasonable alternative is to proceed directly to transsphenoidal surgery (*TSS*).

glucocorticoids are no diagnostic dilemma, although use of steroid creams, inhalers, or intra-articular/soft tissue injections are sometimes not recognized immediately as a significant source of glucocorticoids. In addition, occasionally a patient may conceal glucocorticoid use. Evaluation

of urine for specific glucocorticoids by high-performance liquid chromatography may be necessary in these cases (54). If exogenous glucocorticoid use is excluded, adrenal imaging should be performed in these patients with Cushing's syndrome, low plasma ACTH levels, and no ACTH response to oCRH.

A peak ACTH level greater than 2 pmol/L (> 10 pg/mL) following oCRH indicates ACTH-dependent Cushing's syndrome, and the next step (described in the following section) is to distinguish pituitary from ectopic ACTH sources (55).

It is important for the diagnosis of Cushing's syndrome to be established prior to proceeding with this step. Normal patients or patients with pseudo-Cushing's syndrome will have normal or even high plasma ACTH levels that will stimulate further with oCRH. If one of these patients is erroneously diagnosed as having Cushing's syndrome, the ACTH levels will seem to indicate ACTH-dependent disease, and further evaluation will point to a pituitary source.

Likewise, the biochemical diagnosis of ACTH-dependent or ACTH-independent disease must be established prior to performing imaging procedures because 10% of normal patients will have pituitary or adrenal "incidentalomas" (56, 57). In addition, bilateral hyperplasia is often seen in patients with ACTH-dependent disease and could be mistaken for primary adrenal disease if the principal cause, ACTH oversecretion, is not recognized. Because of these limitations of the diagnostic procedures, it is essential that the evaluation proceed in a stepwise fashion, with a clear diagnosis established at each step before proceeding with further tests.

Step Three: Distinguish Cushing's Disease from Ectopic ACTH Syndrome

Approximately 85 to 90% of patients with ACTH-dependent Cushing's syndrome have Cushing's disease caused by a pituitary corticotroph adenoma. The remainder have ectopic ACTH syndrome caused by any one of a variety of tumors listed in Figure 13.2. Several of these tumors, particularly the malignant ones, manifest symptoms other than Cushing's syndrome and are easily diagnosed with standard tests (e.g., chest radiograph). They may present with a more rapid onset of florid symptoms of Cushing's syndrome and are more likely to have hypokalemia (27). The remaining ectopic tumors are, by definition, occult, and present a challenge to distinguish from pituitary Cushing's disease. The two entities are often clinically and biochemically identical, and imaging modalities for both pituitary and ectopic tumors have suboptimal sensitivity and specificity (56). Given the pretest probability of 90% for Cushing's disease, for any test to be clinically useful, it must demonstrate performance superior to this. A variety of noninvasive tests have been used for many years to try to distinguish these two causes, but, unfortunately, none have a high level of accuracy.

Dexamethasone Suppression Tests

Dexamethasone suppression testing has been used in one form or another in the differential diagnosis of Cushing's syndrome for more than 30 years, since its original description by Grant Liddle in 1960 (58). The basis of these tests is the differential sensitivity to glucocorticoid negative feedback seen in pituitary corticotroph adenomas and ectopic ACTH-secreting tumors. Thus, most pituitary adenomas will suppress ACTH and cortisol secretion with high-dose dexamethasone administration (8.0 mg at bedtime or 2 mg every 6 hours for 2 days) but not with low-dose dexamethasone administration (0.5 mg every 6 hours for 2 days), and most ectopic tumors are resistant to suppression even at the higher dose.

Unfortunately, all variations of dexamethasone suppression tests studied so far (including overnight and 2-day tests and measurement of serum cortisol, UFC, or cortisol metabolites) lack adequate sensitivity and specificity for distinguishing the two causes of ACTH-dependent Cushing's syndrome. Sensitivity is reported at only 60 to 70% when rigorous cutoff values (more than 90% suppression of 24-hour UFC) are set to allow for 100% specificity in diagnosing ectopic tumors (45, 59–62).

Stimulation with metyrapone has also been evaluated for its potential as a diagnostic agent. This drug blocks conversion of 11-deoxycortisol to cortisol and therefore increases levels of 11-deoxycortisol and its metabolites. In this test, pituitary adenomas, which are more responsive to glucocorticoid feedback than ectopic tumors, will respond to the lowered cortisol levels by secreting ACTH, which stimulates adrenal cortisol synthetic pathways. Because of the enzymatic block, increases in 11-deoxycortisol (but not cortisol) levels will be seen. However, when evaluated in a small number of patients, the metyrapone stimulation test demonstrated only slightly better performance (88% sensitivity, 100% specificity) than dexamethasone suppression testing (63).

Similarly, pituitary tumors are more likely to respond to oCRH. However, although ACTH and cortisol responses after stimulation with oCRH were initially found to perform better than with dexamethasone testing (93% sensitivity, 100% specificity), subsequent experience has been less accurate. All of these tests result in an unacceptable false-negative rate (55), and, in our experience, none are particularly helpful in the differential diagnosis of ACTH-dependent Cushing's syndrome because they only minimally increase the posttest probability above pretest probability.

Inferior Petrosal Sinus Sampling (IPSS)

During the past 10 years, IPSS has been studied as a tool to distinguish pituitary-dependent Cushing's disease from ectopic ACTH syndrome (64–67). The basis of this test is selective sampling of the pituitary venous drainage to detect ACTH secretion from the pituitary gland by demonstration of a petrosal sinus:peripheral ACTH gradient. In this test, bilateral catheters are placed fluoroscopically from a femoral approach through the inferior vena cava and the jugular veins into the inferior petrosal sinuses. Baseline blood samples are obtained for ACTH determinations from both catheters as well as from a peripheral site. Ovine CRH (1 μg/kg or 100 μg) is given by intravenous bolus and sampling is repeated at all sites at two or three time points between 3 and 10 minutes after oCRH stimulation. Detection of a central (left or right inferior petrosal sinus):peripheral ACTH gradient greater than or equal to 2.0 in baseline samples or greater than or equal to 3.0 after oCRH stimulation is evidence of a pituitary source of ACTH. Ratios less than this indicate an ectopic ACTH source (64).

Because of the intermittent nature of ACTH secretion from adenomatous cells, oCRH stimulation is required for 100% accuracy in IPSS (44). In addition, bilateral sampling is required, as occasionally central:peripheral gradients will not be detected from lateral tumors if only one catheter is placed and happens to be positioned on the contralateral side (44). When oCRH is used and bilateral sampling is done, this technique has been shown to be highly accurate, correctly classifying 100% of more than 600 patients in several reported series (64–66).

This technique has obvious appeal because of its excellent diagnostic accuracy; however, it is invasive, costly, and not universally available. Although invasive, it can be performed safely by experienced personnel (68). The most serious complication has been brainstem ischemia, reported in a few patients; however, this is believed to have been related to a specific experimental catheter and has not been seen with use of more flexible catheters (4, 69). Because of concerns about its cost, an evaluation of the cost-effectiveness of this procedure has recently been done. In this study, IPSS was found to have higher initial costs but overall was cost-effective because its higher accuracy resulted in fewer inappropriate surgical procedures than biochemical evaluation with dexamethasone testing followed by IPSS if negative (70).

Once again, it is essential that IPSS be undertaken only in patients with definite ACTH-dependent Cushing's syndrome. IPSS studies of patients with pseudo-Cushing's syndrome or of normal subjects clearly demonstrate central:peripheral ACTH gradients that would falsely indicate a pituitary tumor and also almost always demonstrate lateralization (71). In addition, patients with ACTH-independent disease who might have low but detectable ACTH levels would show no gradient on IPSS, falsely indicating the ectopic ACTH syndrome. Finally, there have been reports of two patients with proven ectopic tumors who underwent IPSS with gradients suggesting pituitary disease. In these two cases, the evaluation by IPSS was done at a time when the patients were not hypercortisolemic and therefore did not have pituitary corticotroph suppression. Ovine CRH administration was thus able to stimulate ACTH secretion, falsely indicating a pituitary source (72). Similar to other dynamic evaluations in Cushing's syndrome, IPSS must be performed while the patient is hypercortisolemic.

MRI

MRI is significantly superior to computed tomographic scanning for evaluation of the pituitary gland (73). However, MRI still has poor sensitivity for pituitary microadenomas in Cushing's syndrome, detecting only about 50 to 70% of lesions (73, 74). Despite its poor sensitivity for detecting a lesion, MRI has fairly good specificity of greater than 90% (75) and an approximately 85% positive predictive value (74). This reflects the 10 to 20% incidence of small "pituitary incidentalomas" in patients without pituitary disease (74). Therefore, the authors believe it is a reasonable alternative to begin the evaluation of a patient with ACTH-dependent Cushing's syndrome with MRI scanning. If a definite lesion is seen, one may proceed directly with transsphenoidal surgery (TSS). If no lesion is seen, which will be the case in approximately half of all patients, IPSS with oCRH should be performed. This strategy, however, will correctly identify only 90 to 95% of patients with Cushing's disease because of the problem of specificity of MRI. Again, IPSS is required for 100% accuracy in distinguishing between patients with pituitary Cushing's disease and ectopic ACTH syndrome. However, the decision to proceed with this invasive diagnostic procedure must balance the invasive risk and increased expense with the benefit of the 100% predictive value of the test.

Pituitary Tumor Lateralization

In many centers, if a pituitary adenoma is not readily encountered during TSS, a total hypophysectomy is performed to cure the Cushing's disease (32). Preoperative localization of a tumor within the pituitary gland would allow the neurosurgeon to limit this resection to a hemihypophysectomy in cases in which the tumor is difficult to find, sparing the patient the potential complication of hypopituitarism. After demonstration of limited intercavernous mixing of pituitary venous drainage (76), IPSS was evaluated for its efficacy in predicting pituitary tumor lateralization. To predict lateralization, left:right and right:left inferior petrosal sinus ACTH ratios are calculated. Ratios greater than or equal to 1.4 have a 70 to 87% accuracy rate in predicting tumor lateralization (64, 65, 77, 78). MRI has also been shown to be fairly accurate in lateralizing tumors, if a tumor is seen (79). However, as noted above, half of all proven pituitary adenomas are not seen on MRI scans, limiting its usefulness (74).

The authors have had recent experience at their institution with cavernous sinus sampling (CSS), which samples the pituitary venous effluent more directly than IPSS. Analysis of more than 60 patients with ACTH-dependent Cushing's syndrome who underwent CSS with oCRH stimulation reveals an overall diagnostic accuracy of 100% for distinguishing a pituitary from an ectopic source of ACTH (79; Kathryn E. Graham, unpublished data, 1998), similar to IPSS. The diagnostic accuracy for predicting tumor lateralization was 86%. Lateralization performance was better in patients with lateral tumors (which are seen in approximately 85% of patients) than in patients with midline or bilateral tumors. Further, two-thirds of the inaccurate lateralization could be explained by differences in left and right catheter positions or venous flow asymmetry (80). Further evaluation of this technique with larger patient groups will be needed to verify the increased utility of CSS for predicting lateralization.

TREATMENT OF CUSHING'S DISEASE

The treatment of choice for all causes of endogenous Cushing's syndrome is surgery to remove the autonomous tissue, whether it is an adrenal adenoma producing cortisol, an ectopic ACTH-secreting tumor, or a pituitary corticotroph adenoma. In essentially all cases of Cushing's disease, transsphenoidal microadenomectomy is the procedure of choice, and this is the topic of the following chapter. Rarely, Cushing's disease will be caused by a pituitary macroadenoma that is located in such a position as to warrant a frontal approach, or it may arise in ectopic pituitary tissue (e.g., in the pharynx as a residual from invagination of Rathke's pouch). If the adenoma cannot be clearly identified and resected, hypophysectomy or hemihypophysectomy (if accurate lateralization information is available from MRI, IPSS, or CSS) should be performed.

Cortisol levels fall quickly after successful tumor resection because of suppression of normal pituitary corticotrophs by the prior hypercortisolemia. A cortisol level less than 55 nmol/L (< 2 μg/dL) on the second post-operative day (after withholding exogenous glucocorticoids) is good evidence of complete tumor resection and cure (81, 82). Intraoperative measurement of disappearance of ACTH from the plasma after tumor resection has been shown to be predictive of cure in patients with ectopic ACTH syndrome (83) but has been disappointing in patients with Cushing's disease (84).

MANAGEMENT OF PERSISTENT HYPERCORTISOLEMIA FOLLOWING TSS

Unfortunately, even in the hands of the most experienced surgeon, 10% or more of patients will remain hypercortisolemic after TSS. In patients with macroadenomas or extrasellar tumor extension, or if the tumor is not clearly identified, the failure rate may be as high as 40% (19). In addition, reports of tumor recurrences range from 2 to 50% (32, 85) and should be approached similarly to a primary surgical failure. In cases of residual or recurrent disease, several options may be considered. A second transsphenoidal exploration and repeat tumor resection, hypophysectomy, or hemihypophysectomy may be performed. Success rates are usually lower than with first surgeries, estimated at 30 to 60% (19), and there are higher complication rates, including cerebrospinal fluid leaks and varying degrees of hypopituitarism (86).

A second option is bilateral surgical adrenalectomy to cure the hypercortisolemia. With the advent of a laparoscopic approach to adrenalectomy, the complication rate is much lower than that seen previously with open procedures (87). This option provides complete cure of the physical manifestations of Cushing's syndrome in 90% of patients (19) without the risk of hypopituitarism. However, the patient is subjected to the cost of life-long adrenal insufficiency and dependence on glucocorticoid replacement. In addition, Nelson's syndrome, manifest by rapid and invasive corticotroph tumor growth after removal of the negative feedback of high cortisol levels, occurs in up to 30% of patients (29).

The final option for definitive treatment is pituitary irradiation. Although remission rates vary, pituitary irradiation usually results in control of Cushing's disease (88) and reduces the risk of Nelson's syndrome. Full benefit of radiation may take up to 2 years or longer. It has not been used as commonly in the past 10 years because of concerns about the long-term cognitive and neuropsychiatric effects of irradiation. Anterior pituitary hormone deficiencies occur commonly with pituitary irradiation, including growth hormone deficiency in 67 to 100% of patients, gonadotropin deficiency in 30 to 75%, ACTH deficiency in 37 to 83%, and central hypothyroidism in 0 to 25% of patients assessed 2 to 9 years after treatment (19).

MEDICAL MANAGEMENT OF CUSHING'S DISEASE

Preoperatively, hypertension and hyperglycemia should be controlled as well as possible to decrease operative morbidity and mortality in patients with Cushing's disease. Hypertension often does not respond to treatment with standard medications (89) and may require aggressive, multidrug therapy. Hyperglycemia, if present, responds poorly to administration of oral agents and usually requires insulin therapy. With the recent introduction of metformin and troglitazone, which improve insulin sensitivity, preoperative control of hyperglycemia may be possible without insulin therapy.

Patients with extreme symptoms (psychosis, severe hypertension or hyperglycemia, or active infections) caused by severe hypercortisolemia may benefit from temporary preoperative medical therapy to decrease serum cortisol levels. However, it is the authors' opinion that surgery should not be delayed in such patients. In such cases, medical treatment can provide prompt relief of many of the symptoms and improve the risks associated with surgery.

Medications used to control hypercortisolemia are listed in Table 13.2 with their mechanism of action, efficacy, typical doses, and common toxic effects. The first group is composed of the adrenal enzyme inhibitors and includes ketoconazole, metyrapone, aminoglutethimide, and mitotane, which all act to inhibit adrenocortical steroid synthesis.

Ketoconazole is an antifungal agent that inhibits a number of steroidogenic enzymes involved in the biosynthesis of cortisol. It is highly effective, reducing cortisol levels in nearly 100% of patients. The use of ketoconazole is limited by hepatotoxic effects. Liver function test abnormalities occur in 15% of patients, and serious liver toxic effects occur in 1 of 15,000 patients (19). Hepatitis usually resolves within 3 months of discontinuing the medication. It also commonly causes nausea and vomiting. Gynecomastia occurs because of inhibition of androgen synthesis and an increase in testosterone to estradiol conversion (90). It is a teratogen and is therefore contraindicated during pregnancy. It is the most common medication used in the United States for medical management of Cushing's syndrome because of its efficacy and comparatively low side effect profile.

Metyrapone therapy blocks the final step in cortisol synthesis, the conversion of 11-deoxycortisol to cortisol. This can result in significant elevations of 11-deoxycortisol levels, and there have been occasional reports of hypertensive crisis with its use. The main side effects of metyrapone use are acne and hirsutism, seen in 70% of women secondary to increased androgen production. Lethargy, dizziness, and ataxia occur in 15% of patients, and edema and nausea each in 8%. Although efficacious, with up to 85% of patients responding, dosage increases may be required in 25% of patients because of increased ACTH levels overriding the enzymatic blockade (19).

Table 13.2. _Medications Used to Control Hypercortisolemia_

Medication	Mechanism of Action	Typical Dosage	Efficacy	Common Toxic Effects	Comments
Steroid biosynthesis inhibitors					
Ketoconazole	Blocks multiple steps in cortisol synthesis	200–1200 mg/d	Nearly 100%	Hepatotoxicity, 15%; gynecomastia, 13%; nausea, 8%; edema, 6%; rash, 2%	Hepatitis reverses within 3 months. Risk of severe liver damage in 1/15,000.
Metyrapone	11-β-hydroxylase	500–6000 mg/d	85%	Hirsutism/acne, 70%; lethargy/dizziness/ataxia, 15%; edema, 8%; nausea, 5%; rash, 4%	Increased ACTH may override enzymatic blockade; 25% of patients may require dosage increase.
Aminoglutethimide	Cholesterol to pregnenelone conversion	750–2000 mg/d	> 60%	Lethargy/somnolence; dizziness, 30%; rash/fever, 18%; nausea/anorexia, 12%; hypothyroidism	
Mitotane	Side chain cleavage; adrenolytic	500–12,000 mg/d	83% 30% sustained	Gastrointestinal, 72%; impaired mentation/dizziness, 45%; hypercholesterolemia; gynecomastia; transient rash; LFT abnormalities	Decreased 17-hydroxy corticosteroids because of altered cortisol metabolism.
Centrally acting agents					
Cyproheptadine	Impairs ACTH secretion	24 mg/d	30–50%	Somnolence, hyperphagia; weight gain	
Bromocriptine	Inhibits ACTH secretion	3.75–30 mg/d	42%	Nausea, dry mouth, postural hypotension	
Glucocorticoid receptor antagonist					
Mifepristone	Glucocorticoid receptor antagonist	5–20 mg/kg/d	Symptomatic improvement in small numbers of patients	Nausea/vomiting, irregular menses	Acute symptomatic response; assessment of adrenal insufficiency on clinical grounds only.

ACTH, adrenocorticotropic hormone; LFT, liver function test.

Aminoglutethimide therapy inhibits the conversion of cholesterol to pregnenolone, the initial step of steroid hormone biosynthesis. It therefore decreases estrogen and aldosterone synthesis as well as that of cortisol and can also affect thyroid function. It is effective in more than 60% of patients, but it is commonly associated with rash and fever (18% of patients), as well as dizziness, somnolence, and lethargy in 30% and is generally not well tolerated (19). Its use has declined because of the preferred safety profiles of ketoconazole and metyrapone.

Mitotane is related to the pesticide DTT and blocks 11-β-hydroxylase and cholesterol side chain cleavage and causes adenolysis. In high doses, it induces a remission in 83% of patients, which is sustained after discontinuation in 30% of patients (19). However, in these doses, it is limited by gastrointestinal complaints and neurologic symptoms. In low doses, it is tolerated except for dramatic increases in low-density lipoprotein cholesterol, often up to twofold (90). It also affects cortisol metabolism and reduces urinary 17-hydroxycorticosteroids independent of its effects on cortisol, so clinical efficacy should always be monitored by 24-hour UFC determination.

In addition to agents that act at the adrenal gland, centrally active agents have been used in patients with Cushing's disease. Cyproheptadine is a central antiserotonergic agent that is reported to decrease ACTH secretion by an unknown mechanism (91). It is poorly tolerated because of somnolence, hyperphagia, and weight gain and generally not very efficacious in Cushing's syndrome, improving cortisol levels in only 30 to 50% of patients (19). Another centrally acting agent that has been used is bromocriptine, which has a 42% response rate, but it has been studied in only a few patients.

Mifepristone is a progesterone and glucocorticoid receptor antagonist that acts at the peripheral tissue level to block cortisol action. It has been reported to be highly efficacious in acutely reversing symptoms in a few patients (92). Monitoring for adrenal insufficiency cannot be done by cortisol levels and depends on clinical assessment. Likewise, glucocorticoid administration to treat adrenal insufficiency will be ineffective, and treatment must be with dose reduction.

Medical therapy to control hypercortisolemia is, unfortunately, unsatisfactory in most cases. Response rates can be poor, side effects are common and often limiting. With any of the available medications, the patient must be monitored for signs of adrenal insufficiency and treated with glucocorticoids and/or dosage reduction. Because of this, medical control of hypercortisolemia should be undertaken only in patients who are poor surgical candidates, in preparation for definitive surgery (for relief of extreme symptoms), or while awaiting results from pituitary irradiation. In these cases, ketoconazole or metyrapone are usually the drugs of choice, although mifepristone may be useful when it becomes clinically available.

POSTOPERATIVE MEDICAL MANAGEMENT

Postoperatively, patients who have been cured of Cushing's syndrome manifest profound glucocorticoid deficiency owing to suppression of normal corticotrophs and temporary ACTH deficiency. To avoid clinical adrenal insufficiency, "stress" doses of glucocorticoids are given the day of surgery, usually as intravenous hydrocortisone, 100 mg every 8 hours. This is switched to oral therapy as soon as tolerated and rapidly tapered to maintenance doses, usually 20 mg two to three times a day for the next 2 to 3 days. Patients routinely experience cortisol withdrawal symptoms, including fatigue, arthralgias, depression, and orthostatic symptoms. A more gradual taper of glucocorticoids during the next several weeks to months is done as tolerated by symptoms to allow recovery of the hypothalamic–pituitary adrenal axis. Periodic short ACTH-stimulation tests after withholding hydrocortisone therapy for 24 hours can be helpful to monitor this recovery, with adrenal responsiveness to ACTH recovered first and basal ACTH secretion later.

Acutely, diabetes insipidus may rarely be seen following TSS, and it is treated with free water replacement and subcutaneous desmopressin acetate (DDAVP) (which is switched to intranasal administration when allowed by surgical dressings). Diabetes insipidus is often temporary following TSS, and it is important to watch closely for signs of the "triple phase response" to avoid overtreatment with desmopressin acetate and resultant free water intoxication and hyponatremia.

Other pituitary deficiencies may rarely occur following TSS, and patients should be evaluated approximately 6 weeks after surgery with clinical and biochemical assessment of thyroid and gonadal status (resumption of menses, libido, and erectile function).

CONCLUSIONS

The diagnosis of Cushing's disease requires a careful and thoughtful stepwise approach. It begins with a clinical suspicion of the disease, often based on symptoms that are nonspecific and seen commonly in outpatient medical practices. Because of the low disease prevalence and the nonspecificity of symptoms, most patients suspected of having Cushing's syndrome do not have the disease. However, because of the significant morbidity and mortality associated with the syndrome, the physician must have a high index of suspicion and low threshold for screening.

The first and often most difficult step in the evaluation involves documentation of hypercortisolism and exclusion of pseudo-Cushing's syndrome. Measurement of 24-hour UFC excretion is the most accurate screening test but may be difficult because of patient compliance. The 1 mg dexamethasone overnight suppression test has excellent sensitivity, but suffers from poor specificity, necessitating confirmation of positive test results by a 24-hour UFC determination.

Establishing ACTH-dependent disease is the second step in the evaluation of Cushing's disease and involves measurement of a random plasma ACTH level. In equivocal cases, an ACTH level greater than 2 pmol/L (> 10 pg/mL) during a peripheral oCRH stimulation test clearly separates ACTH-dependent disease from ACTH-independent causes.

The final step involves proving a pituitary source of ACTH. Historically, low- and high-dose dexamethasone suppression tests have been used; however, they suffer from limited sensitivity and specificity. The presence of a pituitary lesion on MRI scanning is highly predictive of pituitary Cushing's disease, but of all the tests evaluated, only IPSS and CSS have demonstrated 100% diagnostic accuracy. In addition, IPSS and CSS provide fairly accurate intrapituitary localization data, which is useful in guiding surgical therapy.

Once diagnosed, the first choice of therapy is transsphenoidal resection, which is usually curative. Medical or surgical adrenalectomy may be temporizing or used in the case of surgical failure. Postoperative medical management involves treatment of secondary adrenal insufficiency and other pituitary deficiencies. These difficult diagnostic and therapeutic decisions are best made by an experienced team of neurosurgeons and endocrinologists.

REFERENCES

1. Reichlin S. Neuroendocrinology. In: Wilson JD, Foster DW, eds. Textbook of Endocrinology. 8th ed. Philadelphia: WB Saunders, 1992.
2. Bertagna X. Proopiomelanocortin-derived peptides. Endocrinol Metab Clin North Am 1994;23:467–485.
3. Holm IA, Majzoub JA. Adrenocorticotropin. In: Melmed S, ed. The Pituitary. Cambridge: Blackwell Science, 1995.
4. Orth DN, Kovacs WJ, DeBold CR. The adrenal cortex. In: Wilson JD, Foster DW, eds. Textbook of Endocrinology. 8th ed. Philadelphia: WB Saunders, 1992.
5. Newell-Price J, Perry L, Medbak S, et al. A combined test using desmopressin and corticotropin-releasing hormone in the differential diagnosis of Cushing's syndrome. J Clin Endocrinol Metab 1997;82:176–181.
6. Malerbi DA, Mendonca BB, Liberman B, et al. The desmopressin stimulation test in the differential diagnosis of Cushing's syndrome. Clin Endocrinol (Oxf) 1993;38:463–472.
7. Orth DN. Cushing's syndrome. N Engl J Med 1995;332:791–803.
8. Moreira AC, Foss MC, Iazigi N, et al. The effect of low-dose naloxone infusion on plasma ACTH and LH in patients with Cushing's and Addison's diseases. Horm Metab Res 1988;20:230–234.
9. Ambrosi B, Bochicchio D, Colombo P, et al. Loperamide to diagnose Cushing's syndrome. JAMA 1993;270:2301–2302.
10. Liu JH, Kazer RR, Rasmussen DD. Characterization of the twenty-four hour secretion patterns of adrenocorticotropin and cortisol in normal women and patients with Cushing's disease. J Clin Endocrinol Metab 1987;64:1027–1034.
11. Samuels MH, Brandon D, Isabel L, et al. Cortisol production rates in patients with suspected Cushing's syndrome. X International Congress of Endocrinology. San Francisco, June 1996.
12. Schlechte JA, Sherman B, Pfol B. A comparison of adrenal cortical function in patients with depressive illness and Cushing's disease. Horm Res 1986;23:1–8.
13. Papanicolaou DA, Yanovski JA, Cutler GB, et al. A single midnight serum cortisol measurement distinguishes Cushing's syndrome from pseudoCushing states. J Clin Endocrinal Metab 1998;83:1163–1167.
14. Wand GS, Dobs AS. Alterations in the hypothalamic-pituitary-adrenal axis in actively drinking alcoholics. J Clin Endocrinol Metab 1991;72:1290–1295.
15. Mortola JF, Liu JH, Gillin JC, et al. Pulsatile rhythms of adrenocorticotropin (ACTH) and cortisol in women with endogenous depression: evidence for increased ACTH pulse frequency. J Clin Endocrinol Metab 1987;65:962–968.
16. Reincke M, Allolio B, Wurth G, et al. The hypothalamic-pituitary-adrenal axis in critical illness: response to dexamethasone and corticotropin-releasing hormone. J Clin Endocrinol Metab 1993;77:151–156.
17. Kapcala LP. Alcohol-induced pseudo-Cushing's syndrome mimicking Cushing's disease in a patient with an adrenal mass. Am J Med 1987;82:849–856.
18. Linkowski P, Mendlewicz J, Kerkhofs M, et al. 24-hour profiles of adrenocorticotropin, cortisol and growth hormone in major depressive illness: effect of antidepressant treatment. J Clin Endocrinol Metab 1987;65:141–152.
19. Miller JW, Crapo L. The medical treatment of Cushing's syndrome. Endocr Rev 1993;14:443–458.
20. Kaye TB, Crapo L. The Cushing syndrome: an update on diagnostic tests. Ann Intern Med 1990;112:434–444.
21. Samuels MH. Cushing's syndrome associated with corticotroph hyperplasia. The Endocrinologist 1993;3:242–247.
22. Asa SL, Kovacs K, Melmed S. The hypothalamic-pituitary axis. In: Melmed S. The Pituitary. Cambridge: Blackwell Science, 1995.
23. Saeger W. Surgical pathology of the pituitary in Cushing's disease. Pathol Res Pract 1991;187:613–616.
24. Yamaji T, Ishibashi M, Teramoto A, et al. Hyperprolactinemia in Cushing's disease and Nelson's syndrome. J Clin Endocrinol Metab 1984;58:790–795.
25. Biller, BMK. Pathogenesis of pituitary Cushing's syndrome. Endocrinol Metab Clin North Am 1994;23:547–554.
26. Samuels MH, Loriaux, L. Cushing's syndrome and the nodular adrenal gland. Endocrinol Metab Clin North Am 1994;23:555–569.
27. Aron DC, Raff H, Findling JW. Effectiveness versus efficacy: the limited value in clinical practice of high dose dexamethasone suppression testing in the differential diagnosis of ACTH-dependent Cushing's syndrome. J Clin Endocrinol Metab 1997;82:1780–1785.
28. Danese RD, Aron DC. Principles of clinical epidemiology and their application to the diagnosis of Cushing's syndrome: Rev. Bayes meets Dr. Cushing. The Endocrinologist 1994;4:339–346.
29. Aron DC, Findling JW, Tyrrell JB. Cushing's disease. Endocrinol Metab Clin Am 1987;16:705–730.
30. Yanovski JA, Cutler GB. Glucocorticoid action and the clinical features of Cushing's syndrome. Endocrinol Metab Clin North Am 1994;23:487–509.
31. Ross EJ, Linch DC. Cushing's syndrome- killing disease: discriminatory value of signs and symptoms aiding early diagnosis. Lancet 1982;2:646–649.
32. Mampalam TJ, Tyrrell JB, Wilson CB. Transsphenoidal microsurgery for Cushing disease. Ann Intern Med 1988;109:487–493.
33. Wajchenberg BL, Bosco A, Marone MM, et al. Estimation of body fat and lean tissue distribution by dual energy X-ray absorptiometry and abdominal body fat evaluation by computed tomography in Cushing's disease. J Clin Endocrinol Metab 1995;80:2791–2794.
34. Adler RA, Rosen CJ. Glucocorticoids and osteoporosis. Endocrinol Metab Clin North Am 1994;23:641–654.
35. Magiakou MA, Mastorakos G, Oldfield EH, et al. Cushing's syndrome in children and adolescents. N Engl J Med 1994;331:629–636.
36. Nosadini R, Prato SD, Tiengo A, et al. Insulin resistance in Cushing's syndrome. J Clin Endocrinol Metab 1983;57:529–536.
37. Ulick S, Wang JZ, Blumenfeld JD, et al. Cortisol inactivation overload: a mechanism of mineralocorticoid hypertension in the ectopic adrenocorticotropin syndrome. J Clin Endocrinol Metab 1992;74:963–967.
38. Starkman MN, Schteingart DE. Neuropsychiatric manifestations of patients with Cushing's syndrome. Arch Intern Med 1981;141:215–219.
39. Graham BS, Tucker WS Jr. Opportunistic infections in endogenous Cushing's syndrome. Ann Intern Med 1984;101:334–338.
40. Saruta T, Suzuki H, Handa M, et al. Multiple factors contribute to the pathogenesis of hypertension in Cushing's syndrome. J Clin Endocrinol Metab 1986;62:275–279.
41. Ross NS. Epidemiology of Cushing's syndrome and subclinical disease. Endocrinol Metab Clin North Am 1994;23:539–546.
42. Etxabe J, Vasquez JA. Morbidity and mortality in Cushing's disease: an epidemiological approach. Clin Endocrinol 1994;40:479–484.
43. Reaven GM. Role of insulin resistance in human disease. Diabetes 1988;38:1495–1607.
44. Findling JW, Doppman JL. Biochemical and radiological diagnosis of Cushing's syndrome. Endocrinol Metab Clin North Am 1994;23:511–537.
45. Crapo L. Cushing's syndrome: a review of diagnostic tests. Metabolism 1979;28:955–977.
46. Sakiyama R, Ashcraft MW, van Herle AJ. Cyclic Cushing's syndrome. Am J Med 1984;77:944–946.
47. Sharp NA, Devlin JT, Rimmer JM. Renal failure obfuscates the diagnosis of Cushing's disease. JAMA 1986;256:2564–2565.
48. Trainer PJ, Grossman A. The diagnosis and differential diagnosis of Cushing's syndrome. Clin Endocrinol 1991;34:317–330.
49. Lu YR, Kuang AK, Chen JL, et al. Radioimmunoassay of salivary cortisol and its clinical applications. Chin Med J 1988;101:703–709.
50. Barrou Z, Guiban D, Maroufi A, et al. Overnight dexamethasone suppression test: comparison of plasma and salivary cortisol measurement for the screening of Cushing's syndrome. Eur J Endocrinol 1996;134:93–96.
51. Deuschle M, Schweiger U, Weber B, et al. Diurnal activity and pulsatility of the hypothalamus-pituitary-adrenal system in male depressed patients and healthy controls. J Clin Endocrinol Metab 1997;82:234–238.

52. Cook DM. Alcohol-induced pseudo-Cushing's syndrome. The Endocrinologist 1994;4:160–166.
53. Yanovski JA, Cutler GB, Chrousos CP, et al. The dexamethasone-suppressed corticotropin-releasing hormone stimulation test differentiates mild Cushing's disease from normal physiology. J Clin Endocrinol Metab 1998;83:348–352.
54. Anderson PW, Galmarini M, Vagnucci A, et al. Factitious Cushing's disease. West J Med 1993;159:487–489.
55. Loriaux DL, Nieman L. Corticotropin-releasing hormone testing in pituitary disease. Endocrinol Metab Clin North Am 1991;20:363–369.
56. Leinung MC, Young WF, Whitaker MD, et al. Diagnosis of corticotropin-producing bronchial carcinoid tumors causing Cushing's syndrome. Mayo Clin Proc 1990;65:1314–1321.
57. Cook DM, Loriaux DL. The incidental adrenal mass. The Endocrinologist 1996;6:4–9.
58. Liddle GW. Tests of pituitary-adrenal suppressibility in the diagnosis of Cushing's syndrome. J Clin Endocrinol Metab 1960;20:1539–1560.
59. Dichek HL, Nieman LK, Oldfield EH, et al. A comparison of the standard high dose dexamethasone suppression test and the overnight 8 mg dexamethasone suppression test for the differential diagnosis of adrenocorticotropin-dependent Cushing's syndrome. J Clin Endocrinol Metab 1994;78:418–422.
60. Tyrrell JB, Findling JW, Aron DC, et al. An overnight high-dose dexamethasone suppression test for rapid differential diagnosis of Cushing's syndrome. Ann Intern Med 1986;104:180–186.
61. Avgerinos PC, Yanovski JA, Oldfield EH, et al. The metyrapone and dexamethasone suppression tests for the differential diagnosis of the adrenocorticotropin-dependent Cushing syndrome: a comparison. Ann Intern Med 1994;121:318–327.
62. Flack MR, Oldfield EH, Cutler GB, et al. Urine free cortisol in the high dose dexamethasone suppression test for the differential diagnosis of the Cushing syndrome. Ann Intern Med 1992;116:211–216.
63. Ashcraft MW, van Herle AJ, Vener SL, et al. Serum cortisol levels in Cushing's syndrome after low- and high-dose dexamethasone suppression. Ann Intern Med 1982;97:21–26.
64. Oldfield EH, Doppman JL, Nieman LK, et al. Petrosal sinus sampling with and without corticotropin-releasing hormone for the differential diagnosis of Cushing's syndrome. N Engl J Med 1991;325:897–905.
65. Landolt AM, Schubiger O, Maurer R, et al. The value of inferior petrosal sinus sampling in diagnosis and treatment of Cushing's syndrome. Clin Endocrinol 1994;40:485–492.
66. Findling JW, Aron DC, Tyrrell JB, et al. Selective venous sampling for ACTH in Cushing's syndrome. Ann Intern Med 1981;94:647–652.
67. McCance DR, McIlrath E, McNeill A, et al. Bilateral inferior petrosal sinus sampling as a routine procedure in ACTH-dependent Cushing's syndrome. Clin Endocrinol 1989;30:157–166.
68. Miller DL, Doppman JL. Petrosal sinus sampling: technique and rationale. Radiology 1991;178:37–47.
69. Miller DL. Neurological complications of petrosal sinus sampling. Radiology 1992;183:878.
70. Midgette AS, Aron DC. High-dose dexamethasone suppression testing versus inferior petrosal sinus sampling in the differential diagnosis of adrenocorticotropin-dependent Cushing's syndrome: a decision analysis. Am J Med Sci 1995;309:162–170.
71. Yanovski JA, Cutler GB, Doppman JL, et al. The limited ability of inferior petrosal sinus sampling with corticotropin-releasing hormone to distinguish Cushing's disease from pseudo-Cushing states or normal physiology. J Clin Endocrinol Metab 1993;77:503–509.
72. Yamamoto Y, Davis DH, Nippoldt TB, et al. False-positive inferior petrosal sinus sampling in the diagnosis of Cushing's disease. J Neurosurg 1995;83:1087–1091.
73. Escourolle H, Abecassis JP, Bertagna X, et al. Comparison of computerized tomography and magnetic resonance imaging for the examination of the pituitary gland in patients with Cushing's disease. Clin Endocrinol 1993;39:307–313.
74. Hall WA, Luciano MG, Doppman JL, et al. Pituitary magnetic resonance imaging in normal human volunteers: occult adenomas in the general population. Ann Intern Med 1994;120:817–820.
75. de Herder WW, Uitterliniden P, Pieterman H, et al. Pituitary tumour localization in patients with Cushing's disease by magnetic resonance imaging: is there a place for petrosal sinus sampling? Clin Endocrinol 1994;40:87–92.
76. Oldfield EH, Girton ME, Doppman JL. Absence of intercavernous venous mixing: evidence supporting lateralization of pituitary microadenomas by venous sampling. J Clin Endocrinol Metab 1985;61:644–647.
77. Colao A, Merola B, Tripodi FS, et al. Simultaneous and bilateral inferior petrosal sinus sampling for the diagnosis of Cushing's syndrome: comparison of multihormonal assay, baseline multiple sampling and ACTH-releasing hormone test. Horm Res 1993;40:209–216.
78. Tabarin A, Greselle JF, San-Galli F, et al. usefulness of the corticotropin-releasing hormone test during bilateral inferior petrosal sinus sampling for the diagnosis of Cushing's disease. J Clin Endocrinol Metab 1991;73:53–59.
79. Graham KE, Samuels MH, Cook DM, et al. Cavernous sinus sampling (CSS) is superior to inferior petrosal sinus sampling (IPSS) in the evaluation of Cushing's syndrome. X International Congress of Endocrinology. San Francisco, June 1996.
80. Nesbit GM, Barnwell SL, Cook DM, et al. Variations in cavernous sinus venous drainage: its implication in petrosal and cavernous sinus sampling for evaluation of Cushing's disease. Western Neuroradiological Society Meeting. Coronado, October 1996.
81. Trainer PJ, Lawrie HS, Veerheist J, et al. Transsphenoidal resection in Cushing's disease: undetectable serum cortisol as the definition of successful treatment. Clin Endocrinol 1993;38:73–78.
82. Bochicchio D, Losa M, Buchfelder M. Factors influencing the immediate and late outcome of Cushing's disease treated by transsphenoidal surgery: a retrospective study by the European Cushing's Disease Survey Group. J Clin Endocrinol Metab 1995;80:3114–3120.
83. Raff H, Shaker JL, Seifert PE, et al. Intraoperative measurement of adrenocorticotropin (ACTH) during removal of ACTH-secreting bronchial carcinoid tumors. J Clin Endocrinol Metab 1995;80:1036–1038.
84. Graham KE, Samuels MH, Raff H, et al. Intraoperative adrenocorticotropin levels during transsphenoidal surgery for Cushing's disease do not predict cure. J Clin Endocrinol Metab 1997;82:1776–1779.
85. Burch W. A survey of results with transsphenoidal surgery in Cushing's disease. N Engl J Med 1983;308:103–104.
86. Laws ER Jr. Pituitary surgery. Endocrinol Metab Clin North Am 1987;6:647–665.
87. Weisnagel SJ, Gagner M, Breton G, et al. Laparoscopic adrenalectomy. The Endocrinologist 1996;6:169–178.
88. Estrada J, Boronat M, Mielgo M, et al. The long-term outcome of pituitary irradiation after unsuccessful transsphenoidal surgery in Cushing's disease. N Engl J Med 1997;336:172–177.
89. Fallo F, Paoletta A, Tona F, et al. Response of hypertension to conventional antihypertensive treatment and/or steroidogenesis inhibitors in Cushing's syndrome. J Intern Med 1993;234:595–598.
90. Trainer PJ, Besser M. Cushing's syndrome. Endocrinol Metab Clin North Am 1994;23:571–584.
91. Suda T, Tozawa F, Mouri T, et al. Effects of cyproheptadine, reserpine, and synthetic corticotropin-releasing factor on pituitary glands from patients with Cushing's disease. J Clin Endocrinol Metab 1983;56:1094–1098.
92. van der Lely AJ, Foeken K, van der Mast RC, et al. Rapid reversal of acute psychosis in the Cushing syndrome with the cortisol-receptor antagonist mifepristone (RU 486). Ann Intern Med 1991;114:143–144.

CHAPTER 14

Cushing's Disease: Operative Management

Marc S. Arginteanu and Kalmon D. Post

INTRODUCTION

The clinical state resulting from a chronic excess of cortisol is known as Cushing's syndrome. The usual manifestations of this endocrinologic imbalance, observed in more than half of the patients affected, includes centripetal obesity, hypertension, hypercholesterolemia, hirsutism, and psychological difficulties. Clinical features occurring in a smaller, but significant, percentage of patients include diabetes mellitus, osteoporosis, "moon" facies, myopathy, menstrual irregularities, atherosclerosis, headache, and dermatologic abnormalities (1–4).

Causes of Cushing's syndrome include ectopic production of adrenocorticotropic hormone (ACTH) or corticotropin releasing hormone (CRH) from various tumors, long-term administration of a supraphysiologic-dose corticosteriods, certain psychiatric illnesses, obesity, alcohol abuse, and inordinate cortisol production directly from the adrenal glands (5). ACTH hypersecretion from an intrasellar source is the most significant cause of Cushing's syndrome, accounting for 50 to 80% of cases, and it has been given the eponym Cushing's disease (6). Some patients with Cushing's disease have diffuse hyperplasia of the corticotropic cells of the pituitary gland. However, the preponderance of patients, between 70 and 90%, harbor a discrete ACTH-secreting pituitary adenoma (4, 6).

Despite recent advances, Cushing's disease remains a diagnostic and therapeutic challenge. The difficulties in diagnosis and medical management of this disorder have been described in a previous chapter. This chapter focuses on diagnostic tests that are required for surgical planning and operative management of Cushing's disease.

INDICATIONS FOR SURGERY

There are several indications for surgery on a lesion involving the pituitary. Chief among these indications are relief of mass effect on critical surrounding structures, establishment of a diagnosis, and control of endocrinopathy.

In the specific case of Cushing's disease, operative intervention is rarely needed for relief of mass effect. Macroadenomas account for few ACTH-secreting tumors. Most series report 5 to 9% of tumors to be greater than 1 cm in maximal diameter (1, 7–9). A few authors report a higher percentage of macroadenomas in their series: 13 to 21% (2, 10). Macroadenomas are in the minority because most

225

lesions become symptomatic, because of endocrinologic effects, while still minuscule in size.

The usual indication for surgery in patients with Cushing's disease is the control of hypercortisolism. The systemic effects of hypercortisolism were discussed earlier. If not abated, chronic hypercortisolism will result in an increased rate of disability and death. Thus, the main indications for operative intervention in patients with Cushing's disease are the inexorable, debilitating, and ultimately deadly effects of hypercortisolism (3). It is now widely accepted that the best chance to induce remission of Cushing's disease is resection of an ACTH-secreting adenoma (2).

PREOPERATIVE EVALUATION

The first step in evaluating a patient with clinical and laboratory evidence of hypercortisolemia is localizing the source of excess hormone production. This evaluation is detailed in a previous chapter, and elsewhere (6). In most cases, the preliminary aspects of this workup are performed before the patient reaches the neurosurgeon's office and the presumed origin of the malady has been localized to the pituitary gland.

Advanced imaging studies allow the characterization of an increasing percentage of pituitary microadenomas and virtually all macroadenomas (which are the minority of ACTH-secreting tumors). In addition, the need for angiography, with its attendant risks, to delineate tumor vascularity or the position of the carotid arteries has been virtually eliminated. The most common diagnostic studies ordered in the evaluation of Cushing's disease are computed tomography (CT) and magnetic resonance imaging (MRI).

High-resolution CT scans were interpreted as showing abnormality in 23 to 59% of cases of Cushing's disease in several series. Precise localization was possible in only 20 to 42% (1, 2, 6, 8–11). More disconcerting is the realization that perceived abnormalities on imaging studies may not represent the position of an adenoma. Incorrect lateralization of microadenomas by CT has been reported to be up to 14% (8). Incidental pituitary tumors have been found in up to 27% of nonselected patients studied at autopsy (4). In one study of 100 normal volunteers, contrast-enhanced MRI was performed to search for sellar lesions that might suggest adenoma. Ten percent of these asymptomatic persons harbored focal pituitary lesions measuring 3 to 6 mm in greatest diameter (12). This may be the cause of some such errors. Not surprisingly, previous operation or radiation renders CT less useful. In one series looking at such patients, adenoma was localized by CT in only 9% (13).

Routine MRI as part of the preoperative workup has improved both sensitivity and specificity for tumor location. Abnormalities seen in the sella are reported in 38 to 81% (2, 8, 10) of patients with Cushing's disease. Precise location may be detected in 33 to 70% of cases (8, 11, 14).

However, caution in interpretation still must be exercised, because incorrect lateralization also occurs with MRI (8, 14). If preoperative localization of the tumor is possible, it is a great aid to the surgeon in the exploration of the gland. However, in our experience, less than half of the patients with confirmed ACTH-secreting pituitary adenomas had definite MRI abnormalities. The indication for transsphenoidal exploration of the pituitary gland frequently must be based on biochemical data indicating a pituitary origin of ACTH hypersecretion causing hypercortisolism (7).

CT and MRI are indispensable for evaluation of structures contiguous with the pituitary gland. Invasion of the cavernous sinus or parasellar tissues by tumor may be noted (Fig. 14.1). This will change the operative plan, as will be discussed later. The anatomy of the sphenoid sinus should be evaluated carefully. An incompletely pneumatized sphenoid sinus is sometimes seen, more frequently in children, and may necessitate some drilling to accomplish a transsphenoidal approach (8). Septations of the sphenoid sinus should also be noted (Fig. 14.2). They may fortuitously act as a guide to a radiographically visible tumor. Conversely, if the intraoperative dissection relative to a sphenoid septation is not carefully noted, the patient's midline may be misinterpreted. One cell of a septated sinus may remain unentered. This could result in opening the anterior wall of the sella in a far lateral position, endangering the cavernous sinus, cranial nerves, and carotid artery. Alternatively, in this situation, the contralateral portion of the sella may remain unexplored, and tumor may be missed (13).

Many patients with ACTH-secreting pituitary adenomas have normal results of imaging studies. In these cases, it is imperative that further tests be performed to confirm the diagnosis of Cushing's disease before surgery is considered. If endocrinologic studies are diagnostic for Cushing's syn-

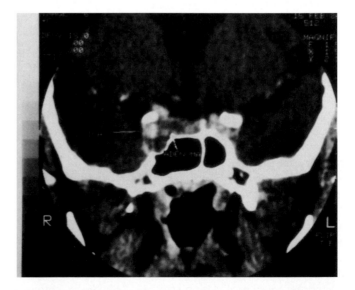

Figure 14.1. Coronal CT scan with intravenous contrast demonstrating an ACTH-secreting pituitary tumor invading the right cavernous sinus.

the pituitary gland in which a tumor is located (Fig. 14.4). IPSS has been reported to give correct lateralization in 54 to 76% of patients (8, 15, 30). This test might help guide the surgeon intraoperatively. If no discrete tumor is found during operative exploration, it may suggest which side of the gland to remove. One caveat is that false lateralization has been reported in 8 to 31% of patients (2, 8) and no lateralization has been reported in 15% of patients (8).

IPSS is also routinely used after a histologically negative exploration of the gland with persistent hypercortisolism, if it was not performed preoperatively, to reassure the physician that a pituitary source for hypercortisolism exists (4, 8).

CRITERIA IN CHOOSING THE APPROACH

The choice of approach is dictated by the radiographically determined location of the tumor. In most cases of Cushing's disease, an adenoma is either not visible on scan or is wholly intrasellar (Fig 14.5). In these cases, transsphenoidal exploration of the gland, with the aim of selective adenomectomy, is the appropriate surgical procedure.

It is unusual, in patients with Cushing's disease, to see a macroadenoma with supradiaphragmatic extension. Most tumors of this type should also be approached via the transsphenoidal route. A debulking, or total resection, should be attempted. Any remaining tumor may descend into the sella during the first few months postoperatively, allowing for completion of resection during a delayed second stage. A suprasellar extension of tumor that the surgeon believes

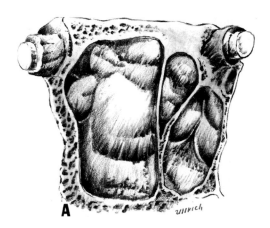
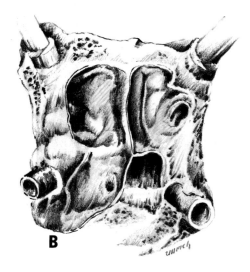

Figure 14.2. Diagrammatic illustration of two different patterns of sphenoid sinus septation that might be encountered during the transsphenoidal approach to a pituitary adenoma.

drome but an adenoma is poorly visualized on CT and MRI, inferior petrosal sinus sampling (IPSS) can be used to corroborate a pituitary source for ACTH hypersecretion (4). In this procedure, bilateral femoral veins are catheterized. Under fluoroscopic guidance, the catheters are then navigated into the inferior petrosal sinuses (Fig. 14.3). The physician thus may sample the effluent from the cavernous sinuses. The ACTH level in this blood sample is compared with the ACTH level in a blood sample drawn at a peripheral site. A central:peripheral ACTH ratio of greater than 2:1 is 86 to 90% sensitive and almost 100% specific for Cushing's disease (2, 30). The accuracy of this test has been improved by adding CRH stimulation to the testing protocol (16, 17). Administration of CRH, with a central: peripheral corticotropin ratio of greater than 3:1, improves the sensitivity to greater than 95% and retains excellent specificity (30). The advanced imaging studies currently available, used in conjunction with IPSS, have reduced the incidence of sellar explorations for the ectopic source of ACTH production (2).

IPSS has also been used to aid in localizing the side of

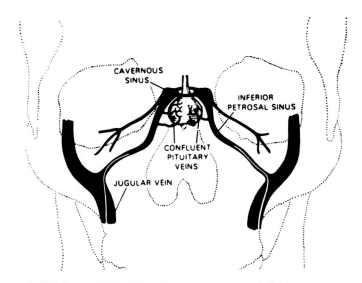

Figure 14.3. Diagrammatic illustration of catheters being guided into bilateral inferior petrosal sinuses for simultaneous blood sampling. (Reproduced with permission from Oldfield EH, Chrousos GP, Schulte HM, et al. Preoperative lateralization of ACTH-secreting pituitary microadenomas by bilateral and simultaneous inferior petrosal sinus sampling. N Engl J Med 1985;312: 100–103.)

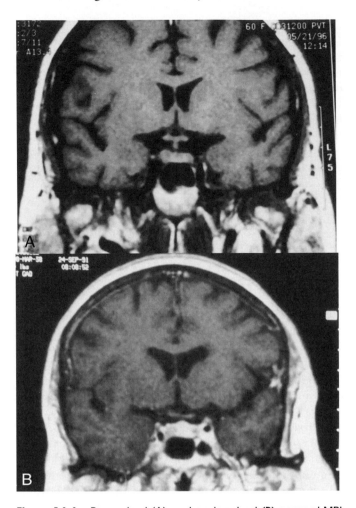

Figure 14.4. Precontrast **(A)** and postcontrast **(B)** coronal MRI demonstrating bilateral microadenomas in a patient with Cushing's disease. IPSS was performed preoperatively and indicated that the ACTH-secreting tumor was on the left side of the gland. This was confirmed pathologically.

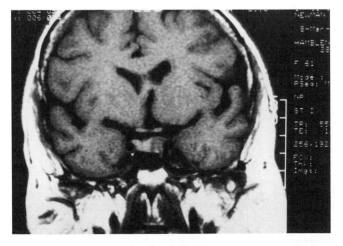

Figure 14.5. Coronal MRI demonstrating a pituitary adenoma that would be amenable to transsphenoidal resection.

will not descend into the sella with time may be approached via a craniotomy, using the pterional or subfrontal route.

Macroadenomas with a large extrasellar component, or any size tumor that invades the bone, dura, or cavernous sinus, are unlikely to be cured by transsphenoidal microsurgery alone (2). In fact, the likelihood of cure from any surgical therapy is low in these cases. If hypercortisolism persists postoperatively, adjuvant therapy needs to be used.

Aggressive surgery is sometimes warranted to achieve maximal cytoreduction (making a lesion more amenable to radiotherapy) or to attempt total resection in the face of failed adjuvant therapy. This strategy involves a craniotomy alone or combined with a transsphenoidal approach. The type of craniotomy is dictated by the location of the extrasellar tumor. For example, a lateral extension of tumor into the cavernous sinus may warrant a staged procedure. The intrasellar component may be resected via the transsphenoidal route followed by a skull base approach for cavernous sinus tumor resection.

Another indication for craniotomy, which is rarely invoked, is technical difficulties precluding successful exploration of the pituitary gland during the attempted transsphenoidal approach (2).

SURGICAL TIPS

The various approaches to the pituitary gland are described elsewhere in this text. Thus, specific details of the procedure and operating room setup are not discussed here.

We carry out our transsphenoidal approach with the patient in the supine position. A sublabial skin incision is usually used. Care should be taken to keep the incision in soft areolar tissue, about 1 cm above the incisors. This will minimize the incidence of numbness of the teeth. A transnasal approach is reserved for patients with previous nasal surgery or complex septal perforations and those with unusual occupations such as musicians who use their lips to play instruments. Fluoroscopy confirms the trajectory to the sella.

Our goal in surgery, during the initial operative intervention, is identification and selective resection of the ACTH-secreting adenoma. The goal during reoperation for recurrence or remission is detailed in the next section. An ACTH-secreting adenoma is usually distinct from the normal pituitary gland, facilitating its identification. It is often pale gray or white in color. In addition, the tumor is usually soft to semiliquid and easily suckable, in contrast to the firm consistency of the normal gland.

The dura is opened by resecting a rectangular window. Often there are troublesome, large venous channels in the dura that must be controlled. This is accomplished either by tamponade with a commercial preparation of oxidized cellulose or by coagulation using a Hardy or Landolt bipolar instrument. These channels may begin to bleed again during further dissection, but patience will allow the sur-

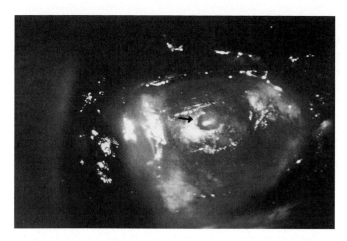

Figure 14.6. A small microadenoma is seen on the surface of the pituitary gland (*arrow*).

geon to obtain good hemostasis. This is essential, as the surgery must be performed under direct visualization.

After dural opening we perform a thorough exploration of the surface of the gland (Fig. 14.6), including the posterior portion of the gland. A painstaking investigation of the gland is mandatory before resection to avoid ablation of normal tissue, if possible. If no tumor is readily apparent on the surface of the gland, vertical incisions are made in the lateral wings of the gland, beginning on the side suggested by IPSS. If tumor is not seen there, a midline vertical incision is made and carried to the posterior gland. The search for tumor might then continue with a horizontal incision across the gland. If the search had thus far been fruitless, the junction of the stalk and the gland is inspected with small dissectors in the search for the tumor. If no tumor can be found, we perform a hemihypophysectomy guided by preoperative imaging or IPSS. If these are conflicting, or nondiagnostic, we often will resect the lateral one-third of the gland on both sides (after the careful midline search outlined above). Although Hardy (18) and Fahlbusch et al. (9) have reported that most tumors arise in the center of the gland, Chandler et al. (1) and Boggan et al. (19) have demonstrated that an adenoma will more often arise in the lateral wings of the pituitary. Recently, some authors have described the use of intraoperative ultrasound to aid in the detection of microadenomas (20, 21). Although not clinically useful at the present time, this technique may prove helpful in the future in locating difficult-to-find microadenomas.

After resection of a discrete adenoma, we carefully evaluate the gland around it visually and with tactile feedback. If there is any suggestion of abnormality, we resect a small cuff of peritumoral tissue. Regrowth of adenoma has been reported in a tumor bed that appeared clean at the time of surgery (5, 22). This suggests that viable tumor cells remain behind in some cases of seemingly noninvasive ACTH-secreting microadenoma. We have, at times, resected an area of normal-appearing tissue around an adenoma. In these cases pathologic examination of the peritumoral tissue did not demonstrate tumor, only Crooke's changes.

A more aggressive or more conservative resection may be indicated, depending on the clinical situation. In an elderly or seriously debilitated patient, without a readily apparent adenoma, it may be appropriate to perform complete hypophysectomy as the primary procedure. This might minimize the number of times a fragile patient would need to undergo general anesthesia. During adenomectomy in the growing child or young woman of childbearing age we try to spare as much normal tissue as possible. The reticence to resect excess pituitary in young adults and children is shared by others (2).

After the resection has been completed without entry into the cerebrospinal fluid space, we use pure ethanol as an aid in hemostasis. A portion of the vomer resected during the approach is used to repair the broached anterior sellar wall. Any evidence of communication of cerebrospinal fluid with the sella mandates intrasellar packing in addition to obliteration of the sphenoid by fat. If the cerebrospinal fluid communication is small (a few drops over the surface of the gland), we use only fat. If the opening is large (as in some cases of hypophysectomy), we use fascia lata in addition to fat, both in the sella and in the sphenoid sinus.

Nasal packing is maintained for 2 days postoperatively. In the perioperative period, corticosteroids and prophylactic antibiotics are administered. Some authors have reported withholding steroids intraoperatively and postoperatively (8). Their goal is to test serum cortisol level the next morning to determine cure or failure. If this strategy is chosen, vigilance for addisonian crisis must be maintained.

We find reports of frozen pathologic specimens to be unreliable, and we usually do not use them to guide our resection. False-negative and false-positive reports on frozen section have been documented to be up to 12 and 6% of cases, respectively (1). A false-positive report may lead the surgeon to do an inadequate sellar exploration, leaving tumor behind. A false-negative report may lead the surgeon to resect normal tissue after the offending lesion, in actuality, had already been ablated. In many cases, the volume of pathologic tissue is so small that we choose not to "waste" it on a frozen section study, protecting all abnormal-appearing tissue for permanent study. Special care is taken not to lose any of the specimen in the suction. We do not rely on suction traps, rather we keep the suction some distance from the specimen.

COMPLICATIONS

The incidence of postoperative complications reported by various authors shows that transsphenoidal resection of ACTH-secreting adenomas is a relatively safe procedure. The mortality ranged from 0 to 3.6%, with most series reporting less than 1% (1, 2, 7–10). Cerebrospinal fluid fistulas occurred in 0 to 8% of patients in series in which it was recorded (7–10). This required surgical repair in less than 2% of cases (2, 8). Meningitis was reported in 2.8 to 5.3% of patients (9, 10). Transient cranial nerve deficits were caused by the procedure in 0 to 1.8% of patients, with permanent deficits reported in none (7, 9).

Permanent endocrinologic complications after primary surgery for adenomectomy, or even hemihypophysectomy, are infrequent. The ability of an affected young woman to successfully become pregnant after operation is frequently noted (9). After attempted selective adenomectomy, partial anterior lobe dysfunction was reported to be 0 to 14%, with panhypopituitarism in 0 to 4% (8, 9). Transient diabetes insipidus has been noted in 30 to 48% (7, 9) of patients. It should be noted that Cushing's disease promotes total body fluid retention. Therefore, patients who undergo successful removal of adenoma may have large urine outputs without having diabetes insipidus (3). Permanent diabetes insipidus is incurred in 1.8 to 18% of patients (1, 2, 8, 9). As expected, patients who were subjected to reoperation had a greater likelihood, up to 45%, of having endocrinologic problems (8). Furthermore, those subjected to complete hypophysectomy require lifelong hormonal replacement.

Some of the problems caused by chronic hypercortisolism put the patient at a higher risk for surgery than individuals undergoing transsphenoidal surgery for other functioning microadenomas (9). The incidence of serious complications such as meningitis or perioperative mortality is higher in patients with Cushing's than in those undergoing transsphenoidal operation for unselected pituitary adenomas (23). The combined clinical manifestations of Cushing's disease puts the patients at a 1 to 2% risk of perioperative myocardial infarction and increased risk for perioperative infection (3). Excessive bleeding is often encountered in this group, preventing adequate exploration in some patients (2, 7).

MANAGEMENT OF RECURRENT AND PERSISTENT DISEASE

After successful removal of a discrete pituitary adenoma, serum and urine cortisol concentrations usually fall to a low level. Many authors have observed that these patients require several months, up to a year, of steroid replacement therapy until they return, gradually, to normal pituitary–adrenal function (9, 10, 22, 24). This protracted period of hypocortisolemia should be looked on as an indication that the surgery was successful in inducing remission of disease. In fact, early recovery of the hypothalamic–pituitary axis is often the harbinger of recurrent disease (10). Postadenomectomy hypocortisolism is accompanied by a hypocorticotropic state, suggesting suppression of the remainder of the pituitary by the excess cortisol that had been produced by the adenoma.

An endocrinologic assessment of the patient should be made between 1 week and a few months after surgery (1, 7, 22). Persistent disease is diagnosed by plasma and urine cortisol levels not being decreased significantly from preoperative values, along with clinical stigmata. Abnormal endocrinologic test results in the first postoperative assessment will usually indicate a significant amount of residual functioning tumor. The surgeon must then review the patient's workup, the operative findings, and the pathologic specimen with the following scenarios in mind:

1. If a hypophysectomy was performed, and the pathologic specimens reveal adenoma cells, there is probably invasion of the cavernous sinus or surrounding dura (in addition to the tumor in the removed specimen) that accounts for the sustained excess of hormone. The surgeon must then review the preoperative films to see if this additional tumor might be removed surgically. This type of two-stage procedure was described earlier. If remaining tumor is seen but is not surgically accessible, radiation therapy should be offered to the patient for disease control. The possibility of metastatic Cushing's disease, although rare, should be kept in mind.

2. If a hypophysectomy was performed, and the pathologic specimens fail to demonstrate any tumor, then one must suspect another cause of Cushing's syndrome. A careful search should be made for a possible ectopic source. If IPSS had not initially been performed, it should be performed at this time. Other causes of Cushing's syndrome related to structures around the sellar region, such as totally supradiaphragmatic pituitary adenomas, have been described (5, 25). Pseudo-Cushing's syndrome caused by alcoholism or depression should also be reconsidered (13).

   In some cases, the hypophysectomy may not be total, and tumor may be left behind with residual gland. Chandler et al. (1) noted the difficulty, on occasion, of assuring complete sellar exenteration. Boggan et al. (19) admonish against incomplete sellar exenteration. They cite the ability of the tumor to grow in unusual locations in the anterior and posterior portions of the gland (1). ACTH hypersecretion from an adenoma in the pars intermedia has been described (26). In addition, a CRH-secreting hypothalamic tumor may be acting on residual normal-appearing tissue (5, 25).

   The patient may be maintained on medical therapy, such as ketoconazole (27). After 6 to 12 weeks, when the initial postoperative changes have settled down, a repeat MRI should be performed to assess the sella and parasellar area. If a clearly accessible tumor is seen, reoperation is indicated. If an ectopic source is found, it should be addressed. If invasive tumor is found, not amenable to surgical extirpation, radiation should be offered to the patient.

3. If a partial hypophysectomy was performed, and tumor is found in the specimen, there is probably tumor left in the sellar area. A few explanations exist. It is possible

that partial resection of a single adenoma was performed. Multiple adenomas (or a multifocal adenoma) may be present (5), only one of which was resected. There may be invasion of surrounding tissue by tumor. The patient should be maintained on medical therapy until adequate images of the area can be performed. If the treating physicians believe that there is surgically accessible tumor remaining, then the patient should undergo reoperation. Most often this would be partial to complete hypophysectomy. If invasion into the contiguous dura or cavernous sinus is seen, radiation therapy is indicated.

4. If a partial hypophysectomy was performed or a presumed microadenoma was removed but results of pathologic examination revealed no tumor, there are two likely possibilities. There may be a distinct adenoma in the remaining portion of the gland. Otherwise, an extrasellar source of ACTH may exist. A reevaluation should proceed as outlined in the section in this chapter entitled "Preoperative Evaluation." In many cases, reexploration of the gland is indicated. Ram et al. (28) reviewed their experience with 222 patients with Cushing's disease focusing on the 13% with persistent hypercortisolism. Their strategy was early reoperation in most of these patients. They were able to induce remission at the second operation in 70% of these patients (28). Thus, a more aggressive resection, i.e., total hypophysectomy, is often warranted in an attempt to induce remission.

5. If an adenoma was removed, proven by pathologic specimen, several possibilities exist: multiple adenomas in the pituitary gland, remaining tumor in the bed, or invasion into surrounding structures. Reevaluation and further therapy should proceed as outlined above.

6. If the removed tissue appears, pathologically, to contain diffuse hyperplasia of corticotrophic cells, the entire gland will probably be involved in this process. The patient should undergo complete hypophysecetomy in an attempt to cure the disease. This is the cause of Cushing's disease in less than 10% of patients (4). Sometimes the intraoperative impression is that of a discrete microadenoma, only later to be proven pathologically to be hyperplasia. Early reoperation in these cases may result in sustained remission (10).

If the early endocrinologic assessment demonstrates low serum and urinary cortisol levels, the patient should be retested at regular intervals postoperatively. A significant percentage of patients, 2 to 14%, initially in remission will have recurrence of disease (2, 4, 7, 10). Recurrence may take place after many years of remission (2). The decision-making process for further therapy is similar to that described above. The additional factor that must be considered, however, is regrowth of adenoma (22). If localized within the sella, re-

growth of adenoma is best treated by reoperation for resection. Invasion of surrounding structures may be found on imaging studies. In these cases, radiation therapy should be used, either alone or in conjunction with reoperation, for resection of accessible tumor.

Reexploration of the sella in the face of recurrent or persistent disease will often be fruitful. Friedman et al. (13), in a study of reoperation for residual or recurrent disease, induced a remission in 73% of 33 patients treated in this manner. If a discrete adenoma is found, selective adenomectomy will likely result in a sustained remission. Friedman et al. were able to induce remission in 95% of this type of patient. Patients do not fare as well if no discrete tumor is found, however. This subgroup of patients had only a 41% rate of remission after reexploration.

Pituitary irradiation is the chief modality of adjuvant therapy used to achieve remission in cases of Cushing's disease not responding to surgical therapy alone. The introduction of stereotactic radiotherapy has increased the efficacy and safety of this treatment. If pituitary irradiation is performed, patients must take adrenostatic medication until the effects are seen (8). The effects of radiotherapy may not be maximally seen for 5 to 10 years (3). Radiotherapy alone will induce remission in about 20% of adults with Cushing's disease using standard techniques (13) and in about 76% using stereotactic radiosurgical techniques. Either type of radiotherapy results in some degree of panhypopituitarism in 50 to 55% of patients (13, 29).

Bilateral adrenalectomy is only used when all other measures fail (2, 8). There is a reported operative mortality of 4% for the procedure, and a 10% incidence of Nelson's syndrome. Nelson's syndrome is characterized by continued growth of a pituitary adenoma after bilateral adrenalectomy, with progressive sellar enlargement and extreme elevations in ACTH levels (31). Patients with Nelson's syndrome have been noted to have worsening headaches, visual field deficits, oculomotor palsies, and hyperpigmentation (31, 32). Even after this procedure, Cushing's syndrome can recur from growth of adrenal rests or remnants (3).

LONG-TERM RESULTS AND OUTCOME

In most large series, a remission of hypercortisolism can be induced in between 70 and 86% of patients (1, 2, 6, 7, 9, 10, 22, 28, 29). If a discrete microadenoma was seen, the results improved further, with a remission rate of 88 to 91% (1, 2, 10). Treatment failures are defined, for the purposes of this discussion, as those patients not cured, and believed not to be curable, by surgery alone. One reported cause for failure is invasive tumor. This was seen in 12% of patients in one series (6). Other common causes cited for treatment failure were an ectopic source of ACTH, seen in 1.6 to 6% of patients (1, 2, 6, 22), and misdiagnosis (e.g., depression or alcoholism masquerading as Cushing's disease [5, 10]). A closer look at some of the recent large series is warranted.

Tindall and coworkers (10) recently reported their results in the management of Cushing's disease between 1977 and 1988. They operated via a transsphenoidal route in all of their patients. They performed selective adenomectomy if possible, otherwise they performed partial or total hypophysectomy. Remission was obtained in 85% of the 53 patients they had good follow-up data on (the preponderance of patients greater than 1 year). On subdivision of the results, they found a remission rate of 91% in patients with presumed microadenomas, 86% with macroadenomas, and none of those patients with diffuse corticotropic hyperplasia. They report recurrence in 2% of their patients, and 13% of patients never achieved normalization of serum cortisol level. The reasons they cited for surgical failure were (a) missing all or part of the tumor and (b) resecting what they initially thought was a tumor but turned out to be hyperplasia. These cases were later treated by complete hypophysectomy. Invasive tumor or an ectopic source of ACTH also resulted in surgical failure. This group relied on bilateral adrenalectomy to address this issue.

Mampalam et al. (2) reviewed a series of 216 patients who had transsphenoidal microsurgery for Cushing's disease between 1974 and 1986. The average length of follow-up in this series was 3.9 years. Of those patients, 2.3% were eventually found to have an ectopic source of ACTH production. One percent of patients had diffuse hyperplasia of the corticotrophs. This group achieved a 79% remission rate overall. In these successful cases, the procedure performed was selective adenomectomy in 87% of cases, total hypophysectomy in 9% of cases, and partial hypophysectomy or biopsy only in 4% of cases. Recrudescence of hypercortisolism was seen in 5% of these cases an average of 3.8 years after primary surgery. The remission rate was better, in a statistically significant fashion, in patients with microadenomas compared with those with macroadenomas, and in tumors totally intrasellar compared with those with extension into the cavernous sinus or parasellar dura. If an adenoma was removed, and pathologically confirmed, their remission rate was 88%.

Carpenter (6) reviewed the series of patients with presumed Cushing's disease operated on at the Mayo Clinic between 1973 and 1986. They had an overall remission rate of about 80% in 183 patients. Three treatment failures (1.6%) were subsequently found to have ectopic ACTH production. Three patients had repeat operations. Two of these had persistent hypercortisolism after the first procedure. The other patient had a recurrence 8 years after the initial surgery. These authors found that two-thirds of the patients who had recurrence or persistence of their disease had invasion of their tumors into adjacent structures. Some patients with persistence of disease had diffuse or nodular hyperplasia of corticotrophic cells. This group treated two documented recurrences with pituitary irradiation, which resulted in sustained remission.

Chandler et al. (1) reviewed their operative experience between 1980 and 1985. During this period, they operated on 34 patients with Cushing's syndrome. Of this group, 26% had been treated previously by irradiation, adrenalectomy, mitotane administration, or previous surgery. Remission was induced in 74% of patients. This was further broken down, with remission in 88% of patients with presumed microadenomas and only 33% of patients harboring macroadenomas. An ectopic source of ACTH was found in 6% of patients subsequent to negative intrasellar explorations.

Guilhaume et al. (7) reviewed their experience with patients suffering from Cushing's disease treated between 1978 and 1985. They had a median follow-up period of 2 years for the 64 patients reviewed. This group reported a 70% initial cure rate. Of the patients who were reported as successes initially, 14% had recurrence during the follow-up period.

Fahlbusch et al. (9) reviewed their experience in treating Cushing's disease. They performed transsphenoidal pituitary exploration on 101 patients, the bulk of which they operated on between 1976 and 1984. Clinical and endocrinologic remission was reported in 74% of patients. Some patients with persistent disease were put into remission by subsequent tumor resection, for an overall rate of 77%. During follow-up, ranging between 8 months and 14 years, 7% of these patients had recurrence. This group relied heavily on adrenalectomy for treatment failures.

Nakane et al. (22) induced a remission in 86% of 100 patients treated for Cushing's disease by transsphenoidal resection of tumor. During follow-up for a mean of 38 months, 9% of these initially cured patients had recurrence. Reoperation for recurrent microadenoma was performed in all cases and was followed by irradiation if invasive tendencies were found. Invasive macroadenomas were treated by attempted resection, followed by irradiation for persistent or recurrent disease. In 7% of cases, no tumor was found on exploration, and partial or total hypophysectomy failed to improve hypercortisolism. In two of these patients, an ectopic source was eventually located.

CUSHING'S DISEASE IN CHILDREN

Pediatric patients with Cushing's disease deserve separate consideration. Children and adolescents account for 13 to 15% of patients undergoing surgery in large series of Cushing's disease (2, 8). The pituitary gland has a central role in a child's normal somatic and sexual growth and development. A finely tuned and poorly understood series of events needs to occur to ensure the success of these processes. Children often present for evaluation with growth retardation, seen in more than 80% of patients, and increase in weight, seen in more than 90% of patients. They will frequently be hypertensive and may have psychiatric disturbances (30).

Transsphenoidal selective adenomectomy, if possible, offers the best chance at cure with the best chance of allowing normal development to proceed. Successful selective removal of tumor may enable "catch-up" growth, or a resumption of normal growth, in 73% of patients (9).

Magiakou et al. (30) reviewed their experience in treating childhood Cushing's disease at the National Institutes of Health between 1982 and 1992. Remission of hypercortisolism was attained in 48 of the 49 patients who underwent transsphenoidal surgery (30). Another group, Knapp and Ludecke (8), recently reported their experience with a series of 55 pediatric patients suffering from Cushing's disease. The patients ranged in age from 4 to 19 years. The primary modality of therapy used by this group was selective surgical extirpation of the tumor. They identified, and removed, discrete adenomas in 88% of their patients and tumorous tissue in another 10%. They failed to find tumor on initial exploration in only one patient. They subsequently brought this child back to surgery for reexploration and successfully removed a tumor. This group believes in early surgical reexploration for persistent hypercortisolism. Practicing the strategy outlined above, they report a remarkable 96% rate of remission of hypercortisolism, with a 100% remission rate when early reexploration is included. Haddad et al. (36) achieved control of hypercortisolism in all five cases of pediatric Cushing's disease treated by their group. The admirable rates of control of hypercortisolism compare favorably to most large series of adult patients with Cushing's disease (1, 2, 6, 7, 9, 10, 22, 29). One group believes that the discrepancy in remission rates suggests that pediatric ACTH-secreting adenomas are more often noninvasive and well localized compared with those of adults (36).

Recurrence of hypercortisolism has been reported in 0 to 32% of patients (8, 24, 30–33). Many tumors recurred after 7 years (24, 33). If possible, a recurrent tumor should be selectively removed. If it is localizable to one part of the gland, but a discrete adenoma is not encountered, a partial hypophysectomy may also be performed. If remission of hypercortisolism is not induced by partial hypophysectomy, consideration should be given to radiation therapy. A complete hypophysectomy in the child or young woman of childbearing age should be avoided.

Some physicians are proponents of radiation therapy as primary treatment for pediatric Cushing's disease. An initial success rate of 80% has been reported (34). Use of stereotactic radiosurgical techniques may increase the remission rate to 88% (35). Delayed onset of hypopituitarism (especially diminished growth hormone) and late recurrences have dampened enthusiasm for the procedure (8, 35–37). We believe that radiation in the child is not a first-line therapy.

Adrenalectomy should be reserved for patients who have failed all other modalities of medical and surgical treatment. Nelson's syndrome, described earlier, has been noted to be a more frequent sequelae of bilateral adrenalectomy in children than in adults (2, 8, 35).

CONCLUSIONS

The treatment of choice for Cushing's disease is transsphenoidal microsurgery for selective resection of a pituitary tumor. This has been demonstrated to be a safe and effective procedure. Remission of hypercortisolism can be attained in most cases. The primary difficulty encountered in achieving this end is localization of the responsible microadenoma. Advances in imaging and adjunctive tests, such as IPSS, have made localization of tumor possible in a larger percentage of cases. Recurrent or persistent disease should be managed with reoperation if surgical cure is a possibility. Radiation therapy should be reserved for invasive tumors and other surgical failures. Adrenalectomy should be performed only as a last resort.

REFERENCES

1. Chandler WF, Schteingart DE, Lloyd RV, et al. Surgical treatment of Cushing's disease. J Neurosurg 1987;66(2):204–212.
2. Mampalam TJ, Tyrrell JB, Wilson CB. Transsphenoidal microsurgery for Cushing's disease: a report of 216 cases. Ann Intern Med 1988;109(6):487–493.
3. Yanovski JA, Cutler GB. Cushing's disease: medical treatment. In: Cooper PR, ed. Neurosurgical Topics: Contemporary Diagnosis and Management of Pituitary Adenomas. Park Ridge, IL: AANS, 1991.
4. Post KD, Habas J. Cushing's disease: results of operative treatment. In: Cooper PR, ed. Neurosurgical Topics: Contemporary Diagnosis and Management of Pituitary Adenomas. Park Ridge, IL: AANS, 1991.
5. Laws ER. Comments on: Nakane T, Kuwayama A, Watanabe M, Takahashi T, Kato T, Ichihara K, Kageyama N. Long term results of transsphenoidal adenomectomy in patients with Cushing's disease. Neurosurgery 1987;21(2):218–222.
6. Carpenter PC. Cushing's syndrome: update of diagnosis and management. Mayo Clin Proc 1986;61(1):49–58.
7. Guilhaume B, Bertagna X, Thomsen M, et al. Transsphenoidal pituitary surgery for the treatment of Cushing's disease: results in 64 patients and long term follow-up studies. J Clin Endocrinol Metab 1988;66(5):1056–1064.
8. Knapp UJ, Ludecke DK. Transnasal microsurgery in children and adolescents with Cushing's disease. Neurosurgery 1996;39:484–493.
9. Fahlbusch R, Buchfelder M, Muller OA. Transsphenoidal surgery for Cushing's disease. J R Soc Med 1986;79(5):262–269.
10. Tindall GT, Herring CJ, Clark RV, et al. Cushing's disease: results of transsphenoidal microsurgery with emphasis on surgical failures. J Neurosurg 1990;72(3):363–369.
11. Buchfelder M, Nistor R, Fahlbusch R, et al. The accuracy of CT and MR evaluation of the sella turcica for detection of adrenocorticotropic hormone-secreting adenomas in Cushing disease. AJNR Am J Neuroradiol 1993;14(5):1183–1190.
12. Hall WA, Luciano MG, Doppman JL, et al. Pituitary magnetic resonance imaging in normal human volunteers: occult adenomas in the general population. Ann Intern Med 1994;120(10):817–820.
13. Friedman RB, Oldfield EH, Nieman LK, et al. Repeat transsphenoidal surgery for Cushing's disease. J Neurosurg 1989;71(4):520–527.
14. Peck WW, Dillon WP, Norman D, et al. High-resolution MR imaging of pituitary microadenomas at 1.5 T: experience with Cushing disease. AJR Am J Roentgenol 1989;152(1):145–151.
15. Landolt AM, Schubiger O, Maurer R, et al. The value of inferior

petrosal sinus sampling in diagnosis and treatment of Cushing's disease. Clin Endocrinol (Oxf) 1994;40(4):485–492.

16. Zarrilli L, Colao A, Merola B, et al. Corticotropin-releasing hormone test: improvement of the diagnostic accuracy of simultaneous and bilateral inferior petrosal sinus sampling in patients with Cushing syndrome. World J Surg 1995;19(1):150–153.

17. Freda PU, Wardlaw SL, Bruce JN, et al. Differential diagnosis in cushing syndrome: use of corticotropin-releasing hormone. Medicine Baltimore 1995;74(2):74–82.

18. Hardy J. Presidential address: XVII Canadian Congress of Neurological Sciences: Cushing's disease: 50 years later. Can J Neurol Sci 1082;9(4):375–380.

19. Boggan JE, Tyrrell JB, Wilson CB. Transsphenoidal microsurgical management of Cushing's disease: report of 100 cases. J Neurosurg 1983;59(2):195–200.

20. Ram Z, Shawker TH, Bradford MH, et al. Intraoperative ultrasound-directed resection of pituitary tumors. J Neurosurg 1995;83(2):225–230.

21. Doppman JL, Ram Z, Shawker TH, et al. Intraoperative US of the pituitary gland: work in progress. Radiology 1994;192(1):111–115.

22. Nakane T, Kuwayama A, Watanabe M, et al. Long term results of transsphenoidal adenomectomy in patients with Cushing's disease. Neurosurgery 1987;21(2):218–222.

23. Black PM, Zervas NT, Candia GL. Incidence and management of complications of transsphenoidal operation for pituitary adenomas. Neurosurgery. 1987;20(6):920–924.

24. Laws ER. Comments on: Knapp UJ, Ludecke DK, Transnasal microsurgery in children and adolescents with Cushing's disease. Neurosurgery 1996;39:484–493.

25. Schteingart DE, Chandler WF, Lloyd RV, et al. Cushing's syndrome caused by an ectopic pituitary adenoma. Neurosurgery 1987;21(2):223–227.

26. Lamberts SW, de Lange SA, Stefanko SZ. Adrenocorticotropin-secreting pituitary adenomas originate from the anterior or the intermediate lobe in Cushing's disease: differences in the regulation of hormone secretion. J Clin Endocrinol Metab 1982;54(2):286–291.

27. Sonino N, Boscaro M, Merola G, et al. Prolonged treatment of Cushing's disease by ketoconazole. J Clin Endocrinol Metab 1985;61(4):718–722.

28. Ram Z, Nieman LK, Cutler GB Jr, et al. Early repeat surgery for persistent Cushing's disease. J Neurosurg 1994;80(1):37–45.

29. Degerblad M, Rahn T, Bergstrand G, et al. Long term results of stereotactic radiosurgery to the pituitary gland in Cushing's disease. Acta Endocrinol Copenh 1986;112(3):310–314.

30. Magiakou MA, Mastorakos G, Oldfield EH, et al. Cushing's syndrome in children and adolescents: presentation, diagnosis, and therapy. N Engl J Med 1994;331(10):629–636.

31. Jennings AS, Liddle GW, Orth DN. Results of treating childhood Cushing's disease with pituitary irradiation. N Engl J Med 1977;297(18):957–962.

32. Thoren M, Rahn T, Hallengren B, et al. Treatment of Cushing's disease in childhood and adolescence by stereotactic pituitary irradiation. Acta Paediatr Scand 1986;75(3):388–395.

33. Cappa M, Stoner E, DiMartino Nardi J, et al. Recurrence of Cushing's disease in childhood after radiotherapy-induced remission. Am J Dis Child. 1987;141(7):736–740.

34. Wara WM, Richards GE, Grumbach MM, et al. Hypopituitarism after irradiation in children. Int J Radiat Oncol Biol Phys 1977;2(5–6):549–552.

35. Partington MD, Davis DH, Laws ER Jr, et al. Pituitary adenomas in childhood and adolescence: results of transsphenoidal surgery. J Neurosurg 1994;80(2):209–216.

36. Haddad SF, VanGilder JC, Menezes AH. Pediatric pituitary tumors. Neurosurgery 1991;29(4):509–514.

37. Mindermann T, Wilson CB. Pediatric pituitary adenomas. Neurosurgery 1995;36(2):259–268.

Growth Hormone–Secreting Adenomas

Mary Lee Vance

ETIOLOGY AND PATHOLOGY OF ACROMEGALY

Studies of the causes of pituitary tumors have revealed several cellular abnormalities in various tumors, including aneuploidy, gene mutations, allele loss (11q13), coproduction of different hormones, and receptor or postreceptor abnormalities. It is commonly accepted that a pituitary adenoma results from an initiating event (e.g., genetic mutation) and a promoting event, which stimulates clonal expansion of the mutated cell. To date, several gene mutations have been described in different types of pituitary adenomas. The most common mutation, the *gsp* mutation, has been described in growth hormone (GH)–producing adenomas and occurs in approximately 40% of GH-secreting adenomas (1). The mutation involves G-proteins, guanosine diphosphate–binding, receptor-coupled membrane proteins, which can change conformation to promote conversion of guanosine diphosphate to guanosine triphosphate after occupying the receptor, which subsequently generates intracellular effec-

tors that may be involved in cell division. This results in increased adenyl cylase activity, with adenylyl cyclase being constitutively activated. This activation of adenylyl cyclase results from a mutation in the α chain of the guanosine triphosphate–binding protein, Gs, which is the adenylyl cyclase–stimulating protein associated with the growth hormone-releasing hormone (GHRH) receptor (2). The end result is that the gene encoding Gs α-subunit is converted into an oncogene, termed *gsp*. α-Gs mutations have also been identified in other types of pituitary adenomas, including 10% of nonfunctioning adenomas (3) and 5% of adrenocorticotropic hormone (ACTH)–producing adenomas (4). Another finding related to GH-producing adenomas includes allele loss of chromosome 11 in association with the *gsp* mutation (5, 6), suggesting that a GH-producing adenoma may result from activation of dominant oncogenes and inactivation of recessive anti-oncogenes (1). In addition to gene mutations, there is likely dysregulation in normal regulatory peripheral hormone feedback mechanisms. The best example is that of aggressive growth of an ACTH-producing adenoma after a patient has undergone bilateral adrenalectomy (Nelson's syndrome). In this situation, elevated serum cortisol levels are reduced to physiologic concentrations, with subsequent increase in ACTH concentrations and expansion of a usually small ACTH-producing pituitary adenoma.

GH-producing adenomas may be monohormonal (produce GH only) or pleurihormonal (produce GH and prolactin with or without α-subunit, or GH and α-subunit). Immunocytochemical studies indicate that pleurihormonal tumors occur in 68% of surgical specimens and monohormonal tumors occur in 32% of specimens. One-third of adenomas produce GH and prolactin. An adenoma that produces both GH and prolactin may contain one or two distinct cell types. A mammosomatotroph adenoma consists of a single cell type that produces both GH and prolactin in the same cell. A mixed GH and prolactin tumor consists of two cell types, one producing GH and the other producing prolactin (7). The clinical significance of these findings resides primarily in the choice of medical treatment in patients with persistent disease after surgery.

CLINICAL FEATURES OF ACROMEGALY

The classical description of a patient with acromegaly is that of enlargement of the hands, feet, and bones of the face, resulting in large, spadelike hands and feet, frontal bossing, dental malocclusion and widened spaces between the teeth, and a large lower jaw. These changes are the result of years of exposure to excessive amounts of GH. Earlier changes include development of carpal tunnel syndrome, arthritis and arthralgias, hypertension, glucose intolerance, including diabetes mellitus in approximately 25% of patients, hyperhidrosis, and oily skin and skin tags. The early facial changes include coarsening of facial features with exaggeration of the nasolabial folds and broadening of the nose and lips, all of which may be attributed by the patient and others to "aging."

Sleep apnea is a common feature in acromegalic patients that may resolve or improve with successful treatment of the acromegaly. In a study of 53 patients with acromegaly, 81% had sleep apnea. Of particular note was the finding that 12 of 20 patients who were *not* thought to have this disorder on clinical grounds were found to have sleep apnea (8). The morbidity and potential adverse effects on cardiac function are compelling reasons to make the diagnosis and institute treatment. It is anticipated that successful treatment of the acromegaly will reverse the sleep apnea, but nighttime continuous positive airway pressure may also be necessary. In consideration of the cost of repetitive sleep studies, it is reasonable to conduct the study after surgery in conjunction with the postoperative endocrine evaluation. If there are symptoms or persistent acromegaly, a sleep study should be performed and treatment with continuous positive airway pressure instituted as indicated.

Acromegalic patients have a 2.4 to 2.7 increased prevalence of colon polyps compared with age- and sex-matched normal subjects (9–15). One study noted that polyps occur at an earlier age in acromegalic patients than in the general population (acromegalics: 50.5 years; nonacromegalics: 59 years) (9). In addition to the increased prevalence of colon polyps, these patients have an increased risk of developing colon cancer (13–15). Colonoscopy should be performed at the time of diagnosis of acromegaly. Because acromegalic patients often have a large and redundant colon, the gastroenterologist will need to take special care to visualize the cecum because polyps may occur in the right colon. If this is not possible, an air contrast barium enema is indicated. Most gastroenterologists recommend repeating the study every 2 or 3 years.

Cardiovascular disease is the most common etiology of premature death in acromegalic patients. Many of these patients have hypertension and diabetes or glucose intolerance, which are risk factors for vascular disease, independent of acromegaly. An acromegalic should be evaluated and treated aggressively for hypertension and diabetes. Serum lipid levels should be measured and treatment with a lipid-lowering agent should be considered, as indicated. Acromegalic patients without symptomatic cardiac disease were found to have an increased left ventricular mass and a reduced ejection fraction during exercise (16). Studies of cardiac function and anatomy are suggested if there is a clinical indication

IMPORTANCE OF EARLY DIAGNOSIS AND SUCCESSFUL TREATMENT OF ACROMEGALY

Although acromegaly is an uncommon condition, it causes considerable morbidity and results in premature mortality in patients who, despite treatment, continue to have excessive GH secretion. Epidemiologic studies have demonstrated that acromegalics have a greater risk of premature death from cardiovascular disease than the rest of the population (17–21). In some series, other causes of premature mortality include respiratory failure and malignancy. This risk of premature mortality persists even with therapy unless GH secretion is adequately suppressed. An outcomes study in which GH was measured several times during the day demonstrated that excessive mortality persisted unless the average daily GH concentration (the mean of five values) was less than 2.5 ng/mL (< 110 pmol/L) (22). Although numerous reports of surgery, radiation, and medical treatment describe a lowering of GH levels (and insulinlike growth factor-1 [IGF-1] levels in some studies), lowering GH concentrations is not adequate unless they are reduced to normal. The study reporting the impact of reducing average GH levels to less than 2.5 ng/mL (< 110 pmol/L) did not include measurement of serum IGF-1 concentrations in all patients, and outcomes were not assessed in relation to IGF-1. However, as expected, serum IGF-1 concentrations were lower in patients who achieved a mean daytime serum GH of less than 2.5 ng/mL (< 110 pmol/L). It is reasonable to surmise that lowering IGF-1 concentrations to those of age- and sex-adjusted normal subjects should reduce the risk of premature mortality.

DIAGNOSIS OF ACROMEGALY

An unfortunate fact about acromegaly is the delay in diagnosis. Most series report that patients have symptoms of the disease for 10 to 20 years before it is recognized. This long interval undoubtedly contributes to the morbidity and premature mortality.

A problem in the early diagnosis of acromegaly is the patient who does not have the classical physical features suggestive of the disease, particularly disease of recent onset. This is especially problematic in young women who present with menstrual disturbance and are found to have hyperprolactinemia. Because of the lack of symptoms and physical findings, these women are usually diagnosed as having a prolactinoma and are treated with a dopamine agonist drug. Use of the medication produces a reduction in prolactin levels and restoration of menses, and only later is the correct diagnosis made, when the magnetic resonance imaging scan does not show reduction in tumor size or when the patient develops symptoms of acromegaly such as dental malocclusion, hyperhidrosis, or arthralgia. Every patient undergoing evaluation for pituitary dysfunction or a pituitary tumor should have a screening serum IGF-1 measured to exclude early acromegaly.

Serum IGF-1 Level: GH action is mediated by production of IGF-1 by the liver and other tissues. This measurement usually provides a reliable indication of overall GH secretion, particularly with excessive GH secretion. Serum IGF-1 level is not helpful in diagnosing GH deficiency because of considerable overlap with normal subjects. In addition, the IGF-1 concentration is influenced by the nutritional state; in malnourished patients, serum IGF-1 levels are reduced. Because total GH secretion is both age and sex dependent (higher in women than men, declines with age), serum IGF-1 values also vary according to age and sex. Some commercial laboratories have a limited database for normal values and do not always report normal values according to age and sex. The lack of an adequate database for normal subjects is a limitation of this measurement that is particularly important in adults older than 50 years. It is prudent to send the sample to a laboratory that reports results in conjunction with normal values for age and sex. Table 15.1 lists how commonly used commercial laboratories report serum IGF-1 concentrations.

IGF-1 circulates in a bound form, and several IGF-binding proteins are under different regulation. The IGF binding protein 3 (IGFBP-3) is the GH-dependent binding protein and has been recommended as an accurate indicator of GH secretion. Unfortunately, this measure does not provide enough discrimination between normal and abnormal subjects to replace IGF-1.

Oral Glucose Tolerance Test: Oral administration of 100 or 75 g of glucose with measurement of serum glucose and GH levels is the definitive test for acromegaly. The normal GH response to glucose administration has changed with development of increasingly sensitive GH assays. In older radioimmunoassay (polyclonal GH antibody) studies, the normal GH response to glucose administration is less than 2 ng/mL. Using immunoradiometric assay (IRMA) (monoclonal GH antibody) method, the normal GH response to glucose is less than 1 ng/mL. The recent development of a more sensitive GH assay using chemiluminescence technology (sensitivity to 0.002 ng/mL compared with conventional IRMA sensitivity of 0.2 ng/mL) has shown that the GH response to glucose (100 mg) is lower in normal subjects than observed previously. The nadir serum GH concentration after ingestion of 100 g of glucose in six women was 0.25 ng/mL and in nine men was 0.029 ng/mL (23). Although the more sensitive chemiluminescence assay is not yet widely available, it is anticipated that it will be used in the future. Thus, as occurred with development of more sensitive thyroid-stimulating hormone assays to define normality, so are there changes in the assessment of normal GH concentrations and the normal GH response to oral glucose therapy.

A recent study of 54 patients with acromegaly and age- and sex-matched normal subjects demonstrated that the GH response to oral glucose administration is the most accurate test for excessive GH secretion. Acromegalics, 41 with active disease (12 untreated, 29 treated but not cured) and 13 considered cured, and 14 normal subjects underwent an oral glucose tolerance test using 100 g of glucose, and GH was measured using an IRMA with a sensitivity of 0.1 ng/mL. Normal patients and cured acromegalics all had nadir GH levels less than 0.9 ng/mL after glucose administration; acromegalics with active disease all had nadir GH levels greater than 1.5 ng/mL after glucose administration. Serum IGF-1, IGFBP-3, and 24-hour urinary

Table 15.1. *Serum Insulinlike Growth Factor-1 Measurements by Commercial Laboratories*

Laboratory	Age-Adjusted Normal Values	Sex-Adjusted Normal Values
Quest (Corning Nichols)	Yes	Yes
Endocrine Sciences	Yes	No
American Medical Laboratories	No	Yes
SmithKline Beecham	No	No
MetPath[a]	Yes	No
Mayo Medical Labs	Yes	Yes
Roche Biomedical[a]	Yes	No

[a] Uses Quest (Corning Nichols) assay.

IGFBP-3 values were also compared; there was overlap among the study groups (untreated acromegalics, treated but not cured acromegalics, cured acromegalics, and normal subjects), particularly those acromegalic patients who had received prior therapy but who were not considered cured by clinical criteria and the oral glucose tolerance test. The serum IGFBP-3 level was the least able to discriminate between normal subjects and patients with active disease (80% overlap) (24). The IGF-1 test is usually a valuable screening test if the level is elevated in a patient in whom there is clinical suspicion of excessive GH secretion. Given the limitations of some laboratory ranges of normal, it is necessary to perform an oral glucose tolerance test for the definitive diagnosis of the disease and to assess response to treatment.

Serum GH Level: A random serum GH level is of little value in diagnosing acromegaly unless the value is extremely elevated (e.g., > 60 ng/mL). GH secretion is pulsatile and is influenced by factors such as food ingestion, exercise, and sleep. Studies comparing 24-hour GH secretory profiles (GH measured every 5 to 10 minutes for 24 hours) in normal subjects and in patients with acromegaly have demonstrated that in normal subjects, most values are below the limit of detection in conventional GH assays (0.28 to 0.5 ng/mL), whereas in acromegalic patients, all values are detectable throughout the 24-hour period. The mean 24-hour GH concentration is likely to be less important than the pattern of GH exposure in promoting the numerous consequences of excessive GH. Measurement of serum GH concentrations every 5 minutes for 24 hours is obviously a research study, but it provides valuable information regarding the pattern of GH secretion. Normal subjects have pulsatile GH secretion interspersed with periods of secretory quiescence with GH values either at the lower end or below detectable levels depending on the GH assay. In patients with acromegaly, the number of secretory pulses in 24 hours is increased, and, probably more importantly, GH values between pulses do not decline to undetectable or close to undetectable levels. Although random GH levels and the mean 24-hour GH concentration may be "normal" in a patient with acromegaly, the continuous exposure to even low levels of GH is pathologic. Figure 15.1 shows 24-hour GH "profiles" in a 70-year-old normal woman and a 62-year-old woman with acromegaly. Growth hormone was assayed using an IRMA with a sensitivity of 0.2 ng/mL. Figure 15.2 shows 24-hour GH profiles in a normal woman and a woman with acromegaly using the more sensitive chemiluminescence assay, illustrating the same principle. The patient is a 66-year-old woman with classical acromegaly, a huge tongue, and severe sleep apnea (177 apnea episodes per night, minimum SaO$_2$: 67%). Her mean 24-hour GH level was 1.93 ng/mL, a value observed in healthy women; serum IGF-1 level was 336 ng/mL (71 to 290 ng/mL is normal for women older than 55 years). After successful surgery, her sleep apnea disappeared and her tongue decreased in size and she had a normal serum IGF-1 level, a normal GH response to

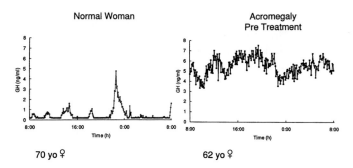

Figure 15.1. Serum GH concentrations measured every 5 minutes for 24 hours in a normal 70-year-old woman (**A**) and in a 62-year-old woman with acromegaly (**B**). GH was assayed with an IRMA with a sensitivity of 0.2 ng/mL.

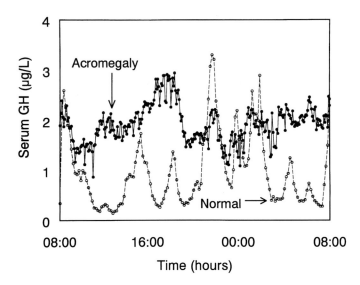

Figure 15.2. Serum GH concentrations measured every 5 minutes for 24 hours in a 68-year-old normal woman (*open circles*) and in a 66-year-old woman with acromegaly (*solid circles*). Growth hormone was assayed with a chemiluminescence assay with a sensitivity of 0.002 ng/mL.

glucose administration and a normal 24-hour GH secretory profile.

Plasma GHRH Level: Ectopic GHRH production by a lung or pancreatic tumor (usually a carcinoid) is a rare cause of acromegaly that should be considered in a patient in whom the pituitary magnetic resonance imaging scan reveals generalized enlargement of the gland and/or no demonstrable tumor. In this circumstance, it is prudent to measure the plasma GHRH concentration before recommending pituitary surgery. This test is available at a commercial laboratory (Quest Laboratory [formerly Corning Nichols], San Juan Capistrano, CA) and requires specimen collection in a special tube containing aprotinin (Trasylol, provided by the laboratory).

Other Diagnostic Tests: Clinical assessments should

include identification of sleep apnea, colon polyps, and cardiac disease. These conditions are associated with significant morbidity and premature mortality (respiratory failure, colon cancer, and cardiovascular disease) and require diagnosis and treatment that may be independent of lowering GH and IGF-1 concentrations to normal.

SURGERY AND RADIATION TREATMENTS: SUMMARY

Surgery: The most important determinants of the surgical outcome are tumor size; extension into the cavernous sinus, dura, and/or bone; and the experience and expertise of the neurosurgeon. The quoted outcomes of surgery are those reported by neurosurgeons who specialize in pituitary surgery. Thus, it is not appropriate to extrapolate these results with those of a surgeon who performs this operation infrequently. Patients should be informed of this before deciding on which neurosurgeon to consult. A difficulty in assessing the reported outcomes of surgery (most commonly performed by the transsphenoidal approach) is the changing criteria for "cure" or remission. In many early reports, lowering of GH to less than 10 ng/mL was considered successful; later, the criterion of lowering GH to less than 5 ng/mL was used (25). More recent publications include the use of the GH response to oral glucose administration to assess effectiveness of surgery. In a series of 214 patients, 117 (54%) had a postoperative GH level of less than 5 ng/mL (25). In 175 patients, a GH response to glucose therapy (< 2 ng/mL) occurred in 28 (52%) of 54 patients studied; the fasting GH level was 2 ng/mL or less in 60 (55%) of 109 patients. However, it should be noted that 25 of the 90 patients considered to be in remission also received postoperative radiotherapy (26). In another report of 25 patients who were followed up for 5 to 11 years after surgery, the postoperative glucose-suppressed GH level was less than 2.5 ng/mL in 21 (84%); however, 3 patients had a relapse 1 to 6 years after surgery, for an overall surgical "cure" rate of 68% (27). It is not known how many patients achieve a normal (for age and sex) serum IGF-1 concentration or a glucose-suppressed GH level of less than 1 ng/mL (IRMA) after surgery. Because serum IGF-1 concentrations decline gradually after successful surgery, this should not be measured until several weeks later. The oral glucose test should also be a part of the postoperative evaluation.

Pituitary Radiation: Radiation as primary therapy is not successful in effecting a *prompt* reduction in serum GH levels or in reducing tumor size. Radiation as primary therapy should not be recommended unless the patient is unable or unwilling to undergo surgery. The widely quoted study from the National Institutes of Health in 1979 of 47 patients treated with fractionated radiotherapy as primary treatment reported that serum GH levels were reduced in 67% of patients to less than or equal to 5 ng/mL within 10 years of treatment (28). Considering what is now known about the importance of lowering GH (and presumably IGF-1) levels to normal to reduce the risk of premature death, all efforts should be made to recommend treatment that has the best chance of accomplishing this goal. Thus, pituitary radiation should be reserved for patients who have residual disease after surgery. Because it usually requires months to years for radiation to be effective in lowering GH and IGF-1 levels to normal, patients should be given medical therapy while awaiting the therapeutic effect of radiation. The conventional manner of delivering radiation to the pituitary is through three ports (bitemporal and frontal) in fractions for 4 to 5 weeks. Other methods include particle beam (protons, deuterons, and helium ions), usually administered in four fractions for 5 days, or the more recently developed stereotactic methods, Gamma Knife and Lineac particle beam radiotherapy. In 220 acromegalic patients, stereotactic methods resulted in lowering of the median GH level to 5 ng/mL or less 4 years after treatment in 169 patients (77%). Another study of 114 patients treated with helium ion radiotherapy resulted in lowering of fasting GH to 5 ng/mL or less 7 years after treatment in 26 patients (23%) (29). Stereotactic radiation with the Gamma Knife involves delivery of focused radiation through 201 ports, usually given in one treatment. The theoretical advantage of this method is minimal exposure of the surrounding brain tissue to radiation and the ability to treat a circumscribed area with minimal exposure to the hypothalamus and optic chiasm. This method is best reserved for patients with a small amount of residual tumor that is not in proximity to the optic chiasm. Gamma Knife radiotherapy in 20 patients resulted in reduction in fasting GH levels to less than 110 pmol/L in 7 patients (35%) 6 months to 7 years after the treatment (30). It is important to note that the technique of planning the radiation field for the Gamma Knife has advanced over the years, from the less precise use of pneumoencephalography to the computed tomographic scan and now to magnetic resonance imaging. Comparison of results among studies using different techniques is difficult.

Anticipated complications of radiation include development of hypopituitarism (31). Deficiency of some or all of the pituitary hormones usually occurs in a progressive fashion, the earliest and most common deficiency being that of the gonadotropins (luteinizing hormone and follicle-stimulating hormone), with consequent gonadal failure. In 35 patients treated with conventional radiotherapy, ACTH deficiency developed in 67%, thyroid-stimulating hormone deficiency in 55%, and gonadotropin deficiency in 67% after a mean follow-up of 4.2 years (32). All patients should be followed regularly (at least every 6 months) with appropriate hormone measurements and prompt institution of replacement therapy as indicated (33). The risk of developing a central nervous system malignancy is low but is a consideration. Prospective studies detailing intellectual function before and after radiotherapy are not available. The incidence of pituitary failure after stereotactic radiation

(Gamma Knife, Lineac) is not yet known, and careful monitoring of these patients is mandatory.

MEDICAL TREATMENT OF ACROMEGALY

There are two classes of drugs that lower GH concentrations in acromegalic patients: dopamine agonists and somatostatin analogs. Initially, the only drugs available were the dopamine agonists (e.g., bromocriptine, pergolide, lisuride, and cabergoline). Although clinical improvement occurred in 80 to 90% of patients, less than 20% had a reduction in GH or IGF-1 concentrations to a normal or near normal level (33). Some patients have greater reduction in GH and IGF-1 levels with a combination of a dopamine agonist and a somatostatin analog, but as a single agent, a dopamine agonist is not the most effective medical therapy.

The 8 amino acid somatostatin analog, octreotide, was the first agent designed specifically to lower GH concentrations; it is more suppressive of GH than its native somatostatin and more suppressive of GH than insulin, thus making it an ideal agent to treat acromegaly (34). The limiting factor in responsiveness to somatostatin analog treatment is the number of tumor somatostatin receptors (35); thus, increasing the dose of an analog may not be more effective.

In several large trials of octreotide, usually given as 100 μg every 8 h by subcutaneous injection, 80 to 90% of patients have a reduction in serum GH and IGF-1 concentrations. Lowering of GH and IGF-1 levels to normal occurred in 42 to 60% of patients (36–40). Because the limiting factor in responsiveness seems to be the number of somatostatin receptors on the tumor, increasing the total daily dose above 300 μg is not usually more efficacious. Although octreotide is effective in reducing serum GH and IGF-1 concentrations, reduction in tumor size occurs in only about 30% of patients, and the reduction in tumor size is usually less than 30%. Thus, treatment of large tumors with octreotide as the primary therapy is not recommended. Some investigators have suggested that octreotide treatment prior to surgery may improve the outcome of surgery. There are no published results of controlled trials of preoperative octreotide, but historical comparison suggests that better surgical results are achieved when the patient is given octreotide before surgery (41).

Long-acting somatostatin analogs have also been developed and, depending on the formulation, are administered every 10, 14, or 28 days as a single intramuscular injection. A long-acting octreotide formulation, octreotide LAR, given to eight patients, 20 to 40 mg every 28 to 42 days by intramuscular injection, decreased mean GH concentrations from 10.7 ± 2.8 ng/mL to 2.6 ± 0.4 ng/mL after 12 injections (42). In 14 patients who had responded previously to multiple daily octreotide injections, octreotide LAR was given every 28 days for 18 injections; all patients had improvement in clinical symptoms. Mean serum GH level was reduced to less than 2 ng/mL in 9 patients (64%), to less than 5 ng/mL in 3 patients (21%), and to less than

10 ng/mL in 2 patients (14%); serum IGF-1 level was reduced to normal in 9 patients (64%) (43). Four patients who had received no prior treatment had a greater than 20% reduction in tumor size during 16 months of octreotide LAR therapy; there was no change in residual tumor size in 7 patients who had prior surgery (43).

Lanreotide is an octapeptide somatostatin analog in encapsulated microspheres of polylactide-polyglycolide copolymers that provides a slow-release formulation that suppresses GH levels for 10 to 14 days. In 19 patients treated with the long-acting somatostatin analog lanreotide, 6 months of treatment with 30 mg intramuscularly every 10 or 14 days, serum IGF-1 concentration decreased to normal in 16 (84%), and the mean GH level (mean of eight daytime values) was 4.9 ± 1.3 ng/mL. Improvement in clinical symptoms occurred in 18 of 19 patients, and tumor shrinkage of 25 to 75% occurred in 3 of 8 patients treated for 1 year (44). Fifty acromegalic patients, unselected regarding prior octreotide responsiveness, were treated with lanreotide, 30 mg intramuscularly every 2 weeks for 6 months. After 6 months of treatment, mean daytime serum GH levels decreased to less than 1 ng/mL in 21 patients (45%), to less than 2 ng/mL in 10 patients (21%), to less than 5 ng/mL in 9 patients (19%), and to greater than 5 ng/mL in 7 patients (15%). Serum IGF-1 levels decreased to normal in 38% of patients (45). In another study of 10 patients treated with lanreotide for 6 months, 5 achieved a normal serum IGF-1 level; 1 patient developed asymptomatic gallstones (46). Long-term lanreotide treatment of 22 patients, 1 to 3 years, resulted in persistent suppression of GH and IGF-1 levels; serum IGF-1 concentration remained in the normal range in 63% of patients. A reduction in tumor size was observed in 3 patients (13%) (47).

Side effects of somatostatin analog therapy include abdominal discomfort and diarrhea in a few patients. Development of cholelithiasis or gall bladder sludge occurs in 18% of patients treated chronically with octreotide (38–40); only a minority of these patients developed symptomatic gall bladder disease requiring cholecystectomy. In 52 acromegalic patients, 16% had asymptomatic biliary sludge or gallstones prior to treatment with lanreotide, over the course of 6 months of treatment 20% had asymptomatic sludge or gallstones (45). Lanreotide therapy for 1 to 3 years was associated with gallstone formation in 4 of 22 patients (18%) (47).

The development of somatostatin analogs has been the most effective medical therapy for acromegaly. A limitation of this therapy is that GH secretion is controlled only as long as the somatostatin analog is taken. In addition, this is an expensive treatment, from $10,000 to $13,00 per year for octreotide. Thus, medical therapy should be viewed as an adjunctive treatment after surgical resection and while awaiting the curative effects of pituitary radiation.

A potential new development for the treatment of acromegaly is a modification of the GH molecule that acts as a GH receptor antagonist. Preliminary information indicates that this antagonist lowers circulating IGF-1 concentrations by 50% in normal subjects. Studies in patients with acromegaly are ongoing, the results of which should be informative. One theoretical difficulty with a GH receptor antagonist is the potential for increasing circulating GH concentrations and tumor growth if IGF-1 has any substantial negative feedback effect on the regulation of GH secretion from a GH-producing adenoma.

SUMMARY

Acromegaly is a treatable and potentially curable disease. The importance of early diagnosis and early and aggressive treatment cannot be overemphasized. Once the diagnosis is ascertained, prompt treatment should be given; surgery remains the first choice. However, as noted, surgery is not curative in the majority of patients, which emphasizes the need for multimodality therapy including surgery, pituitary radiation, and medical therapy for excessive GH secretion. In addition, conditions such as hypertension, diabetes, hyperlipidemia, sleep apnea, colon polyps, and osteoarthritis should be treated aggressively to reduce the morbidity and potential for premature mortality.

REFERENCES

1. Faglia G. Genesis of pituitary adenomas. In: Landolt AM, Vance ML, Reilly PL, eds. Pituitary Adenomas. New York: Churchill Livingstone, 1996:3–11.
2. Landis C, Masters SB, Spada A, et al. GTPase inhibiting mutations activate the alpha chain of Gs and stimulate adenylyl cyclase in human pituitary tumors. Nature 1989;340:692–696.
3. Tordjman K, Stern N, Ouaknine G, et al. Activating mutations of the Gs alpha gene in nonfunctioning pituitary tumors. J Clin Endocrinol Metab 1993;77:765–769.
4. Williamson EA, Harrison D, Ince PG, et al. Mutations of Gs-alpha in human pituitary adrenocorticotrophin hormone (ACTH)-secreting adenomas (abstract). J Endocrinol Invest 1993;16(suppl 1):22.
5. Thakker RV, Pook MA, Wooding C, et al. Association of somatotropinomas with loss of alleles on chromosome 11 and with gsp mutations. J Clin Invest 1993;91:2815–2821.
6. Boggild MD, Jenkinson S, Pistorello M, et al. Molecular genetic studies of sporadic pituitary tumors. J Clin Endocrinol Metab 1994;78:387–392.
7. Trouillas J, Girod C. Pathology of pituitary adenomas. In: Landolt AM, Vance ML, Reilly PL, eds. Pituitary Adenomas. New York: Churchill Livingstone, 1996:27–46.
8. Grunstein RR, Ho KY, Sullivan CE. Sleep apnea in acromegaly. Ann Intern Med 1991;115:527–532.
9. Terzolo M, Tappero G, Borretta G, et al. High prevalence of colonic polyps in patients with acromegaly: influence of sex and age. Arch Intern Med 1994;154:1271–1276.
10. Vasen HFA, van Erpecum KJ, Roelfsema F, et al. Increased prevalence of colonic polyps in patients with acromegaly. Eur J Endocrinol 1994;131:235–237.
11. Klein I, Pareveen G, Gavaler JS, et al. Colonic polyps in patients with acromegaly. Ann Intern Med 1982;97:27–30.
12. Ituarte EA, Petrini J, Hershman JM. Acromegaly and colon cancer. Ann Intern Med 1984;101:627–628.
13. Pines A, Rozen P, Ron E, et al. Gastrointestinal tumors in acromegalic patients. Am J Gastroenterol 1985;80:266–269.
14. Barzilay J, Heatley GJ, Cushing GW. Benign and malignant tumors in patients with acromegaly. Arch Intern Med 1991;151:1629–1632.
15. Ron E, Gridley G, Hrubec Z, et al. Acromegaly and gastrointestinal cancer. Cancer 1991;68:1673–1677.
16. Fazio S, Cittadini A, Cuocolo A, et al. Impaired cardiac performance is a distinct feature of uncomplicated acromegaly. J Clin Endocrinol Metab 1994;79:441–446.
17. Wright AD, Hill DM, Lowery C, et al. Mortality in acromegaly. QJM 1970;39:1–16.
18. Alexander L, Appleton D, Hall R, et al. Epidemiology of acromegaly in the Newcastle region. Clin Endocrinol (Oxf) 1980;12:71–79.
19. Ritchie CM, Atkinson AB, Kennedy AL, et al. Ascertainment and natural history of treated acromegaly in Northern Ireland. Ulster Med J 1990;59:55–62.
20. Etxabe J, Gaztambide S, Latorre P, et al. Acromegaly: an epidemiologic study. J Endocrinol Invest 1993;16:181–187.
21. Rajasoorya C, Holdaway IM, Wrightson P, et al. Determinants of clinical outcome and survival in acromegaly. Clin Endocrinol (Oxf) 1994;41:95–102.
22. Bates AS, Van't Hoff W, Jones JM, et al. An audit of outcome of treatment in acromegaly. QJM 1993;86:293–299.
23. Chapman IM, Hartman ML, Struame, et al. Enhanced sensitivity of growth hormone (GH) chemiluminescence assay reveals lower post glucose nadir GH concentrations in men than women. J Clin Endocrinol Metab 1994;78:1312–1319.
24. Stoffel-Wagner B, Springer W, Bidlingmaier D, et al. A comparison of the different methods for diagnosing acromegaly. Clin Endocrinol 1997;46:531–537.
25. Ross DA, Wilson CB. Results of transsphenoidal microsurgery for growth hormone-secreting pituitary adenoma in a series of 214 patients. J Neurosurg 1988;68:854–867.
26. Davis DH, Laws ER, Ilstrup DM, et al. Results of surgical treatment for growth hormone-secreting pituitary adenoma. J Neurosurg 1993;79:70–75.
27. Serri O, Somma M, Comtois R, et al. Acromegaly: biochemical assessment of cure after long term follow-up of transsphenoidal selective adenomectomy. J Clin Endocrinol Metab 1985;61:1185–1189.
28. Eastman RC, Gorden P, Roth J. Conventional supervoltage irradiation is an effective treatment for acromegaly. J Clin Endocrinol Metab 1979;48:931–940.
29. Levy RP, Fabrikant JI, Frankel KA. Particle-beam irradiation of the pituitary gland. In: Alexander E, Woffler JS, Lunsford CD, eds. Stereotactic Radiosurgery. 1993:157–165.
30. Thoren M, Rahn T, Gou WY, et al. Stereotactic radiosurgery with the cobalt-60 gamma unit in the treatment of growth hormone-producing pituitary tumors. Neurosurgury 1991;29:663–668.
31. Vance ML. Medical progress: hypopituitarism. N Engl J Med 1994;330:1651–1662.
32. Synder PJ, Fowble BF, Shatz NJ. Hypopituitarism following radiation therapy for pituitary adenomas. Am J Med 1986;81:457–462.
33. Barkan AL. Acromegaly: diagnosis and therapy. Endocrinol Metab Clin North Am 1989;18:277–310.
34. Plewe G, Beyer J, Krause U, et al. Long-acting and selective suppression of growth hormone secretion by somatostatin analogue SMS 201–995 in acromegaly. Lancet 1984;2:782–784.
35. Reubi JC, Landolt AM. The growth hormone responses to octreotide in acromegaly correlate with adenoma somatostatin receptor status. J Clin Endocrinol Metab 1989;68:844–850.
36. Quabbe HJ, Plockinger U. Dose-response study and long-term effects of the somatostatin analog octreotide in patients with therapy-resistant acromegaly. J Clin Endocrinol Metab 1989;68:873–881.
37. McKnight JA, McCance DR, Sheridan B, et al. A long-term dose-response study of somatostatin analogue (SMS 201–995, octreotide) in resistant acromegaly. Clin Endocrinol 1991;34:119–125.
38. Vance ML, Harris AG. Long term treatment of 189 acromegalic patients with the somatostatin analog octreotide. Arch Intern Med 1991;151:1573–1578.
39. Ezzat S, Snyder PJ, Yourn WF, et al. Octreotide treatment of acromegaly: a randomized multicenter trial. Ann Intern Med 1992;117:711–718.
40. Newman CB, Melmed S, Snyder PJ, et al. Safety and efficacy of long-term octreotide therapy of acromegaly: results of a multicenter trial in 103 patients. J Clin Endocrinol Metab 1995;80:2768–2775.
41. Lucas-Morante T, GarcRa-UrRa J, Estada J, et al. Treatment of invasive growth hormone pituitary adenomas with long-acting so-

matostatin analog SMS 201–995 before transsphenoidal surgery. J Neurosurg 1994;81:10–14.

42. Stewart PM, Kane KF, Stewart SE, et al. Depot long-acting somatostatin analog (Sandostatin-LAR) is an effective treatment for acromegaly. J Clin Endocrinol Metab 1995;80:3267–3272.

43. Flrgstad AK, Halse J, Bakke S, et al. Sandostatin LAR in acromegalic patients: long term treatment. J Clin Endocrinol Metab 1997;82:23–28.

44. Morange I, DeBoisvilliers F, Chanson P, et al. Slow release lanreotide treatment in acromegalic patients previously normalized by octreotide. J Clin Endocrinol Metab 1994;79:145–151.

45. Giusti M, Gussoni G, Cuttica CM, et al. Effectiveness and tolerability of slow release lanreotide treatment in active acromegaly: six-month report on an Italian multicenter study. J Clin Endocrinol Metab 1996;81:2089–2097.

46. Al-Maskari M, Gebbie J, Kendall-Taylor P. The effect of a new slow-release, long-acting somatostatin analogue, lanreotide, in acromegaly. Clin Endocrinol 1996;45:415–421.

47. Caron P, Morange-Ramos I, Cogne M, et al. Three year follow-up of acromegalic patients treated with intramuscular slow-release lanreotide. J Clin Endocrinol Metab 1997;82:18–22.

CHAPTER 16

Growth Hormone–Secreting Pituitary Tumors: Operative Management

Kamal Thapar and Edward R. Laws Jr.

INTRODUCTION

Of clinically significant primary pituitary tumors, about 15 to 20% will arise from growth hormone (GH)–producing cells of the pituitary (1, 2). For this group of neoplasms, the menu of potential therapeutic options is broader than that available for any other type of pituitary tumor. Surgical resection, receptor-mediated pharmacotherapy, conventional irradiation, and sterotactic radiosurgery are each effective to varying degrees in various situations, and all afford the treating physician some latitude in providing a comprehensive plan of management for these tumors (3). In the overwhelming majority of instances, operative treatment has been, and continues to be, a major component of the overall management plan. In this chapter, we review the operative management of GH-secreting pituitary tumors.

HISTORICAL CONSIDERATIONS

Arguably the most spectacular of the endocrine hypersecretory states, acromegaly is the eventual and often dramatic result of pathologic GH excess. In all but the rarest of instances, the cause will be a GH-secreting pituitary tumor. So distinctive is the transformation that acromegalics and related giants have been subjects of seemingly mythical reference throughout history, legend, and literature as keepers of great strength and power. This, however, was seldom the case, and, particularly during the later, debilitating phases of the disease, afflicted individuals were often consumed by the many metabolic, musculoskeletal, and cardiovascular complications that typify active acromegaly.

As a clinical entity, the earliest description of acromegaly was introduced to the medical literature by Noel in 1779. Thereafter, additional examples were reported by Magendie (1839), Verga (1864), Brigidi (1877), and Fritsche and Klebs (1886) (as reviewed by Danowski [4]). It was, however, Pierre Marie (1886) who, in reviewing previously reported cases and after adding two cases of his own, coined the term "acromegaly" and provided the detailed clinical descriptions that captured the attention of the academic mainstream (5, 6). Whereas pituitary enlargement was recognized as a regular feature of the generalized acromegalic state, uncertainty and controversy surrounded the role of the pituitary in the genesis of the condition. The first, but still somewhat equivocal, suggestion that acromegaly resulted from dysfunction of the pituitary was made by Minkowski (7) in 1887, in describing a patient with headache and hemianopia. In 1900, Benda recognized that the enlarged pituitaries of acromegalic patients consisted primarily of eosinophilic adenohypophyseal cells (8). Not only did he regard these cells as being etiologically relevant, but he further proposed them to be neoplastic and hyperfunctioning. The demonstration by Cushing in 1909, that partial hypophysectomy was accompanied by regression of acromegalic features, together with the studies by Evans and Long that pituitary extracts injected into rodents produced gigantism, established the synaptic link between a hyperfunctioning pituitary adenoma and acromegaly (9, 10). In doing so, acromegaly came to be the earliest example of a pituitary disorder that could be clinically and pathologically recognized and appropriately treated.

Almost from the beginning, surgery has maintained a central role in the management of the GH-secreting tumors. The first operation, a salvage transcranial decompressive procedure, was performed in 1893 by Paul in an acromegalic patient for relief of increased intracranial pressure (11). Transcranial procedures for pituitary tumors, including some in acromegalic patients, were performed by Horsely between 1889 and 1906 using both subfrontal and temporal approaches. Thereafter, and until the 1920s, one or another variation of the transsphenoidal approach became the preferred route for somatotroph adenomas. Hochenegg was the first to do so, using Schloffer's transsphenoidal approach (12). During the same era, Cushing perfected the sublabial transseptal submucosal approach, operating on about 60 acromegalics in this fashion. For the next 40 to 50 years, with the development of transcranial surgery, transsphenoidal approaches to the sella were overlooked in favor of various transcranial approaches. In a few centers, however, the concept of the transsphenoidal approach was sustained, eventually to be repopularized by Guiot et al. (13) and Hardy (14) in the 1960s. With the introduction of the operating microscope and microsurgical technique, the transsphenoidal microsurgical method has ultimately become the current standard for approaching somatotroph and other tumors of the sella.

GENERAL CONSIDERATIONS AND THERAPEUTIC GOALS

Once the diagnosis of a somatotroph adenoma has been confirmed on the basis of the clinical examination, endocri-

nologic profile, and imaging studies (see Chapter 5), several general issues deserve careful consideration in formulating a treatment plan. First, it is of fundamental importance to recognize that acromegaly is a complex, multisystem disorder and that any successful treatment strategy should be sufficiently comprehensive to encompass all aspects of the condition, including the obvious neurologic, oncologic, and endocrinologic issues, but also the established secondary complications of the condition (e.g., cardiovascular, respiratory, and musculoskeletal). To do so often requires multidisciplinary expertise, and, not infrequently, will also require multimodal therapy if the desired reductions in acromegaly-associated morbidity are to be realized.

A second, but related consideration concerns the recognition that GH excess of any degree is truly a life-threatening condition and that any therapeutic intervention must ultimately have an impact on the high mortality present in the acromegalic population (15). That acromegaly is associated with a reduced life expectancy has been validated by three detailed epidemiologic studies (16–18). Over the period of one study, Wright et al. (16) observed the death rate among acromegalic patients to be more than twice that of a control population. Cardiovascular disease, cerebrovascular disease, malignant tumors, and respiratory disease accounted for 24.0%, 15.0%, 15.5%, and 15.5% of deaths, respectively. Comparable results were obtained from a second English study from the Newcastle region wherein the mortality rates among male and female acromegalics were 4.8 and 2.4 times, respectively, those of a control population (17). In the Götenborg region of Sweden, acromegalic patients suffered a threefold increase in mortality. Again, vascular disease and malignancy figured prominently as causes of premature death (18). These data are important and indicate that whatever treatment strategy is used for GH-secreting tumors, it must favorably affect acromegaly-associated mortality. This issue was addressed in a series of 79 acromegalic patients, all of whom had their tumors treated with one or another form of therapy. In follow-up, the most important factor associated with reduced mortality was a mean GH level of less than 110 pmol/L (< 2.5 ng/mL) (15). Accordingly, partial reduction of GH excess cannot be considered adequate treatment for these patients because their mortality rate continues to be at least twice that of normal individuals (19).

Goals of Therapy

Based on the foregoing, an effective management strategy for acromegaly-associated pituitary tumors should comprehensively address the following specific goals:

1. Elimination of mass effects and restoration of normal neurologic function;

2. Normalization of GH hypersecretion;

3. Preservation of residual anterior and posterior pituitary function;

4. Reduction of risk for oncologic or biochemical recurrence; and

5. Management of acromegaly-associated complications (cardiovascular, musculoskeletal).

SURGICAL CONSIDERATIONS

For the overwhelming majority of patients presenting with acromegaly, surgical resection will represent the initial treatment of choice. The effectiveness of surgery will depend on several factors, including tumor size and invasion status and preoperative GH levels. In the most favorable circumstances, such as those involving noninvasive intrasellar microadenomas with basal GH levels less than 2200 pmol/L (< 50 ng/mL), surgery alone can prove curative. In other instances, such as those involving some invasive macroadenomas and those with preoperative GH levels in excess of 2200 pmol/L (> 50 ng/mL), curative resection may still represent a reasonable operative goal, although the possibility of inaccessible tumor remnants, persistent GH hypersecretion, and the potential need for eventual adjuvant therapy are recognized from the outset. Finally, in the least favorable situation, one is confronted with a tumor whose size and invasiveness have clearly exceeded the limits of surgical resectability. For such tumors, surgical resection is undertaken primarily for the relief of mass effects. In doing so, tumor burden is also reduced, thus possibly enhancing the effectiveness of adjuvant pharmacologic and/or radiation therapies.

Surgical Indications

Indications for operative management of GH-secreting tumors are several, and these can be considered endocrinologic, neurologic, and/or ophthalmologic in nature (20, 21). In most instances, the primary indication will be endocrinologic; such patients will have clinical and biochemical findings of active acromegaly, and a pituitary tumor will be demonstrable radiologically. For a significant proportion of these patients, additional neurologic and/or ophthalmologic surgical indications may also coexist. Because it is well recognized that most somatotroph adenomas will have already progressed to the macroadenoma stage by the time of detection, symptomatic mass effects are commonly an indication for surgical intervention (1, 22–25). Chiasmal compression with progressive visual loss is the most common of these, having been variably reported in 9 to 30% of patients with somatotroph adenomas (26–31). Cavernous sinus invasion/compression also occurs with some regularity and in some instances may be a source of facial pain or ophthalmoplegia. Another mass-related surgical indication is seizure activity; it is usually of complex partial type and relates to tumor growth into the middle fossa with resultant temporal lobe irritation. An uncommon but emergent surgical indication for somatotroph adenomas is pituitary apoplexy. As is true for all pituitary tumors, acute hemorrhagic infarction of a pituitary tumor constitutes a true neurosurgical emergency for which prompt recognition, glucocorticoid replacement, and timely surgical decompression cannot only restore neurologic function but, in some instances, will also be lifesaving (32). A final surgical indication for somatotroph adenomas is failure of pharmacologic therapy in the form of resistance to, intolerance of, or patient preference against somatostatin analogs and/or dopamine agonists.

Surgical contraindications are few. In the occasional acromegalic patient, medical complications such as hypertension, cardiovascular disease, and diabetes may so significantly elevate operative risks so as to effectively contraindicate surgical intervention; these patients ordinarily become candidates for primary somatostatin analog therapy. As is true for all transsphenoidal procedures, active sinus infection will occasionally contraindicate surgery.

PREOPERATIVE EVALUATION

In contemplating surgery for somatotroph adenomas, several issues deserve careful attention.

Endocrine Issues

The endocrine diagnosis of acromegaly must be secure. Although the clinical phenotype is often characteristic, pathologic GH excess must be documented on careful endocrine testing. Our endocrine criteria include (a) elevated basal GH level (> 220 pmol/L [> 5 ng/mL]), (b) insufficient GH suppressibility on oral glucose tolerance testing (> 88 pmol/L [> 2 ng/mL]), and (c) elevation of serum insulinlike growth factor-1 (IGF-1) levels. Whereas fulfilling these criteria does establish a state of GH excess that, in the overwhelming majority of instances, will imply the presence of a somatotroph adenoma, one is often wise not to automatically make this assumption, even in the presence of a radiologically evident sellar mass. As a rule, one should always consider the remote possibility of ectopic acromegaly wherein GH excess is the result of a rare extrapituitary growth hormone-releasing hormone (GHRH) producing tumor. Although numerically insignificant in the broader context of acromegaly, this rare cohort of GHRH-producing lesions is diagnostically important. These include GHRH-producing carcinoid tumors in the gastrointestinal tract or lung; pancreatic islet cell tumors; small cell carcinoma of the lung; and, rarely, pheochromocytomas (33). As a result of their GHRH production, these lesions induce somatotroph hyperplasia with resultant sellar enlargement, GH excess, and clinical acromegaly that is phenotypically indistinguishable from that caused by a somatotroph adenoma. Failure to consider and exclude these ectopically secreting variants as potential causes of acromegaly can lead to inappropriate therapy, delaying recognition of an underlying and potentially aggressive neoplasm for which acromegaly may be the only early manifestation (33). If suspected, the diagnosis of an ectopic GHRH-producing lesion can be confirmed by radioimmunoassay; such lesions will produce measurable elevations in plasma GHRH levels (34).

The endocrine evaluation must also assess other elements of pituitary function, specifically the basal and reserve capacities of adrenal, thyroid, and gonadal axes. This will identify those patients in need of preoperative hormone replacement therapy and will also serve as a baseline for future hormonal replacement. Hormone deficiencies, particularly those involving cortisol and thyroid hormones, should be corrected prior to any elective procedure to minimize perioperative catastrophes related to inadequate pituitary reserve. Given the universal use of perioperative glucocorticoids for operative procedures in the region, adequacy of thyroid reserve tends to be the issue most often neglected. Preexisting hypothyroidism can present acutely in the early postoperative period. Accordingly, normalization of thyroid function, which may require a week of replacement therapy, should be attained prior to the procedure. In approximately one-third of patients, modest elevations of serum prolactin (PRL) levels will also be seen. In some instances, these elevations represent a "stalk section effect," whereas in others, they reflect hypersecretion from one of several plurihormonal somatotroph adenomas that actively cosecrete PRL, GH, and, occasionally, thyroid-stimulating hormone. Finally, because somatotroph adenomas are a well-known component of the autosomal-dominant multiple endocrine neoplasia type 1 syndrome (pituitary, parathyroid, and pancreatic islet cell tumors), the endocrine evaluation should be directed at identifying or excluding this condition (35, 36).

Imaging

As is true for all pituitary tumors, magnetic resonance imaging provides the most precise information on the size and extent of somatotroph adenomas. Important relationships between the adenoma and its surrounding structures should be clearly delineated. Magnetic resonance imaging is especially helpful in assessing chiasm compression, cavernous sinus invasion and/or compression, the extent of extrasellar growth, and the position of the carotid arteries. Such knowledge not only facilitates surgical planning, but also adds to the safety of the procedure. Given that overgrowth of soft tissues and bone are common accompaniments to acromegaly, particular attention should be given to the status of paranasal sinuses and potential distortions in the bony anatomy that may be encountered along the transsphenoidal route. Both plain skull radiographs and computed tomographic scans may be helpful in this regard.

Neuro-ophthalmologic Evaluation

Because visual dysfunction frequently complicates the course of many somatotroph adenomas, a complete ophthalmologic evaluation is mandatory in all patients with visual complaints and for those whose tumors exhibit suprasellar extension. In addition to the asymmetrical bitemporal hemianopic defect classically associated with pituitary tumors, other forms of visual dysfunction also occur. Depending on the anatomic status of the chiasm (prefixed, normal, or postfixed), the size of the tumor, its precise direction of growth, and the chronicity of the process, junctional scotomas, various monocular field defects, impaired acuity, afferent pupillary defects, papilledema, and optic atrophy may all be observed. Assessment of visual fields and acuity on a serial basis are often necessary to document disease progression and response to therapeutic intervention.

Special Problems in the Acromegalic Patient

Compared with patients with other types of pituitary tumors, several perioperative issues are unique to the acromegalic patient (37). Given that acromegaly is a complex, multisystem disease, a variety of medical problems frequently coexist in this patient population, all of which can serve to complicate operative management. Hypertension, ischemic heart disease, cardiomyopathy, peripheral vascular disease, and thyroid dysfunction together with diabetes and its protean complications all occur with some regularity in patients with acromegaly, and each adds an element of risk to the operative procedure. Whereas these medical problems will seldom be of such severity to contraindicate surgery, they are problems that must be recognized and carefully managed throughout the perioperative period.

The enlargement of the jaw and tongue that accompanies acromegaly can complicate perioperative airway management. Because acromegalics commonly suffer from dental malocclusion and temporal mandibular joint problems, jaw excursion may be severely limited. Macroglossia, goiter, and kyphosis further complicate the issue of airway management, sometimes necessitating fiberoptic endotracheal tube placement. In one series, difficulties with intubation were encountered in one-third of acromegalic patients (38).

Musculoskeletal problems are common in patients with acromegaly, particularly degenerative osteoarthritis of the spine. This can compromise ideal positioning of the neck. The overgrowth of soft tissues and bone in the skull and paranasal sinuses can complicate technical aspects of the procedure. In the transsphenoidal approach, the distance from the maxillary crest or the pyriform aperture of the nose to the sella is often sufficiently long that special lengthened instruments are required if successful surgery is to be performed. The nasal spine and the bony structures encountered during transsphenoidal exposure can be unusually stout and tend to bleed more when dissected. This is also true of the mucosal surfaces of the nose and sinuses, which are commonly hypertrophied and prone to hemorrhage during dissection. Tortuous, atherosclerotic carotid arteries are common in acromegalic patients, and their tendency to bulge into the operative field during sellar entry and intrasellar dissection render them prone to injury. In the few patients who require a transcranial approach, additional problems may exist. The scalp tends to be thick, corrugated, highly vascular, and unusually mobile. Because the skull is thick and not easily perforated, elevating a bone flap can be difficult. The air sinuses are exuberant, and often a frontal sinus must be violated to gain adequate exposure.

Preoperative Somatostatin Analog Therapy

Recognizing that endocrine remission is not uniformly achieved in somatotroph adenomas, particularly in the setting of large and invasive examples, there has been interest in the preoperative use of somatostatin analogs as a means of reducing tumor size and perhaps improving surgical outcome (39–41). Tumor softening has been reported in response to these agents, a change that, according to some, may facilitate tumor resection and perhaps even improve surgical outcome as well (39, 40). Whereas the concept has theoretical appeal, the number of rigorously evaluated patients so treated have been few, and whether this strategy actually improves operative outcomes in either the short or long-term remains to be established. In our experience, the results of pretreatment have not been sufficiently dramatic to warrant its adoption as routine.

OPERATIVE MANAGEMENT

Having decided to intervene surgically, consideration is then given to the choice of surgical approach. Currently, more than 95% of pituitary tumors, including those associated with acromegaly, can be approached by one or another variation of the transsphenoidal route (21). In most instances, this will imply a standard microsurgical submucosal transseptal transsphenoidal procedure. The virtues of the transsphenoidal approach are well recognized. It represents the most physiologic corridor of surgical access to the sella, providing direct and superior visualization of the pituitary gland and of the sellar pathologic findings, and does so in a minimally traumatic fashion. The surgical exposure is performed by the traditional sublabial rhinoseptal route, or, given the typically capacious nostrils of the acromegalic patient, through an endonasal approach. Current practice favors both approaches in equal proportions. Details of our approach have been presented elsewhere (20). Variations of the transsphenoidal approach, including transethmoidal, lateral rhinotomy, transnasal septal displacement, transantral, and transpalatal procedures, can occasionally be helpful in certain situations, most frequently in the setting of repeat surgery for recurrence. Endoscopic transsphenoidal approaches have also been described and have been successfully employed in resecting GH-secreting pituitary tumors.

Fewer than 5% of patients require a transcranial (pterional, subfrontal, or subtemporal) approach. The primary features considered in deciding between a transsphenoidal and a transcranial approach are those related to the anatomy of the sellar region. These include the size of the sella, its degree of mineralization, and the size and pneumatization of the sinuses. Of tumors with extrasellar extensions, the extent and direction of the extension are also taken into account. As a rule, a transsphenoidal approach is preferred in all but the following circumstances: (*a*) a tumor with significant anterior extension into the anterior cranial fossa or lateral and/or posterior extension into the middle cranial fossa; (*b*) a tumor with suprasellar extension and an hourglass configuration suggestive of a small diaphragmatic aperture; and (*c*) when there is reason to believe that the consistency of a tumor having suprasellar extension is sufficiently fibrous to prevent its collapse and descent into the sella when resected from below.

RESULTS OF SURGERY

In evaluating the results of surgery, one must consider the clinical response from the standpoint of presenting symptoms, the biochemical response with regard to restoration of GH secretory dynamics, and the long-term response in terms of prevention of tumor recurrence. The latter issue is considered later (see Tumor Recurrence).

Acromegalic Symptoms and Mass Effects

In the overwhelming majority of acromegalic patients, including all those in whom biochemical remission has been achieved, as well as those in whom GH levels have been significantly reduced but not normalized, prompt regression of several symptoms can be expected postoperatively. Headache frequently improves immediately. Over the next few days, this is followed by improvements in hyperhydrosis and paresthesias and by regression of soft tissue swelling. Such responses tend to be the rule, being observed to some degree in 97% of surgically treated patients (21). Diabetes mellitus also responds to surgery in a predictable, favorable fashion; for patients in whom GH levels are normalized, resolution of diabetes and/or glucose intolerance have been reported in up to 80 to 100% of cases (42, 43). Significant improvements in glucose tolerance can also be expected in patients in whom surgery reduces, but fails to normalize, GH levels. Hypertension tends to be considerably less responsive to surgery than are the other acromegalic features (42, 43). Although some improvement in blood pressure has been noted postoperatively, hypertension often persists, sometimes even after successful surgery, probably because of chronic structural changes in the heart and vessels.

Hyperprolactinemia, accompanying about 40 to 50% of somatotroph adenomas, is frequently the result of a bihormonal tumor capable of both GH and PRL hypersecretion. Of acromegalic women of childbearing age, approximately half will have amenorrhea (23). We previously reported a series of six such amenorrheic women, four of whom experienced postoperative resumption of menses; two of these eventually conceived (28). A comparable response has been reported by others (44).

Symptomatic mass effects can be expected to respond to surgery in most instances. Improvements or stabilization in visual fields occurs in 90 to 100% of patients (28, 29, 45).

Defining Endocrinologic Remission

Although it has been recognized for some time that the completeness of surgical resection must ultimately be judged on the basis of measurable endocrinologic parameters, there has been a distinct lack of uniformity in the specific endocrinologic criteria that investigators have used to define remission or "cure." It is now clear that the criteria used to define remission in earlier series, such as reduction of basal GH levels to less than 440 pmol/L (< 10 ng/mL), may have been too liberal; patients thought to have been "cured" on this basis were in fact not cured and continued to have active acromegaly (19, 46, 47). As a result, and particularly during the past decade, the concept of "cure" in acromegaly has evolved considerably, and some consensus now exists as to the minimum biochemical criteria that must underlie its definition. First, it is preferable to speak in terms of remission rather than "cure" because the long-term outcome of surgically treated somatotroph adenomas is still not definitively known and no endocrinologic criteria, however stringent, can absolutely guarantee that the patient will remain free of disease in the future. Currently, and in addition to a favorable clinical response, the operational definition of endocrinologic remission in acromegaly requires (*a*) suppression of GH levels to less than 88 pmol/L (< 2 ng/mL) during an oral glucose tolerance test and (*b*) normalization of plasma IGF-1 levels (3, 19, 26, 47–49). In virtually all instances, patients fulfilling these criteria will also have basal GH levels of less than 220 pmol/L (< 5 ng/mL), but because the converse is often, but not necessarily always, true, there has been a move away from using this, or for that matter, any, specific basal or random GH level as the sole remission criterion. Moreover, it can be argued that the value of GH level less than 220 pmol/L (< 5 ng/mL), despite its widespread use in reporting surgical results, is still a somewhat arbitrary therapeutic endpoint. If remission is to be based on any critical GH level, the only prognostically justifiable criterion is a mean GH level less than 110 pmol/L (< 2.5 ng/mL). As discussed previously, reductions of mean GH levels below this threshold have been identified as the most important factor associated with reducing mortality in patients with acromegaly (15). Accordingly, if lowering of GH levels is to be used as a measure of surgical success, reduction below this value would, in this context, represent a reasonable therapeutic end point. Other endocrinologic outcome criteria have been proposed, such as postoperative normalization of a previously paradoxical response to thyrotropin-releasing hormone or the somewhat laborious verification that the 24-hour integrated GH level has normalized (19, 50). Whereas some have found a persistent paradoxical GH response to thyrotropin-releasing hormone to be indicative of residual tumor and a higher risk for biochemical recurrence (50), others have questioned the prognostic merits of this test and the necessity of its inclusion in the definition of postoperative remission (26, 51).

Reported Rates of Endocrine Remission

Despite the difficulties in defining postoperative endocrinologic remission in acromegaly and the variations in remission criteria used by different investigators, a large body of data does exist for evaluating the results of operative therapy for somatotroph adenomas. Using a postoperative GH level of less than 220 pmol/L (< 5 ng/mL) as the remission criterion, Ross and Wilson (31) analyzed the results of 30 published surgical series and identified an overall endocrine remission rate of 60% in 771 patients. Similar results were reported by Zervas (52) in a multicenter survey. Of 1256 acromegalic patients in which the minimum of several remission criteria included basal GH level less than 220 pmol/L (< 5 ng/mL), an overall rate of endocrine remission was 66% (52). These composite data also compare with the results of individual series from the literature (26, 27, 29–31, 48, 51, 53–57). When surgery is used as the sole primary therapy and in the absence of any prior therapy, endocrine remission can be expected in 42 to 84% of patients (Table 16.1). Understandably, with the application of more rigorous remission criteria, such as those outlined above, rates of surgical success are lower. This is illustrated in the 222-patient series of Fahlbusch et al. (26) in which a 71% remission rate was observed when GH level less than 220 pmol/L (< 5 ng/mL) was used but which dropped to 57% when remission was defined on the basis of suppressibility of GH to less than 88 pmol/L (< 2 ng/mL) on an oral glucose tolerance test. Similarly, Losa et al. (56) reported a remission rate of 55% when GH less than 44 pmol/L (< 1 ng/mL) and normal IGF-1 levels were used to define remission.

As discussed below, tumor size and invasion status have a clear influence on surgical outcome. Understandably, remission rates will be highest for microadenomas, tending to drop somewhat for diffuse macroadenomas, and dropping significantly for invasive macroadenomas and those with extrasellar extension. For microadenomas, postoperative endocrine remission has been variably reported in 66 to 100% of somatotroph microadenomas (Table 16.1). When all macroadenomas are considered, including all grades of invasion and extrasellar extension, postoperative remission has been reported in 49 to 77% of patients. When remission rates of diffuse (i.e., grade II) and invasive (i.e., grades III and IV) macroadenomas are separated, however, the outcome among the latter is considerably less favorable. Among grade II, III, and IV tumors, Tindall et al. (27) reported remission rates of 60%, 23%, and 0%, respectively. Interestingly, a relationship between tumor size/grade and

Table 16.1. *Results of Primary Transsphenoidal Surgery for GH-Secreting Pituitary Adenomas*

Series	Number	Total Series	Remission Rates		Remission Criteria
			Microadenomas	Macroadenoma	
Teasdale et al. 1982 (53)	28	19/28 (68%)	N/A	N/A	GH < 5.0 ng/mL
Serri et al. 1985 (54)	25	21/25 (84%)	8/8 (100%)	13/17 (77%)	GH < 5.0 ng/mL; and GH < 2.5 ng/mL on OGTT
Roelfsema et al. 1985 (55)	60	37/60 (62%)	6/9 (67%)	31/51 (61%)	GH ≤ 2.5 ng/mL
Grisoli et al. 1985 (29)	100	60/100 (60%)	N/A	N/A	GH < 5.0 ng/mL
van't Verlaat et al. 1988 (30)	25	14/25 (56%)	N/A	N/A	GH < 5.0 ng/mL and GH ≤ 2.0 ng/mL on OGTT
Ross and Wilson 1988 (31)	153	86/153 (56%)	N/A	N/A	GH < 5.0 ng/mL
Losa et al. 1989 (56)	29	16/29 (55%)	N/A	N/A	GH < 1.0 ng/mL on OGTT *and* normal IGF-1 level
Valdemarsson et al. 1991 (51)	38	28/38 (74%)	11/13 (85%)	17/25 (68%)	GH < 5.0 ng/mL and/or GH < 3.0 ng/mL on OGTT
Fahlbusch et al. 1992 (26)	222	126/222 (57%)	53/74 (72%)	73/150 (49%)	GH < 2.0 ng/mL during OGTT
		158/222 (71%)	60/74 (81%)	98/150 (65%)	GH < 5.0 ng/mL
Tindall et al. 1993 (27)	291	75/91 (82%)	N/A	N/A	GH < 5.0 ng/mL and/or normal IGF-1 level
Davis et al. 1993 (57)	174	(52%)	N/A	N/A	GH ≤ 2.0 ng/mL (basal or during OGTT)
Sheaves et al. 1996 (48)	100	42/100 (42%)	4 (61%)	(23%)	GH ≤ 2.5 ng/mL
Authors series (1988–97)	117	64/117 (55%)	16/22 (73%)	48/95 (50.5%)	GH ≤ 2.5 ng/mL *and* GH ≤ 2.0 ng/mL during OGTT; *and* IGF-1 level normal

[1] Results from 153 patients who did not have prior therapy from a total series of 214 patients are included here.
[2] Results from 91 patients who did not have prior therapy from a total series of 103 patients are included here.
[3] 25% of patients in this series had postoperative radiation therapy.
[4] 6 patients achieving surgical remission were also give postoperative radiation therapy.

Table 16.2. *Results of Transsphenoidal Microsurgery in the Management of Acromegaly (1988-1997; n = 117)*

Tumor Category	Mean Preoperative GH Level (ng/mL)	Remission Rate (%)[a]
Microadenoma	29	73
Noninvasive macradenoma (diffuse)	56	58
Invasive macroadenoma	65	46

[a] Remission criteria: Basal GH ≤ 2.0 ng/mL; and GH ≤ 2.5 ng/mL on OGTT; and normalized IGF-1 level.

outcome was less obvious in the series of Ross and Wilson (31). Aside from grade IV tumors, which had a remission rate of 23%, the remission rates for grade II and III tumors in that series were similar (57%). In our 1988 to 1997 series of 117 acromegalic patients using GH, less than 110 pmol/L (< 2.5 ng/mL), surgical remission rates for microadenomas, diffuse macroadenomas, and invasive macroadenomas were 73%, 58%, and 46%, respectively (Table 16.2).

Complications

The spectrum of complications associated with the operative management of somatotroph adenomas tends, for the most part, to parallel the spectrum of complications associated with the transsphenoidal procedure in general (20, 58) (Table 16.3). Ross and Wilson (31), in their review of operative complications in 30 published surgical series involving a total of 1360 acromegalic patients, identified an overall operative mortality rate of 1.04%. Most operative deaths stem from direct operative trauma to the carotid arteries or the hypothalamus, perioperative medical complications, and, less frequently, meningitis. The major categories of nonfatal operative complications include vascular complications, cerebrospinal fluid leak, meningitis, visual complications, injury to other cranial nerves, new anterior pituitary deficits, permanent diabetes insipidus, complications relating to the nasal/extracranial aspect of the procedure, perioperative medical complications, and, of course, failure to achieve control of GH hypersecretion. Fortunately, major morbidity is uncommon in the transsphenoidal management of these tumors (27, 28, 31, 42, 43, 48, 55, 57, 59). Excluding for the moment the failure to control GH hypersecretion, which is discussed separately below, the most frequent major complication is the development of new anterior pituitary deficits, having been reported in 5 to 19% of patients. The reported frequencies of other major complications are summarized in Table 16.4. With the exception of vascular complications, which tend to be somewhat more frequent in the acromegalic patient, no other category of complication seems especially unique to this population of pituitary tumor patients. Three main reasons seem to account for acromegalic patients having a slightly higher risk of vascular complications. Perhaps most important is the fact that these patients tend

to have ectactic atherosclerotic carotid arteries, particularly in the region of the cavernous sinus, wherein a tortuous loop may bulge into the operative field, putting it at risk for operative injury. Second, during the extracranial dissection, the bone and mucosal tissues encountered during the transsphenoidal exposure tend to be heavily vascularized and are therefore more prone to hemorrhage. This can be sufficiently severe that the procedure may have to be abandoned at an early stage. Finally, because cavernous sinus invasion/extension occurs with some regularity in somatotroph adenomas, it is recognized that the surgeon may be required to work within one or another cavernous sinus to achieve total removal; venous bleeding of this type can be troublesome but usually responds to gentle tamponade.

When viewed from that standpoint of individual major complication rates, as depicted in Table 16.4, it is true that major operative complications are uncommon in the management of these tumors. Often overlooked and not reflected in these figures, however, is the case complication rate for these tumors, which, when meticulously analyzed, tends to be considerably higher than might be expected. For example, in the series of Ross and Wilson (31), one or more complications occurred in 44 (19.6%) of 224 operative procedures for somatotroph adenomas. Thus, although it is acknowledged that mortality and major morbidity are uncommon, it must be recognized that complications of one form or another are not rare in the individual acromegalic patient.

Most complications are preventable, others can be anticipated, and some will be unavoidable; however, all must be promptly recognized and appropriately treated. Hypothalamic injuries, intracavernous carotid injuries, and damage to the optic apparatus, usually the result of blind curetting attempts or application of undue traction to adherent tumor fragments, can be avoided with careful dissection techniques. Once encountered, arterial bleeding from a

Table 16.3. Complications of Transsphenoidal Surgery for Somatotroph Adenomas (n = 450 Patients)

Complication	Number
Deaths	0
Hypothalamic injury	0
Intracranial hemorrhage	0
Carotid artery injury	2
Anterior cerebral artery injury	1
Vascular occlusion with stroke	0
Hemorrhage, intraoperative	3
CSF rhinorrhea	4
Meningitis	0
Visual loss	1
Cranial nerve injury	0
Permanent diabetes insipidus	4
SIADH, symptomatic	6
Nasal septal injury	1
Infection (lip, sinus, nose)	3
Postoperative dementia	1
Angiographic complication	1
New hypopituitarism	18
Total	**45**
Overall case complication rate (45/450)	**10.0%**

Table 16.4. Complications of Transsphenoidal Surgery for Somatotroph Adenomas

Series	No. of Patients	Deaths	Vascular[1]	Meningitis	CSF Leak	Visual Defect (Worsening)	Cranial Nerve Injury	New Hypopituitarism	DI (Permanent)
Laws et al. 1979 (28)	82	0	1	0	1	0	0	15/80[2] (19%)	0
Tucker et al. 1980 (43)	32	0	0	1	1	0	0	4/32 (13%)	1
Balagura et al. 1981 (42)	132[3]	5	1	3	8	0	0	N/A	1
Quabbe 1982 (59)	152	0	1	5	4	0	1	26/152 (17%)	8
Teasdale et al. 1982 (53)	28	0	0	0	0	0	0	5/28 (18%)	2
Roelfsema et al. 1985 (55)	60	0	0	1	3	0	2	9/60[4] (15%)	3
Ross & Wilson 1988 (31)	214	0	5[5]	4	11	0	3	9/172[6] (5%)	0
Davis et al. 1993 (57)	175	0	1[7]	0	0	3	0	22/175 (13%)	0
Tindall et al. 1993 (27)	103	0	0	0	7	1	0	6/103 (6%)	1
Sheaves et al. 1996 (48)	100	0	1	8	9	0	0	21/100 (21%)	8
Total	**1078**	**5/1078 (0.46%)**	**10/1078 (0.92%)**	**22/1078 (2.0%)**	**45/1078 (4.2%)**	**4/1078 (0.37%)**	**6/1078 (0.56%)**	**117/902 (13.0%)**	**24/1078 (2.2%)**

[1] Includes patients with intra- and/or postoperative hemorrhage and/or vascular injury.
[2] 2 patients excluded for lack of follow-up.
[3] 7 patients in this series had a transcranial procedure.
[4] Reported as the proportion of new anterior pituitary deficits requiring replacement therapy.
[5] 2 patients had carotid artery injury and 3 patients had severe intraoperative bleeding.
[6] Patients with postoperative radiotherapy excluded.
[7] Refers to a delayed intracranial hematoma 11 months postoperatively.

damaged segment of the cavernous carotid can be difficult to control. A small piece of fat or microfibrillar collagen strategically placed over the bleeding site can often control bleeding better than vigorous overpacking, which may only serve to enlarge the tear. Because carotid occlusion, vasospasm, false aneurysm, and carotid-cavernous fistulae are potential sequelae to such injuries, immediate postoperative angiography will always be required in suspected carotid injuries. Gentle intrasellar dissection, together with a thorough awareness of the position of the carotid arteries, as determined by the preoperative magnetic resonance imaging scan, will minimize such complications. Injuries to the visual apparatus can also arise from technical factors related to packing of the sella. Overzealous packing can lead to chiasmal compression, whereas underpacking can predispose to chiasmal prolapse. Injuries to the cranial nerves within the cavernous sinus, due again to aggressive instrumentation or packing, are generally neuropraxic in nature; permanent damage can occur, but transient and self-limited dysfunction is the rule. Intraoperative cerebrospinal fluid leaks will necessitate some form of tissue graft, usually fat, followed by careful sellar reconstruction. Of cerebrospinal fluid leaks in the postoperative period, most are best treated by prompt reexploration and repair. Although not life threatening, complications relating to the nasofacial aspect of the procedure (nasal septal perforations, nasal deformities, fractures of the hard palate or cribiform plate, dental denervation, sinusitis, and mucoceles) can be troublesome and persist for some time. Often related to technical errors in tissue handling during the exposure, most of these can be avoided with careful technique.

PREDICTORS OF SURGICAL OUTCOME

A number of clinicopathologic factors have been recognized as having some bearing on surgical outcome and remission likelihood. In the broadest sense, these can be categorized as those factors relating to the patient and those relating to the tumor. Of the latter, the size, growth characteristics, invasion status, secretory activity, and ultrastructural morphologic characteristics of the tumor can each have some impact on the outcome of surgery.

Patient-Related Factors

Of the factors predictive of surgical outcome, comparatively few will be directly referable to patient-related factors. It has been suggested that an early age of presentation, particularly age younger than 25 years (60), may be an adverse prognostic factor; however, a relationship between age and surgical outcome has not been borne out of other studies (27, 61). Patients suffering from gigantism, compared with acromegaly, are well recognized as a potentially refractory group of patients in whom remission is not routinely achieved (28). Why they should be less responsive

to surgical resection is unclear. One explanation, stemming from the occasional finding of primary mammosomatotroph hyperplasia rather than a typical adenoma in these patients, is that hypothalamic dysfunction may underlie GH excess in some of these patients, a phenomenon that would not be remedied by surgery.

Patients with multiple endocrine neoplasia type 1 syndrome are predisposed to pituitary tumor development, of which about 20% will be of somatotrophic type (35, 36). The basis of this autosomal-dominant disorder has been linked to a tumor suppressor gene mapped to the 11q13 region (62). Despite the theoretical possibility that these patients may be more prone to the development of aggressive or multicentric pituitary tumors, or that somatotroph tumors in this setting may be more refractory to surgical remission or subject to increased rates of recurrence, this does not seem to be the case (35).

Of the patient-related factors, the most important adverse prognostic factor is a history of previous treatment, especially unsuccessful prior surgery (63). That transsphenoidal surgery following unsuccessful prior transcranial or transsphenoidal surgery, and to a lesser extent, following radiation or pharmacotherapy, is associated with a less favorable endocrinologic outcome and a higher rate of complications is well recognized for all types of pituitary tumors. In this setting of unsuccessful prior therapy, we reported an overall remission rate of 42% for acromegaly-associated pituitary tumors (63). Similar results were reported by Ross and Wilson (31) in that surgical remission was achieved in 56% of acromegalics without prior surgery but in only 44% of patients with prior surgery (31). A similar trend was evident in the series of Tindall et al. in which the remission rates of previously untreated patients were considerably more favorable than those subject to prior bromocriptine therapy or radiation; the remission rates in these three groups were 82%, 75%, and 64%, respectively (27).

Tumor-Related Factors

Both the secretory activity and growth characteristics (i.e., size, invasion status, and extrasellar growth) of the tumor can influence responsiveness to surgical outcome. Although these are discussed separately, they tend to be somewhat interrelated factors, because larger tumors also tend to be those associated with higher preoperative GH levels and are also those more prone to invasive and extrasellar growth.

Secretory Activity

In many surgical series, an inverse relationship between preoperative GH levels and the likelihood of postoperative remission has been observed (26, 27, 31, 48, 56, 57, 61). This relationship can be characterized in several ways. First, when comparing the mean preoperative GH levels of patients in whom remission has and has not been achieved, virtually all surgical series have found that of the latter group to be significantly higher. Second, this inverse relationship tends to be somewhat linear, wherein progressive increments in preoperative GH levels are associated with a stepwise decline in the likelihood of postoperative remission. This has been shown in the series of Fahlbusch et al. (26) in which remission rates for tumors with preoperative GH levels of less than 440, 440 to 1320, 1320 to 2200, 2200 to 4400, 4400 to 8800, and greater than 800 pmol/L ($<$ 10, 10 to 30, 30 to 50, 50 to 100, 100 to 200, and $>$ 200 ng/mL) were 73%, 57%, 51%, 46%, 35%, and 25%, respectively (26). Third, a threshold preoperative GH level can be identified, below and beyond which remission is more and less likely, respectively. Various threshold values between 1760 and 3080 pmol/L (40 and 70 ng/mL) have been proposed, although 2200 pmol/L (50 ng/mL) tends to be the most frequently used. In general, tumors associated with preoperative GH values of less than 2200 pmol/L ($<$ 50 ng/mL) are most amenable to postoperative remission. For tumors with preoperative GH levels below this threshold, Ross and Wilson (31) achieved a remission rate of 83%, differing significantly from the 57% remission rate in tumors with preoperative GH levels in excess of 2200 pmol/L ($>$ 50 ng/mL). An even wider difference was demonstrated by Davis et al. (57): the likelihood of remission for tumors with a GH level less than 2112 pmol/L ($<$ 48 ng/mL) was 62%, whereas the remission rate for tumors with higher GH levels was only 22%. Similarly, Sheaves et al. (48) observed remission in 65% and 18% of patients with preoperative GH levels below and above 2200 pmol/L (50 ng/mL), respectively. Although the preoperative GH level does provide a practical prognostic index, it is important to recognize that the preoperative GH level is to some degree dependent on the size and invasiveness of the tumor. As shown in Table 16.2, the preoperative GH levels tends to increase with increasing size and invasiveness. The issue was more precisely illustrated in the outcome analysis of Tindall et al. (27) wherein preoperative GH level was a significant univariate predictor of postoperative remission; however, when subject to multivariate analysis in the presence of other more robust predictors, such as Hardy grade and tumor stage, the predictive significance of preoperative GH level was no longer apparent.

As discussed previously, hyperprolactinemia is present in approximately 20 to 30% of acromegalic patients. The prognostic significance of PRL cosecretion by somatotroph adenomas from the standpoint of surgical responsiveness is unsettled. In one report, the preoperative PRL level was significantly higher in patients failing to achieve postoperative remission (61); however, this has not been a universal finding (27).

Tumor Size, Grade, Stage, and Invasiveness

Of the various clinicopathologic predictors of surgical outcome, tumor size, invasiveness, and, particularly, the degree of extrasellar extension have generally been re-

garded as being the most important. With regard to tumor size, the fact that microadenomas have a more favorable outcome than macroadenomas has been discussed previously. As an alternative to the conventional comparison of micro- and macroadenomas based on the 10 mm size criterion, Stevenaert et al. (41) used 16 mm as a cutoff value to compare outcomes of small and large tumors. Using GH levels less than 88 pmol/L ($<$ 2 ng/mL) as the remission criterion, 68% of tumors less than 16 mm in diameter had a successful result compared with a 37% remission rate in larger tumors (41). The adverse effect of increasing tumor size on outcome was also apparent in the study of Delalande et al. (60). In comparing tumors less than 15, less than 25, and greater than 25 mm in size, the rates of remission dropped from 82%, to 50%, to 30%, respectively (60).

The growth characteristics of pituitary tumors are classified on the five-grade classification of Hardy (grades 0 through IV) and further stratified into one of five stages (stages A through E), depending on the degree and direction of extrasellar extension (64, 65) (Fig. 16.1). Progressive increments in tumor grade and stage are both associated with reductions in remission likelihood. The adverse effect of increasing tumor grade on outcome has been discussed previously. Although tumor grade and stage tend to be related, tumor stage seems to be the most important prognostic factor. In the outcome analysis of Tindall et al. (27), tumor stage was the strongest outcome predictor. Whereas remission was achieved in 73% of tumors without extrasellar extension, it was achieved in only 27% of tumors with extrasellar extension (stages A through E). Similarly, in the series of Ross and Wilson (31), tumor stage was a more convincing predictor of postoperative outcome than was the Hardy grade alone.

One of the main reasons for the less favorable outcomes that accompany increases in tumor size, grade, and stage is the fact that larger tumors and those with extrasellar extension are more prone to invasive growth (24, 66). Invasion is a major problem for all pituitary tumors and is particularly so in the case of somatotroph adenomas because a larger proportion of these tumors are invasive macroadenomas at presentation compared with other secretory types of pituitary tumors (1, 22). Invasion of surrounding dura or bone may be evident histologically in the surgical specimen or grossly on the basis of intraoperative inspection and/or preoperative imaging. Both gross and microscopic evidence of invasion adversely affect surgical success in patients with acromegaly. Using the criterion of microscopic invasion, Landolt et al. (67) reported an 84% remission rate among noninvasive tumors, differing significantly from the 46% remission rate present among invasive tumors. More frequently, investigators tend to define invasion grossly, on the basis of intraoperative or radiologic findings. Numerous reports have indicated that remission rates for grossly invasive tumors are significantly lower than those for noninvasive tumors (26, 29, 41, 42).

Tumor Pathology

Although unified by their hypersecretion, the pituitary tumors underlying acromegaly are a morphologically di-

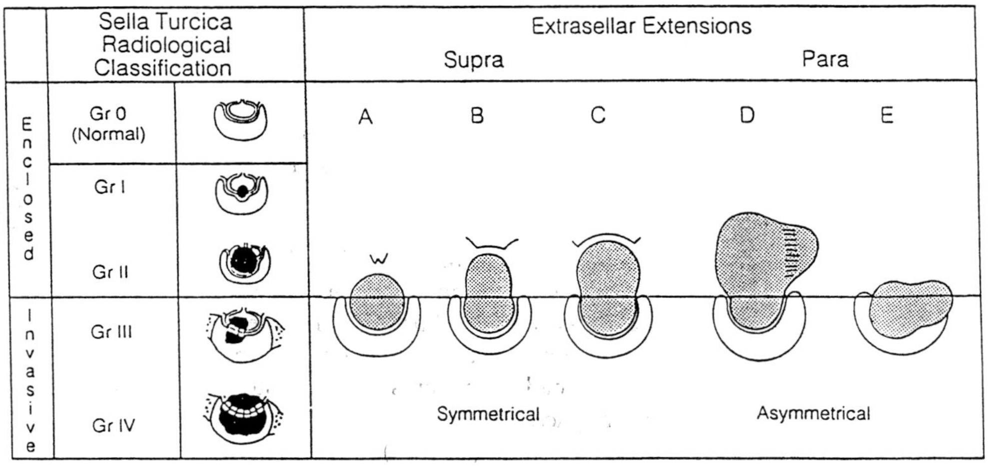

	Sella Turcica Radiological Classification		Extrasellar Extensions				
			Supra			Para	
E n c l o s e d	Gr 0 (Normal)		A	B	C	D	E
	Gr I						
	Gr II						
I n v a s i v e	Gr III						
	Gr IV		Symmetrical			Asymmetrical	

Hardy Classification of Pituitary Tumors[a]

Radiologic	Anatomic	Surgical
Sella Turcica		
Grade 0	Intact, normal contour	Micro enclosed
Grade I	Intact, focal bulging	Micro enclosed
Grade II	Intact, enlarged	Macro enclosed
Grade III	Destroyed, partially	Macro invasive
Grade IV	Destroyed, totally	Macro invasive
Grade V[b]	Distant spread via CSF or blood	Macro carcinoma

Extrasellar Extensions

Suprasellar (Symmetrical)

A	Suprasellar cistern
B	Recesses of III ventricle
C	Whole anterior III ventricle

Parasellar (Asymmetrical)

D	Intracranial intradural
	Anterior
	Midline
	Posterior
E[b]	Extracranial extradural (lateral cavernous sinus)

[a]Radiologic classification of pituitary tumors as originally proposed by Jules Hardy (ref. 65) with subsequent modification by C.B. Wilson (64).

[b]Additional grades as proposed by Wilson (64). Hardy Classification system.

Figure 16.1. Hardy classification system.

verse collection of neoplasms. On the basis of ultrastructural morphology, five main somatotroph adenoma subtypes have been identified. These include densely granulated GH cell adenomas, sparsely granulated GH cell adenoma, mixed somatotroph-lactotroph adenomas, mammosomatotroph adenomas, and the acidophil stem cell adenomas (1, 68). Data concerning the relationship between tumor subtype and postoperative outcome are limited. In a recent analysis of 100 acromegaly-associated pituitary tumors, we were unable to isolate a significant statistical effect of ultrastructural pathology on postoperative outcome (69). Others have, however, demonstrated that some variants seem to be more aggressive than others. For example, Yamada et al. (70) reported that surgical remission could be achieved in only 13% of sparsely granulated tumors, whereas it could be achieved in 65% of densely granulated tumors. The wide difference seemed to reflect the greater tendencies of the former toward aggressive and invasive growth, a feature that has been recognized for some time. A second group of tumors that seems to have a less favorable outcome are those that immunohistochemically coexpress both PRL and GH. Compared with the 83% remission rate present in tumors immunoreactive for GH only, the remission rate of tumors that also coexpressed PRL was only 21% (71). Finally, we recently demonstrated that somatotroph adenomas that overexpress the GHRH gene tend to have a more aggressive clinical phenotype (69). These tumors were associated with higher preoperative GH levels, were more likely to be invasive, had higher tumor growth fractions, and were significantly less likely to achieve postoperative remission.

ADJUVANT THERAPY

Overall, in about 50 to 70% of acromegalic patients, surgery alone can be expected to induce a durable endocrine remission. Although these patients will require periodic follow-up and, in some instances, hormone replacement therapy, no additional adjuvant therapy will be required. For the substantial proportion of patients that remain, however, surgery alone will not be entirely successful and persistence of active acromegaly will necessitate the use of one or more forms of adjuvant therapy. In most instances, mass effects will have been effectively ameliorated by surgery, and attention generally turns to the goals of reducing GH hypersecretion and preventing regrowth. As discussed previously, an immediate therapeutic end point will be reduction of GH levels to less than 110 pmol/L (< 2.5 ng/mL) as a means of eliminating the premature mortality associated with acromegaly. To achieve these goals, the options can include medical therapy with somatostatin analogs and/or dopamine agonists, conventional radiation therapy, or stereotactic radiosurgery. Although each of these options is effective to various degrees in various situations, little consensus is reached as to what constitutes the "best" strategy. The selection of adjuvant therapies will depend on the specific situation at hand, as well as the preferences of both the patient and the treating physician. Not infrequently, multimodal adjuvant therapy will be required. Medical and radiation therapies for acromegaly are discussed in detail elsewhere in this text.

In deciding between pharmacologic and radiation therapies, a key consideration will be the extent of residual tumor. In some instances, usually in the context of invasive macroadenomas in which inaccessible and macroscopic tumor remnants remain, symptomatic regrowth will represent a major long-term threat. For such patients, it has been our practice to recommend radiation therapy because it is the most effective means of forestalling tumor regrowth. While awaiting a radiotherapeutic response, octreotide and, to a lesser extent, bromocriptine therapy can prove effective in reducing GH levels. In other instances, the amount of residual tumor will be small. Typically, this will be represented by the patient in whom gross total resection has been achieved but in whom GH levels have not normalized. For such patients, adjuvant medical therapy with octreotide and/or bromocriptine is often a reasonable first step. In such settings, radiation therapy would be reserved for an inadequate response to medical therapy or radiologically evident tumor regrowth. Although it is true that the great majority of patients (80 to 90%) will have a clinical and biochemical response to octreotide administration, the enthusiasm for octreotide therapy must be tempered with the realization that only about half of all octreotide-treated patients will have suppression of GH levels below the desired therapeutic end point of 110 pmol/L (2.5 ng/mL) (72–74).

TUMOR RECURRENCE
Frequency

In considering the problem of recurrence, an initial distinction should be made between the genuine recurrence of a previously removed tumor and the regrowth of a persistent, incompletely excised tumor. In this context, we strictly adopt the former definition and consider recurrence as new tumor growth after gross total removal and/or the relapse of active acromegaly after a sustained and well-documented period of endocrine remission. Understandably, the rate of recurrence in acromegaly will depend on the stringency of the criteria with which remission was originally defined, as well as the period of follow-up. When strict criteria are used to define remission, such as suppression of GH levels to less than 88 pmol/L (< 2 ng/mL) on an oral glucose tolerance testing and normalization of IGF-1 levels, a durable remission is usually achieved and recurrence tends to be infrequent. As outlined in Table 16.5, the rate of recurrence in several large series has ranged from 0 to 18% during mean follow-up periods of 2.9 to 8.9 years; in aggregate, the rate of recurrence in these 10 series was approximately 6% (29–31, 48, 54, 57, 67, 75). Of surgically treated acromegalic patients in whom endocrine remission had been achieved, we encountered an 8% recurrence rate during a 10-year follow-up period (76). The series of Davis et al. (57) emphasizes the importance of long-term follow-up and the tendency of recurrences to increase with time. In that report, the cumulative probability of recurrence at 1 and 5 years was 11% and 32%, respectively (57).

Management

The goals of management for recurrent somatotroph adenomas are identical to those described for virgin somatotroph adenomas; however, realization of these goals tends to be more difficult in the setting of recurrence. Management options include repeat surgery, a trial of medical therapy, and/or radiation therapy.

Table 16.5. *Rates of Somatotroph Adenoma Recurrence After Prior Successful Surgery*

Series	No. of Patients in Remission	Recurrence Rate	Mean Follow-up (Years)	Original Remission Criteria
Serri et al. 1985 (54)	21	14.3%	8.9	GH < 2.5 ng/mL during OGTT
Grisoli et al. 1985 (29)	60	10.0%	N/A	GH < 5.0 ng/mL
Ross et al. 1988 (31)	117	4.3%	6.3	GH < 5.0 ng/mL
Landolt et al. 1988 (67)	169	2.4%	4.1	GH < 5.0 ng/mL
van't Verlaat et al. 1988 (30)	14	0.0%	3.5	GH < 2.0 ng/mL during OGTT
Losa et al. 1989 (56)	16	0.0%	2.9	GH < 1.0 ng/mL during OGTT *and* normal IGF-1 level
Buchfelder et al. 1991 (75)	61	6.6%	6.0	GH < 5.0 ng/mL
Buchfelder et al. 1991 (75)	63	0.0%	6.5	GH < 2.0 ng/mL during OGTT
Davis et al. 1993 (57)	90[1]	17.8%	5.8	GH < 2.0 ng/mL (fasting or on OGTT)
Sheaves et al. 1996 (48)	32[2]	3.1%	3.8	GH < 2.5 ng/mL

[1] 25% of patients in this series had postoperative radiation therapy.
[2] Includes only those patients in whom surgery was the only treatment.

Many recurrent acromegalics will be candidates for repeat surgery; however, the need for reoperation and its role among the alternatives of surgical management should be carefully individualized. In contemplating reoperation for acromegaly, several basic considerations apply. The first fundamental principle is that a surgical target must be clearly identifiable. This implies the presence of radiologically evident intrasellar and/or suprasellar abnormality on magnetic resonance imaging. Proceeding with surgical exploration of the sella in the absence of clear imaging findings, even with biochemical evidence of active acromegaly, is generally ill-advised in patients with acromegaly, will seldom produce the desired result, and may be a source of unnecessary complications. A second principle that must be understood by both the patient and the surgeon relates to the risks of surgical intervention. It is generally true in neurosurgery and certainly true for pituitary tumors that reoperations carry complication rates somewhat higher and outcomes somewhat less favorable than initial operations (77). This issue was carefully studied in a series of 158 patients, most of whom had pituitary tumors and all of whom required secondary transsphenoidal surgery for recurrence, persistent disease, or treatment of complications relating to unsuccessful prior therapy of one form or another (63). Although the scope of that study extended beyond the single issue of repeat surgery for recurrent pituitary tumors, many of the conclusions are still applicable in the current context. Of the 158 patients treated with repeat transsphenoidal surgery, operative mortality was 2.5% and the new complication rate was 29%; this contrasts with the 0.5% mortality and 2.2% morbidity rates that are frequently quoted of initial transsphenoidal operations (78). Furthermore, half of all patients treated with repeat transsphenoidal surgery still required additional measures (radiation, medical therapy, or additional surgery) to achieve disease control. In a recent study, the risks and benefits of repeat surgery were specifically analyzed in patients with acromegaly (79). In a series of 16 acromegalic patients, of which 15 had

persistent or progressive disease and 1 had a genuine recurrence, reoperation was associated with a 19% major complication rate and new hypopituitarism involving one or more axes in 63% of patients. Moreover, in only 19% of patients did reoperation induce endocrine remission. It should be emphasized that most patients in this series had persistent refractory disease, rather than true recurrence. Collectively, these data indicate that the decision for repeat surgical exploration of the sella can never be taken lightly in the patient with recurrent acromegaly. Although these issues should not dissuade the surgeon against reoperation for recurrent acromegaly when indicated, their consideration is important in establishing realistic expectations of the procedure, both for the patient and for the physician.

Having made the decision to intervene surgically, consideration will then turn to the surgical approach. In all but a few instances, the transsphenoidal route, with its direct surgical access to the pituitary and its superior intrasellar visualization, will represent the approach of choice for recurrent pituitary tumors. For most recurrent pituitary tumors, a previous transseptal procedure will have been performed, the reexposure of which may prove extraordinarily difficult (63, 77). The septal mucosa may be scarred with adhesions, septal perforations may be present, portions of the bony septum may be absent, and the usual midline landmarks used for navigation may be significantly distorted or absent. On occasion, the sinus cavities may have also been affected by prior surgery, with the development of postoperative mucoceles, cysts, or retained areas of packing material. As a result of these difficulties, some versatility with technical variations of the transsphenoidal approach will be highly desirable. For example, if the original procedure was a standard sublabial transseptal approach, careful reexposure through the same route can be attempted, although a transnasal septal displacement "pushover" approach, an external rhinoplasty approach, or a transethmoidal–transsphenoidal or transantral–transsphenoidal approach may provide an alternative and easier route of access. For most, if not all, of these reoperative approaches, assistance from ear, nose, and throat colleagues is routinely recommended. Details of our operative approach for recurrent pituitary tumors have been recently reviewed (80).

Because of the tendency to consider both recurrent and persistent acromegaly under the general category of "recurrence," few data are available concerning the surgical outcomes of genuinely recurrent somatotroph adenomas. Of 29 acromegalic patients with recurrent tumors, we recently reported a 48% rate of secondary remission with reoperation (76). Similar results were reported by Nicola et al. (81) in their operative series of 10 patients with recurrent tumors. For tumors in which remission cannot be achieved surgically, adjuvant radiotherapy has been and continues to be the usual next step, even with the availability of somatostatin analog therapy. In a recent report of postoperative radiotherapy for somatotroph adenomas, biochemical remission (i.e., suppressibility of GH levels to < 88 pmol/L [< 2 ng/mL]) was achieved in 62% of 57 acromegalic patients (82). In general, the response of these tumors to radiotherapy is fairly predictable; GH levels drop to 50% of baseline in the first 2 years; to 75% of baseline after 5 years; and further tumor growth is virtually always halted (83). Preliminary results of stereotactic radiosurgery seem to be comparable but not necessarily superior (84).

Some latitude exists for the use of somatostatin analogs for recurrent tumors. They may be used as an alternative to either surgery or radiotherapy, or as an adjuvant to both. Although these agents are being used as primary therapy for recurrences, they are frequently used as an interim measure in anticipation of a radiotherapeutic response. Further studies are required to more precisely define their role in this setting.

LONG-TERM RESULTS OF OPERATIVE MANAGEMENT

In summarizing the surgical series reviewed in this chapter, it seems that endocrine remission can be achieved in approximately 50 to 70% of somatotroph adenomas. As previously discussed, this figure will vary depending on the size, invasiveness, stage, and secretory activity of the tumor, as well as the criteria used to define remission and the length of the follow-up period. In the analysis of Davis et al. (57), the actuarial probability of remission (GH level < 88 pmol/L [< 2 ng/mL]) at 5 years was approximately 63%. A more encouraging long-term picture was provided by Tindall et al. (27). In their series of 103 patients with a mean follow-up period of 8.5 years, 88% of patients ultimately achieved endocrine control, as defined by GH levels less than 220 pmol/L [< 5 ng/mL]. This includes 18 patients in whom postoperative adjuvant therapy of one form or another was used. In another analysis of long-term outcome, we previously evaluated the status of 100 surgically treated acromegalic patients during a follow-up period of 10 years or more: 74% of patients are well and remain in remission; 11% of patients continue to live with active acromegaly; 7% of patients have suffered recurrence; and 8% of patients have died during the follow-up period (85).

A frequent long-term problem in the management of these patients is hypopituitarism of some degree. In one long-term analysis, hypopituitarism involving one or more axes was present in 78% of surgically treated patients, some of whom had also received adjuvant radiotherapy (86). Accordingly, vigilant long-term endocrine surveillance, early diagnosis of pituitary insufficiency, and adequate hormone replacement therapy will represent a crucial part of the management of these lesions.

REFERENCES

1. Thapar K, Kovacs K, Muller P. Clinical-pathologic correlations of pituitary tumors. Baillieres Clin Endocrinol Metab 1995;9(2):243–270.
2. Kovacs K, Horvath E. Tumors of the Pituitary Gland. Atlas of Tumor Pathology, Fascile 21, 2nd Series. Washington, DC: Armed Forces Institute of Pathology, 1986:1–269.
3. Klibanski A, Zervas NT. Diagnosis and management of hormone-secreting pituitary adenomas. N Engl J Med 1991;324(12):822–831.
4. Danowski T. Clinical Endocrinology. Baltimore: Williams & Wilkins, 1962:99–112.
5. Marie P. Sur deux cas d'acromegalie, hypertrophie singulière, non-congénitale des extrémités supérieures, inferieures, et céphalique. Rev Med 1886;6:297–333.
6. Marie P, Souza-Leite J. Essays on Acromegaly. London: The New Sydenham Society, 1891.
7. Minkowski O. gber einen Fall von Akromegalie. Berl Klin Wochnschr 1887;24:371.
8. Benda C. Beitr<aul>age zur normalen and pathologischen Histologie der menschlichen Hypophysis cerebri. Berl Klin Wochenschr 1900;36:1205.
9. Evans H, Long J. The effect of the anterior lobe of the pituitary administered intra-peritoneally upon growth, maturity, and oestrus cycle of the rat. Anat Rev 1921;21:62.
10. Cushing H. Partial hypophysectomy for acromegaly. Ann Surg 1909;50:1002–1017.
11. Caton R, Paul F. Notes on a case of acromegaly treated by operation. BMJ 1893;2:1421–1423.
12. Schloffer H. Erfolgreiche Operation eines Hypophysentumor auf nasalem Wege. Wien Klin Wochenschr 1907;20:621–624.
13. Guiot G, Arfel G, Brion S, et al. Adenomes Hypophysaires. Paris: Masson, 1958:1–276.
14. Hardy J. Transsphenoidal surgery of the normal and pathological pituitary. Clin Neurosurg 1969;16:185–217.
15. Bates A, Van't Hoff W, Jones J, et al. An audit on the outcome of acromegaly. QJM 1993;86:293–299.
16. Wright AD, Hill DM, Lowy C, et al. Mortality in acromegaly. QJM 1970;39:1–16.
17. Alexander L, Appleton D, Hall R, et al. Epidemiology of acromegaly in the Newcastle region. Clin Endocrinol 1980;12:71–79.
18. Bengtsson B-A, Eden S, Ernest I, et al. Epidemiology and long-term survival in acromegaly. Acta Med Scand 1988;223:327–335.
19. Melmed S. Acromegaly. In: Melmed S, ed. The Pituitary. Cambridge: Blackwell Science, 1995:413–442.
20. Laws ER Jr. Transsphenoidal approach to pituitary tumors. In: Schmidek HH, Sweet WH, eds. Operative Neurosurgical Techniques. Philadelphia: WB Saunders, 1995:283–292.

21. Laws ER Jr. Neurosurgical management of acromegaly. In: Cooper PR, ed. Contemporary Diagnosis and Management of Pituitary Adenomas. Park Ridge, IL: American Association of Neurological Surgeons, 1990:53–59.
22. Molitch ME. Clinical manifestations of acromegaly. Endocrinol Metab Clin North Am 1992:21(3):597–614.
23. Nabarro JDN. Acromegaly. J Clin Endocrinol 1987;26:481–512.
24. Scheithauer B, Kovacs K, Laws ER Jr, et al. Pathology of invasive pituitary tumors with special reference to functional classification. J Neurosurg 1986;65:733–744.
25. Wilson C. A decade of pituitary microsurgery: The Herbert Olivecrona Lecture. J Neurosurg 1984;61:814–833.
26. Fahlbusch R, Honegger J, Buchfelder M. Surgical management of acromegaly. Endocrinol Metab Clin North Am 1992;21:669–692.
27. Tindall G, Oyesiku N, Watts N, et al. Transsphenoidal adenomectomy for growth hormone secreting pituitary adenomas in acromegaly: outcome analysis and determinants of failure. J Neurosurg 1993; 78:205–215.
28. Laws ER Jr, Piepgras D, Randall R, et al. Neurosurgical management of acromegaly. J Neurosurg 1979;50:454–461.
29. Grisoli F, Leclercq T, Jaquet P, et al. Transsphenoidal surgery for acromegaly: long-term results in 100 patients. Surg Neurol 1985; 23:513–519.
30. van't Verlaat J, Nortier J, Hendriks M, et al. Transsphenoidal microsurgery as primary treatment in 25 acromegalic patients: results and follow-up. Acta Endocrinologica (Copenh) 1988;117:154–158.
31. Ross DA, Wilson CB. Results of transsphenoidal microsurgery for growth hormone-secreting pituitary adenoma in a series of 214 patients. J Neurosurg 1988;68:854–867.
32. Ebersold MJ, Laws ER Jr, Scheithauer BW, et al. Pituitary apoplexy treated by transsphenoidal surgery: a clinicopathological and immunocytochemical study. J Neurosurg 1983;58:315–320.
33. Faglia G, Arosio M, Bazzoni N. Ectopic acromegaly. Endocrinol Metab Clin North Am 1992;21(3):575–595.
34. Thorner MO, Vance ML, Horvath E, et al. The anterior pituitary. In: Wilson JD, Foster DW, eds. Williams Textbook of Endocrinology. Philadelphia: WB Saunders, 1992:221–310.
35. O'Brien T, O'Riordan DS, Gharib H, et al. Results of treatment of pituitary disease in multiple endocrine neoplasia, type 1. Neurosurgery 1996;39:273–279.
36. Scheithauer B, Laws ER Jr, Kovacs K, et al. Pituitary adenomas of the multiple endocrine neoplasia type 1 syndrome. Semin Diagn Pathol 1987;4:205–211.
37. Laws ER Jr, Randall R, Abboud C. Special problems in the therapeutic management of acromegaly. In: Lhdecke D, Tolis G, eds. Growth Hormone, Growth Factors, and Acromegaly. New York: Raven Press, 1987:259–266.
38. Mhchler H, Renz D, Lhdecke D. Anesthetic management of acromegaly. In: Lhdecke D, Tolis G, eds. Growth Hormone, Growth Factors, and Acromegaly. New York: Raven Press, 1987:267–271.
39. Fahlbusch R, Giovanelli M, Buchfelder M, et al. Consensus statement: advances in the medical and surgical treatment of pituitary adenomas: the role of long-acting somatostatin analogs. J Endocrinol Invest 1993;16:449–460.
40. Barkan AL, Lloyd RV, Chandler WF, et al. Preoperative treatment of acromegaly with long-acting somatostatin analog SMS 201–995: shrinkage of invasive pituitary macroadenomas and improved surgical remission rate. J Clin Endocrinol Metab 1988;67(5): 1040–1048.
41. Stevenaert A, Harris A, Kovacs K, et al. Presurgical octreotide treatment in acromegaly. Metabolism 1992;41(suppl 2):51–58.
42. Balagura S, Derome P, Guiot G. Acromegaly: analysis of 132 cases treated surgically. Neurosurgery 1981;8:413–416.
43. Tucker H, Grubb S, Wigand J, et al. The treatment of acromegaly by transsphenoidal surgery. Arch Intern Med 1980;140:795–802.
44. Arafah B, Brodkey J, Kaufman B, et al. Transsphenoidal microsurgery in the treatment of acromegaly and gigantism. J Clin Endocrinol Metab 1980;50:578–585.
45. Laws ER Jr, Trautmann JC, Hollenhorst RW. Transsphenoidal decompression of the optic nerve and chiasm: visual results in 62 patients. J Neurosurg 1977;46:717–722.
46. Melmed S. Acromegaly. N Engl J Med 1990;322:966–977.
47. Newman C, Kleinberg D. Acromegaly: how do you define cure? In: Cooper P, ed. Contemporary Diagnosis and Management of Pituitary Adenomas. Park Ridge: American Association of Neurological Surgeons, 1990:47–52.
48. Sheaves R, Jenkins P, Blackburn P, et al. Outcome of transsphenoidal surgery for acromegaly using strict criteria for surgical cure. Clin Endocrinol 1996;45:407–413.
49. Lindholm J, Giwercman BAG, Astrup J, et al. Investigation of the criteria for assessing the outcome of treatment in acromegaly. Clin Endocrinol 1987;27:553–562.
50. Arafah B, Rosenzweig J, Fenstermaker R, et al. Value of growth hormone dynamics and somatostatin C (insulin-like growth factor1) levels in predicting the long-term benefit after transsphenoidal surgery for acromegaly. J Lab Clin Med 1987;109:346–354.
51. Valdemarsson S, Bramnert M, Cronquist S, et al. Early postoperative basal serum GH level and the GH response to TRH in relation to the long-term outcome of surgical treatment for acromegaly: a report on 39 patients. J Intern Med 1991;230:49–54.
52. Zervas N. Multicenter surgical results in acromegaly. In: Lhdecke D, Tolis G, eds. Growth Hormone, Growth Factors, and Acromegaly. New York: Raven Press, 1987:253–257.
53. Teasdale G, Hay I, Beasttall G, et al. Cryosugery or microsurgery in the management of acromegaly. JAMA 1982;247:1289–1291.
54. Serri O, Somma M, Comtois R, et al. Acromegaly: biochemical assessment of cure after long term follow-up of transsphenoidal selective adenomectomy. J Clin Endocrinol Metab 1985;61: 1185–1189.
55. Roelfsema F, van Dulken H, Frölich M. Long-term results of transsphenoidal pituitary microsurgery in 60 acromegalic patients. Clin Endocrinol 1985,23:555–565.
56. Losa M, Oeckler R, Schopohl J, et al. Evaluation of selective transsphenoidal adenomectomy by endocrinological testing and somatostatin-C measurement in acromegaly. J Neurosurg 1989;70: 561–567.
57. Davis D, Laws ER Jr, Ilstrup D, et al. Results of surgical treatment for growth hormone-secreting pituitary adenomas. J Neurosurg 1993;79:70–75.
58. Laws ER Jr, Kern EB. Complications of transsphenoidal surgery. In: Laws ER Jr, Randall RV, Kern EB, Abboud CF, eds. Management of Pituitary Adenomas and Related Lesions with Emphasis on Transsphenoidal Microsurgery. New York: Appleton Century Crofts, 1982:329–346.
59. Quabbe H-J. Treatment of acromegaly by transsphenoidal operation. 90-yttrium implantation and bromocriptine: results in 230 patients. Clin Endocrinol 1982;19:107–119.
60. Delalande O, Peillon F, Maestro J, et al. Results a moyen et longe terme de l'adenomectomie sélective hypophysaire dans l'acromegalie. Éléments de pronostic. Ann Endocrinol (Paris) 1985;46: 321–323.
61. Oyen W, Pieters G, Meijer E, et al. Which factors predict the results of pituitary surgery in acromegaly? Acta Endocrinol (Copenh) 1988; 117:491–496.
62. Bystrom C, Larsson C, Blomberg C, et al. Localization of the MEN1 gene to a small region within chromosome 11q13 by deletion mapping in tumors. Proc Natl Acad Sci U S A 1990;87:1968–1972.
63. Laws ER Jr, Fode NC, Redmond MJ. Transsphenoidal surgery following unsuccessful prior therapy: an assessment of benefits and risks in 158 patients. J Neurosurg 1985;63:823–829.
64. Wilson CB. Neurosurgical management of large and invasive pituitary tumors. In: Tindall G, Collins W, eds. Clinical Management of Pituitary Disorders. New York: Raven Press, 1979:335–342.
65. Hardy J. Transsphenoidal surgery of hypersecreting pituitary tumors. In: Kohler P, Ross G, eds. Diagnosis and Treatment of Pituitary Tumors. Amsterdam: Excerpta Medica, 1973:179–194.
66. Selman WR, Laws ER Jr, Scheithauer BW, et al. The occurrence of dural invasion in pituitary adenomas. J Neurosurg 1986;64: 402–407.
67. Landolt AM, Illig R, Zapf J. Surgical treatment of acromegaly In: Lamberts SWJ, ed. Sandostatin in the Treatment of Acromegaly. Berlin: Springer-Verlag, 1988:23–35.
68. Thapar K, Kovacs K, Scheithauer B, et al. Classification and pathology of sellar and parasellar tumors. In: Tindall G, Cooper P, Barrow D, eds. The Practice of Neurosurgery. Baltimore: Williams & Wilkins, 1996:1021–1070.
69. Thapar K, Kovacs K, Stefaneanu L, et al. Overexpression of the growth hormone-releasing hormone gene in acromegaly associated pituitary tumor: an event associated with neoplastic progression and aggressive behavior. Am J Pathol 1997;151.
70. Yamada S, Tadishi A, Sano T, et al. Growth hormone producing

pituitary adenomas: correlation between clinical characteristics and morphology. Neurosurgery 1993;33:20–27.

71. Nyquist P, Laws ER Jr, Elliot E. Novel features of tumors that secret both growth hormone and prolactin in acromegaly. Neurosurgery 1994;35:179–184.

72. Vance M, Harris A. Long term treatment of 189 acromegalic patients with the somatostatin analog octreotide: results of the International Multicenter Acromegaly Study Group. Arch Intern Med 1991;151:1573–1578.

73. Vance M. Acromegaly: Medical treatment. In: Landolt A, Vance M, Reilly P, eds. Pituitary Adenomas. Edinburgh: Churchill Livingstone 1996:409–415.

74. Ezzat S, Snyder PJ, Young WF, et al. Octreotide treatment of acromegaly: a randomized, multicenter study. Ann Intern Med 1992; 117(9):711–718.

75. Buchfelder M, Brockmeier S, Fahlbusch R, et al. Recurrence following transsphenoidal surgery for acromegaly. Horm Res 1991;35: 113–118.

76. Laws ER Jr, Chenelle AG, Thapar K. Recurrence after transsphenoidal surgery for pituitary adenomas: clinical and basic science aspects. In: von Werder K, Fahlbusch R, eds. Pituitary Adenomas: From Basic Research to Diagnosis and Therapy. Amsterdam: Elsevier, 1996:3–9.

77. Laws ER Jr. Pituitary tumors. In: Little JR, Awad IA, eds. Reoperative Neurosurgery. Baltimore: Williams & Wilkins, 1992:106–112.

78. Zervas NT. Surgical results for pituitary adenomas: results of an international survey. In: Black PM, Ridgeway EC, Martin JB, Zervas NT, eds. Secretory Tumors of the Pituitary Gland. New York: Raven Press, 1984:377–385.

79. Long H, Beauregard H, Somma M, et al. Surgical outcome after repeated transsphenoidal surgery in acromegaly. J Neurosurg 1996; 85:239–247.

80. Thapar K, Laws ER Jr. Transsphenoidal surgery for recurrent pituitary tumors. In: Kaye AH, Black PM, eds. Operative Neurosurgery. Edinburgh: Churchill Livingstone, 1997.

81. Nicola GC, Tonnarelli G, Griner AC, et al. Surgery for recurrence of pituitary adenomas. In: Faglia G, et al., eds. Pituitary Adenomas: New Trends in Basic and Clinical Research. Amsterdam: Excerpta Medica, 1991:329–338.

82. Caruso M, Shaw E, Davis D. Radiation treatment of growth hormone secrering pituitary adenomas. Int J Radiol Oncol Biol Phys 1993;21:121–122.

83. Eastman RC, Gorden P, Glatstein E, et al. Radiation therapy of acromegaly. Endocrinol Metab Clin North Am 1992;21(3): 693–713.

84. Ganz JC. Gamma knife treatment of pituitary adenomas. In: Landolt A, Vance M, Reilly P, eds. Pituitary Adenomas. Edinburgh: Churchill Livingstone, 1996:461–474.

85. Laws ER Jr, Carpenter S, Scheithauer B, et al. Long-term results of transsphenoidal surgery for the management of acromegaly. In: Robbins R, Melmed S, eds. Acromegaly: A Century of Scientific and Clinical Progress. New York: Plenum Press, 1987:241–248.

86. Jenkins D, O'Brien I, Johnson A, et al. The Birmingham pituitary database: auditing the outcome of the treatment of acromegaly. Clin Endocrinol 1995;43:517–522.

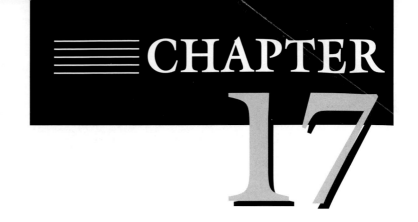

CHAPTER 17

Gonadotroph Pituitary Adenomas

Rita M. Chidiac, Warren R. Selman, and
Baha M. Arafah

INTRODUCTION

Gonadotropin-secreting or gonadotroph pituitary adenomas were first recognized as a distinct entity approximately 20 years ago (1). Until a few years ago, these adenomas were considered a rare medical curiosity (2, 3). Currently, these tumors are easier to recognize, and they account for approximately 10 to 15% of all clinically diagnosed pituitary adenomas. The advent of newer techniques such as immunocytochemistry and, more recently, molecular biology have shed light on many facets of this pathologic entity. Although they are considered among the functioning pituitary tumors, gonadotroph adenomas are typically inefficient in secreting their hormonal products (2, 4). It is therefore easy to appreciate why patients with gonadotroph adenomas do not have a distinct clinical or phenotypic presentation, even when gonadotropin secretion is truly excessive. Furthermore, the heterogeneous nature of these adenomas with respect to hormonal secretion and ultrastructural characteristics have made it difficult to define criteria for the diagnosis of this disease entity.

In this review, the definition, prevalence, and pathophysiologic characteristics of the clinical as well as the hormonal manifestations of these adenomas are discussed. The review also addresses currently available treatment approaches as well as potential future therapeutic interventions.

HISTORICAL BACKGROUND

Results of reports in the late 1970s and early to mid-1980s showed that nonfunctioning tumors composed 30% of all pituitary adenomas. Since then, however, most tumors previously characterized as being nonfunctional have been subsequently recognized to secrete, at least a fraction of (α-subunit [α-SU]) or an intact molecule of, any of the glycoprotein hormones (5–8). The routine use of immunocytochemical techniques on most resected tumor tissue in addition to advances in other research tools such as cell culture, free-subunit radioimmunoassay, and mRNA analysis have facilitated the recognition of gonadotroph adenoma as a distinct entity (4, 9).

Before the development of radioimmunoassay, several case reports, including two published by Cushing in 1912, suggested the presence of gonadotroph tumors. In 1974, Woolf and Schenk (1) reported on a follicle-stimulating hormone (FSH)–secreting pituitary tumor and documented elevated serum as well as tumoral FSH levels. Initial reports postulated that at least some gonadotroph adenomas are caused by prolonged stimulation from chronic primary hypogonadism (1). However, after 1975, Snyder (2, 4) was one of the first authors to recognize macroadenomas associated with elevated FSH levels as a distinct clinical entity, unrelated to primary hypogonadism. Since then, the number of recognized or reported cases of gonadotroph adenomas has steadily increased, accounting for approximately 10 to 15% of all pituitary adenomas.

DEFINITION

Gonadotropin-secreting or gonadotroph adenomas encompass broad clinical and pathologic features that depend on the investigational techniques used. When studied in vivo, these adenomas are identified on the basis of hypersecretion of FSH, luteinizing hormone (LH), α-SU, or β-subunit (β-SU), in the basal state as well as after dynamic stimulation (10–14). In vitro studies performed on surgically resected tumor tissue (immunocytochemistry, cell culture, or Northern blot analysis) have allowed the broader characterization of these adenomas (6, 9, 15–17). Silent gonadotroph adenomas are those that are discovered by immunocytochemistry without the associated elevation of serum gonadotropin levels. The degree of LH, FSH, and α-SU immunoreactivity within the adenoma varies from less than 5% to more than 50% of adenomatous cells. A reasonably acceptable criterion would be to have at least 10% of cells within the adenoma stain positively for the hormone or the subunit.

A third, less commonly observed form of manifestations of these tumors includes occasional tumors that are nonsecreting in vivo and that, despite having negative immunostaining studies, have the capacity to secrete gonadotropins in cell cultures.

From a practical standpoint, we believe that the most reasonable criterion for defining gonadotroph adenomas would be one that is based on immunocytochemical studies performed on resected tumor tissues. Such criterion will therefore include tumors that are silent as well as those secreting gonadotropins.

INCIDENCE

The actual incidence or prevalence of gonadotroph cell adenomas is difficult to determine given the different criteria used in various published series. Based on excessive hormonal secretion in vivo, the incidence of gonadotroph adenomas ranges from 3 to 17% of all pituitary tumors. Using immunostaining techniques as the criterion for diagnosis, a higher number of gonadotroph adenomas can be identified, with most series reporting an incidence of approximately 10 to 15%.

NORMAL PHYSIOLOGIC CHARACTERISTICS OF GONADOTROPIN SECRETION

Normal gonadotropin production requires coordinate synthesis, processing, and dimerization of α-SU and β-SU with subsequent hormone-regulated secretion. In normal pituitary as well as placental tissue, the peptide concentration and mRNA levels of α-SU are greater than the respective levels of β-SU. Hence, it has been suggested that production of β-SU is the rate-limiting step in intact heterodimer synthesis. Testicular as well as ovarian function are primarily under the control of LH and FSH.

FSH, LH, thyroid-stimulating hormone (TSH), and human chorionic gonadotropin (hCG) are structurally similar, each composed of two glycopeptide chains (α and β). The α chains of all these glycoproteins have the common sequence of 96 amino acids. The β chain is unique to each and confers receptor binding specificity. A terminal sialic acid is present on the carbohydrate chains of hCG-β and FSH-β. Sialic acid decreases the metabolic clearance of these hormones and, consequently, the plasma half-lives of FSH and hCG are longer than that of LH. Furthermore, LH and, to a lesser extent, FSH are secreted in a pulsatile fashion. Their secretion is regulated by the episodic stimulation of pituitary gonadotrophs by gonadotropin-releasing hormone (GnRH) as well as by the negative feedback mechanism of gonadal steroids.

CLINICAL AND IMAGING CHARACTERISTICS

Most published series have reported a variable degree of male:female preponderance, with ratios as high as 3:1 and as low as 1.5:1. The exact cause for male predilection in this disease is not known. Patients' ages at presentation vary from 30 to 85 years in both men and women, with a mean of approximately 60 years. This relatively late age at diagnosis is probably related to the slow growth rate of the adenomas and also the lack of specific phenotypic features and clinical manifestations (18).

The most common clinical presentation has been related to the mechanical effects of the expanding macroadenoma (18). These manifestations include visual complaints (diminished vision, visual field deficits, and alterations in eye motility), headaches, and hypopituitarism. Up to 20% of patients diagnosed as having gonadotroph adenoma present for medical care after the adenomas were discovered incidentally. In rare cases, apoplexy of the adenoma was the first and only presenting clinical picture.

Endocrine manifestations vary with the sex and age of the patient. Because these tumors are inefficient in hormone secretion, symptoms of excessive hormone secretion are rare and are seen in occasional patients with increased LH production. Male patients with these features present with elevated serum testosterone levels and increased libido. Similarly, the occasional woman with LH hypersecretion can present with ovarian hyperstimulation syndrome, including supranormal estradiol concentrations, multiple ovarian cysts, and endometrial hyperplasia (16, 19, 20).

However, because of the large size of these tumors, most patients present with various signs and symptoms of hypopituitarism (18, 21, 22). Diminished libido and impotence were found in most male patients presenting with this type of tumor. Many patients also have variable degrees of other pituitary hormone deficits, such as TSH, adrenocorticotropic hormone, and growth hormone. In premenopausal women, amenorrhea, oligomenorrhea, and/or galactorrhea were reported in many cases. After menopause, the most common form of presentation is usually related to mass effects of the adenoma. The latter manifestations include headaches, visual complaints, and variable signs and symptoms of hypopituitarism. By the time most of these tumors are clinically recognized they are large (> 10 mm) and often have extension beyond the confines of the sella turcica. Only an occasional patient can be diagnosed with a small (< 10 mm) gonadotroph adenoma.

HORMONAL STUDIES IN PATIENTS WITH GONADOTROPH ADENOMAS

Basal Hormone Secretion

As stated earlier and for unknown reasons, gonadotroph adenomas are generally inefficient in hormone secretion. Furthermore, their secretory characteristics vary from one tumor to another. Recent studies suggest that only 30 to 40% of patients with gonadotroph adenomas, as documented on immunocytochemical staining of resected tissue, have elevated basal serum levels of the intact or the α-SU of gonadotropins (4, 9, 18). For reasons that are not clear, men represent the vast majority of patients with documented elevation of serum gonadotropin levels. In the latter group of patients, intact FSH is the glycoprotein most commonly secreted in excess, occurring in up to 60% of such patients. Cosecretion of FSH and LH occurs in up to 30% of such patients. Much less commonly (< 5%), isolated LH secretion with normal or decreased FSH levels were reported. Basal elevation of gonadotropin levels occurs with similar frequency and distribution in premenopausal women. However, most postmenopausal women with this type of adenoma have, in general, decreased serum FSH and LH levels, and only a few have truly excessive gonadotropin secretion.

Results of earlier studies suggest that measurement of the α-SU is a useful marker for these adenomas. However, elevation of the α-SU lacks specificity because it can be increased in 10% of other pituitary tumors, secreted alone or with growth hormone, TSH, and prolactin (5, 7). Hence, one has to interpret elevated α-SU levels with caution, particularly because of the possibility of ectopic secretion from other, nonpituitary malignancies capable of secreting hCG, such as lung, stomach, and placenta. In addition to direct measurements of serum α-SU levels, determination of the molar ratio of α-SU to FSH and LH has been recommended as an additional marker in the diagnosis of gonadotroph adenomas. This would be particularly valuable in postmenopausal women who normally have a ratio that ranges between 1.4 and 3.3.

Measurements of β-SU levels of FSH or LH have been found to be valuable in the evaluation of these patients (11–13). Secretion of FSH-β and/or LH-β is increased in such tumors. FSH-β levels in women with gonadotroph adenomas were found to be roughly twofold higher than those seen in patients with primary hypogonadism with similarly elevated intact FSH levels. The imbalanced secretion of FSH-β relative to the α-SU in neoplastic tissue has been demonstrated in about one-third of the tumors (23). Based on these findings, it was advocated that FSH-β might be a more specific, though less sensitive, marker of gonadotroph adenomas.

Dynamic Testing

Evaluating FSH and LH responses to stimulation with different hypothalamic hormones (e.g., thyrotropin-releasing hormone [TRH]) was another approach used by many investigators in studies of patients with nonsecreting pituitary tumors as well as those with gonadotroph adenomas (10–13). Results of earlier reports in a small number of patients with elevated basal gonadotropin levels suggested that TRH testing was helpful in that it resulted in a rise in serum FSH as well as LH levels. Contrary to results of earlier studies, results of subsequent reports suggested that normal people as well as those who have different types of pituitary adenomas can have nonspecific increases in serum gonadotropin and/or α-SU levels after TRH administration. Results of additional studies, however, have shown that the increase in β-SU of LH following TRH stimulation was a more specific as well as frequent finding in men and women with gonadotroph adenoma. Results of published reports indicate that the rise in the β-SU level in response to TRH stimulation can be used as a diagnostic tool to identify patients with gonadotroph adenomas with normal basal hormone levels. The clinical significance of the latter testing is not clear and is likely to be limited by the absence of widely available reliable assays for β-SU.

Another approach used by some investigators was evaluation of FSH and LH responses to stimulation with the hypothalamic hormone GnRH (9, 18, 24). Several studies have shown no consistent findings because the observed responses were heterogeneous (24, 25). Similar observations were made when responses to exogenous steroid administration were evaluated in these patients. Some studies suggested that the heterogeneous response to GnRH administration in these patients could reflect biosynthetic defects in GnRH receptors in some of the adenomatous tissue.

Despite the fact that FSH and LH in these patients are produced by adenomatous cells, secretion of these hormones remains pulsatile (26). Results of studies in patients with gonadotroph adenoma have demonstrated normal pulse frequency compared with normal men or premenopausal and postmenopausal women. However, the pulse amplitude was elevated in the patients with baseline elevated basal hormone levels. It is not clear whether the preservation of pulsatile hormone secretion reflects the presence of intrinsic properties, commonly seen in other hormone-secreting adenomas, or whether it represents some degree of hypothalamic control (26).

Biologic Activity of Secreted Glycoproteins

Using gel filtration chromatography, several studies have demonstrated that most FSH immunoreactivity eluted as intact FSH rather than α- or β-SU (2). Similarly, subunit elevation that occurs in such tumors was also demonstrated by gel filtration to elute, almost exclusively, in the subunits' position (16).

Results of most studies have shown that FSH secreted by adenoma cells retains its biologic activity, as demonstrated by granulosa cell bioassay. Results of some studies have even demonstrated a higher biologic:immunologic ratio than those of normal FSH.

The normal pituitary secretes multiple species of FSH with varying degrees of glycosylation depending on the hormonal milieu. These oligosaccharides are critical for FSH biologic activity because deglycosylated FSH retains receptor binding potential but lacks the ability to stimulate downstream responses. The high serum concentrations of bioactive FSH found in some patients with adenomas suggests that the cellular machinery for biosynthesis and processing of FSH remains functional, despite aberrant cellular growth.

STUDIES ON RESECTED TUMOR TISSUE

Ultrastructural Studies

Before the introduction of the newer classification of pituitary tumors, most gonadotroph adenomas were considered chromophobe. A few occasional tumors would, however, be considered acidophilic if they demonstrate oncocytic transformation.

Several studies have reported the ultrastructural features of these adenomas using electron microscopy. Studies by Horvath and Kovacs described a gender-related ultrastructural dimorphism in these tumors (6, 18). In men, gonadotroph cell adenomas are often composed of small cells with moderately developed cytoplasm that contains few endoplasmic reticulum and Golgi membranes and a variable number of secretory granules. In women, the cells of gonadotroph adenomas contain highly distinctive vesicular dilatation of the Golgi complex, well-developed endoplasmic reticulum with dilated cisternae, and sparse small secretory granules. These and other gender-related differences in ultrastructural findings were not reported by other investigators.

Oncocytic changes within the gonadotroph adenomas were reported by several groups. These are characterized by cytoplasmic accumulation of mitochondria. It follows that tumors exhibiting these findings are termed "oncocytomas." Some tumors are classified as null cell because they lack specific immunocytochemical, ultrastructural, or biochemical markers. Cytoplasmic organelles involved in hormone synthesis and release may be present, but they are typically scant. The cellular origin of null-cell adenomas is obscure. Null-cell adenomas and oncocytomas may contain small numbers of TSH, FSH, LH, or α-SU. It is not clear, therefore, whether null cells represent undifferentiated precursors of gonadotrophs, capable of multidirectional differentiation not only toward glycoprotein-producing cells but also other cell types.

Immunohistochemistry

In earlier studies, this technique was performed using polyclonal antibodies directed against FSH, LH, α-SU, or β-SU. One of the serious limitations with the latter approach was the lack of specificity of the antibodies used. To eliminate the cross-reaction between the subunits and their intact hormones, absorption tests were performed by incubating the antibodies with the appropriate antigen and also other antigens. For the diagnosis of gonadotroph adenoma to be made, most studies have suggested that an arbitrary figure of 5 to 10% of immunoreactive cells, with at least one gonadotropin with or without α-SU, are required. In addition, staining with prolactin, growth hormone, and adrenocorticotropic hormone should be negative.

In general, the degree of immunocytochemical reaction does not correlate with plasma concentrations of LH and FSH or with tumor size. Also, comparison of immunocytochemical and morphologic studies showed no evidence of morphologic differences related to the type of immunoreactivity. On the ultrastructural level, the most differentiated gonadotroph adenomas are related to tumors displaying the highest degree of immunoreactive cells.

The use of more specific monoclonal antibodies in recent studies and the improvement in immunocytochemical techniques have both contributed to increasing recognition of glycoprotein hormone–containing adenomas among null-cell adenomas and oncocytomas. In earlier studies, only 15 to 20% of null-cell adenomas were found to be immunoreactive for glycoprotein hormones. Later reports, however, showed that approximately 80% of null-cell adenomas and oncocytomas showed some degree of immunoreactivity (6,18). Thus, it is believed that a substantial majority of clinically nonfunctioning adenomas are ultrastructurally distinct lesions that exhibit ultrastructural and immunocytochemical similarities to gonadotroph adenomas.

Thus, immunocytochemistry of resected adenomas plays a major role in the diagnosis of gonadotroph adenomas. One has to correlate clinical characteristics with morphologic, ultrastructural and immunocytochemical features before a definitive categorization of gonadotroph adenomas can be made.

Cell Culture Studies

In general, gonadotroph adenomas demonstrate significant in vitro secretion of hormones. Gonadotropins and their subunits were released by most adenomas in vitro, and there was a variable proportion of α-SU to free β-SU. In vitro cell culture studies allow evaluation of hormonal release related to specific stimuli such as activin and GnRH. However, many discrepancies in basal and stimulated hormone levels between in vivo and in vitro secretory behavior were noted by many investigators. Thus, routine in vitro testing does not improve diagnostic accuracy because this approach presents many difficulties that would limit clinical application.

Northern Blot Analysis

Several recent studies have used this approach in defining gonadotroph adenomas. In some series, at least one gonadotropin subunit mRNA was demonstrated in up to 75% of gonadotroph adenomas. The mRNA for FSH β-SU was present in excess of that of the α-SU in about one-third of tumors. Investigators in some studies were able to quantitate imbalanced biosynthesis of free-subunits in human pituitary tumors. In most cases, there was often a good correlation between steady state free-subunit mRNA levels and the detection of the corresponding subunit. In general, results of studies have shown that Northern blot analysis is less sensitive than immunostaining in the detection of glycoprotein hormones.

DIAGNOSIS OF GONADOTROPH ADENOMAS

Given the limitations of available in vivo as well as in vitro testing, and the discrepancies seen in the results of different studies, it is recommended that the basal serum hormone levels of intact FSH, intact LH as well as α-SU be measured (4, 12). If specific assays are available for the β-SU, then FSH-β as well as LH and LH-β should be determined preoperatively in any patient with clinically nonfunctioning pituitary adenoma. GnRH stimulation testing is not generally indicated given the heterogeneous response seen as well as the lack of correlation between a positive response preoperatively and the effect of therapy with GnRH agonists or antagonist. More than 10% of the cells of resected adenoma tissue should stain positively for intact FSH, LH, and/or the α-SU. Tumors that demonstrate isolated α-SU immunostaining or secretion would be classified to be gonadotroph adenomas when appropriate morphologic characteristics are demonstrated at the ultrastructural level. The accurate classification of nonfunctioning adenomas as gonadotroph tumors is necessary because this might affect future medical treatments of recurrent or residual tumors.

PATHOPHYSIOLOGIC CHARACTERISTICS OF GONADOTROPH ADENOMAS

Recent studies used newer techniques and methods in molecular biology and clonal analysis in examining pituitary adenomas. Using these techniques, it became apparent that clinically functioning as well as nonfunctioning pituitary adenomas are monoclonal in origin. These observations support the hypothesis that pituitary adenomas originate from mature adenohypophyseal cells or precursor cells that undergo somatic mutations and are capable of differentiating not only toward gonadotrophs but also toward other cell types. Several factors have been implicated in the neoplastic development and multidirectional differentiation of these tumors, including (a) factors related to abnormalities inherent to neoplastic cells caused by genetic alteration, (b) hypothalamic disturbances, and (c) gonadal peptides.

Imbalance in biosynthetic pathways could be related to abnormalities inherent to neoplastic cells. Nonfunctioning pituitary adenomas are monoclonal, and this is consistent with the hypothesis that one or more genetic alterations could lead to clonal proliferation. Subsequent changes in receptor-mediated or independent second messenger systems could lead to both tumor growth and altered gonadotropin subunit regulation.

Some investigators speculate that hypothalamic peptides may play a role in augmentation of potential biosynthetic imbalances found in clinically nonfunctioning adenomas. Chronic GnRH administration may lead to dissociation of gonadotropin subunits production by pituitary tumors with altered GnRH receptors. Also, there is a paradoxical response of gonadotroph adenomas to stimulation by TRH, suggesting the presence of TRH receptors. It is not known how clinically nonfunctioning adenomas acquire TRH receptors or what role these receptors may play in tumor pathogenesis.

A few recent studies suggest that gonadal peptides such as activin might play a role in subunit dysregulation, specifically FSH-β (17). Normally, activin selectively stimulates FSH-β mRNA synthesis and intact FSH release by pituitary gonadotrophs. In contrast to findings in normal tissue, it has been demonstrated that activin can induce synthesis of FSH-β in vitro without secretion of intact FSH dimer. Activin, therefore, could be playing a role in intact gonadotropin secretion in these tumors. Also, by producing a differential regulation of FSH β-SU synthesis, activin may have its effect at the posttranslational processing level whereby dimerization of gonadotropin subunits by adenomatous cells is prevented.

The previously discussed factors are speculative mechanisms that could play a role in the pathogenesis of gonadotroph cell adenomas. Abnormal glycosylation of gonadotropins secreted by these tumors has been postulated, although not substantiated, by objective studies. The biologic activity of the hormones secreted seems preserved. However, there is no correlation with gonadal steroid hypersecretion, probably because of postreceptor defective second messenger mechanisms.

THERAPY OF GONADOTROPH ADENOMAS

Primary Treatment

The primary treatment for gonadotroph adenomas is surgical adenomectomy. This therapeutic approach is effective and safe, with low morbidity and mortality. Normal pituitary function is most often preserved (27), and recovery of lost function is common (21, 22). Most of these adenomas are large at presentation and are complicated by visual symptoms, headaches, and variable degrees of hypopituitarism. Despite the enormous size of some of these tumors, the transsphenoidal approach is preferred by most neurosurgeons (18, 28). A subsequent craniotomy may be necessary in some patients with residual suprasellar tumor that did not descend during the transsphenoidal approach. Surgical treatment results in improvement of visual symptoms in at least 70% of patients. The incidence of additional visual loss postoperatively varies between 2 and 11%.

Complete tumor removal can be achieved in most, but not all patients. The outcome of surgery is determined by the surgeon's experience, the size of the adenoma, and the degree of its extension beyond the sella turcica. Recurrence of pituitary adenoma after apparent complete surgical resection is reported to occur in 10 to 25% of patients, usually within the first 4 years. However, recurrences and continued tumor growth have been seen after long-term follow-up. Therefore, periodic hormonal testing as well as repeat imaging studies are recommended annually.

The hypopituitarism, found in most patients at presentation can often be reversible (21, 22). Studies have demonstrated that the dominant pathophysiologic mechanism for loss of pituitary function in this setting is compression of the pituitary stalk and portal vessels by the expanding adenoma. Tumor growth causes increased intrasellar pressure that is likely to decrease blood flow in portal vessels and diminish the availability of hypothalamic hormones to the normal pituitary. Following transsphenoidal decompression, normal hypothalamic control of pituitary function is restored, and, as a result, normal pituitary hormone secre-

tion is established. Thus, recovery of pituitary function can be documented to occur immediately postoperatively. An additional contributing mechanism for hypopituitarism that may limit potential recovery of pituitary function is the ischemic necrosis of anterior pituitary cells as a result of decreased blood supply and compression by the adenoma. It is therefore important to monitor pituitary function after surgery and assess the potential for recovery. A detailed approach is described elsewhere in this review. It is important to point out that loss of anterior pituitary hormone secretion can also occur after surgery, with a reported incidence of 5 to 10%.

Radiation therapy has been advocated as a treatment option for different reasons. In earlier studies that preceded recent advances in neurosurgical techniques, radiation therapy was recommended as a primary treatment for all types of pituitary tumors, particularly in patients who were poor surgical risks. The use of radiation therapy has since diminished because of the noted advances in neurosurgical techniques and the availability of additional forms of medical treatments for most types of adenomas.

At present, radiation therapy is rarely recommended as a primary form of therapy for pituitary tumors in general. It is, however, used as an adjunctive therapy in patients with functioning as well as those with nonfunctioning adenomas. In patients with gonadotroph tumors, radiation therapy can be used in patients whose adenomas could not be removed completely at surgery or those with recurrent tumors that are not compressing the optic chiasm. Every attempt should be made to exclude the optic chiasm from the field of irradiation even if an additional surgical decompression procedure becomes necessary. Although the standard fractionated delivery using the linear accelerator is still commonly used, other approaches are now available, including heavy particle irradiation and stereotactic delivery. A promising approach that is being currently tested in a few centers is the fractionated stereotactic method.

Complications caused by radiation therapy itself are many, and some are serious. One of the serious complications seen in some patients within a short period of time is worsening visual symptoms. Several potential mechanisms can cause progressive and rapid visual loss, including edema, tumor hemorrhage, and optic nerve necrosis. Chiasmal herniation can, at times, be seen following radiation therapy and more often years after transsphenoidal surgery. Most patients with chiasmal herniation have minimal or no visual symptoms. The risk of malignant brain tumors is increased compared with the rest of the population. Brain necrosis and dementia are also rare but serious complications of radiation therapy.

Progressive loss of pituitary function is a frequent chronic complication of radiation therapy. The primary initial damage from radiation is at the level of the hypothalamus and is associated with a slight increase in serum prolactin level. Anterior pituitary cells are subsequently damaged by the cumulative effects of radiation. It is estimated that after 10 years of follow-up, more than 90% of patients have at least two or more deficient hormones.

Although pituitary radiation is associated with a substantial number of side effects, it is still needed as a second line of therapy in recurrent gonadotroph adenomas. It is fairly effective in controlling pituitary adenoma growth, preventing regrowth after surgery and causing tumor shrinkage in most patients. The beneficial effects of radiation therapy are not immediate and are often delayed for years.

Medical Therapy of Gonadotroph Adenomas

Currently, there is no standard medical therapy for gonadotroph adenomas. Most published data are based on case reports and anecdotal experiences. Early reports described the presence of dopamine receptors in clinically nonfunctioning and gonadotroph adenomas. Dopamine agonists can suppress the release of gonadotropins and their subunits from most gonadotroph tumors, both in vivo and in vitro (29). Suppression of the secretory activity of the adenoma is, occasionally, accompanied by improvement of visual field defects or tumor shrinkage. Dopamine agonist therapy should be attempted when surgical resection is incomplete. The optimal dose of dopamine agonist (e.g., bromocriptine) is unknown, but 10 to 15 mg/day of the latter drug seems reasonable. Treatment should continue as long as it is shown to be effective or until the benefits of other therapeutic modalities used simultaneously (e.g., radiation therapy) are appreciated.

Therapy with GnRH agonists has, in general, been disappointing (24). Long-acting GnRH analogs usually produce an initial agonist effect on normal gonadotroph cells, followed by reduction in gonadotropin secretion and bioactivity, leading to clinical and biochemical hypogonadism. When these drugs are used in gonadotroph adenomas, however, they are reported to produce sustained hormonal elevation and, at times, increase in tumor size. Hence, they are not recommended as a diagnostic or therapeutic modality. In contrast, GnRH antagonists (Nal-Glu GnRH) have shown more promising results in patients with gonadotroph adenomas. At this point, treatment with GnRH antagonists is still investigational and as such is not available for clinical use. However, based on preliminary studies, the drug may emerge as an adjuvant therapy in patients with gonadotroph adenomas.

Another potential approach in medical treatment is the use of the hypothalamic hormone somatostatin or one of its analogs. Somatostatin receptors have been demonstrated on nonfunctioning adenomas both in vivo and in vitro (30). Somatostatin was demonstrated to inhibit gonadotropin and/or α-SU secretion both in vivo and in vitro (30, 31). The influence of this drug on inhibiting tumor growth seems to be less predictable and less common as minimal to moderate reductions in size were reported in less than 10 to 15% of treated patients. Because the response to this drug does not correlate with the presence of somatostatin receptor, imaging studies using radiolabeled octreotide are not necessary as a screening test to predict the presence of octreotide-responsive nonfunctioning adenomas. Until more experience is acquired using large numbers of patients, octreotide cannot be recommended for routine use.

Tamoxifen is a potent antiestrogen that has been shown to have significant in vitro inhibitory effects on the growth of various human pituitary adenomas (32). There are currently no in vivo studies on the use of tamoxifen in patients with gonadotroph adenomas. It might prove to be a promising agent as a potential adjuvant therapy. The detection of estrogen receptors in most gonadotroph adenomas supports the potential beneficiary effects of antiestrogens or other pharmacologic agents that could affect secretion of estrogen or its binding to the receptor (32).

CONCLUSIONS

Gonadotroph adenomas account for approximately 15% of all pituitary tumors. The newer advances in immunocytochemistry and immunoradiometric assays have made it easier to recognize these tumors as a distinct clinical and pathologic entity that is different than those considered to be nonfunctioning. Therapy for gonadotroph adenomas is primarily surgical, with adjuvant radiation and medical therapy in selected patients.

ACKNOWLEDGMENTS

We thank all referring physicians and the staff of The Clinical Research Center of the University Hospitals of Cleveland, Cleveland, OH, for their help in conducting the clinical studies; Paul Hartman and Elizabeth Smith for their technical help; and Robert Myers for his help in preparing the manuscript.

REFERENCES

1. Woolf PD, Schenk EA. An FSH-producing pituitary tumor in a patient with hypogonadism. J Clin Endocrinol Metab 1974;38:561–568.
2. Snyder PJ. Gonadotroph cell adenomas of the pituitary. Endocr Rev 1985;6(4):552–563.
3. Whitaker MD, Prior JC, Scheithauer B, et al. Gonadotrophin-secreting pituitary tumor: report and review. Clin Endocrinol 1985;22:43–48.
4. Snyder PJ. Extensive personal experience: gonadotroph adenomas. J Clin Endocrinol Metab 1995;80:1059–1061.
5. Ridgway EC, Klibanski A, Ladenson P, et al. Pure alpha-secreting pituitary adenomas. N Engl J Med 1981;304:1254–1259.
6. Asa SL, Gerrie BM, Singer W, et al. Gonadotropin secretion in vitro by human pituitary null cell adenomas and oncocytomas J Clin Endocrinol Metab 1986;62:1011–1019.
7. Demura R, Jibiki K, Kubo O, et al. The significance of alpha-subunit

as a tumor marker for gonadotropin-producing pituitary adenomas. J Clin Endocrinol Metab 1986;63:564–569.

8. Alamo PG, Petterson KSI, Saccomanno K, et al. Abnormal response of LH beta subunit to TRH in patients with non-functioning pituitary adenoma. Clin Endocrinol 1994;41:661–666.

9. Kwekkeboom DJ, De Jong FH, Lamberts SWJ. Gonadotropin release by clinically nonfunctioning and gonadotroph pituitary adenomas in vivo and in vitro: relation to sex and effects of TRH, GnRH, and bromocriptine. J Clin Endocrinol Metab 1989;68:1128–1135.

10. Snyder PJ, Muzyka R, Janice J, et al. Thyrotropin-releasing hormone provokes abnormal FSH and LH responses in men who have pituitary adenomas and FSH hyper secretion. J Clin Endocrinol Metab 1980;51:744–748.

11. Daneshdoost L , Gennarelli TA, Bashey HM, et al. Recognition of gonadotroph adenomas in women. N Engl J Med 1991;324:589–594.

12. Molitch ME. Gonadotroph-cell adenomas (editorial). N Engl J Med 1991;324:626–627.

13. Daneshdoost L, Gennarelli TA, Bashey HM, et al. Identification of gonadotroph adenomas in men with clinically nonfunctioning adenomas by the luteinizing hormone beta subunit response to TRH. J Clin Endocrinol Metab 1993;77:1352–1355.

14. Blanco C, Lucas T, Alcaniz J, et al. Usefulness of TRH test, SMS 201–995, and bromocriptine in the diagnosis and treatment of gonadotropin-secreting pituitary adenomas. J Endocrinol Invest 1994;17:99–104.

15. Friend KE, Chiou YK, Lopes MBS, et al. Estrogen receptor expression in human pituitary: correlation with immunohistochemistry in normal tissue, and immunohistochemistry and morphology in macroadenomas. J Clin Endocrinol Metab 1994;78:1497–1504.

16. Galway AB , Hsueh AJW, Daneshdoost L, et al. Gonadotroph adenomas in men produce biologically active FSH. J Clin Endocrinol Metab 1990;71:907–912.

17. Alexander JM, Jameson JL, Bikkal HA, et al. The effects of Activin on FSH secretion and biosynthesis in human glycoprotein hormone-producing pituitary adenomas. J Clin Endocrinol Metab 1991;72:1261–1267.

18. Young WF, Scheithauer BW, Kovacs KT, et al. Gonadotroph adenoma of the pituitary gland: a clinicopathologic analysis of 100 cases. Mayo Clin Proc 1996;71:649–656.

19. Zarate A, Fonesca ME, Mason M, et al. Gonadotropin-secreting pituitary adenoma with concomitant hyper secretion of testosterone and elevated sperm count: treatment with LRH agonist. Acta Endocrinologica (Copenh) 1986;113:29–34.

20. Klibanski A, Deutsch P, Jameson JL, et al. Luteinizing hormone-secreting pituitary tumor: biosynthetic characterization and clinical studies. J Clin Endocrinol Metab 1987;64:536–542.

21. Arafah BM. Reversible hypopituitarism in patients with large nonfunctioning pituitary adenomas. J Clin Endocrinol Metab 1986;62:1173–1179.

22. Arafah BM, Kailani SH, Nekl KE, et al. Immediate recovery of pituitary function following transsphenoidal resection of pituitary macroadenomas. J Clin Endocrinol Metab 1994;79:348–354.

23. Katznelson L, Alexander JM, Bikkal HE, et al. Imbalanced FSH beta-subunit hormone biosynthesis in human pituitary adenomas. J Clin Endocrinol Metab 1992;74:1343–1351.

24. Chanson PH, Lahlou N, Warnet A, et al. Responses to GnRH agonist and antagonist administration in patients with gonadotroph cell adenomas. J Endocrinol Invest 1994;17:91–98.

25. Alexander J, Klibanski A. Gonadotropin-releasing hormone receptor mRNA expression by human pituitary tumors in vitro. J Clin Invest 1993;93:2332–2339.

26. Samuels MH , Henry P, Kleinschmidt-Demasters BK, et al. Pulsatile glycoprotein hormone secretion in glycoprotein-producing pituitary tumors. J Clin Endocrinol Metab 1991;73:1281–1288.

27. Hout WM, Arafah BM, Salazar R, et al. Evaluation of the hypothalamic-pituitary-adrenal axis immediately following pituitary adenomectomy: is perioperative steroid therapy necessary. J Clin Endocrinol Metab 1988;66:1208–1212.

28. Ebersold MJ, Quast LM, Laws ER, et al. Long-term results in transsphenoidal removal of nonfunctioning pituitary adenomas. J Neurosurg 1986;64:713–719.

29. Kwekkeboom DJ, Lamberts SWJ. Long-term treatment with the dopamine agonist CV 205–502 of patients with a clinically nonfunctioning, gonadotroph, or alpha-subunit secreting pituitary adenoma. Clin Endocrinol 1992;36:171–176.

30. Plockinger U, Reichel M, Fett U, et al. Preoperative Octreotide treatment of GH secreting and clinically nonfunctioning pituitary macroadenomas: effect on tumor volume and lack of correlation with Immunohistochemistry and Somatostatin receptor scintigraphy. J Clin Endocrinol Metab 1994;79:1416–1423.

31. Vos P , Croughs RJM, Thijssen JHH, et al. Response of luteinizing hormone secreting pituitary adenoma to a long-acting Somatostatin analogue. Acta Endocrinol (Copenh) 1988;118:587–590.

32. Caronti B, Palladini G, Bevilacqua MG, et al. Effects of 17-beta estradiol, progesterone and tamoxifen on in vitro proliferation of human pituitary adenomas: correlation with specific cellular receptors. Tumor Biol 1993;14:59–68.

Thyroid-Stimulating Hormone–Secreting Pituitary Tumors

Ian E. McCutcheon and Edward H. Oldfield

INTRODUCTION

Pituitary adenomas that secrete thyroid-stimulating hormone (TSH) are the least common of the major categories of pituitary tumors. Traditionally, these adenomas have formed less than 1% of major series (1, 2). The incidence of these tumors has been increasing, however, during the past 10 years (Fig. 18.1) for several reasons. Better radiologic imaging has improved detection of small tumors. Sensitive immunoradiometric assays of TSH introduced in the 1980s provide more complete profiles of thyroid hormone function in patients with hyperthyroidism (3). Finally, endocrinologists have increasingly recognized the concept of hyperthyroidism of pituitary origin.

Because thyrotrophs represent 5% of the cells in the anterior lobe of the pituitary (4), the higher, later incidence seems closer to what might be expected for the true prevalence of such tumors. It seems unlikely that thyrotrophs would have a less inherent tendency to neoplasia than other cell types in the pituitary, and the high incidence of null-cell adenomas in all large series makes each secretory tumor type less common than its cell of origin. Although pituitary tumors were suspected as the cause of some cases of thyroid excess in the 1950s (5, 6), the first proven case was documented by bioassays of serum TSH in 1960 (7). As radioimmunoassays were developed, the sensitivity and specificity of TSH measurement increased. The first case of a TSH-secreting tumor proven by radioimmunoassay was reported in 1970 (8). Since then, approximately 300 cases have been reported. As the ability to detect and diagnose these tumors biochemically and radiologically has improved, the efficacy of our therapeutic strategies also has improved.

PITUITARY-THYROID AXIS

Patients with TSH-secreting tumors present with disordered balance in the pituitary–thyroid axis because of overproduction of TSH. Like other hormones produced by the anterior lobe, TSH production and release is under hypothalamic control. Thyrotropin-releasing hormone (TRH) was the first hypothalamic releasing factor isolated (9). It has since become apparent that thyroid hormone and other molecules not only inhibit TRH secretion but also act at the level of the thyrotroph to impede TSH release directly. TRH is produced in the periventricular nucleus of the hypothalamus and travels to the anterior lobe of the pituitary gland in the portal venous plexus of the pituitary stalk (Fig.

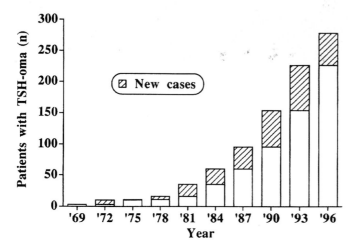

Figure 18.1. Cumulative sum of all reported patients with TSH-secreting pituitary adenoma. The number of reported cases tripled during the last 9 years as a result of the introduction of TSH-ultrasensitive immunometric assays as the first line test for the evaluation of thyroid function. (Reprinted with permission from Beck-Peccoz et al.)

18.2). It is also produced in several other locations inside and outside the central nervous system; circulating TRH is derived largely from extrahypothalamic sites. Its measurement in peripheral venous blood is therefore of little clinical use in assessing thyroid disorders.

TSH is a 28-kd glycoprotein composed of two subunits, each coded by separate genes (10) (Fig. 18.3). It shares a common α-subunit with such other glycoprotein hormones as luteinizing hormone (LH), follicle-stimulating hormone (FSH), and human chorionic gonadotropin. Its β-subunit, which provides its biologic specificity, binds noncovalently to the α-subunit in an equimolar ratio.

TSH release is stimulated by TRH and inhibited by dopamine, somatostatin, and some neuropeptides (e.g., serotonin and cholecystokinin) and steroid hormones (estrogen and cortisol). The binding of TSH to its target receptor on the surface of cells in the thyroid gland is influenced by the degree of glycosylation of the α- and β-subunits. For this reason, TSH molecules exhibit diverse bioactivities; although some are relatively ineffective in provoking thyroid hormone secretion, other isoforms are more effective. Thus, clinical hyperthyroidism can occur with minor or no increases in basal TSH level, and some patients are more (or less) hyperthyroid than others with similar serum levels of TSH.

TSH induces enlargement of thyroid follicular cells and promotes the synthesis and release of both tetraiodothyronine (thyroxine [T4]) and triiodothyronine (T3). T4 is the predominant hormone produced in the thyroid, whereas most measurable T3 is produced by deiodination of T4 in the periphery, where T3 is the active hormone. T3 binds to nuclear receptors in such target organs as muscle, liver, and adipose tissue. Its primary function is to promote and regulate cell growth and metabolic rate.

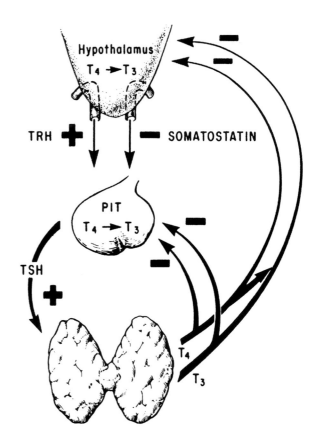

HYPOTHALAMIC – PITUITARY – THYROID AXIS

Figure 18.2. Hypothalamic-Pituitary-Thyroid Axis. TSH from the pituitary stimulates the secretion of both T4 and T3. These act at the pituitary level to control secretion of TSH by a negative feedback mechanism. In addition, T4 is degraded to the much more potent T3 within the pituitary by a monoiodinase. Secretion of TSH is stimulated by TRH from the hypothalamus and inhibited by somatostatin and, to a lesser extent, dopamine. Hypothalamic factors thus interact at the pituitary level to determine the secretion rate. Thyroid hormone acts at the hypothalamus to stimulate secretion of somatostatin (this stimulating effect acts as a negative signal to the pituitary). The effect of thyroid hormones on secretion of TRH has not been determined precisely. Finally, within the hypothalamus, T4 is also degraded to T3, and this degradation may play a role in feedback control. (Reprinted with permission from Reichlin S. Neuroendocrinology. In: Wilson JD, Foster DW, eds. Williams Textbook of Endocrinology. 8th ed. WB Saunders, 1992.)

The pituitary–thyroid axis is a self-regulating system through a negative feedback mechanism operative primarily in the pituitary but also in the hypothalamus (Fig. 18.2). T3 inhibits pituitary TSH production and release and similarly inhibits TRH in the hypothalamus.

SYNDROMES OF INAPPROPRIATE TSH SECRETION

Most patients with hyperthyroidism have a primary disorder of the thyroid gland. In these conditions, such as

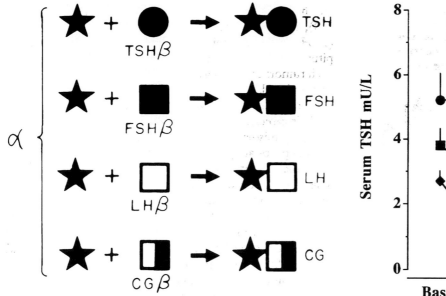

Figure 18.3. Subunit nature of the glycoprotein hormones. Each glycoprotein hormone is comprised of two different glycopeptide subunits called alpha and beta, which are products of separate genes. The common α-subunit (*star*) associates with a specific β-subunit in a noncovalent fashion to yield the biologically active dimer. The four hormones in this family are TSH, FSH, LH, and CG. (Reprinted with permission from Chinn WW. Biosynthesis of glycoprotein hormones. In: Black PM, Zervas NT, Ridgeway EC, eds. Secretory Tumors of the Pituitary Gland. NY: Raven Press, 1984.)

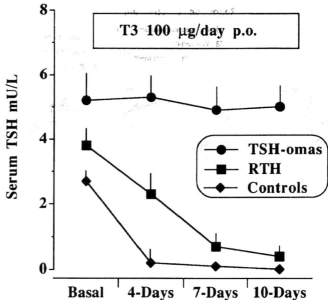

Figure 18.4. Results of T3 suppression test (Werner's test, T3 being administered orally at a dose of 100 μg/day for 10 days) in 14 patients with TSH-secreting tumors, in 16 with resistance to thyroid hormones (RTH), and in 13 normal controls. This test is accurate in documenting the autonomy (TSH-secreting tumors) or with the refractoriness (RTH) of pituitary thyrotrophs to the thyroid hormone feedback mechanism. Note that TSH inhibition in RTH patients is qualitatively, but not quantitatively, normal. (Reprinted with permission from Beck-Peccoz et al.)

Graves' disease and toxic multinodular goiter, T4 and T3 levels are high, but the serum TSH level is appropriately suppressed and does not rise after TRH administration. In secondary (central) hyperthyroidism, the TSH level remains elevated (or measurable) despite the presence of high levels of T4 and T3, which in a healthy patient would push TSH levels below the level of detectability with current assays (Fig. 18.4). This syndrome of inappropriate TSH secretion was first described by Gershengorn and Weintraub in 1975 (11).

Patients with inappropriate TSH secretion and hyperthyroidism usually have either of two diseases. Most have a TSH-secreting pituitary tumor with hyperactivity of the pituitary–thyroid axis by neoplastic hypersecretion. One-quarter of such patients, however, do not have a pituitary tumor but instead have isolated pituitary resistance to negative feedback by thyroid hormone (12, 13). This resistance is caused by polymorphic point mutations in the thyroid hormone receptor that are expressed only in the pituitary gland. The distinction between the two conditions is difficult to make clinically because both of the clinical entities are associated with evidence of excess thyroid hormone and goiter is typically present. Total and free thyroid hormone levels are increased in both conditions, and basal TSH level is not suppressed (i.e., it remains > 0.1 μIU/L [> 100 μIU/mL]). However, the two conditions can be distinguished in several ways. The most obvious test is magnetic resonance imaging (MRI) of the sella. The presence of a

pituitary tumor strongly suggests a neoplastic cause. However, patients with inappropriate TSH secretion may harbor incidental pituitary adenomas that are unrelated to their hyperthyroid state. Occult microadenomas are found fairly frequently in the general population (14, 15). In a series of 10 patients with inappropriate TSH secretion reported by the Mayo Clinic, 6 had a pituitary tumor; 5 of the tumors were responsible for the TSH excess but 1 tumor was a null-cell adenoma possibly unrelated to the patient's hyperthyroid state (16).

A biochemical distinction can be made in several ways. Dynamic testing with TRH stimulates a significant increase of TSH in patients with isolated pituitary resistance, but little or no increase occurs in those with a pituitary tumor secreting TSH (Fig. 18.5). Hormone secretion by TSH-secreting tumors is usually, although not invariably, autonomous. Administration of exogenous thyroid hormone typically fails to suppress TSH secretion in a patient with a TSH-secreting tumor but will suppress TSH in patients with isolated pituitary resistance (Fig. 18.4).

One of the most useful biochemical tests for confirming the presence of a TSH-secreting tumor, and for distinguishing it from pituitary resistance, is the molar ratio of α-subunit to TSH (Fig. 18.6). This ratio, equimolar in patients with pituitary resistance or Graves' disease, is disordered in the passage of tumor. It should always be measured in patients suspected of having central hyperthyroidism.

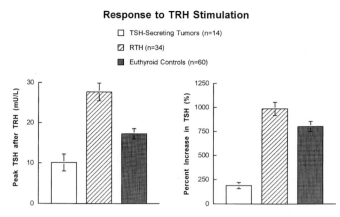

Figure 18.5. Results of TRH stimulation testing (500 ug iv) in patients with TSH-secreting tumors, resistance to thyroid hormones (RTH), and euthyroid control subjects. (Data reprinted with permission from Brucker-Davis F, Oldfield EH, Skarulis MC, Doppman JL, Weintraub BD. TSH-secreting pituitary tumors: diagnostic criteria, thyroid hormone sensitivity and treatment outcome in 25 patients followed prospectively at the NIH. J Clin Endocrinol Meta 1998. In press.)

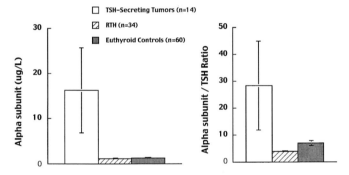

Figure 18.6. Levels of α-subunit and the α-subunit/TSH molar ratio in patients with TSH-secreting tumors, resistance to thyroid hormones (RTH), and euthyroid control subjects. (Data reprinted with permission from Brucker-Davis F, Oldfield EH, Skarulis MC, Doppman JL, Weintraub BD. TSH-secreting pituitary tumors: diagnostic criteria, thyroid hormone sensitivity and treatment outcome in 25 patients followed prospectively at the NIH. J Clin Endocrinol Metab, 1998. In press.)

Patients with generalized resistance to thyroid hormone are also occasionally described (17). These patients are easily distinguished from those with tumors or isolated pituitary resistance because they present with increased serum TSH levels but are euthyroid or hypothyroid. This disorder tends to be familial, and the biochemical findings otherwise mirror those of isolated pituitary resistance. Patients with pituitary resistance may actually be a subset of those with generalized resistance. Thus, these may simply be two forms of the same disease.

CLINICAL DESCRIPTION OF TSH-SECRETING TUMORS

Although some small series of TSH-secreting pituitary tumors have been published (1, 18–21), the two largest

are the series by Beck-Peccoz, which contains 17 patients (20), and the series from the National Institutes of Health (NIH), which contains 25 patients (22). TSH-secreting pituitary tumors are so rare that most authors describing such tumors reported a single case, and only surgeons who accumulate large series of pituitary tumors can expect to see more than one or two TSH-secreting pituitary tumors in their careers. Further difficulty arises because many patients are misdiagnosed with primary hyperthyroidism and are inappropriately treated with one or more forms of thyroid ablation long before a pituitary tumor is discovered. This elimination of normal negative feedback by thyroid hormone may alter the natural history of the disease (1). Of the 280 cases collected from the literature by Beck-Peccoz et al. (23), one-third had been treated previously with thyroid ablation. In their own 17 patients, 9 had had therapy directed at the thyroid (surgical thyroidectomy, ^{131}I administration, or methimazole administration). An average delay of 8 years occurred before the diagnosis of a pituitary tumor in these inappropriately treated patients (24). It is tempting to speculate that the frequent use of such measures could encourage the growth of a preexisting but unrecognized adenoma or even induce an adenoma when none existed before. Loss of end-organ function in other hormonal axes under pituitary control does have such an effect. For example, approximately 10% of patients with intractable Cushing's disease who are treated with bilateral adrenalectomy develop Nelson's syndrome, in which a fulminant pituitary adenoma secreting adrenocorticotropic hormone (ACTH) grows because of a loss of constraint by negative feedback from cortisol (25, 26).

Animal studies dating back to the 1950s support the idea that a similar stimulus to pituitary neoplasia may exist in thyroid-ablated patients. Thyrotroph hyperplasia occurs after thyroid ablation by thyroidectomy (27), ^{131}I administration (28), and propylthiouracil therapy (29). Hyperplasia and progression to frank adenoma occur in these animals by 6 to 10 months (30). The thyrotrophic tumor cell lines thus created, most notably one called TtT-97, have been used in many in vitro studies of TSH tumor biology. Such tumors must be passaged in thyroidectomized mice to maintain their vitality (31). If the mice are given T4, the tumor involutes (32), a process that may involve up-regulation of somatostatin receptor isoforms (33). In these hypothyroid animals, a switch of phenotype by somatotrophs contributes to the thyrotroph hyperplasia (34). Of particular interest is a report by Faller et al. (35) of a patient with congenital thyroid hypoplasia who showed both nodular thyrotroph hyperplasia and microadenoma formation in the pituitary. An autopsy series of 64 patients with primary hypothyroidism showed diffuse thyrotroph hyperplasia in 69% and nodular hyperplasia in 25% (36). Adenomas were found in 12 patients, 5 of which stained for TSH. Other cases linking primary hypothyroidism with thyrotroph adenoma formation have also been reported (37–39).

Patients with primary hypothyroidism and pituitary enlargement mimicking a pituitary tumor also are not uncommon (23, 36, 39–42). A few even present with visual field defects from chiasmatic compression, and amenorrhea and galactorrhea with associated hyperprolactinemia are common. These patients must be recognized before an unnecessary operation is performed because the pituitary enlargement regresses if the hypothyroidism is medically corrected. Improvement should occur within 2 months; persistence of the mass beyond that interval suggests either an incidental tumor of nonthyrotroph origin or an autonomous adenoma induced by long-standing deficiency. In one series, radiographic abnormalities persisted in 5 of 11 hypothyroid patients despite thyroid replacement therapy (43). Most patients, however, do not have a true pituitary adenoma, and surgery should be performed only if medical therapy fails to shrink the tumor. Increases in prolactin (PRL) in this setting that are caused by TRH release stimulated by decreased negative feedback by thyroid hormone are typically mild, i.e., within two to three times normal (40).

CLINICAL PRESENTATION

The typical clinical presentation of a TSH-secreting tumor includes long standing thyroid dysfunction. In patients with an intact thyroid gland, typical clinical features of hyperthyroidism are present, including heat intolerance, tachyarrhythmias, diarrhea, weight loss, tremor, and emotional lability. The symptoms, which may be more subtle in the elderly, are often progressive in severity. Patients who mistakenly undergo thyroid ablation have less severe symptoms for a period of time after the ablation, but the improvement is temporary and contributes to a stuttering course. Most patients have a goiter, usually diffuse, although one patient had a follicular carcinoma of the thyroid (44), and several patients with coincident Graves' disease have been identified (45, 46). In the patient with thyroid cancer, the thyroid tumor was removed first to allow nuclear imaging for metastatic disease without exogenous TSH administration. In another patient, autonomously functioning nodules were found in the thyroid, again suggesting causation by excess TSH (47). In most patients, however, the goiter resolves if the pituitary tumor is completely removed.

Visual deficits often occur because of suprasellar extension of tumor and compression of the visual pathways. Because microadenomas are still relatively uncommon (presumably because of delays in diagnosis), compression of the visual system still occurs in more than half of the patients. Although cavernous sinus involvement has not been emphasized, it frequently occurs (1, 22, 48), as can direct orbital invasion (49). The bilateral exophthalmos typical of Graves' disease is only infrequently seen.

As in other types of pituitary tumors, hypopituitarism owing to direct compression of the normal pituitary gland occurs commonly with larger tumors. Menstrual disorders in women, impotence in men, and decreased libido in both sexes are often seen.

Several of these tumors have been reported in children, with the youngest patient to date aged 11 years (50, 51). The only reported presentation of diabetes insipidus associated with a TSH-secreting tumor occurred in a 13-year-old boy (52).

Although pituitary resistance to thyroid hormone is often familial, TSH-secreting tumors occur sporadically in most cases, although four cases have been reported in which such a TSH-secreting tumor was diagnosed in patients with multiple endocrine neoplasia type 1 (MEN-1) (16, 53, 54). In MEN-1, autosomal-dominant transmission of a mutant gene on chromosome 11q13 leads to variable penetrance of pancreatic, pituitary, and parathyroid neoplasms. In this condition, the pituitary adenomas usually secrete PRL or growth hormone (GH), but patients with TSH-secreting tumors should be asked about a family history of endocrine neoplasia to rule out the occasional association with MEN-1 (55).

The severity of the symptoms of hyperthyroidism varies widely, even in patients with similar TSH levels. Although most patients are hyperthyroid to some degree, some are hypothyroid by biochemical criteria (and have never been hyperthyroid) (56–58). Others are biochemically euthyroid (59–61). Thus, the absence of hyperthyroidism, either historically or by current testing, does not exclude a pituitary tumor as the cause of inappropriate TSH elevation.

This variability in thyroid function is caused by disordered TSH synthesis and posttranslational processing by some tumors. Some patients may have normal levels of TSH and increased levels of T3 and T4 (20, 62, 63), and others may have high TSH levels but no excess thyroid hormone (56, 64, 65). Carbohydrate branching and sialylation vary for the TSH moieties produced in different thyroid diseases. Each tumor secretes heterogeneous isoforms of TSH that differ in the extent of exposed galactose residues, the degree of sialylation, and the degree of core fucosylation. In general, tumors tend to have increased fucosylation and decreased or normal sialylation, but this profile differs among individual tumors (66). Gesundheit et al. (67) studied the ratio of biologic:immunologic activity in TSH-secreting tumors and found a relatively high ratio for tumor TSH. These changes in posttranslational processing may explain why up to one-third of patients have serum TSH levels in the normal range but still have hyperthyroidism. In the series by Losa et al. (20), 10 of 14 patients had normal TSH levels (< 5 μIU/L [< 5 μIU/mL]), yet all were clinically hyperthyroid. Isoforms of TSH within the adenoma have profiles similar to those in the normal gland. Thus, a mechanism of disproportionate release of the more bioactive forms of TSH may be operative in many tumors.

LABORATORY DIAGNOSIS
Static Testing

The initial effort should be to confirm the presence of detectable TSH levels in the presence of elevated T3 and T4 levels (Fig. 18.4). Although most patients will have a true syndrome of inappropriate TSH secretion, other conditions can provoke this combination of hormone excess. These conditions include an increase in TSH transport proteins such as thyroxine-binding globin, albumin, and transthyretin; familial dysalbuminemia; acute psychiatric disease; and the effects of certain drugs (most notably amphetamines and amiodarone). The misleading values caused by changes in transport proteins can be easily dealt with by measuring free T4 and free T3 levels, which also avoids testing errors introduced by the presence of anti-T4 or anti-T3 antibodies. Several patients with a TSH-secreting tumor have been described who had normal levels of total T4 but high levels of free T4, which more accurately reflects the inappropriate TSH secretion (66–70). If the T4 level is normal, the free T4 level should be measured; if it too is normal, T3 and free T3 levels also should be measured.

When a TSH-secreting tumor is suspected, α-subunit should always be measured so that the α-subunit:TSH molar ratio can be calculated (Fig. 18.6). The absolute level of α-subunits is high in approximately two-thirds of patients; calculation of the molar ratio increases the sensitivity to 80%. The ratio is unity or less in patients with primary hyperthyroidism or selective pituitary resistance to TSH. Interpreting the ratio can be tricky given that molar ratios greater than 1 can be found in some euthyroid individuals, and the ratio varies if TSH is normal but other glycoprotein hormones (e.g., LH and FSH) are elevated (71). Thus, some normal individuals have an α-subunit:TSH molar ratio greater than 1, and some patients with tumors (about one in five) have a "normal" molar ratio compared with appropriate controls. In fact, some patients with tumors have a molar ratio less than 1 (1, 72–74). In one of seven patients described in the series by Beckers et al. (18), α-subunit was not secreted in a measurable quantity.

TSH and α-subunit diverge because of excess secretion of the subunit by individual cells or because of the presence in the tumor of some cells that secrete both TSH-β and α-subunit and others that secrete α-subunit alone. Localization of α-subunit and TSH-β has been studied by immunohistochemistry by several authors (63, 75, 76). This technique frequently colocalizes TSH-β and α-subunit within the same cells, but some cells contain only α-subunit and some contain only TSH-β (75). In general, in any given tumor there are more α-positive than β-positive cells. Other studies that use double gold particle immunostaining demonstrate two cell types: one containing α-subunit only and one containing both α-subunit and TSH-β (77, 78). Similar patterns of hormone segregation among cell types have been reported by Jacquet et al. (79) and Beck-Peccoz et al. (63) in plurihormonal tumors that secrete TSH and other hormones. Although such cases do not rule out the possibility of differential release of the two subunits from tumor cells, they support the presence of diverse populations of cells within the tumor that are responsible for the discordance between α-subunit and TSH-β secretion.

Several other measurements, the results of which reflect the effects of excess TSH action, occasionally prove useful in distinguishing neoplastic hypersecretion of TSH from selective pituitary resistance to thyroid hormone. Sex hormone–binding globulin, a marker of peripheral hormone action, which is elevated in more than 80% of patients with a TSH-secreting tumor, is much lower with inappropriate TSH secretion of nonneoplastic origin (80). The two groups show some overlap in values, which disappears when age- and sex-matched controls are used for comparison. The binding globulin level is not elevated in the nonneoplastic syndrome because resistance to thyroid hormone is not truly limited to thyrotrophs in the pituitary but also involves the globulin-synthesizing cells of the liver. For similar reasons, serum levels of carboxyl terminal cross-linked telopeptide of type 1 collagen can also be used to distinguish a TSH-secreting tumor from selective pituitary resistance. In tumors, levels of this marker of osteoclast function are significantly elevated, with levels greater than 5 mg/mL usually signifying the presence of a TSH-secreting tumor (81).

Other pituitary hormones (e.g., ACTH, GH) are released in pulsatile fashion, even by tumors exhibiting relative autonomy from hypothalamic stimuli. In healthy patients, TSH has a circadian variation, with moderately pulsatile release and a nocturnal surge between 8 PM and 4 AM (82, 83). In patients with tumors, the nocturnal pulse disappears, and little diurnal variation in TSH release occurs (18, 77, 84–86). However, pulsatile release remains, with a higher mean pulse amplitude and normal pulse frequency relative to controls (87). As always, exceptions exist, and at least one patient with a tumor has been described with a normal circadian rhythm (85). Because normal TSH pulses are smaller than those that occur with other pituitary hormones, random interphase measurement of TSH is unlikely to prevent a diagnosis of thyroid excess in these patients.

Dynamic Testing

Dynamic testing also is to be performed in patients suspected of having a TSH-secreting tumor. Most patients (> 90%) have autonomous TSH secretion with no response to stimulation with exogenous TRH (Fig. 18.5) or inhibition by T3 administration (Fig. 18.4). Discordant responses to stimulation or suppression are possible when α-subunit and TSH-β are measured simultaneously. After TRH is given, TSH levels show little response, whereas levels of α-subunit rise (but they do not usually fall after T3 administration) (17, 18, 20, 63, 70, 77). These tests are unlikely to affect the diagnosis except in equivocal cases, but they have contributed significantly to the understanding of the pathophysiologic process associated with this tumor. These tests are also useful in providing a benchmark before treatment begins because normalization of dynamic responses seems to be the best predictor of long-term cure (20, 22).

Reasons for the relative autonomy of TSH-secreting tumors remain unclear. Early reports suggested that the TRH receptor is simply absent (88). The preponderance of evi-

Side effects arose in one-third of the patients and included abdominal discomfort with loose stools, carbohydrate intolerance, and cholelithiasis. Restoration of normal TSH dynamics is also induced by octreotide treatment, with reappearance of the nocturnal surge typically lost in patients with tumors (87). Tumors that do not respond to octreotide therapy may respond to dopamine agonist therapy, but such patients are exceptional (115).

The main drawbacks of octreotide therapy are its subcutaneous route of administration (up to 750 mg three times a day) and its cost. Because of the need for self-injection, patient compliance may be difficult to achieve, and a longer-acting analog requiring less frequent doses has been developed. This drug, known as lanreotide, can be given twice a month. A single dose normalizes T4 and T3 for 9 to 20 days. The effect on TSH-secreting tumors can be maintained for many months by two or three monthly doses. In the only study of this drug that has been published, tumor size continued to diminish for up to 6 months but not after that point, in contrast to the more rapid shrinkage of tumors noted with octreotide therapy (116). The side effects of lanreotide therapy include abdominal pain and diarrhea, and approximately one in four study patients stopped taking the drug because of such discomfort.

If the therapy induces a profound fall in TSH levels, patients may become hypothyroid and require exogenous T4. Reducing the dose of octreotide to restore euthyroidism is unwise because it might allow tumor escape and recurrence of hyperthyroidism. It is not known whether or when somatostatin analog administration can be stopped. Permanent tumor regression is achieved in some cases, but most patients require permanent treatment in the absence of side effects.

RADIOTHERAPY

Because these are rare tumors, no specific study of the efficacy of radiotherapy in the treatment of TSH-secreting tumors has been undertaken. It is also difficult to verify the specific effects of sellar irradiation from retrospective review of the literature given that most patients have undergone surgery as well. Because of the long delays in hormone normalization seen after irradiation of other secretory pituitary tumors, and the deleterious effects of ongoing hyperthyroidism, irradiation is best used as a postoperative adjunct when surgical excision of the tumor fails to restore euthyroidism. Because most TSH-secreting tumors are macroadenomas that extend into the suprasellar cistern, they typically do not meet the criteria for safe use of stereotactic radiosurgery (Fig. 18.9). One patient in the NIH series underwent stereotactic irradiation after postoperative relapse, but no other patients have been described in whom this technique has been used (22).

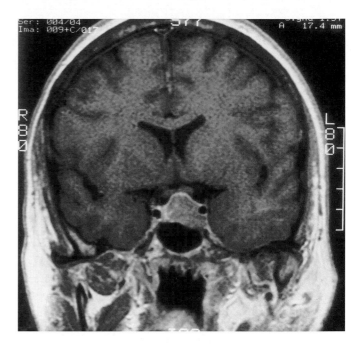

Figure 18.9. MRI of the sella after contrast infusion in a 38-year-old with prior ablative therapy of the thyroid gland for treatment of hyperthyroidism reveals a macroadenoma originating in the left half of the pituitary and extending above the sella to reach the optic chiasm and into the left cavernous sinus.

SURGICAL TREATMENT

Surgical excision is the first treatment to consider when a TSH-secreting tumor has been identified. The optimal approach depends on tumor size, but most tumors are best removed by a transsphenoidal route. As in other types of pituitary tumors, craniotomy should be reserved for patients with persistent suprasellar tumor after transsphenoidal exploration or for patients with significant lateral extension of tumor that is not accessible by a midline approach. Those with cavernous sinus or skull base extension are unlikely to be cured by surgery, but such tumors should still be debulked because this establishes the diagnosis and will at least partially ameliorate the disease.

TSH-secreting tumors pose several difficulties of a technical nature. They are often fibrous and firmer than the more typical soft pituitary adenomas, and several patients have had extensive calcification (21, 99, 100). In addition, several authors have commented on the relatively high incidence of postoperative complications in such patients (1, 21). In the NIH series, 2 of 25 patients died in the early postoperative period (1, 22). Deaths only occurred in patients with macroadenomas greater than 2.5 cm in diameter, i.e., in those in whom a long delay in diagnosis (and the use of inappropriate thyroid ablation) was associated with a large and invasive tumor. Before the introduction of somatostatin analog therapy, radical surgical approaches were deemed necessary for such patients and carried concomitantly higher risk. No deaths were reported in the 17 patients described by Losa et al. (20). In that series, 7 of

17 patient tumors were confined to the sella, suggesting that earlier diagnosis helped prevent the development of invasive behavior by the tumor. In the larger series of 25 patients at the NIH, cavernous sinus invasion was present in most patients; only 5 patients had tumors confined to the sella (22). Early recognition of this disease is associated with smaller tumors, which makes surgery easier, safer, and more effective.

The effect of previous thyroid ablation on surgical outcome is unclear, with some series that contain relatively low percentages of thyroid ablation (21) having higher morbidity than series in which thyroid ablation was more common (20). Nonlethal complications included transient or permanent diabetes insipidus, symptomatic inappropriate secretion of antidiuretic hormone, and permanent central hypothyroidism. After surgical cure, it generally takes 3 to 12 months for the remaining thyrotrophs to recover normal function (22). The rate of minor complications, such as transient cerebrospinal fluid leakage, is similar to that seen after surgery for other pituitary tumor subtypes.

The chance of achieving surgical cure depends on several factors. Patients with long-standing symptoms, larger tumors, invasive tumors, and significant elevations in TSH and α-subunit have less chance of surgical remission. In the NIH series, the mean TSH level for cured patients was 5.8 μIU/L (5.8 μIU/mL), but the mean TSH level for patients in whom cure was not achieved was 75 μIU/L (75 μIU/mL) (22). The analogous values for α-subunit were 4 mg/L and 29 mg/L, respectively. All patients who were cured in that series had a mean tumor diameter of 13 mm, whereas those who were not cured had a mean tumor diameter of 37 mm.

Estimates of cure rate are inversely related to how strictly cure is defined. Return of thyroid hormone levels to normal and absence of tumor on postoperative scans does not, per se, indicate that the tumor has been eliminated. Microscopic disease may persist with subsequent biochemical and radiologic relapse as the tumor remnant regrows. An undetectable TSH level measured within 7 days of surgery has been proposed as a predictor of success (20); normal thyrotrophs are still fully suppressed during that interval, so TSH measurements reflect tumor secretion only. In the series by Losa et al. (20), normalization of thyroid hormones and sex hormone–binding globulin was achieved after surgery in 86% of patients, and normal α-subunit:TSH molar ratios occurred in 58%; normal α-subunit levels were present in 54%; and complete removal by imaging was documented in 47%. It is, therefore, possible to have persistent tumor that is evident on postoperative scans yet achieve one or more measures of biochemical normalization.

A return of the various dynamic test results to normal provides the most secure index of cure (Fig. 18.10). Normal suppression of TSH secretion by T3 was achieved in 40% of patients, but only 2 of the 11 patients were tested after surgery, for normalization of the TRH stimulation test (20). Dynamic testing should be done no sooner than

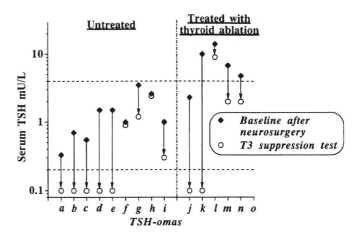

Figure 18.10. Results of a T3 suppression test carried out after pituitary surgery in 14 apparently cured patients either untreated or treated with thyroid ablation before neurosurgery. The *horizontal dashed lines* indicate the upper and lower limits of TSH normal range. Note that only five of nine untreated patients and two of five previously thyroid-ablated patients could be judged truly cured, as their serum TSH levels were completely suppressed. (Reprinted with permission from Beck-Peccoz et al.)

1 year after surgery to allow time for full recovery of function of the normal thyrotrophs. Of course, if cosecretion of another hormone occurs because the tumor is plurihormonal, the criteria for cure also needs to include criteria for the cosecreted hormone. A true calculation of the rate of cure, as opposed to remission, depends on long-term follow-up. No series had a mean follow-up longer than 4 years (22). Applying the most rigorous criteria of cure to that series gives a rate of apparent surgical cure of 35% overall (1982 to 1997).

If inappropriate TSH secretion persists after surgery, the chances are still excellent for achieving control of both tumor growth and hypersecretion. In the NIH series, a judicious combination of postoperative radiotherapy and somatostatin analog treatment controlled tumor in all patients except one, who, after multiple surgeries and radiotherapy, ultimately developed a pituitary carcinoma and died of distant metastasis (22, 48). Nevertheless, long-term follow-up is essential for all these patients to allow early treatment should relapse occur. Initially, this should include yearly MRI of the sella, measurement of T3 and T4 levels, and basal and dynamic testing of TSH and α-subunit.

PATHOLOGIC CHARACTERISTICS

Although TSH-secreting tumors are often invasive, they generally have a benign histologic appearance that is similar to that of other pituitary tumors by light microscopy. Pleomorphic cells with large nuclei and prominent nucleoli are common, and reticulin deposition is disorganized. Mitotic figures are occasionally seen but do not denote frank malignancy. The hallmark of a pituitary carcinoma is the presence of distant metastasis, a phenomenon that has been reported only twice with TSH-secreting tumors (48, 117). Electron microscopy shows characteristic small secretory granules and sparse rough endoplasmic reticulum.

TSH-β can be demonstrated by immunohistochemical staining in most patients. Indeed, its absence might suggest that the tumor is not truly TSH secreting, or (as has been proposed in one patient who otherwise met rigid biochemical criteria for such a tumor) lack of immunolabeling may be caused by sampling error (16). The presence of TSH staining by immunohistochemistry does not guarantee, however, that a tumor is functionally TSH secreting. Several authors have reported such staining in clinically nonfunctional adenomas (118–121). Saccomanno et al. (121) compared staining characteristics of 10 nonfunctional tumors with those of 3 TSH-secreting tumors; 10 to 30% of cells in each TSH-secreting tumor stained positively for TSH-β but failed to stain for other hormones. Half of the nonfunctional tumors showed positive staining for TSH-β, but fewer (5 to 30%) of the cells were labeled. The likelihood of positive staining for TSH varies from series to series, which implies that nonfunctional tumors either produce the hormone but do not secrete it or secrete the hormone in quantities insufficient to ensure detection by standard tests.

Although most TSH-secreting tumors produce only TSH, one-quarter to one-third of them also have positive staining for other hormones. The most common of these other hormones is GH, followed by PRL, and then by FSH and LH. The percent of tumors that stain for hormones other than TSH is greater than the percent of patients with clinical symptoms and biochemical abnormalities associated with hypersecretion of the additional hormone. For example, in one series reporting eight tumors, only two stained for TSH alone. Of the remaining tumors, one also stained for GH, one also stained for PRL, and four also stained for both GH and PRL. However, only one of the five patients with positive staining for GH had clinical acromegaly (75). The symptoms of acromegaly can, in some instances, overshadow those of thyroid excess; in some patients, the true hormonal profile is recognized only in retrospect.

This frequent cosecretion of GH, PRL, and TSH in some combination suggests that thyrotrophs and somatomammotrophs derive from a common stem cell, as does the observation that TSH-secreting tumors are monoclonal (122). An animal model of pituitary tumor development in mice transgenic for GH-releasing hormone also supports this concept (123). These mice develop pituitary tumors between the ages of 10 and 24 months; the tumors are invariably positive for GH and usually stain for PRL but are also positive for TSH about 40% of the time. Further, demonstration of cosecretion depends on the technique used. In one series, immunohistochemistry showed four of five tumors positive for GH and PRL as well as for TSH (76). The same tumors were all positive for all these hormones by in situ hybridization. This implies either that

some tumors have a block to translation, but not transcription, at the genomic level or that immunohistochemical techniques were insensitive to the true extent of polypeptide synthesis.

Colocalization of GH and TSH makes sense in light of the experimental evidence favoring a common progenitor stem cell. However, some tumors are plurihormonal for TSH and ACTH (21), and it seems that corticotroph tumors are more plurihormonal than previously believed. Desai et al. (124) found that 6 of 13 ACTH-secreting tumors also stained positively for TSH. However, in none of the patients described was excess TSH detectable in the serum, and none of the patients were clinically hyperthyroid (124). A tumor should be classified as a TSH-secreting adenoma only if there is appropriate evidence for inappropriate excess activity of the pituitary–thyroid axis on clinical and/or biochemical grounds.

Equally, hyperthyroidism in the presence of a pituitary tumor does not confirm that the tumor is TSH secreting. In an autopsy study of 33 hyperthyroid patients, Scheithauer et al. (125) showed that 6 had adenomas; however, none of the tumors stained positive for TSH-β. In addition, no thyrotroph hyperplasia was seen that, if present, might have caused a central hyperthyroid state. The hypothyroid patient has also been studied at autopsy; diffuse thyrotroph hyperplasia was found in 69%, nodular hyperplasia in 25%, and true adenomas in 12 patients, 5 of which stained positive for TSH (36). The stages of adenoma formation occur sequentially in thyroidectomized mice, from the induction of hyperthyroidism, through hyperplasia, focal adenoma formation at 6 months, and frank adenoma after 10 months (30). Although hypersecretion of pituitary hormones has been associated with hyperplasia of other secretory cell types (most notably with corticotroph hyperplasia), central hyperthyroidism caused by thyrotroph hyperplasia has not been noted. If hyperplasia is found in a patient suspected preoperatively of having an adenoma, the likely diagnosis is reactive thyrotroph enlargement secondary to end-organ failure. However, the clinical scenario must always be considered when interpreting pathologic findings. Longstanding thyroid ablation may allow the coexistence of reactive hyperplasia as well as the secreting pituitary adenoma, which was the cause of the original hyperthyroidism in the same patient.

CONCLUSIONS

TSH-secreting tumors, considered the rarest of the functional adenomas, are becoming more common as diagnostic methods improve. Often described as intrinsically more invasive than other pituitary tumors, their typical presentation as invasive macroadenomas may simply reflect delays in diagnosis and prior inappropriate ablation of the thyroid. When detected early, these tumors can be cured with the same success as other types of pituitary tumor. Rigorous evaluation—including measurements of thyroid hormones, TSH, and α-subunit and dynamic stimulation and suppression tests—is imperative to accurately assess therapeutic outcome. Standard transsphenoidal approaches are useful in most patients, and although cure is achieved in less than 40% of patients by surgery alone, somatostatin analog therapy and postoperative radiother-apy control tumor growth and hormonal excess in almost all patients. The keys to successful treatment are early recognition of inappropriate TSH secretion, early detection of an associated pituitary tumor, and collaboration in the care of the patient by both a neurosurgeon and an endocrinologist skilled in the treatment of pituitary disease.

REFERENCES

1. McCutcheon IE, Weintraub BD, Oldfield EH. Surgical treatment of thyrotropin-secreting pituitary adenomas. J Neurosurg 1990; 73:674–683.
2. Wilson CB. A decade of pituitary microsurgery: the Herbert Olivecrona lecture. J Neurosurg 1984;61:814.
3. Spencer CA. Clinical utility and cost-effectiveness of sensitive thyrotropin assays in ambulatory and hospitalized patients. Mayo Clin Proc 1988;63:1214–1222.
4. Phifer RF, Spicer SS. Immunohistochemical and histologic demonstration of thyrotropic cells of the human adenohypophysis. J Clin Endocrinol Metab 1973;36:1210–1221.
5. Albeaux-Fernet M, Guiot J, Braun S, et al. Results of surgical hypophysectomy in a case of malignant edematous exophthalmos. J Clin Endocrinol Metab 1955;15:1239–1245.
6. Werner SC, Stewart WB. Hyperthyroidism in a patient with a pituitary chromophobe adenoma and a fragment of normal pituitary. J Clin Endocrinol Metab 1958;18:266–270.
7. Jailer JW, Holub DA. Remission of Graves' disease following radiotherapy of a pituitary neoplasm. Am J Med 1960;28: 497–500.
8. Hamilton C, Adams LC, Maloof F. Hyperthyroidism due to thyrotropin-producing pituitary chromophobe adenoma. N Engl J Med 1970;283:1077–1080.
9. Burgus R, Dunn TF, Desiderio D, et al. Characterization of ovine hypothalamic hypophysiotropic TSH-releasing factor. Nature 1970;226:321–325.
10. Magner JA. Thyroid-stimulating hormone: biosynthesis, cell biology, and bioactivity. Endocr Rev 1990;11:354–385.
11. Gershengorn MC, Weintraub BD. Thyrotrophin-induced hyperthyroidism caused by selective pituitary resistance to thyroid hormone: a new syndrome of inappropriate secretion of TSH. J Clin Invest 1975;56:633–642.
12. Kourides IA, Ridgway EC, Weintraub BD, et al. Thyrotropin-induced hyperthyroidism: use of alpha and beta subunit levels to identify patients with primary tumors. J Clin Endocrinol Metab 1977;45:534–543.
13. Weintraub BD, Gershengorn MC, Kourides IA, et al. Inappropriate secretion of thyroid-stimulating hormone. Ann Intern Med 1981;95:339–351.
14. Hall WA, Luciano MG, Doppman JL, et al. Pituitary magnetic resonance imaging in normal human volunteers: occult adenomas in the general population. Ann Intern Med 1994;120:817–820.
15. Saeger W, Ludecke DK. Pituitary adenomas with hyperfunction of TSH: frequency, histological classification, immunocytochemistry and ultrastructure. Virchows Arch A Pathol Anat Histopathol 1982;394:255–267.
16. Wynne AG, Gharib H, Scheithauer BW, et al. Hyperthyroidism due to inappropriate secretion of thyrotropin in 10 patients. Am J Med 1992;92:15–24.
17. Kourides IA. Inappropriate secretion of thyroid-stimulating hormone. Curr Ther Endocrinol Metab 1997;6:52–56.
18. Beckers B, Abs R, Mahler C, et al. Thyrotropin-secreting pituitary adenomas: report of seven cases. J Clin Endocrinol Metab 1991; 72:477–483.
19. Grisoli F, Leclercq T, Winteler JP, et al. Thyroid-stimulating hormone pituitary adenomas and hyperthyroidism. Surg Neurol 1986; 25:361–368.
20. Losa M, Giovanelli M, Persani L, et al. Criteria of cure and follow-up of central hyperthyroidism due to thyrotropin-secreting pituitary adenomas. J Clin Endocrinol Metab 1996;81:3084–3090.
21. Mindermann T, Wilson CB. Thyrotropin-producing pituitary adenomas. J Neurosurg 1993;79:521–527.
22. Brucker-Davis F, Oldfield EH, Skarulis MC, et al. TSH-secreting pituitary tumors: diagnostic criteria, thyroid hormone sensitivity and treatment outcome in 25 patients followed prospectively at the NIH. J Clin Endocrinol Metab 1998 (in press).
23. Beck-Peccoz P, Brucker-Davis F, Persani L, et al. Thyrotropin-secreting pituitary tumors. Endocr Rev 1996;17:610–638.
24. Losa M, Magnani P, Mortini P, et al. Indium-111 pentetreotide single-photon emission tomography in patients with TSH-secreting pituitary adenomas: correlation with the effect of a single administration of octreotide on serum TSH levels. Eur J Nucl Med 1997;24:728–731.
25. Kelly WF, MacFarlane IA, Longson D, et al. Cushing's disease treated by total adrenalectomy: long-term observations of 43 patients. Q J Med 1983;52:224–231.
26. Nelson DH, Meakin JW, Dealy JBJ, et al. ACTH-producing tumor of the pituitary gland. N Engl J Med 1958;259:161–164.
27. Doniach I, Williams ED. The development of thyroid and pituitary tumours in the rat two years after partial thyroidectomy. Br J Cancer 1962;16:222–231.
28. Gorbman A. Tumorous growths in the pituitary and trachea following radiotoxic dosages of ^{131}I. Proc Soc Exp Biol Med 1949; 71:237–240.
29. Moore GE, Brackney EL, Bock FG. Production of pituitary tumors in mice by chronic administration of thiouracyl derivative. Proc Soc Exp Biol Med 1953;82:643–645.
30. Halmi NS, Gude WD. The morphogenesis of pituitary tumors induced by radiothyroidectomy in the mouse and the effects of their transplantation on the pituitary body of the host. Am J Pathol 1954;30:403–419.
31. Furth J, Moy P, Hershman JM, et al. Thyrotropic tumor syndrome. Arch Pathol 1973;96:217–226.
32. Sarapura VD, Wood WM, Gordon DF, et al. Effect of thyroid hormone on T_3-receptor mRNA levels and growth of thyrotropic tumors. Mol Cell Endocrinol 1993;91:75–81.
33. James RA, Sarapura VD, Bruns C, et al. Thyroid hormone-induced expression of specific somatostatin receptor subtypes correlates with involution of the TtT-97 murine thyrotrope tumor. Endocrinology 1997;138:719–724.
34. Horvath E, Lloyd RV, Kovacs K. Propylthiouracil-induced hypothyroidism results in reversible transdifferentiation of somatotrops into thyroidectomy cells: a morphologic study of the rat pituitary including immunoelectron microscopy. Lab Invest 1990;63: 511–520.
35. Faller G, Hensen J, Thierauf P, et al. Thyreotropinproduzierende hypophysenadenome in einem fall mit kongenitaler schilddrusenhypoplasie. Pathologe 1994;15:242–245.
36. Scheithauer BW, Kovacs K, Randall RV, et al. Pituitary gland in hypothyroidism; histologic and immunocytologic study. Arch Pathol Lab Med 1985;109:499–504.
37. Katz MS, Gregerman RI, Horvath E, et al. Thyrotroph cell adenoma of the human pituitary gland associated with primary hypothyroidism: clinical and morphological features. Acta Endocrinol 1980;95:41–48.
38. Leong ASY, Chawla JC, Teh E-C. Pituitary thyrotropic tumour secondary to long standing primary hypothyroidism. Pathol Eur 1976;11:49–55.
39. Samaan NA, Osborne BM, MacKay B, et al. Endocrine and morphologic studies of pituitary adenomas secondary to primary hypothyroidism. J Clin Endocrinol Metab 1977;45:903–911.
40. Chan AW, Macfarlane IA, Foy PM, et al. Pituitary enlargement and hyperprolactinaemia due to primary hypothyroidism: errors and delays in diagnosis. Br J Neurosurg 1990;4:107–112.

41. Grubb MR, Chakeres D, Malarkey WB. Patients with primary hypothyroidism presenting as prolactinomas. Am J Med 1987;83: 765–769.
42. Pioro EP, Scheithauer BW, Laws ERJ, et al. Combined thyrotroph and lactotroph cell hyperplasia simulating prolactin-secreting pituitary adenoma in long-standing primary hypothyroidism. Surg Neurol 1988;29:218–226.
43. Thomas DJB, Touzel R, Charlesworth M, et al. Hyperprolactinaemia and microadenomas in primary hypothyroidism. Clin Endocrinol 1987;27:289–295.
44. Calle-Pascual AL, Yuste E, Martin P, et al. Association of a thyrotropin-secreting pituitary adenoma and a thyroid follicular carcinoma. J Endocrinol Invest 1991;14:499–502.
45. Frandsen NJ, Transbol I. Coexisting Graves' disease and TSH-producing pituitary adenoma. Ugeskr Laeger 1991;153:854–855.
46. Kamoi K, Mitsuma T, Sato H, et al. Hyperthyroidism caused by a pituitary thyrotropin-secreting tumour with excessive secretion of thyrotropin-releasing hormone and subsequently followed by Graves' disease in a middle-aged woman. Acta Endocrinol 1985; 110:373–382.
47. Abs R, Stevenaert A, Beckers A. Autonomously functioning thyroid nodules in a patient with a thyrotropin-secreting pituitary adenoma: possible cause-effect relationship. Eur J Endocrinol 1994;131:355–358.
48. Mixson J, Friedman TC, Katz DA, et al. Thyrotropin-secreting pituitary carcinoma. J Clin Endocrinol Metab 1993;76:529–533.
49. Yovos JG, Falko JM, O'Dorisio TM, et al. Thyrotoxicosis and a thyrotropin-secreting pituitary tumor causing unilateral exophthalmos. J Clin Endocrinol Metab 1981;53:338–343.
50. Avramides A, Karapiperis A, Triantafyllidou E, et al. TSH-secreting pituitary macroadenoma in an 11-year-old girl. Acta Paediatr 1992; 81:1058–1060.
51. Suntornlohanakul S, Vasiknanont P, Mo SL, et al. TSH-secreting pituitary adenoma in children: a case report. J Med Assoc Thai 1990;73:175–178.
52. Phillip M, Hershkovitz E, Kornmehl P, et al. Hypopituitarism and diabetes insipidus in an adolescent boy. J Ped Endocrinol Metab 1995;8:47–50.
53. Burgess JR, Shepherd JJ, Greenaway TM. Thyrotropinomas in multiple endocrine neoplasia type 1 (MEN-1). Aust N Z J Med 1994;24:740–741.
54. Lamberg BA, Ripatti J, Gordin A, et al. Chromophobe pituitary adenoma with acromegaly and TSH-induced hyperthyroidism associated with parathyroid adenoma. Acta Endocrinol 1969;69: 157–172.
55. McCutcheon IE. Management of individual tumor syndromes: pituitary neoplasia. Endocrinol Metab Clin North Am 1994;23: 37–52.
56. Dickstein G, Barzilai D. Hypothyroidism secondary to biologically inactive thyroid-stimulating hormone secretion by a pituitary chromophobe adenoma. Arch Intern Med 1982;142:1544–1545.
57. Fatourechi V, Gharib H, Scheithauer BW, et al. Pituitary thyrotropic adenoma associated with congenital hypothyroidism: report of two cases. Am J Med 1984;76:725–728.
58. Wajchenberg BL, Tsanaclis AMC, Marino RJ. TSH-containing pituitary adenoma associated with primary hypothyroidism manifested by amenorrhoea and galactorrhoea. Acta Endocrinol 1984; 106:61–66.
59. Girod C, Trouillas J, Claustrat B. The human thyrotropic adenoma: pathologic diagnosis in five cases and critical review of the literature. Semin Diagn Pathol 1986;3:58–68.
60. Koide Y, Kugai N, Kimura S, et al. A case of pituitary adenoma with possible simultaneous secretion of thyrotropin and follicle-stimulating hormone. J Clin Endocrinol Metab 1982;54: 397–403.
61. Scanlon MF, Howells S, Peters JR, et al. Hyperprolactinaemia, amenorrhoea and galactorrhoea due to a pituitary thyrotroph adenoma. Clin Endocrinol 1985;23:35–42.
62. Beck-Peccoz P, Persani L. Variable biological activity of thyroid-stimulating hormone. Eur J Endocrinol 1994;131:331–340.
63. Beck-Peccoz P, Piscitelli G, Amr S, et al. Endocrine, biochemical, and morphological studies of a pituitary adenoma secreting growth hormone, thyrotropin (TSH), and α-subunit: evidence for secretion of TSH with increased bioactivity. J Clin Endocrinol Metab 1986;62:704–711.
64. Felix I, Asa SL, Kovacs K, et al. Recurrent plurihormonal biomor-
65. Waldhausl W, Brautsch-Marrain P, Nowotony P, et al. Secondary hyperthyroidism due to thyrotropin hypersecretion: study of pituitary tumor morphology and thyrotropin chemistry and release. J Clin Endocrinol Metab 1979;49:879–887.
66. Magner JA, Kane J. Binding of thyrotropin to lentil lectin is unchanged by thyrotropin-releasing hormone administration in three patients with thyrotropin-producing pituitary adenomas. Endocr Res 1992;18:163–173.
67. Gesundheit N, Petrick PA, Nissim M, et al. Thyrotropin-secreting pituitary adenomas: clinical and biochemical heterogeneity. Ann Intern Med 1989;111:827–835.
68. Comi RJ, Gesundheit N, Murray L, et al. Response of thyrotropin-secreting pituitary adenomas to a long-acting somatostatin analogue. N Engl J Med 1987;317:12–17.
69. Dunne FPM, Feely MP, Ferriss JB, et al. Hyperthyroidism, inappropriate plasma TSH and pituitary adenoma in three patients, two receiving long-term phenothiazine therapy. Q J Med 1990; 75:345–354.
70. Samuels MH, Wood WM, Gordon DF, et al. Clinical and molecular studies of a thyrotropin-secreting pituitary adenoma. J Clin Endocrinol Metab 1989;68:1211.
71. Beck-Peccoz P, Persani L, Faglia G. Glycoprotein hormone α-subunit in pituitary adenomas. Trends Endocrinol Metab 1992;3: 41–45.
72. Caron P, Gerbeau C, Pradayrol L, et al. Successful pregnancy in an infertile woman with a thyrotropin-secreting macroadenoma treated with somatostatin analog (octreotide). J Clin Endocrinol Metab 1996;81:1164–1168.
73. Korn EA, Gaich G, Brines M, et al. Thyrotropin-secreting adenoma in an adolescent girl without increased serum thyrotropin-alpha. Horm Res 1994;42:120–123.
74. Ozata M, Ozturk E, Narin Y, et al. A case of thyrotropin-secreting pituitary microadenoma with normal thyrotropin alpha-subunit level. Thyroid 1997;7:441–447.
75. Sanno N, Teramoto A, Matsuno A, et al. Clinical and immunohistochemical studies on TSH-secreting pituitary adenoma: its multi-hormonality and expression of pit-1. Mod Pathol 1994;7: 893–899.
76. Sanno N, Teramoto A, Matsuno A, et al. GH and PRL gene expression by nonradioisotopic in situ hybridization in TSH-secreting pituitary adenomas. J Clin Endocrinol Metab 1995;80: 2518–2522.
77. Kuzuya N, Inoue K, Ishibashi M, et al. Endocrine and immunohistochemical studies on thyrotropin (TSH)-secreting pituitary adenomas: responses of TSH, a-subunit, and growth hormone to hypothalamic releasing hormones and their distribution in adenoma cells. J Clin Endocrinol Metab 1990;71:1103–1111.
78. Terzolo J, Orlandi F, Bassetti M, et al. Hyperthyroidism due to a pituitary adenoma composed of two different cell types, one secreting a-subunit alone and another cosecreting a-subunit and thyrotropin. J Clin Endocrinol Metab 1991;72:415–421.
79. Jacquet P, Hassoun J, Delori P, et al. A human pituitary adenoma secreting thyrotropin and prolactin: immunohistochemical, biochemical, and cell culture studies. J Clin Endocrinol Metab 1984; 59:817–824.
80. Beck-Peccoz P, Roncoroni R, Mariotti S, et al. Sex hormone-binding globulin measurement in patients with inappropriate secretion of thyrotropin (IST): evidence against selective pituitary thyroid hormone resistance in nonneoplastic IST. J Clin Endocrinol Metab 1990;71:19–25.
81. Persani L, Preziati D, Matthews CH, et al. Serum levels of carboxy-yterminal cross-linked telopeptide of type I collagen (ICTP) in the differential diagnosis of the syndromes of inappropriate secretion of TSH. Clin Endocrinol 1997;47:207–214.
82. Custron-Schelione R. Surcadian rhythm of TSH in adult men and women. Acta Endocrinol 1980;95:465–471.
83. Vanhaelst L, Van Cauter E, Degaute JP, et al. Circadian variations of serum thyrotropin levels in man. J Clin Endocrinol Metab 1972; 35:479–482.
84. Brabant G, Prank K, Ranft U, et al. Circadian and pulsatile TSH secretion under physiological and pathophysiological conditions. Horm Metab Res Suppl 1990;23:12–17.
85. Levy A, Eckland DJA, Gurney AM, et al. Somatostatin and thyrotropin-releasing hormone response and receptor status of a thyro-

tropin-secreting pituitary adenoma: clinical and in vitro studies. J Neuroendocrinol 1989;1:321–326.

86. Samuels MH, Henry P, Kleinschmidt-Demasters BK, et al. Pulsatile glycoprotein hormone secretion in glycoprotein-producing pituitary tumors. J Clin Endocrinol Metab 1991;73:1281–1288.

87. Adriaanse R, Brabant G, Endert E, et al. Pulsatile thyrotropin and prolactin secretion in a patient with a mixed thyrotropin- and prolactin-secreting pituitary adenoma. Eur J Endocrinol 1994;130:113–120.

88. Chanson P, Li JY, Le Dafniet M, et al. Absence of receptors for thyrotropin (TSH)-releasing hormone in human TSH-secreting pituitary adenomas associated with hyperthyroidism. J Clin Endocrinol Metab 1988;66:447–450.

89. Filetti S, Rapoport B, Aron DC, et al. TSH and TSH-subunit production by human thyrotropic tumour cells in monolayer culture. Acta Endocrinol 1982;99:224–231.

90. Le Dafniet M, Brandi AM, Kujas M, et al. Thyrotropin-releasing hormone (TRH) binding sites and thyrotropin response to TRH are regulated by thyroid hormones in human thyrotropic adenomas. Eur J Endocrinol 1994;130:559–564.

91. Dong Q, Brucker-Davis F, Weintraub BD, et al. Screening of candidate oncogenes in human thyrotroph tumors: absence of activating mutations of the Ga$_q$, Ga$_{11}$, Ga$_s$, or thyrotropin-releasing hormone receptor genes. J Clin Endocrinol Metab 1996;81:1134–1140.

92. Faccenda E, Melmed S, Bevan JS, et al. Structure of the thyrotrophin-releasing hormone receptor in human pituitary adenomas. Clin Endocrinol 1996;44:341–347.

93. Akiyoshi F, Okamura K, Fujikawa M, et al. Difficulty in differentiating thyrotropin secreting pituitary microadenoma from pituitary-selective thyroid hormone resistance accompanied by pituitary incidentaloma. Thyroid 1996;6:619–625.

94. Stadnik T, Stevenaert A, Beckers A, Luypaert R, Osteaux M. Diagnosis of primary thyrotrophin-secreting microadenoma by 1.5 T MR. Eur J Radiol 1992;14:18–21.

95. Bartynski WS, Lin L. Dynamic and conventional spin-echo MR of pituitary microlesions. Am J Neuroradiol 1997;18:965–972.

96. Kucharczyk W, Bishop JE, Plewes DB, et al. Detection of pituitary microadenomas: comparison of dynamic, keyhole, fast spin-echo, unenhanced, and conventional contrast-enhanced MR imaging. Am J Roentgenol 1994;163:671–679.

97. Magnali S, Frezza F, Longo R, et al. Assessment of pituitary microadenomas: comparison between 2D and 3D MR sequences. Magn Reson Imaging 1997;15:21–31.

98. Kurki T, Lundbom N, Valtonen S. Tissue characterization of intracranial tumours: the value of magnetization transfer and conventional MRI. Neuroradiology 1995;37:515–521.

99. Sato M, Kanai N, Kanai H, et al. TSH-secreting fibrous pituitary adenoma showing calcification: a case report. No Shinkei Geka 1995;23:259–263.

100. Webster J, Peters JR, John R, et al. Pituitary stone: two cases of densely calcified thyrotrophin-secreting pituitary adenomas. Clin Endocrinol 1994;40:137–143.

101. Watanabe K, Kameya T, Yamauchi A, et al. Thyrotropin-producing microadenoma associated with pituitary resistance to thyroid hormone. J Clin Endocrinol Metab 1993;76:1025–1030.

102. Boni G, Ferdeghini M, Bellina CR, et al. [^{111}In-DTPA-D-Phe]-Octreotide scintigraphy in functioning and non-functioning pituitary adenomas. Q J Nucl Med 1995;39:90–93.

103. Frank SJ, Gesundheit N, Doppman JL, et al. Preoperative lateralization of pituitary microadenomas by petrosal sinus sampling: utility in two patients with non–ACTH-secreting tumors. Am J Med 1989;87:679–682.

104. Itagaki Y, Yoshida K, Sakurada T, et al. A case of refetoff syndrome: selective venous sampling for TSH is useful in differentiating thyroid hormone resistance from TSH secreting tumor. Tohoku J Exp Med 1989;157:69–78.

105. Wolansky LJ, Leavitt GD, Elias BJ, et al. MRI of pituitary hyperplasia in hypothyroidism. Neuroradiology 1996;30:50–52.

106. Gup RS, Sheeler LR, Maeder MC, et al. Pituitary enlargement and primary hypothyroidism: a report of two cases with sharply contrasting outcomes. Neurosurgery 1982;11:792–794.

107. Wood DF, Johnston JM, Johnston DG. Dopamine, the dopamine D2 receptor and pituitary tumours. Clin Endocrinol 1991;35:455–466.

108. Bevan JS, Burke CW, Esiri MM, et al. Studies of two thyrotrophin-secreting pituitary adenomas: evidence for dopamine receptor deficiency. Clin Endocrinol 1989;31:59–70.

109. Chanson P, Orgiazzi J, Derome PJ, et al. Paradoxical response of thyrotropin to L-Dopa and presence of dopaminergic receptor in a thyrotropin-secreting pituitary adenoma. J Clin Endocrinol Metab 1984;59:542–546.

110. De Rosa G, Testa A, Giacomini D, et al. Escape phenomenon after successful bromocriptine and octreotide treatment in thyroid stimulating hormone secreting pituitary adenoma residual tissue. Eur J Cancer 1994;30A:247–248.

111. Wollesen F, Andersen T, Karle A. Size reduction of extrasellar pituitary tumors during bromocriptine treatment. Quantitation of effect on different types of tumors. Ann Intern Med 1982;96:281–286.

112. Bertherat J, Brue T, Enjalbert A, et al. Somatostatin receptors on thyrotropin-secreting pituitary adenomas: comparison with the inhibitory effects of octreotide upon in vivo and in vitro hormonal secretions. J Clin Endocrinol Metab 1992;75:540–546.

113. Guillausseau PJ, Chanson P, Timsit J, et al. Visual improvement with SMS 201–995 in a patient with a thyrotropin-secreting adenoma [Letter]. N Engl J Med 1987;317:53.

114. Warnet A, Lajeunie E, Gelbert F, et al. Shrinkage of a primary thyrotropin-secreting pituitary adenoma treated with the long-acting somatostatin analogue octreotide (SMS 201–995). Acta Endocrinol 1991;124:487–491.

115. Karlsson FA, Burman P, Kampe O, et al. Large somatostatin-insensitive thyrotropin-secreting pituitary tumour responsive to D-thyroxine and dopamine agonists. Acta Endocrinol 1993;129:291–295.

116. Gancel J, Vuillermet P, Legrand A, et al. Effects of a slow-release formulation of the new somatostatin analogue lanreotide in TSH-secreting pituitary adenomas. Clin Endocrinol 1994;40:421–428.

117. O'Brien DP, Phillips JP, Rawluk DR, et al. Intracranial metastases from pituitary adenoma. Br J Neurosurg 1995;9:211–218.

118. Heshmati HM, Turpin G, Kujas M, et al. The immunocytochemical heterogeneity of silent pituitary adenomas. Acta Endocrinol 1988;118:533–537.

119. Hitchcock E, Morris CS. Thyroid stimulating and gonadotrophic hormones in pituitary adenomas without clinical or serological abnormality. Histochem J 1986;18:317–320.

120. Jameson JL, Klibanski A, Black PM, et al. Glycoprotein hormone genes are expressed in clinically nonfunctioning pituitary adenomas. J Clin Invest 1987;80:1472–1478.

121. Saccomanno K, Bassetti M, Lania A, et al. Immunodetection of glycoprotein hormone subunits in nonfunctioning and glycoprotein hormone-secreting pituitary adenomas. J Endocrinol Invest 1997;20:59–64.

122. Mantovani S, Beck-Peccoz P, Saccomanno K, et al. TSH-secreting pituitary adenomas are monoclonal in origin. Proceedings of the 77th Annual Meeting of the Endocrine Society, 1995:412.

123. Asa SL, Kovacs K, Stefaneanu L, et al. Pituitary adenomas in mice transgenic for growth hormone-releasing hormone. Endocrinology 1992;131:2083–2089.

124. Desai B, Burrin JM, Nott CA, et al. Glycoprotein hormone alpha-subunit production and plurihormonality in human corticotroph tumours: an in vitro and immunohistochemical study. Eur J Endocrinol 1995;133:25–32.

125. Scheithauer BW, Kovacs KT, Young WF, et al. The pituitary gland in hyperthyroidism. Mayo Clin Proc 1992;67:22–26.

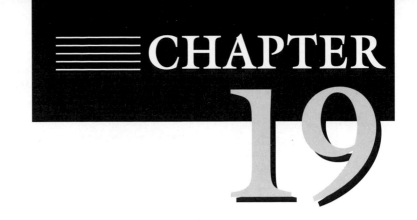

Nonfunctional Pituitary Adenomas

Rudolf Fahlbusch, Michael Buchfelder,
Jurgen Honegger, and Panos Nomikos

DEFINITION

Nonfunctioning pituitary adenomas are also called "endocrine inactive" or "nonsecreting" adenomas because they do not cause specific clinical syndromes of hormone excess. However, most of these tumors are endocrinologically active. This can be demonstrated in cell explant cultures and in immunohistochemical examinations. In cell explant cultures, expression of gonadotropins can be determined mainly in older patients. Results of immunohistochemical examinations are positive for gonadotropins (α- and β-subunits included) in about 80% of tumors. Fourteen percent of these tumors are positive for hormones other than gonadotropins, including the so-called "silent somatotroph" adenomas, "silent corticotroph" adenomas, and "silent gonadotroph" adenomas. Only 6% of pituitary nonfunctional adenomas are negative for all pituitary hormones (1). However, the produced subunits have no endocrine activity and no known clinical significance yet. Unlike other pituitary hormones (2, 3), presently they are not use-

ful as tumor markers to indicate complete tumor removal, tumor residual, or tumor recurrence.

DIAGNOSIS

Nonfunctioning pituitary adenomas usually present with symptoms related to their mass effect: endocrinologic deficiencies (partial or complete anterior pituitary deficiency) and/or impairment of vision. The diagnosis is made by magnetic resonance imaging (MRI) (or computed tomography) demonstrating the tumor size, location, and relationship to adjacent anatomic structures. These tumors can be associated with hyperprolactinemia secondary to compression of the pituitary stalk (stalk effect). The prolactin level in this case is usually less than 150 μg/L (< 150 ng/mL).

INDICATION FOR SURGERY

Surgery is indicated when there is evidence of compression and mass effect. This is usually manifested with visual

281

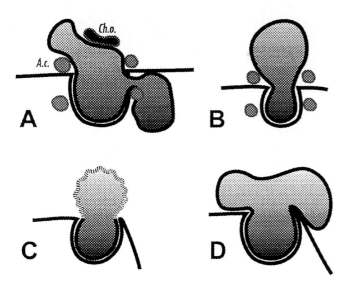

Figure 19.1. Contraindications for primary transsphenoidal surgery: suprasellar asymmetric and parasellar extension (**A; coronal view**), smaller parts in the sella turcica, small sella entrance (**B; coronal view**), invasive tumor with no capsule and no adequate loss of vision (**C; sagittal view**), and subfrontal, retrosellar extension (**D; sagittal view**). *Ch.o.*, optic chiasm; *A.c.*, carotid artery.

impairment and/or hypopituitarism. Because operative morbidity is low, even smaller suprasellar and parasellar tumors should be operated on. Functional disturbances of the anterior pituitary lobe are frequently observed in large intrasellar tumors, tumors with suprasellar extension and visual compromise, and tumors with parasellar extension causing extraocular cranial neuropathy and palsies. Surgery is not indicated in the so-called "incidentalomas," small adenomalike lesions found incidentally on MRI (or computed tomographic scan) with no clinical symptoms. Surgery is contraindicated in patients with poor general health.

APPROACHES

Our series of 2391 operations done in 2193 patients with pituitary adenomas from 1982 to 1997 includes a total of 963 patients with nonfunctional pituitary adenomas. Of those, 822 (85%) underwent transsphenoidal surgery and 141 (15%) underwent transcranial surgery. To achieve radical and complete resection, 74 patients were operated on using both approaches. Transsphenoidal surgery is indicated in all microadenomas and macroadenomas that extend into the sellar area, into the sphenoidal area, and symmetrically into the central suprasellar region. Transcranial surgery is indicated in most suprasellar tumors with asymmetric extension, with retrosellar or subfrontal extension (Figs. 19.1 and 19.2). If the major part of the tumor mass is located in the suprasellar region and the sella turcica is not enlarged, then tumor removal by the transsphenoidal route cannot be as complete and carries a higher surgical risk. Another contraindication for transsphenoidal surgery is in tumors with

suprasellar extension with evidence that they lack the tumor capsule. The latter are recognized by the fact that despite their large suprasellar extension, the visual deficit is remarkably minimal.

RESULTS

Mortality and morbidity decreased tremendously in the microsurgical era. In our series of patients with pituitary adenomas, the mortality was 0.27%. Among the 133 patients with nonfunctional adenomas who were operated on by the transcranial approaches, 1 died as a result of hemorrhage into a suprasellar tumor remnant that led to hypothalamic dysfunction. Following transsphenoidal surgery, meningitis and cerebrospinal fluid leak occurred in *less than 1%* of patients.

Selective adenomectomy without causing additional hormonal deficits was achieved in almost all the microadenomas and small macroadenomas (Figs. 19.3 and 19.4). In up to 20% of the large tumors, hormonal replacement therapy was necessary. This rate increased to 30% after transcranial surgery. After transsphenoidal surgery, ophthalmologic symptoms improved in up to 80% of patients. In nearly 75% of patients, normalization of vision can be expected after 3 to 6 months. Deterioration of vision was the exception. After transcranial operations, the rate of complete normalization of vision fell to 40%, but amaurosis was the exception.

Invasive adenomas were encountered during operative treatment in 129 (24.5%) of 527 transsphenoidal cases and in 43 (43.8%) of 98 transcranial cases (Fig. 19.5). As expected, invasion was *more* frequent in larger, especially the giant, adenomas with parasellar extension compared with the smaller adenomas (4, 5).

FURTHER ADJUVANT THERAPY

Cases in which tumor residual was left and/or invasiveness was found were closely followed up. Patients harboring large invasive tumors with aggressive features were treated with radiotherapy following surgical treatment. Between 1983 and 1990, 50 of our patients were treated with external beam radiation: 61% after transsphenoidal surgery, 24% after transcranial surgery, and 15% after combined operations. The mean radiation dose was 48 Gy (46 to 63 Gy). Forty-seven of 50 patients had good control of their tumor, with tumor progression-free course. Side effects from radiation were reported in 8% of patients. Three patients developed optic neuropathy and one patient developed temporal lobe necrosis (6). Progressive hypopituitarism secondary to the radiation treatment is expected to develop within 3 to 5 years in up to 40% of patients. In another series, patients were treated between 1962 and 1986 (7) and were found to have a progression-free interval of 94% within 10 years and 88% within 20 years. However, only a few of these patients underwent complete tumor removal.

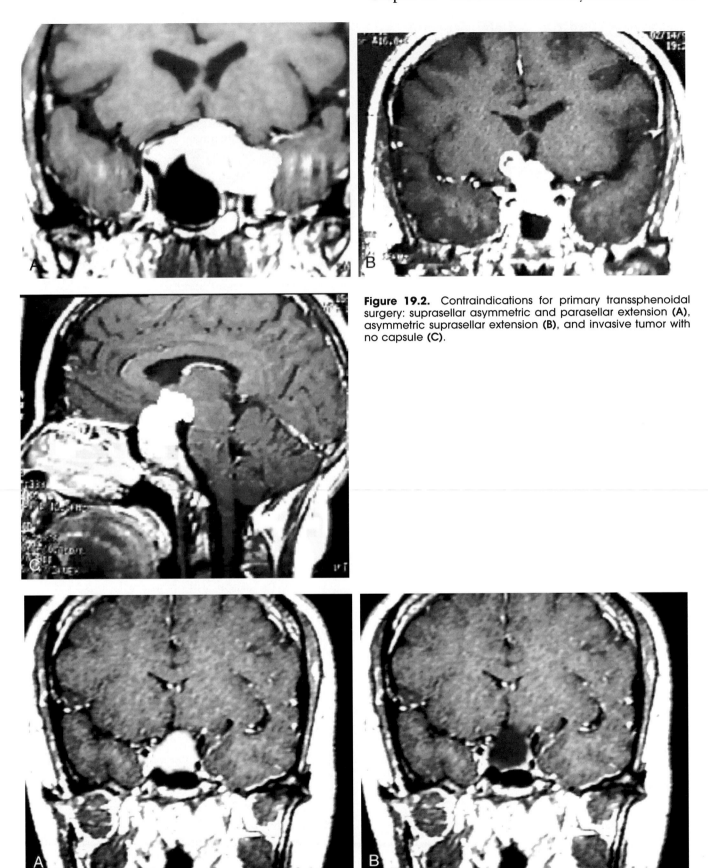

Figure 19.2. Contraindications for primary transsphenoidal surgery: suprasellar asymmetric and parasellar extension **(A)**, asymmetric suprasellar extension **(B)**, and invasive tumor with no capsule **(C)**.

Figure 19.3. Complete removal of an intrasellar and suprasellar adenoma in a 67-year-old man with secondary hypogonadism, which resolved after transsphenoidal surgery.

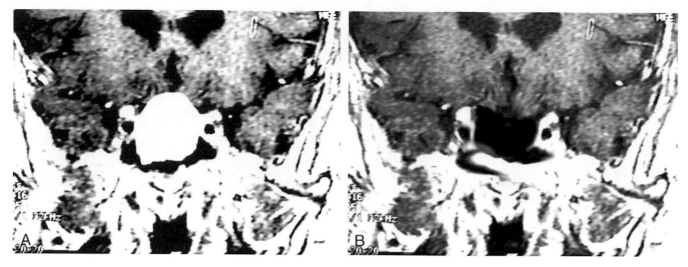

Figure 19.4. Complete removal of a giant adenoma by the transsphenoidal route.

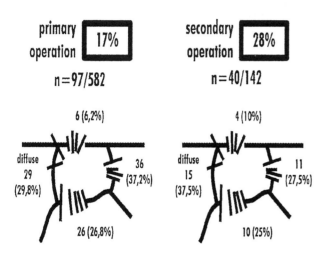

Figure 19.5. Site of invasion for primary and secondary operation.

RECURRENCES

Diagnosis of recurrent adenoma depends on the surgeon's impression of compete tumor resection and the absence of residual tumor in postoperative sophisticated imaging. Computed tomography is much less reliable than MRI. However, even today it is not easy to differentiate on MRI between tissue suspicious of tumor recurrence and normal sellar structures. This fact as well as the fact that the duration of follow-up has been reported differently in different series explains why the percentage of recurrence reported in the literature varies considerably between 5 and 27% (8–10). In our series, recurrence was observed in 7% of patients (21 of 311 patients) after complete tumor resection and during 5-year follow-up. Most of the reoperations

for the recurrences in the 21 patients were performed between the third and fifth year after the first operation (Fig. 19.5). If we include cases with suspicious postoperative tumor remnants, this percentage increases to 20% (63 of 311 patients). Reoperations were performed in 63 patients. In 48%, complete tumor removal could be achieved. However, half of these patients underwent radiotherapy for control of tumor growth. Although transsphenoidal reoperations are more difficult than the primary surgery (11), only a minor increase in morbidity was observed. The chance of tumor recurrence is significantly decreased with use of more radical resections, such as those achieved with the help of two-stage surgeries and when aids of better assessment of the extent of tumor resection are used, like endoscopy and intraoperative MRI guidance (12). Recurrences also can be prevented by postoperative radiotherapy. Histologic proof of invasion and the determination of the cell proliferation activity may help predict the potential for tumor recurrence and guide further treatment plans accordingly.

CONCLUSIONS

Most nonfunctional adenomas can be resected completely, selectively, and safely via the transsphenoidal approach. More difficulties are expected in cases of large tumors, which require transcranial surgery that should be performed by experienced surgeons. Unlike the case with some of the hormone-secreting tumors, medical treatment for inhibition of hormone release and tumor growth is still lacking. Close long-term follow-up with MRI is necessary, especially when a high recurrence rate of up to 25% can be expected and in the absence of tumor markers to help predict the possibility of recurrence.

REFERENCES

1. Sano T, Yamada S. Histologic and immunohistochemical study of clinically non-functioning pituitary adenomas: special reference to gonadotropin-positive adenomas. Pathol Int 1994;44:697–703.
2. Colombo P, Ambrosi B, Saccomanno K, et al. Effects of long-term treatment with the gonadotropin-releasing hormone analog nafarelin in patients with non-functioning pituitary adenomas. Eur J Endocrinol 1994;130:339–345.
3. Lamberts SW, de HW, Van KP, et al. Somatostatin receptors: clinical implications for endocrinology and oncology. Ciba Found Symp 1995;190:222–236.
4. Fahlbusch R, Buchfelder M. Current management of invasive pituitary adenomas. Contemp Neurosurg 1989;1:1–6.
5. Fahlbusch R, Buchfelder M. Transsphenoidal surgery of parasellar pituitary adenomas. Acta Neurochir 1988;92:93–99.
6. Grabenbauer GG, Fietkau R, Buchfelder M, et al. Hormonally inactive hypophyseal adenomas: the results and late sequelae after surgery and radiotherapy. Strahlenther Onkol 1996;172:193–197.
7. Brada M, Rajan B, Traish D, et al. The long-term efficacy of conservative surgery and radiotherapy in the control of pituitary adenomas. Clin Endocrinol (Oxf) 1993;38:571–578.
8. Bradley KM, Adams CB, Potter CP, et al. An audit of selected patients with nonfunctioning pituitary adenoma treated by transsphenoidal surgery without irradiation. Clin Endocrinol (Oxf) 1994;41:655–659.
9. Jaffrain RK, Derome P, Bataini JP, et al. Influence of radiotherapy on long-term relapse in clinically non-secreting pituitary adenomas: a retrospective study (1970–1988). Eur J Med 1993;1:398–403.
10. Petruson B, Jakobsson KE, Elfverson J, et al. Five-year follow-up of nonsecreting pituitary adenomas. Arch Otolaryngol Head Neck Surg 1995;121:317–322.
11. Laws ER, Fode NC, Redmond MJ. Transsphenoidal surgery following unsuccessful prior therapy. J Neurosurg. 63:823–829, 1985.
12. Fahlbusch R, Heigl T, Huk W, et al. The role of endoscopy and intraoperative MRI in transsphenoidal pituitary surgery. In: Werder Kv, Fahlbusch R, ed. Pituitary Adenomas: From Basic Research to Diagnosis and Therapy. Amsterdam: Elsevier, 1996.

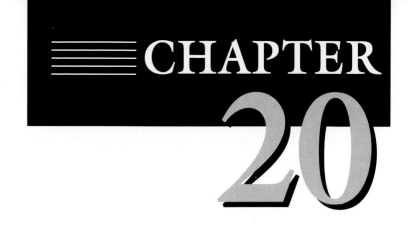

CHAPTER 20

Giant Invasive Pituitary Adenomas

Ali F. Krisht

INTRODUCTION

Pituitary adenomas are the most common intrasellar tumors and account for up to 13% of intracranial tumors (1). Our ability to adequately replace the anterior pituitary hormones and recent surgical advances, especially refinements in the transsphenoidal approach, have made the outcome of these tumors favorable. About 5% of pituitary adenomas become invasive and may grow to gigantic sizes (> 4 cm in diameter). This subgroup of giant invasive adenomas has a more aggressive clinical course and seems to have a different biologic behavior. Treatment with conventional surgical approaches is associated with a high recurrence rate (2–6). By the time these tumors present, they have acquired one or more of the following invasive features:

1. Extensive invasion of the cavernous sinus.

2. Extensive suprasellar extension with lateralization.

3. Extensive erosion of the skull base and invasion of the sphenoid sinus.

Although these tumors look histologically benign, they have an aggressive and rather malignant clinical course (7–34).

MOLECULAR BIOLOGY OF INVASIVE PITUITARY ADENOMAS

Based on the histopathologic features, microadenomas and giant invasive adenomas were considered to be the same tumor but at different stages of growth (7, 12). This led to the conclusion that any microadenoma has the potential to become an invasive pituitary adenoma. It was later realized that this is not always the case. The overall majority of microadenomas remain small, and for a long time. Electron microscopic pictures indicated that histopathologically similar pituitary adenomas have different ultrastructural features (35, 36). In some adenomas, these differences account for the differences in the tumor's potential to grow and invade. Growth hormone (GH) pituitary adenomas, which can be either densely or sparsely granulated, are a good example of this. Tumors with densely granulated cells on electron microscopy have a more benign course, whereas tumors with sparsely granulated cells have a more aggressive clinical behavior.

Recently introduced molecular biology techniques are helping to shed light on the possible reasons for the differences in growth and aggressive potentials of this subgroup of pituitary adenomas. Results of these studies suggest that invasive pituitary adenomas have a genetic makeup that is different than that of the more benign adenoma, although histologically they look the same. Seventeen patients with pituitary adenomas were tested for the loss of heterozygosity of a locus around the retinoblastoma gene, on the long arm of chromosome 13, by Pei et al. (37). They found loss of heterozygosity in highly invasive adenomas and no loss of heterozygosity in benign pituitary adenomas. In their study, Pei et al. suggest that a genetic mutation occurring on chromosome 13 at a location different than the retinoblastoma gene may play a role in the pathogenesis of invasive adenomas. The expression of P-53 gene products was studied by Thapar et al. (38) in 70 adenomas and 7 pituitary carcinomas. The expression of P-53 gene products was identified in 12 of the tumors that were either invasive or carcinomas. The P-53 expression was present in 100% of the carcinomas, 15.2% of the invasive adenomas, and none of the noninvasive tumors (38). Although the occurrence of P-53 mutations in pituitary adenomas was rare, in general the results were different when studies focused on more aggressive adenomas (39). Results of these studies suggest that the P-53 gene, a tumor suppressor gene, may play a role in the pathogenesis of more aggressive and invasive pituitary adenomas and that the P-53 gene can clinically be used as a predictor of their aggressive course. NM-23 is a metastasizing suppressive gene the activity of which, when reduced, indicates a high metastatic potential of a tumor. The activity of this gene was studied in 22 pituitary adenomas by Takino et al. (40). The expression of the NM-23 gene was significantly reduced in the invasive adenomas and showed a high correlation with invasion into the cavernous sinus.

The high proliferative potential of aggressive and invasive pituitary adenomas has also been the subject of several studies. Dural infiltration with tumor correlated with a higher KI-67 labeling index in studies by Kitz et al. (41) and Knsop et al. (42). The activity of the protein kinase C, which has a role in transmembrane signaling and cell proliferation, was studied in pituitary adenomas by Alvaro et al. (43). The protein kinase C alpha-isoform was overexpressed in invasive compared with noninvasive pituitary tumors.

It is becoming clear that invasive pituitary adenomas have a more aggressive proliferating potential and a different genetic makeup than the more commonly encountered microadenomas and small macroadenomas. These tumors should not be underestimated and should be treated aggressively.

CLINICAL PRESENTATION

The initial clinical presentation of patients with giant invasive pituitary adenomas continues to be related to visual loss. In up to 70% of patients, the visual field deficits are consistent with a chiasmal syndrome with bitemporal hemianopia. Unilateral progressive or sudden blindness is not an infrequent occurrence in patients with giant invasive adenomas. This differential loss of function in the optic nerves is thought to be caused by ischemia or infarction from compression and stretching of the small arterioles supplying blood to the optic nerves and optic chiasm, especially those arising from the medial aspect of the internal carotid artery and belonging to the superior hypophyseal artery complex (47). This loss of function could also be caused by sudden expansion of the tumor mass as a result of an apoplectic event such as hemorrhage in the tumor bed or infarction (45–47).

Weakness of the extraocular muscles secondary to intracavernous cranial neuropathy is not infrequent with invasive pituitary adenomas. Unlike intracavernous and invasive meningiomas of the sellar and parasellar region, it is rare for pituitary adenomas to present with extraocular cranial neuropathy before the onset of visual loss. In addition, the occurrence of extraocular cranial neuropathies with invasive pituitary adenomas is less common than what is seen with other tumors of the cavernous sinus. This is thought to be because of the less compressive nature of pituitary adenomas, which are softer in texture compared with the other, more solid, tumors of the cavernous sinus, such as meningiomas.

Pituitary adenomas rarely present with diabetes insipidus in the preoperative period, in contradistinction to the craniopharyngiomas, in which diabetes insipidus is common at presentation. The exact cause of this phenomenon is not known. The presence of a dural barrier between the tumor mass and the overlying stretched pituitary stalk in pituitary adenomas and its absence in craniopharyngiomas, resulting in more direct compression of the blood supply to the pituitary stalk in the latter, may account for this difference in presentation. In some cases, extensive invasion and erosion of the skull base may lead to nasal obstruction and/or spinal fluid leakage presenting as rhinorrhea (9, 48). Exophthalmus may occasionally be seen as a result of tumor invasion into the orbit or secondary to compromise of the venous drainage of the orbit owing to cavernous sinus invasion (49, 50).

Most giant invasive pituitary adenomas are grouped under the nonfunctional adenomas. As discussed in Chapter 17, most nonfunctional tumors are gonadotroph adenomas. Because of the lack of biochemically active hormones, giant invasive pituitary tumors present with symptoms related to mass effect, as described above. Amenorrhea and galactorrhea are common with prolactin-producing giant invasive adenomas. The serum prolactin level in these cases is usually greater than 1000 μg/L (> 1000 ng/mL). Higher serum prolactin levels are encountered more often with tumors invading the cavernous sinus, and this is thought to be because of the direct access of the secreted prolactin to the venous system (51, 52). The GH-producing adenomas present with signs and symptoms of acromegaly (for a detailed account refer to Chapter 15). Most adrenocorticotropic hormone (ACTH)–producing adenomas are small microadenomas, and they occasionally present with invasive features and are associated with Cushing's syndrome.

TREATMENT PLAN

Refinement of the transsphenoidal approach and availability of replacement therapy for anterior pituitary hormones have resulted in a favorable outcome in most patients with pituitary adenomas. Treatment of invasive pituitary adenomas in the conventional way, using transsphenoidal tumor resection and adjuvant radiation therapy, resulted in a high recurrence rate. Tumors with significant suprasellar extension (> 2 cm) were reported with a 42% recurrence rate by Ciric et al. (53). In a series of 77 giant pituitary adenomas reported by Mohr et al. (5), the occurrence of residual or recurrent tumor was present in 40% of the cases. Although visual improvement can be achieved in a good number of patients with invasive adenomas treated with the transsphenoidal approach, the long-term outcome of these patients, especially if they are young and have a long life expectancy, is not satisfactory. Radiation therapy, no doubt, improves the recurrence rate (54–61). However, the side effects of radiation therapy, including radiation-induced neoplasia, occlusive vascular disease, delayed optic neuropathy, hypopituitarism, and the possibility of cognitive dysfunctions, are difficult to ignore (62–72). On the positive side, the introduction of effective medical therapy for some invasive adenomas, such as prolactinomas, and the recent advances in skull base surgery and microsurgical techniques resulted in a more favorable outcome and even biochemical cures in some patients with invasive adenomas (73). When a giant invasive adenoma is diagnosed, the treatment plan is chosen based on two important factors: (*a*) the hormonal activity of the tumor and (*b*) the presence or absence of acute clinical symptoms (Fig. 20.1 shows an algorithm for a proposed treatment plan for giant and invasive pituitary adenomas).

GIANT INVASIVE PROLACTINOMAS

Bromocriptine or other dopamine agonist therapy is the treatment of choice for patients with giant invasive prolactin-producing adenoma, unless they present with progressive visual or other neurologic deterioration. Giant prolactinomas can have a dramatic response to dopamine agonist therapy, with a 1- to 2-log decrease in the prolactin level within hours of starting treatment. Visual improvement can be seen as early as the first week of therapy. A follow-up magnetic resonance image (MRI) of the sella is performed within 2 to 3 weeks to radiologically confirm tumor shrinkage. Lack of response to treatment with bromocriptine may be seen in 18 to 20% of prolactinomas. Lack of response should be recognized early, preferably within the first 4 weeks of treatment. This becomes an indication for surgical intervention. This plan avoids a prolonged waiting period during which visual or other neurologic deterioration may occur, and it also provides an early window for surgical intervention before the possible transformation of the tumor into a more fibrosed, and difficult to remove, mass, which has previously been documented as a result of previous treatment with bromocriptine (73).

In patients with giant invasive prolactinomas who present with rapid visual or neurologic deterioration, immediate surgical intervention is indicated. In these cases, the surgical approach is decided based on the tumor configuration. If the MRI suggests that the bulk of the tumor is more centrally located, and a good decompression of the optic apparatus can be achieved through the transsphenoidal approach, the latter approach becomes a favorable option with the plan to follow with dopamine agonist therapy in the postoperative period (see Case Example 1). If the bulk of the tumor is laterally located, a cranial approach becomes indicated. Evidence of lack of response to bromocriptine and other dopamine agonist therapy is another indication for a cranial approach aimed at radical tumor resection.

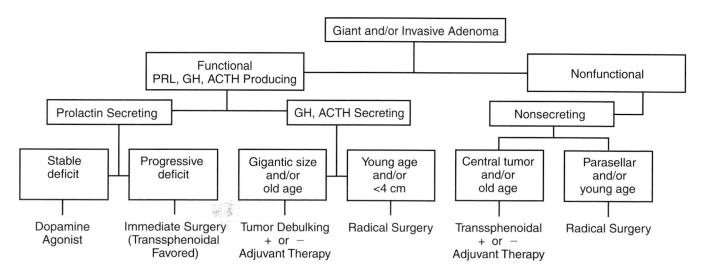

Figure 20.1. Treatment plan for giant and invasive pituitary adenomas.

Undoubtedly, decision-making should continue to be individualized. In an older patient with a centrally located tumor, a transsphenoidal approach with or without postoperative radiation therapy may be adequate. On the other hand, a more radical surgical approach is indicated in the younger population with longer life expectancy.

GH- AND ACTH-PRODUCING GIANT INVASIVE ADENOMAS

Giant invasive GH- and ACTH-producing adenomas continue to be a treatment challenge. Patients with such tumors have a shorter life expectancy and significant morbidity. Based on this, we maintain an aggressive approach to GH- and ACTH-producing invasive adenomas. The classic teaching suggests that a hormonal cure cannot be achieved in such tumors and that they should all be treated with partial or no resection followed by radiation therapy. Unfortunately, this leads to a poor outcome in a good number of patients with low cure rates. The more gigantic these tumors are, the less likely they will be cured. However, in our experience, cures were achieved, especially in invasive tumors of moderate size (< 4 cm in diameter) (see Case Example 2). The recent advances in skull base techniques allow safe access to the different corners of the sellar and parasellar region, which were previously considered inaccessible. A detailed account of the surgical techniques is given in Chapter 30.

Somatostatin analog (octreotide) has been tried in large GH-secreting adenomas. Tumor shrinkage was achieved in 60% of patients. However, the extent of shrinkage was less than 30% of the total tumor mass. This may lead to improvement in visual and other symptoms in some patients, but it rarely leads to long-term tumor control and never

leads to a cure. The treatment of giant and/or invasive tumors with octreotide is of benefit in the perioperative period, especially in patients with significant symptoms related to the overproduction of GH and in whom there is high surgical risk because of the presence of secondary congestive heart failure.

Although we recommend an aggressive approach to biochemically active GH- and ACTH-producing invasive pituitary tumors, decision-making regarding the treatment option should continue to be individualized. Older patients who are considered high-risk surgical candidates could be treated with transsphenoidal debulking of the tumor to relieve the mass effect and improve vision. They can also be considered for preoperative or postoperative radiation therapy.

NONFUNCTIONAL INVASIVE PITUITARY ADENOMAS

The absence of the harmful side effects of hormonal overproduction seen with GH- and ACTH-producing adenomas leads to a relatively more benign course in nonfunctional invasive pituitary adenomas. Despite this fact, radical surgical resection continues to be relevant in most patients, especially in the younger population. In older patients, a transsphenoidal approach with or without postoperative radiation therapy may be more relevant and sufficient. In our experience, a good number of patients with small residual tumors in the region of the cavernous sinus were followed up for several years without evidence of tumor regrowth even when no radiation therapy was given. These patients could be followed up with interval MRIs and visual field evaluations and further treatment decided accordingly (see Case Example 3).

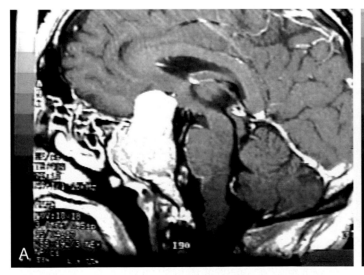
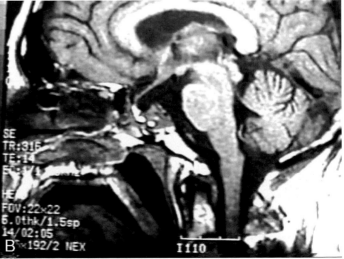

Figure 20.2. **A.** T1-weighted sagittal MRI of a giant invasive prolactin-producing pituitary adenoma. **B.** Postoperative follow-up MRI after partial transsphenoidal tumor resection and bromocriptine therapy.

CASE EXAMPLES

Case Example 1: Giant Invasive Prolactinoma

Clinical Findings

A 52-year-old man presented with a rapidly progressive visual loss during a 24-hour period. He was lethargic and weak on admission and had a history of decreased libido. Results of his examination revealed a dense bitemporal hemianopia with decreased visual acuity. The prolactin blood level was 27,000 μg/L (27,000 ng/mL). An MRI of the brain (Fig. 20.2A) revealed a giant and invasive pituitary adenoma eroding the skull base into the sphenoid sinus and extending into both cavernous sinuses.

Treatment Options

Plan 1.   The treatment of choice if this patient presented with a stable and nonprogressive visual deficit should be dopamine agonist therapy (bromocriptine).

Plan 2.   Because of the patient's rapidly progressive visual deficit, surgical debulking and decompression of the optic apparatus became indicated. Transsphenoidal tumor debulking was done, and the patient was later treated with bromocriptine. His follow-up MRI (Fig 20.2B) 2 years after surgery showed no evidence of recurrent tumor. The patient is still taking bromocriptine, 2.5 mg/day, and his prolactin serum level is undetectable.

Plan 3.   If plan 1 was done and there was no significant clinical or radiologic response to bromocriptine or other dopamine agonist therapy, surgical resection becomes indicated. The surgical approach is chosen with consideration of the tumor configuration and the patient's age. In a younger patient with a tumor with significant parasellar extension, a cranial approach with a plan for radical tumor

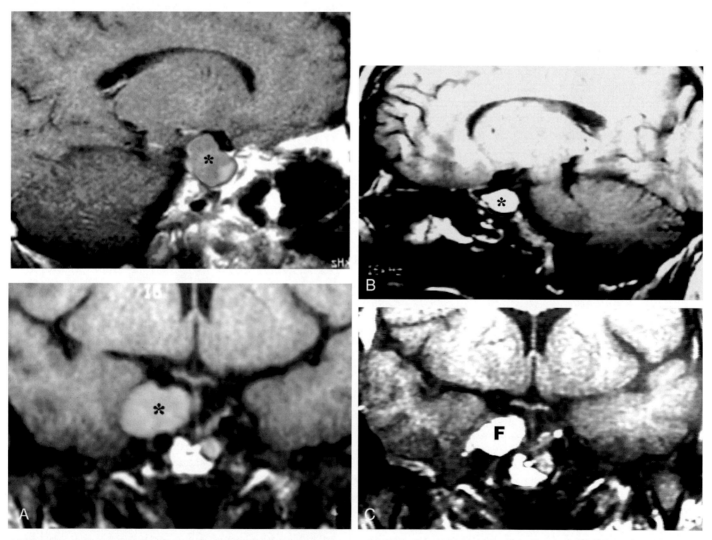

Figure 20.3.   A. A cavernous sinus invasive ACTH-producing adenoma (*). B. Postoperative follow-up sagittal T1-weighted MRI showing the white fat in the tumor cavity within the cavernous sinus (*). C. Coronal T1-weighted image showing the fat (*F*) within the cavity of the resected tumor in the right cavernous sinus.

resection is favored. In an older patient with a more centrally located tumor, a transsphenoidal approach may be sufficient.

Case Example 2: Invasive Hormonally Active Pituitary Adenoma

Clinical Findings

A 42-year-old female presented with a history of insulin-dependent diabetes mellitus, hypertension, obesity, myopathy, and right retro-orbital pain and double vision. Results of clinical examination revealed physical changes consistent with Cushing's syndrome and right extraocular muscle weakness consistent with oculomotor and abducent cranial neuropathies. Her biochemical workup results were consistent with Cushing's disease. MRI of the brain revealed a suprasellar and parasellar tumor predominantly in the right cavernous sinus (Fig. 20.3*A*).

Treatment Options

Plan 1. If this tumor was gigantic in size (> 4 cm), then aiming at surgical cure would not be a realistic expectation. In that case, surgical debulking to alleviate the tumor mass followed by radiation therapy would be a more reasonable option.

Plan 2. In a tumor with much smaller size, although it is predominantly within the cavernous sinus, there is a high possibility of cure with radical surgical resection. This case was approached through an extradural cranio-orbital zygomatic approach, and radical surgical resection was achieved, as shown in the postoperative MRI (Fig. 20.3*B*, *C*). The patient's diabetes mellitus resolved within 2 weeks of surgery, and she became normotensive 4 weeks later. She lost 50 lb within 2 months, and her myopathy resolved. This patient achieved clinical and biochemical cure from her Cushing's syndrome. (The same treatment plan would apply if this patient had a GH-secreting invasive adenoma.)

Case Example 3: Invasive Hormonally Inactive Pituitary Adenoma

Clinical Findings

A 45-year-old man presented with a history of headaches and progressive visual deficit and recent onset of double vision. His clinical evaluation revealed a bitemporal hemianopia and an oculomotor cranial neuropathy. Results of his hormonal workup were consistent with a nonfunctional pituitary adenoma. An MRI of the brain (Fig. 20.4*A*) showed an invasive pituitary tumor with suprasellar extension and invasion of the right cavernous sinus.

Treatment Options

Plan 1. In an older patient with high surgical risk, transsphenoidal surgical debulking of the tumor is a relevant option. However, surgical debulking may not resolve his right oculomotor cranial neuropathy and the residual tumor. In this case, radiation therapy may need to be considered.

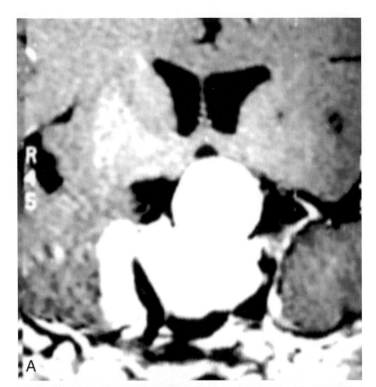

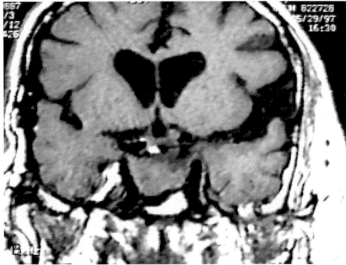

Figure 20.4. **A.** Coronal T1-weighted images of a large and invasive nonfunctional pituitary adenoma with suprasellar extension and invasion into the right cavernous sinus. **B.** Coronal T1-weighted images 3 years after surgery with no evidence of tumor recurrence. Subcutaneous fat graft seen in the tumor bed within the cavernous sinus (*F*).

Plan 2. In a younger patient, radical surgical resection using a skull base approach aimed at total removal of both the intracavernous and suprasellar portions of the tumor is recommended. The patient in this case elected to proceed with radical surgical resection. Three years after surgery, he continues to have no evidence of tumor recurrence (Fig. 20.4*B*), and he had complete resolution of his visual field deficit and cranial neuropathy. Should this tumor recur, further surgery or radiation therapy are to be considered.

SUMMARY

Giant and invasive pituitary adenomas compose up to 5% of all pituitary adenomas. They seem to have a different genetic makeup, which may account for their different and more aggressive clinical behavior. The recent advances in adjuvant medical therapy and surgical approaches have made their outcome more favorable. The giant invasive prolactinomas are best treated with dopamine agonist therapy in most cases. The biochemically active GH- and ACTH-producing invasive adenomas should be treated aggressively with radical surgical resection aimed at the possibility of a cure. This is justified by the lack of effective adjuvant medical therapies and the significant morbidity and shorter life expectancy caused by the hormones produced by these tumors. Nonfunctional invasive pituitary adenomas should be treated with radical surgical resection aimed at cure in the younger population. In older patients, transsphenoidal debulking of the tumor, with or without postoperative radiation therapy, may be sufficient.

REFERENCES

1. Bakay L. The results of 300 pituitary adenoma operations (Prof. Herbert Olivecrona's series). J Neurosurg 1950;7:240–255.
2. Landolt AM, Shibata T, Kleihues P. Growth rate of human pituitary adenomas. J Neurosurg 1987;67:803–806.
3. Hashimoto N, Handa H, Yamashita J, et al. Long-term follow-up of large or invasive pituitary adenomas. Surg Neurol 1986;25:49–54.
4. Martins AN, Hayes GJ, Kempe LG. Invasive pituitary adenomas. J Neurosurg 1965;22:268–276.
5. Mohr G, Hardy J, Comtois R, et al. Surgical management of giant pituitary adenomas. Can J Neurol Sci 1990;17:62–66.
6. Symon L, Jakubowski J, Kendall B. Surgical treatment of giant pituitary adenomas. J Neurol Neurosurg Psychiatry 1979;42:973–982.
7. Symon L, Jakubowski J. Transcranial management of pituitary tumors with suprasellar extension. J Neurol Neurosurg Psychiatry 1979;42:123–233.
8. Ahmadi J, North CM, Segall HD, et al. Cavernous sinus invasion by pituitary adenomas. AJR Am J Roentgenol 1986;146:257–262.
9. Davis J, Sheppard M, Heath DA. Giant invasive prolactinoma: a case report and review of nine further cases. QJM 1980;275:227–238.
10. Dent JA, Rickhuss PK. Invasive pituitary adenoma presenting with nasal obstruction. J Laryngol Otol 1989;103:605–609.
11. Falbusch R, Buchfelder M, Schrell U. Short time preoperative treatment of macroprolactinomas by dopamine agonists. J Neurosurg 1987;67:807–815.
12. Falbusch R, Buchfelder M. Transphenoidal surgery of parasellar pituitary adenomas. Acta Neurochir 1988;92:93–99.
13. Grote E. Characteristics of giant pituitary adenomas. Acta Neurochir 1982;60:141–153.
14. Hashimoto N, Kikuchi H. Transsphenoidal approach to intrasellar tumors involving the cavernous sinus. J Neurosurg 1990;73:513–517.
15. Jefferson G. Extrasellar extensions of pituitary adenomas: President's address. Proc R Soc Med 1940;33:433–458.
16. Jefferson G. The invasive adenomas of the anterior pituitary (The Sherrington Lectures III): selected papers of Sir Geoffrey Jefferson. Springfield, IL: Charles C Thomas, 1960.
17. Knosp E, Kitz K, Steiner E, et al. Pituitary adenomas with parasellar invasion. Acta Neurochir Suppl (Wien) 1991;53:65–71.
18. Knosp E, Steiner E, Kitz K, et al. Pituitary adenomas with invasion of the cavernous sinus space: a magnetic resonance imaging classification compared with surgical findings. Neurosurgery 1993;33:610–618.
19. Kojima T, Waga S, Moroka Y. Huge invasive pituitary adenoma with involvement of middle and posterior fossa. Neurol Med Chir (Tokyo) 1980;20:95–99.
20. Laws ER Jr, Kern EB. Complications of transsphenoidal surgery. Clin Neurosurg 1976;23:401–416.
21. Lundburg PO, Drettner B, Hemmingsson A, et al. The invasive pituitary adenoma: a prolactin-producing tumor. Arch Neurol 1977;34:742–749.
22. Margo CE, Gonzalvo AA. Extracranial manifestation of invasive pituitary adenoma. South Med J 1987;80:381–383.
23. Martin NA, Hales M, Wilson CB. Cerebellar metastasis from a prolactinoma during treatment with bromocriptine: case report. J Neurosurg 1981;55:615–619.
24. Nicola G. Transsphenoidal surgery for pituitary adenomas with extrasellar extension. Prog Neurol Surg 1975;6:142–199.
25. Scheithauer BW, Kovacs KT, Laws ER, et al. Pathology of invasive pituitary tumors with special reference to functional classification. J Neurosurg 1986;65:733–745.
26. Scotti G, Yu CY, Dillon WP, et al. MR imaging of cavernous sinus involvement by pituitary adenomas. AJR Am J Roentgenol 1988;151:799–806.
27. Srivastava VK, Narayanaswamy KS, Rao TV. Giant pituitary adenoma. Surg Neurol 1983;20:379–382.
28. Trumble HC. Pituitary tumours: observations on large tumours which have spread widely beyond the confines of the sella turcica. Br J Surg 1951;39:7–24.
29. Virapongse C, Bhimani S, Sarwar M, et al. Prolactin-secreting pituitary adenomas: CT appearance in diffuse invasion. Radiology 1984;152:447–451.
30. White JC, Warren S. Unusual size and extension of a pituitary adenoma: case report of a chromophobe tumour with unusually extensive compression of the base of the brain, and a review of the literature on the pathways of extension of these tumours. J Neurosurg 1945;2:126–139.
31. Wilson CB. A decade of pituitary microsurgery: the Herbert Olivecrona lecture. J Neurosurg 1984;61:814–834.
32. Wilson CB. Neurosurgical management of large and invasive pituitary tumors. In: Tindall GT, Collin WF, eds. Clinical Management of Pituitary Disorders. New York: Raven Press, 1979:335–342.
33. Yasargil MG. Microneurosurgery, Vol II. Stuttgart: George Thieme Verlag, 1984.
34. Zorub DS, Martinex AJ, Nelson PB, et al. Invasive pituitary adenoma with abscess formation: case report. Neurosurgery 1979;5:718–722.
35. Landolt AM. Ultrastructure of human sellar tumours: correlation of clinical finding and morphology. Acta Neurochir (Wien) 1975; Suppl 22:1–167.
36. Robert F, Hardy J. Prolactin-secreting adenomas: a light and electron microscopical study. Arch Pathol 1975;99:625–633.
37. Pei L, Melmed S, Scheithamer B, et al. Frequent loss of heterozygosity at the retinoblastoma susceptibility gene (RB) focus in aggressive pituitary tumors: evidence for a chromosome 13 tumor suppressor gene other than RB. Cancer 1995;55:1616.
38. Thapar K, Scheithaner W, Kovacs K, et al. P53 expression in pituitary adenomas and carcinomas: correlation with invasiveness and tumor growth fractions. Neurosurgery 1996;38:763–770.
39. Levy A, Hall L, Yeudall WA, et al. P53 gene mutations in pituitary adenomas: rare events. Clin Endocrinol 1994;41(6):809–814.
40. Takino H, Herman V, Weiss M, et al. Purine-binding factor (nm23) gene expression in pituitary tumors: marker of adenoma invasiveness. J Clin Endocrinol Metab 1995;80:1733–1738.
41. Kitz K, Knosp E, Koos WT, et al. Proliferation in pituitary adenomas: measurement by Mab Ki-67. Acta Neurochir Suppl (Wien) 1991;53:60–64.
42. Knosp E, Kitz K, Pernecsky A. Proliferation activity in pituitary adenomas: measurement by monoclonal antibody Ki-67. Neurosurgery 1989;25:927–930.
43. Alvaro V, Levy L, Dubray C, et al. Invasive human pituitary tumors express a point-mutated alpha-protein kinase-C. J Clin Endocrinol Metab 1993;77:1125–1129.

44. Mohanty S, Tandon PN, Banerjee AK, et al. Hemorrhage into pituitary adenomas. J Neurol Neurosurg Psychiatry 1977;40:987–991.
45. Lyle TK, Clover P. Ocular symptoms and signs of pituitary tumors. Proc R Soc Med 1961;54:611.
46. Melmed S. The Pituitary. Cambridge: Blackwell Science, 1995:432.
47. Krisht AF, Barrow DL, Barnett DW, et al. The microsurgical anatomy of the superior hypophyseal artery. Neurosurgery 1994;35:899–903.
48. Summers GW. Nasal obstruction caused by a pituitary adenoma. Laryngoscope 1976;86:1718–1721.
49. Daita G, Yonemasu Y, Hashizume A. Unilateral exophthalmos caused by an invasive pituitary adenoma: case report. Neurosurgery 1987;21:716–718.
50. Sammartino A, Bonaiotonta G, Pattinato G, et al. Exophthalmos caused by an invasive pituitary adenoma in a child. Ophthalmologica 1979;179:83–89.
51. Barrow DL, Minuzo J, Tindall GT. Management of prolactinomas associated with very high serum prolactin levels. J Neurosurg 1988;68:554–558.
52. Shucart WA. Implications of very high serum prolactin levels associated with pituitary tumors. J Neurosurg 1980;52:226–228.
53. Ciric I, Mikhael M, Stafford T, et al. Transsphenoidal microsurgery of pituitary macroadenomas with long-term follow-up results. J Neurosurg 1983;59:395–401.
54. Fisher BJ, Gaspar LE, Noone B. Giant pituitary adenomas: role of radiotherapy. Int J Radiat Oncol Biol Phys 1993;25:677–681.
55. Grisby PW, Simpson JR, Emami BN, et al. Prognostic factors and results of surgery and postoperative irradiation in the management of pituitary adenomas. Int J Radiat Oncol Biol Phys 1989;16:1411–1417.
56. Grisby PW, Stokes S, Marks JE, et al. Prognostic factors and results of radiotherapy alone in the management of pituitary adenomas. Int J Radiat Oncol Biol Phys 1988;15:1103–1110.
57. Halberg FE, Sheline GE. Radiotherapy of pituitary tumors. Endocrinol Metab Clin North Am 1987;16(3):667–684.
58. Hughes MN, Llamas KJ, Yelland ME, et al. Pituitary adenomas: long-term results for radiotherapy alone and post-operative radiotherapy. Int J Radiat Oncol Biol Phys 1993;27:1035–1043.
59. Kramer S. Indication for, and results of treatment of pituitary tumors by external radiation. In: Kohler PO, Ross GT, eds. Diagnosis and Treatment of Pituitary Tumors. New York: Excerpta Medica/American Elsevier, 1973:217–229.
60. Rush SC, Newall J. Pituitary adenomas: The efficacy of radiotherapy as the sole treatment. Int J Radiat Oncol Biol Phys 1989;17:165–169.
61. Sheline GE. Conventional radiation therapy in the treatment of pituitary tumors. In: Tindall GT, Collins WF, eds. Clinical Management of Pituitary Disorders. New York: Raven Press, 1979:303–336.
62. Ahmad K, Fayos JV. Pituitary fibrosarcoma secondary to radiation therapy. Cancer 1978;42:107–110.
63. Al-Mefty O, Kersh JE, Routh A, et al. The long-term side effects of radiation therapy for benign brain tumors in adults. J Neurosurg 1990;73:502–512.
64. Albert RE, Omran AR, Brauer EW, et al. Follow-up study of patients treated by x-ray for tinea capitis. Am J Public Health 1966;56:2114–2120.
65. Almquist S, Dahlgren S, Notter G, et al. Brain necrosis after irradiation of the hypophysis in Cushing's disease: report of a case. Acta Radiol 1964;2:179–188.
66. Aloia JF, Archambeau JO. Hypopituitarism following pituitary irradiation for acromegaly. Horm Res 1978;9:201–207.
67. Atkinson AB, Allen IV, Gordon DS, et al. Progressive visual failure in acromegaly following external pituitary irradiation. Clin Endocrinol 1979;10:469–479.
68. Conomy JP, Kellermeyer RW. Delayed cerebrovascular consequences of therapeutic radiation: a clinico-pathologic study of a stroke associated with radiation-related carotid arteriopathy. Cancer 1975;36:1762–1768.
69. Darmody WR, Thomas LM, Gurdjian ES. Postirradiation vascular insufficiency syndrome: case report. Neurology 1967;17:1190–1192.
70. Fukamachi A, Wakao T, Akai J. Brain stem necrosis after irradiation of pituitary adenoma. Surg Neurol 1982;18:343–350.
71. Haward RH. Arteriosclerosis induced by radiation. Surg Clin North Am 1972;52:359–366.
72. Snyder PJ, Fowble BF, Schatz NJ, et al. Hypopituitarism following radiation therapy of pituitary adenomas. Am J Med 1986;81:457–462.
73. Landolt AM, Keller PJ, Froesch ER, et al. Bromocriptine: does it jeopardize the result of later surgery for prolactinomas? Lancet 1982;2:657–658.

Pituitary Apoplexy

Ali F. Krisht, Michael Vaphiades,
and Muhammad Husain

INTRODUCTION

The term pituitary apoplexy has been used to describe different clinical and pathophysiologic conditions related to an apoplectic event of the pituitary gland. The definition of pituitary apoplexy has been used in multiple ways (1–9). The apoplectic event is usually related to either hemorrhage or infarction in the pituitary gland. It was initially described at the end of the 19th century, and its first description as a clinical entity was made by Brougham et al. in 1950 (10–12). They described the acute onset of a severe headache associated with diplopia and followed by drowsiness and/or coma and gave it the name "pituitary apoplexy." Their paper helped identify a large number of cases that were later reported in the literature (13–24). The recent advances in radiologic studies, especially magnetic resonance imaging (MRI), have shown that hemorrhage in pituitary adenomas can occur without the associated clinical syndrome of pituitary apoplexy. For this reason, apoplexy should be used in the context of an acute, pituitary-related event with a clinical syndrome in which patients present with the acute onset of a headache associated with visual or other neurologic impairment, with or without alterations in their mental and/or hemodynamic status related to hypothalamic and/or endocrinologic abnormalities.

INCIDENCE

Hemorrhage in a pituitary tumor not necessarily associated with a clinical apoplectic event has been seen in up to 25% of several series of pituitary tumors (5, 8, 19, 21, 22, 25–27). Pituitary apoplexy as a syndrome has been reported to occur with an incidence from as low as 1% (22) to as high as 20% (15). There seems to be a slight male predilection, with a male:female ratio of 1.3:1 (28). Age at occurrence ranged from 6 to 88 years, with a mean age of 46.7 years (28).

PATHOPHYSIOLOGIC AND PATHOLOGIC CHARACTERISTICS OF PITUITARY APOPLEXY

The pathophysiologic changes that lead to pituitary apoplexy are still open to speculation. The fact that the clinical syndrome can occur with hemorrhage or necrosis in the gland, and the fact that in most patients a pituitary tumor and an enlarged sella are present, leads to a hypothesis suggesting that acute and rapid growth of the intrasellar contents predisposes to the occurrence of such an event. In their paper, Brougham et al. (10) suggested that the rapid growth of a pituitary adenoma leads to the outstripping of its vascular supply, resulting in either hemorrhage or necrosis. Bailey (29), conversely, suggested that an endarteritis of the hypophysis is the source of the hemorrhage. Results of other studies suggested that the thrombosis seen within the sinusoids of a pituitary adenoma presenting with apoplexy is caused by compression of the pituitary stalk and compromise of the blood flow from the portal vessels, leading to ischemia of the gland and the tumor (16, 30). However, if this is the case, further explanation is needed to account for the hemorrhages and infarctions that occur in small pituitary adenomas (31, 32). This hypothesis has been challenged and refuted by others based on studies of the blood supply to pituitary adenomas and the normal pituitary gland. Cerebral angiography of pituitary tumors showed the main blood supply to these tumors to arise from inferior hypophyseal branches arising from the meningohypophyseal trunk originating from the intracavernous internal carotid artery. Occasionally blood supply arises from the superior hypophyseal artery complex (34–39).

Results of anatomic studies of the opening in the diaphragma sellae revealed a large amount of variations, which speaks against the theory of compression of the portal vessels (40, 41). Gorczyca and Hardy (42), in a study of the pituitary vasculature in microadenomas, proposed that the blood supply of pituitary adenomas arising from a high-pressure system through the inferior hypophyseal arteries leads to spontaneous hemorrhages within the low-pressure adenohypophyseal sinusoids.

After the original description in 1898 by Bailey (29) of a fatal hemorrhage in a patient with pituitary adenoma and another case described by Bleibtreu in 1905 (43), the first comprehensive study was done by Brougham et al. (10) in 1950, when they reviewed the literature and coined the term "pituitary apoplexy." Since then, numerous individual case reports, retrospective case reviews, and literature reviews have been published (14, 25, 30, 33, 44, 45). The association of a particular type of tumor with apoplexy is not well established. The syndrome has been seen in cases of chromophobe, eosinophilic, basophilic, and mixed-cell adenomas. Pituitary apoplexy in the three types of histologic patterns of pituitary adenomas—diffuse, sinusoidal, and papillary—show the same distribution as that of pituitary adenomas without hemorrhage. The diffuse adenomas have the highest incidence of hemorrhage despite abundant vascularity in the sinusoidal type (8). Eosinophilic and basophilic adenomas were thought to have higher incidences of apoplexy; however, others found no such relationship (8, 21). Many authors have pointed out that the distribution of apoplexy was similar in the different histologic types of pituitary tumors (33). Among the functional adenomas, prolactinomas have the highest incidence of apoplexy (25) probably because this is the most frequent type of tumor (46). However, nonfunctioning and null-cell adenomas have

the highest incidence of apoplexy of all pituitary adenomas. Fraioli et al. (25) described 8 (61.5%) of 13 patients with pituitary apoplexy who had nonfunctioning adenomas, whereas Bills et al. (14) demonstrated that 54% of apoplectic pituitary adenomas are of null-cell type.

Most authors have found no correlation between the size of adenomas and the occurrence of hemorrhage (21) or could not correlate between the two because of absence of previous history in many patients with tumor (8). However, Fraioli et al. (25) found in their series a definite relationship between size and pituitary hemorrhage, with 84% of apoplectic tumors and asymptomatic pituitary hemorrhages being large adenomas with suprasellar extension.

Most cases of pituitary apoplexy show hemorrhage, necrosis, or both. However, necrosis and hemorrhage also occur in normal or nonadenomatous pituitary. As mentioned earlier, hemorrhage in a pituitary adenoma may also occur with no clinical syndrome of apoplexy. Also, asymptomatic pituitary hemorrhage has been found at surgery (8, 14, 25, 33).

Both recent and old hemorrhage may be found in surgically removed specimens. According to Peillon et al. (47), a definite sign of hemorrhage in tumor before surgery is the dissociation of the adenomatous parenchyma by partly lysed erythrocytes. Increase in tumor vascularization may be found (25) with a variable degree of hemorrhage, liquefaction and softening, corresponding to the rapidity and severity of the clinical course (30) (Fig. 21.1). Sometimes the coagulation type of necrosis is seen as ghost cells with no significant hemorrhage seen (Fig. 21.2). Occasionally, patients with the syndrome of pituitary apoplexy show no hemorrhage at surgery but xanthochromic fluid in the

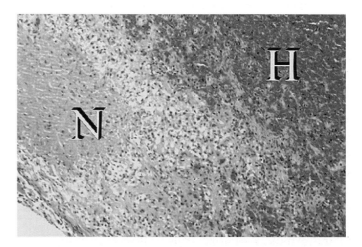

Figure 21.1. A specimen obtained from a patient presenting with pituitary apoplexy syndrome. The picture is hematoxylin and eosin stained, showing a hemorrhagic portion of the tumor (H) with adjacent necrosis (N) and scattered necrotic cells with pyknotic nuclei.

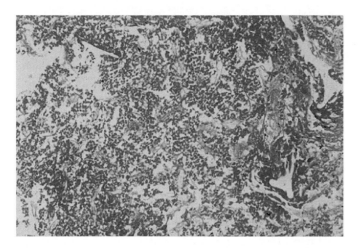

Figure 21.2. A hematoxylin and eosin stain of necrotic tissue obtained from an enlarged sella in a patient with a clinical history of pituitary apoplexy. Note the absence of nuclei, and what is left are residual (ghost) cells of a necrotic tumor.

tumor, empty sella, or solid tumor that is soft in consistency (8).

Long-term pathologic change in few cases of pituitary apoplexy showed replacement of the necrotic tissue by an intrasellar cyst, empty sella, or squamous metaplasia (15, 48–51). Chiasmal arachnoiditis has also been described (5, 21).

The cause of propensity for hemorrhage in pituitary adenomas is not well understood. Some have postulated that a rapid growth of tumor outstrips its blood supply, producing ischemic necrosis followed by hemorrhage (10, 52). Cardoso and Peterson (33) objected to this hypothesis based on the finding that the vessels supplying the pituitary adenoma originate from the inferior hypophyseal artery and that compression of the superior hypophyseal artery would lead to ischemia of adenohypophysis rather than hemorrhagic necrosis of adenoma; also, intentional occlusion of hypophyseal portal vessels in animals leads to ischemic infarction and not to hemorrhage of the adenohypophysis. Fraioli et al. (25) described a cluster of tumor cells bulging into vessel lumen with apparent disruption of endothelial lining in one of their cases of large invasive adenoma and so postulated direct invasion of vessel wall by the tumor and consequent vessel rupture. Findings of asymptomatic multiple hemorrhages in some tumors may indicate intrinsic tumor factors causing hemorrhage (25). Differences in the vasculature of pituitary adenoma and normal adenohypophysis may play a part in the hemorrhage in adenomas. The vessels in adenomas are variable in number and caliber (33). Electron microscopically, the normal adenohypophyseal capillary endothelium is richly fenestrated, whereas the endothelium of adenoma vessels shows incomplete maturation, poor fenestration, and, often, fragmentation with ruptured basal membranes (53, 54). Cholesterol embolus was observed by Sussman and Porro (55).

Most cases of pituitary apoplexy are not associated with any predisposing factors. However, pituitary apoplexy has been described in association with a variety of conditions, although the reason for most of these associations is not clear. The syndrome of pituitary apoplexy has also been described with other intracranial tumors (e.g., meningioma, malignant tumor, craniopharyngioma) (56, 57); intrasellar malignant teratoma (58); hypothalamic astrocytoma (59); and metastatic endometrial (60), prostate (61), and small cell carcinoma of the pituitary (62). Pituitary apoplexy has been observed following radiotherapy (9). Vessel proliferation with thickening and hyalinization of vessel wall occurs following radiotherapy (63, 64), but the association between radiotherapy and pituitary apoplexy has not been observed consistently (33). Apoplexy has been documented during procedures like angiography; following lumbar puncture and pneumoencephalography (33, 65, 66); during cardiac surgery (23, 67–69); during hemodialysis (70); following cholecystectomy (71); and following subtotal thyroidectomy in a case of acromegaly (72). Other conditions associated with pituitary apoplexy described in the literature include repetitive coughing secondary to respiratory infection (73); head trauma (74, 75); hyperestrone states, including pregnancy and estrogen administration causing apoplexy in a normal gland (76); anticoagulant states, including thrombocytopenia and administration of anticoagulants (77, 78); administration of isosorbide and chlorpromazine (79, 80); following dynamic testing of the pituitary using gonadotropin-releasing hormone or triple bolus test (81); bromocriptine therapy for pituitary adenoma (8, 70, 82); shortly after administration of leuprolide, a gonadotropin-releasing hormone analog, to treat prostate carcinoma in a patient who possibly had gonadotrophadenoma (83); 5 months after shock syndrome in a pituitary gland (84); secondary to dissection of internal carotid artery (85); and in pituitary abscess in a patient who had chronic lymphocytic leukemia associated with hypogammaglobulinemia (86). Infarction of normal pituitary has been described in diabetes (87) and apoplexy in adenomatous gland was reported in diabetic ketoacidosis (88, 89). Apoplectic syndrome secondary to narcotizing hypophysitis due to mycobacterial infection was reported by Leech et al. (90).

It is evident that a lot of speculation has been made about the possible pathophysiologic mechanisms leading to pituitary apoplexy. We know that hemorrhage alone is not sufficient to cause an apoplectic event. In addition, most full-blown apoplexies are associated with necrosis, which probably comes as a later phase of the initial hemorrhage. This is supported by the fact that early treatment of apoplexy may lead to recovery and improvement of pituitary functions (72). We hereby introduce a parameter that, if factored into the equation, may explain and account for a lot of the data relevant to the apoplectic event: this factor is *intrasellar pressure*. In a small sella with a competent diaphragma sellae and a small pituitary adenoma thriving to establish a larger size, its fragile neovascularization may result in a hemorrhage that can cause an acute increase in the *intrasellar pressure*, leading to vascular compression, ischemia, and necrosis of both the tumor and the normal pituitary gland. In the same fashion, a large pituitary macroadenoma growing through a wide diaphragma sellae may not cause significant symptoms, and the hemorrhage that occurs from the vascular tumor bed and the fragile neovascularity leads to a variable clinical presentation after a hemorrhagic event, depending on the extent of *intrasellar pressure* buildup. This accounts for the symptoms of headaches and occasional double vision seen in several patients with radiologic or surgical evidence of intratumoral hemorrhage, without the full-blown pituitary apoplexy clinical syndrome.

CLINICAL PRESENTATION

The most common presenting symptom of pituitary apoplexy is sudden onset of severe headache or acute exacerbation of previous headaches. The headache is usually associated with nausea and vomiting and is followed by symptoms related to the dysfunctions in the visual apparatus. The headache is usually described as retro-orbital, and it is apoplectic in its onset and similar to aneurysmal subarachnoid hemorrhage. It is thought to be caused by either stretching of the pain-sensitive dura of the sellar and parasellar skull base and/or spillage of blood into the subarachnoid space, resulting in meningeal irritation associated with neck stiffness and photophobia (10, 90–97).

Ocular paresis (78%) results from compression of the cavernous sinus, making cranial nerves III, IV, and VI vulnerable to compression (14, 98). If consciousness is maintained, diplopia is present. Of the cranial nerves, the oculomotor nerve is most commonly involved, resulting in a unilateral dilated pupil, ptosis, and a globe that is deviated inferiorly and laterally (98). Less commonly involved is cranial nerve IV (98). A fourth cranial nerve palsy typically manifests as vertical diplopia that worsens when the patient gazes in an opposite direction, tilts the head toward the direction of the hypertropic (affected) eye, or gazes downward. Sixth cranial nerve palsies are least common, perhaps because of the sheltered position of cranial nerve VI in the cavernous sinus (99). Defects produce horizontal diplopia, which results from inability to abduct the involved eye. By virtue of its existence in the cavernous sinus, trigeminal nerve involvement may produce facial pain or sensory loss (98). A Horner's syndrome may develop from damage to the sympathetic fibers (98). Visual acuity (52%) and visual field (64%) defects result from upward expansion of the tumor compressing the optic chiasm, optic tracts, or optic nerve (14, 98). The classic visual field defect from compression of the optic chiasm from below is a bitemporal superior quadrant defect; optic tract involvement from a "prefixed chiasm" is less common and results in a homonymous hem-

ianopia (100). Optic nerve compression from a "postfixed chiasm" is rare and may mimic optic neuritis, with pain on eye movement, monocular visual acuity, and a central scotoma on visual field testing (101). Hemispheric deficits may also develop, and vasospasm from subarachnoid blood may lead to stroke (98). Leakage of blood and necrotic tissue into the subarachnoid space may lead to meningismus and, in more severe cases, stupor and coma (98, 102). The meningismus is usually associated with photophobia, occasionally fever, and alteration in mental status. The cerebrospinal fluid is frequently marked by an increase in pleocytosis (even in the absence of hemorrhage) and an increase in the number of red blood cells and/or xanthochromia. The protein level is often elevated (73, 103–110).

When hypothalamic involvement occurs, patients may present with hypotension, fever, cardiac dysrhythmias, and other hypothalamic-related dysfunctions (10, 20, 48, 75, 77, 91, 111–115). The hemodynamic instability could be related to hypopituitarism and secondary adrenal insufficiency owing to absence of the adrenocorticotropic hormone.

Another less common presentation is hemiparesis, which has been attributed to cerebral ischemia as a result of occlusion of cerebral vessels by either tumor expansion or secondary vasospasm, as mentioned above. Cerebral ischemia could also explain why some patients present with speech difficulties and seizures (10, 15, 52, 116–122).

RADIOLOGIC STUDIES

The radiologic features of patients presenting with pituitary apoplexy are similar to those of patients with pituitary lesions in general. This aspect is well described in Chapter 8, Neuroradiologic Evaluation of Pituitary Disorders. In brief, use of computed tomography (CT) improved our ability to achieve an early and preoperative diagnosis of pituitary apoplexy. The hemorrhage is shown as a hyperdense area on the noncontrasted axial sections, usually associated with an enlarged sella and occasionally with erosion into the sphenoid sinus (Fig. 21.3). There may be extension of the hemorrhage into the suprasellar region and into the subarachnoid space. A more severe hemorrhage may extend into the ventricular system and occasionally into the brain tissue itself (4, 13, 16, 32, 123). A CT scan performed with contrast injection may or may not show an increased enhancement in the residual tumor tissue. When the apoplectic event is associated with necrosis, a noncontrasted CT scan shows a hypodense or isodense sellar mass, with enhancement of a surrounding ring when contrast is given (13, 117, 123).

MRI is the most sensitive test for evaluating lesions of the pituitary gland. Hemorrhage within the sella is isointense or slightly hypointense when checked on the T1-weighted images in the acute phase (within the first 3 to 5 days). On T2-weighted images, the blood is seen as hypointense. In the subacute phase, the blood becomes hyperin-

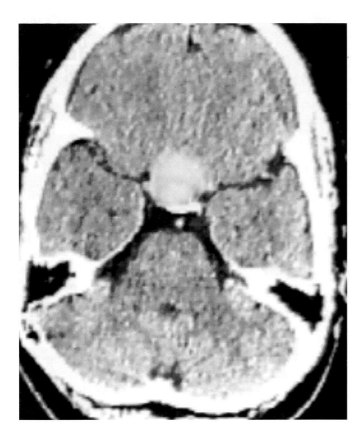

Figure 21.3. A CT scan showing a hyperdense suprasellar hemorrhagic lesion in a patient presenting with clinical syndrome of pituitary apoplexy.

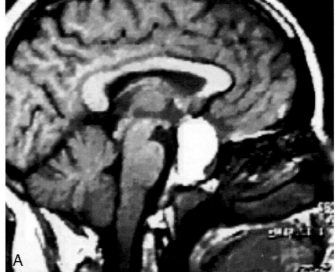

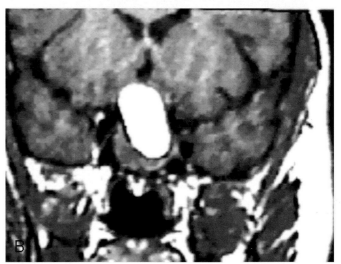

Figure 21.4. **A.** Sagittal T1-weighted MRI of the brain showing a hyperintense suprasellar mass extending to the third ventricular region in a patient presenting with pituitary apoplexy syndrome with significant visual impairment. Note the contrast between the hyperintense hemorrhagic component of the tumor and the isointense and hypointense tumor tissue located both anterior and posterior to the hemorrhagic component. **B.** Coronal MRI of the same patient showing the hyperintense hemorrhagic component of the tumor mass. The tumor component is the isotense portion shown on the inferior and lateral aspects of the mass.

tense on T1-weighted images (Fig. 21.4*A, B*) and starts changing and becomes isointense or hyperintense on T2-weighted images (93, 124–126). However, when cystic changes take place, the T1-weighted images vary, and the intensity is higher with a higher protein content of the intrasellar fluid. The T2-weighted images, conversely, are always hyperintense in the cystic areas. Hemorrhage in pituitary tumors may be visualized on the MRI without being seen on the CT scan even in the early days after the hemorrhage.

MANAGEMENT OF PITUITARY APOPLEXY

The management of patients with pituitary apoplexy should focus on two main aspects of their problem: (*a*) the associated endocrinopathy and (*b*) the acute neurologic deficits resulting from the tumor mass. Although many consider pituitary apoplexy to be an emergency, it should not be managed with a premature decision for surgical intervention in a medically unstable patient. The initial management should focus on the overall medical condition of the patient and should be guided by the clinical presentation. Patients who present in a comatose condition should first be stabilized, and the possible cause of their coma

analyzed, before surgical intervention is decided. However, in a patient who presents fully alert with rapidly progressive visual loss, emergency surgical intervention is indicated.

High-dose steroids are given to all patients at presentation because most patients presenting with apoplexy have hypopituitarism (127). Steroid administration is followed by immediate evaluation of all the pituitary hormones. Blood electrolyte levels and glucose levels are measured. Although diabetes insipidus is not commonly seen with pituitary apoplexy, it may transiently occur in a small percentage of patients (127). Intravenous fluids are administered, taking into consideration the hemodynamic status, the presence or absence of diabetes insipidus, and the possible presentation of some patients with the syndrome of inappropriate antidiuretic hormone secretion caused by affection of the hypothalamic–pituitary axis (26, 102).

Once the patient is medically stabilized, surgical decompression is planned. As mentioned above, visual loss or other neurologic deficits are factors that favor a more urgent intervention, within hours of presentation. Urgent surgical decompression does not seem to influence the outcome related to the extraocular cranial neuropathies (33, 73, 128–131). Results of some studies recommend early surgical intervention as part of the effort to save the severely compressed residual functioning normal gland. Arafah et al. (91) and Harrington et al. (100) reported recovery of pituitary function after urgent decompression for pituitary apoplexy. Although this is important knowledge to keep in mind, it should not be the reason for premature intervention in a medically unstable patient.

Because most patients with pituitary apoplexy present with pathologic evidence of necrosis in the gland and clinical evidence of hypopituitarism, the argument was made in several reports that spontaneous recovery of cranial neuropathies and adequate hormonal replacement is an indication to follow a conservative treatment plan without surgical intervention. Although this may be adequate in several patients, long-term follow-up of conservatively treated pituitary apoplexy may lead to either recurrent apoplexy or tumor recurrence, which can occur several years after the initial event (13, 97, 112, 119, 128, 132–143). The above reasons are why surgical intervention should always be considered. Surgery increases the chances of recovery of residual normal gland tissue and prevents the possibility of recurrence of the tumor and/or the apoplectic event.

OUTCOME AND PROGNOSIS

A lethal outcome as a result of pituitary apoplexy is becoming a less frequent event. The previously reported higher mortality is predominantly caused by the delay in diagnosis and the lack of adequate medical therapy, especially hormonal replacement therapy with steroids (12, 51, 89, 117, 122, 134, 144, 145). The recent technologic advances in radiologic studies and the availability of adequate medical and hormonal therapy has dramatically improved on the mortality and morbidity associated with pituitary apoplexy (4, 17, 26). In most patients, the extraocular cranial neuropathy resolves with time. The timing of surgical intervention did not seem to affect the course of recovery. Patients operated on within 72 hours of onset of symptoms had a similar outcome as those operated on afterward (14). Although several reports indicated a similar long-term outcome of vision in both the early and the delayed surgical groups (83, 146–148), other reports indicated a more favorable outcome of the visual field deficits in the group that was operated on early. Hence, unless patients present with a rapidly progressive visual or neurologic deficit, urgent but not emergent intervention is recommended (14). In a way similar to other pituitary adenomas, the extent of recovery of the visual deficits depends on the extent of the deficit prior to surgical intervention and on its chronicity. McFadzean et al. (20) suggested that even the duration of symptoms and the severity of the visual deficits did not affect the extent of visual recovery, and they put more weight on the status of the optic disc as an indicator of the potential for visual recovery.

REFERENCES

1. Glick RP, Tiesi JA. Subacute pituitary apoloexy: clinical and magnetic resonance imaging characteristics. Neurosurgery 1990;27:214.
2. Jeffcoate WJ, Birch CR. Apoplexy in small pituitary tumours. J Neurol Neurosurg Psychiatry 1986;49:1077.
3. Kaplan B, Day AL, Quisling R, et al. Hemorrhage into pituitary adenomas. Surg Neurol 1983;20:280.
4. Onesti ST, Wisniewski T, Post KD. Clinical versus subclinical pituitary apoplexy: presentation, surgical management, and outcome in 21 patients. Neurosurgery 1990;26:980.
5. Symon L, Mohanty S. Hemorrhage in pituitary tumours. Acta Neurochir 1982;65:41.
6. Tsitsopoulos P, Andrew J, Harrison MJP. Pituitary apoplexy and hemorrhage into adenomas. Postgrad Med J 1986;62:623.
7. Uihlein A, Balfour WM, Donovan PF. Acute hemorrhage into pituitary adenomas. J Neurosurg 1957;14:140.
8. Wakai S, Fukushima T, Teramoto A, et al. Pituitary apoplexy: its incidence and clinical significance. J Neurosurg 1981;55:187.
9. Weisberg LA. Pituitary apoplexy: association of degenerative change in pituitary adenoma with radiotherapy and detection by cerebral computed tomography. Am J Med 1977;63:109.
10. Brougham M, Heusner AP, Adams RD. Acute degenerative changes in adenomas of the pituitary body with special reference to pituitary apoplexy. J Neurosurg 1950;7:421.
11. Henderson WR. The pituitary adenomata: a follow-up study of the surgical results in 338 cases (Dr. Harvey Cushing's series). Br J Surg 1939;26:811.
12. Dingley LA. Sudden death due to a tumour of the pituitary gland. Lancet 1932;2:183.
13. Ahmed M, Rifai A, Al-Jerf M, et al. Classical pituitary apoplexy presentation and a follow-up of 13 patients. Horm Res 1989;31:125.
14. Bills DC, Meyer FBM, Davis DH, et al. A retrospective analysis of pituitary apoplexy. Presented at the LX Annual Meeting of the American Association of Neurological Surgeons, San Francisco, CA, 1992.
15. Dastur HM, Pandya SK. Haemorrhagic adenomas of the pituitary gland: their clinical and radiological presentations and treatment. Neurology (India) 1971;19:4.
16. Ebersold MJ, Laws ER Jr, Scheithauer BW, et al. Pituitary apoplexy treated by transsphenoidal surgery: a clinicopathological and immunocytochemical study. J Neurosurg 1983;58:315.
17. Laws ER Jr, Ebersold MJ. Pituitary apoplexy: an endocrine emergency. World J Surg 1982;6:686.
18. Liu SS, White W, Sonntag VKH. Pituitary apoplexy: a 10 year review (abstract). Presented at the Rocky Mountain Neurological Society Meeting, Lake Tahoe, NV, 1988.
19. Lunardi P, Rizzo A, Missori P, et al. Pituitary apoplexy in an acromegalic woman operated on during pregnancy by transsphenoidal approach. Int J Gynecol Obstet 1991;34:71.

20. McFadzean RM, Doyle D, Rampling R, et al. Pituitary apoplexy and its effect on vision. Neurosurgery 1991;29:669.
21. Mohanty S, Tandon PN, Banjeri AK, et al. Haemorrhage into pituitary adenomas. J Neurol Neurosurg Psychiatry 1977;40:987.
22. Muller W, Pia HW. Zur Klinik und Atiologic der Massenblutungen in Hypophysenadenoma. Deutsche Zeitschrift Nervenheilkunde 1953;170:S326.
23. Peck V, Lieberman A, Pinto R, et al. Pituitary apoplexy following open-heart surgery. N Y State J Med 1980;80:641.
24. Rachlin JR, Wilson CB, Hoyt W, et al. Pituitary apoplexy: a review of surgical results in 32 cases. Presented at the annual meeting of the American Association of Neurological Surgeons, Washington, DC, 1989.
25. Fraioli B, Esposito V, Palma L, Cantore G. Hemorrhagic pituitary adenomas: clinicopathological features and surgical treatment. Neurosurgery 1990;27:741.
26. Hickstein DD, Chandler WF, Marshall JCL. The spectrum of pituitary adenoma hemorrhage. West J Med 1986;144:433.
27. Muller-Jensen A, Ludecke D. Clinical aspects of spontaneous necrosis of pituitary tumors (pituitary apoplexy). J Neurol 1981;224:267.
28. White W, Liu SS. Pituitary apoplexy. In: Carter LP, Spetzler RF, eds. Neurovascular Surgery. New York: McGraw-Hill, 1995:497–519.
29. Bailey P. Pathological report of a case of akromegaly, with especial reference to the lesions in the hypophysis cerebri and in the thyroid gland; and a case of hemorrhage into the pituitary. Philadelphia Med J 1898;1:789.
30. Rovit RL, Fein JM. Pituitary apoplexy: a review and reappraisal. J Neurosurg 1972;37:280.
31. Alhajje A, Lambert M, Crabbe J. Pituitary apoplexy in an acromegalic patient during bromocriptine therapy. J Neurosurg 1985;63:288.
32. L'Huillier F, Combes C, Martin N, et al. MRI in the diagnosis of so-called pituitary apoplexy: seven cases. J Neuroradiol 1989;16:221.
33. Cardoso ER, Peterson EW. Pituitary apoplexy: a review. Neurosurgery 1984;14:363.
34. Baker HL Jr. The angiographic delineation of sellar and parasellar masses. Radiology 1972;104:67.
35. Numaguchi Y, Kishikawa T, Ikeda J, et al. Neuroradiological manifestations of suprasellar pituitary adenomas, meningiomas and craniopharyngiomas. Neuroradiology 1981;21:67.
36. Powell DF, Baker HL Jr, Laws ER Jr. The primary angiographic findings in pituitary adenomas. Radiology 1974;110:589.
37. Westberg G, Ross RJ. The vascular supply of chromophobe adenomas. Acta Radiol (Stockh) 19676:475.
38. Krisht AF, Barrow DL, Barnett D, et al. The microsurgical anatomy of the superior hypophyseal artery. Neurosurgery 1994;35:899–903.
39. Krisht AF, Barnett D, Barrow D, et al. The microsurgical anatomy of the blood supply to the intracavernous cranial nerves. Neurosurgery 1994;34:899–903.
40. Ouaknine GE, Hardy J. Microsurgical anatomy of the pituitary gland (hypophysis cerebri) and the sellar region, 3: the meninges. Clin Anat 1988;1:33.
41. Renn Wh, Rhoton AL Jr. Microsurgical anatomy of the sellar region. J Neurosurg 1975;43:288.
42. Gorczyca W, Hardy J. Microadenomas of the human pituitary and their vascularization. Neurosurgery 1988;22:1.
43. Bleibtreu L. Ein fall von Akromegalic (Zerstorung der Hypophysis durch Blutung). Munch Med Wochenschr 1905;52:2079–2080.
44. Markowitz S, Sherman L, Kolodny HD, et al. Acute pituitary vascular accident (pituitary apoplexy). Med Clin North Am 1981;65:105–116.
45. Rolih CA, Ober KP. Pituitary apoplexy. Endocrinol Metab Clin North Am 1993;22:291–302.
46. Kovacs K, Horvath E. Pathology of pituitary adenomas. In: Givens J, ed. Hormone-Secreting Pituitary Tumors. Chicago: Year Book Medical Publishing, 1982:97.
47. Peillon F, Vila-Porcile E, Olivier L, et al. L'action des oestrogenes sur les adenomes hypophysaires chez l'homme: documents histopathologiques en microscopie optique et electronique et apport de l'experimentation. Ann Endocrinol 1970;31:259–270.
48. Pelkonen R, Kuusisto A, Salmi J, et al. Pituitary function after pituitary apoplexy. Am J Med 1978;65:773–778.
49. Weinberger LM, Adler FH, Grant FC. Primary pituitary adenoma and the syndrome of the cavernous sinus: a clinical and anatomic study. Arch Ophthalmol 1940;24:1197–1236.
50. Gutin PH, Cushard WG Jr, Wilson CB. Cushing's disease with pituitary apoplexy leading to hypopituitarism, empty sella and spontaneous fracture of the dorsum sellae. J Neurosurg 1979;51:866–869.
51. Kepes JJ, Sayler J, Hiszczynskyj R. Squamous metaplasia following necrosis of the adenohypophysis and of a chromophobe adenoma of the pituitary. Virchows Arch [Pathol Anat] 1982;395:69–76.
52. Epstein S, Pimstone BL, de Villiers JC, et al. Pituitary apoplexy in five patients with pituitary tumors. BMJ 1971;2:267.
53. Hirano A, Tomiyasu U, Zimmerman HM. The fine structure of blood vessels in chromophobe adenoma. Acta Neuropathol 1972;22:200–207.
54. Landolt AM. Ultrastructure of human sella tumors: correlations of clinical findings and morphology. Acta Neurochir Suppl (Wien) 1975;22:1–167.
55. Sussman EB, Porro RS. Pituitary apoplexy: the role of atheromatous emboli. Stroke 1974;5:318–323.
56. Lloyd MH, Belchetz PE. The clinical features and management of pituitary apoplexy. Postgrad Med J 1977;53:82–85.
57. Lopez IA. Pituitary apoplexy. J Oslo City Hosp 1970;20:17–27.
58. Fernandez-Real JM, Villabona C, Acebes JJ, et al. Pituitary apoplexy into nonadenomatous tissue: case report and review. Am J Med Sci 1995;310:68–70.
59. Glew WB. Simulated pituitary apoplexy: report of an unusual case due to hemorrhage into hypothalamic astrocytoma. Ann Ophthalmol 1977;9:139–142.
60. Lieschke GJ, Tress B, Chambers D. Endometrial adenocarcinoma presenting as pituitary apoplexy. Aust N Z J Med 1990;20:81–84.
61. Anderson DF, Afshar F, Toma N. Metastatic prostatic adenocarcinoma presenting as complete ophthalmoplegia from pituitary apoplexy. Br J Ophthalmol 1994;78:315–316.
62. Chandra V, McDonald LW, Anderson RJ. Metastatic small cell carcinoma of the lung presenting as pituitary apoplexy and Cushing's syndrome. J Neurooncol 1984;2:59–66.
63. Chang CH, Pool JL. The radiotherapy of pituitary chromophobe adenomas. Radiology 1967;89:1005–1016.
64. Doron Y, Schwartz A. The significance of the angiographic demonstration of tumour vessels in pituitary neoplasms. Br J Radiol 1965;38:356–359.
65. Reichenthal E, Manor RS, Shalit MN. Pituitary apoplexy during carotid angiography. Acta Neurochir (Wien) 1980;54:251–255.
66. Perpetuo FO. Pituitary apoplexy after pneumoencephalogram. Arq Neuropsiquiatr 1976;34:298–301.
67. Cooper DM, Bazaral MG, Furlan AJ, et al. Pituitary apoplexy: a complication of cardiac surgery. Ann Thorac Surg 1986;41:547.
68. Kovacs K, Yao J. Pituitary necrosis following major heart surgery. Z Kardiol 1975;64:52.
69. Absalom M, Rogers KH, Moulton RJ, et al. Pituitary apoplexy after coronary artery surgery. Anesth Analg 1993;76:648–649.
70. Mohr G, Hardy J. Hemorrhage, necrosis and apoplexy in pituitary adenomas. Surg Neurol 1982;18:181–189.
71. Yahagi N, Nishikawa A, Matsui S, et al. Pituitary apoplexy following cholecystectomy. Anaesthesia 1992;47:234–236.
72. Kato K, Nobori M, Miyauchi Y, et al. Pituitary apoplexy after subtotal thyroidectomy in an acromegalic patient with a large goiter. Intern Med 1996;35:472–477.
73. Dawson BH, Kothandram P. Acute massive infarction of pituitary adenomas: a study of five patients. J Neurosurg 1972;37:275.
74. Holness RO, Ogundimu FA, Langille RA. Pituitary apoplexy following closed head trauma. J Neurosurg 1983;59:677.
75. Tamasawa N, Kurahashi K, Baba T, et al. Spontaneous remission of acromegaly after pituitary apoplexy following head trauma. J Endocrinol Invest 1987;11:429.
76. Nagulesparan M, Roper J. Hemorrhage into the anterior pituitary during pregnancy after induction of ovulation with clomiphene: a case report. Br J Obstet Gynaecol 1978;85:153.
77. Nourizadeh AR, Pitts FW. Hemorrhage into pituitary adenoma during anticoagulant therapy. JAMA 1965;193:623.
78. Tiwary CM. Thrombocytopenia and pituitary necrosis associated with rubella [letter]. Proc R Soc Med 1962;62:908.
79. Bevan JS, Oza AM, Burke CW. Pituitary apoplexy following isorbide administration [letter]. J Neurol Neurosurg Psychiatry 1987;50:636.

80. Silverman VE, Boyd AE, McCrary JA, et al. Pituitary apoplexy following chlorpromazine stimulation. Arch Intern Med 1978; 138:1738.

81. Arafah BM, Taylor HC, Salazar R, et al. Apoplexy of a pituitary adenoma after dynamic testing with gonadotropin-releasing hormone. Am J Med 1989;87:103.

82. Yamaji T, Ishibashi M, Kosaka K, et al. Pituitary apoplexy in acromegaly during bromocriptine therapy. Acta Endocrinol Copenh 1981;98:171–177.

83. Morsi A, Jamal S, Silverberg JD. Pituitary apoplexy after leuprolide administration for carcinoma of the prostate. Clin Endocrinol (Oxf) 1996;44:121–124.

84. Mauerhoff T, Leveque P, Lambert AE. Spontaneous pituitary apoplexy with transient panhypopituitarism and diabetes insipidus. Acta Clin Belg 1991;46:30–36.

85. Provenzale JM, Hacein-Bey L, Taveras JM. Internal carotid artery dissection associated with pituitary apoplexy: MR findings. J Comput Assist Tomogr 1995;19:150–152.

86. Kingdon CC, Sidhu PS, Cohen J. Pituitary apoplexy secondary to an underlying abscess. J Infect 1996;33:53–55.

87. Brennan CF, Malone RGS, Weaver JA. Pituitary necrosis in diabetes mellitus. Lancet 1956;2:12.

88. Lufkin EG, Reagan TJ, Doan DH, et al. Acute cerebral dysfunction in diabetic ketoacidosis: survival followed by panhypopituitarism. Metabolism 1977;26:363.

89. Gurling KJ. Diabetic coma and pituitary necrosis in an acromegalic patient: a case report. Diabetes 1955;4:138–140.

90. Leech RW, Goodkin D, Obert G, et al. Etiology of pituitary apoplexy: review and case presentation. Clin Neuropathol 1987;6: 7–11.

91. Arafah BM, Harrington JF, Madhoun ZT, et al. Improvement of pituitary function after surgical decompression for pituitary tumor apoplexy. J Clin Endocrinol Metab 1990;71:323.

92. Jefferson M, Rosenthal FD. Spontaneous necrosis in pituitary tumours (pituitary apoplexy). Lancet 1959;1:342.

93. Kyle CA, Laster RA, Burton EM, et al. Subacute pituitary apoplexy: MR and CT appearance. J Comput Assist Tomogr 1990; 14:40.

94. Meadows SP. Unusual clinical features and modes of presentation in pituitary adenoma, including pituitary apoplexy. In: Smith JL, ed. Neuroophthalmology, IV. St. Louis: Mosby, 1968:178–189.

95. Rogolosi RS, Schwartz E, Glick SM. Occurrence of growth-hormone deficiency in acromegaly as a result of pituitary apoplexy. N Engl J Med 1968;279:362.

96. Ruiz AE, Mazzaferri EL, Skillman TG. Silent reversal of acromegaly: pituitary apoplexy resulting in panhypopituitarism. Ohio State Med J 1969;65:1017.

97. Sachdev Y, Garg VK, Gopal K, et al. Pituitary apoplexy (spontaneous pituitary necrosis). Postgrad Med J 1981;57:289.

98. Reid RL, Quigley ME, Yen SSC. Pituitary apoplexy: a review. Arch Neurol 1985;42:712.

99. Wray SH. Neurol-ophthalmologic manifestations of pituitary and parasellar lesions. Clin Neurosurg 1976;34:86–117.

100. Harrington JF Jr, Selman WR, Arafah N. Improvement in pituitary function after urgent surgical decompression on patients with pituitary apoplexy. Presented at the annual meeting of the American Association of Neurological Surgeons, Washington, DC, 1989.

101. Peterson P, Christiansen KH, Lindholm J. Acute monocular disturbances mimicking optic neuritis in pituitary apoplexy. Acta Neurol Scand 1988;78:101.

102. Conomy JP, Ferguson JH, Brodkey JS, et al. Spontaneous infarction in pituitary tumors: neurologic and therapeutic aspects. Neurology 1975;25:580.

103. Cooperman D, Malarkey WB. Pituitary apoplexy. Heart Lung 1978;7:450.

104. Fong LP, Fabinyi GCA. Ophthalmic manifestations of pituitary apoplexy. Med J Aust 1985;142:142.

105. Goodman JM, Gilson M, Shapiro B. Pituitary apoplexy: a cause of sudden blindness. J Indiana State Med Assoc 1973;66:320.

106. Guarnaschelli JJ, Talalla A. Pituitary apoplexy: a case report. Bull Los Angeles Neurol Sci 1972;37:12.

107. Keane JR. Pituitary apoplexy presenting with epistaxis. J Clin Neurol Ophthalmol 1984;4:7.

108. List CF, Williams JR, Balyeat GW. Vascular lesions in pituitary adenomas. J Neurosurg 1952;9:177.

109. Powell DF, Baker HL Jr, Laws ER Jr. The primary angiographix findings in pituitary adenomas. Radiology 1974;110:589.

110. Winer JB, Plant G. Stuttering pituitary apoplexy resembling meningitis. J Neurol Neurosurg Psychiatry 1990;53:440.

111. Lacomis D, Johnson LN, Mamourian AC. Magnetic resonance imaging in pituitary apoplexy. Arch Ophthalmol 1988;106:207.

112. Sachdev Y, Evered DC, Hall R. Spontaneous pituitary necromas. BMJ 1976;1:942.

113. David NJ, Gargano FP, Glaser JS. Pituitary apoplexy in clinical perspective. In: Glaser TS, Smith JL, eds. Neuroophthalmology, VII. St. Louis: Mosby, 1975:140–165.

114. Jolley FL, Mabon RL. Pituitary apoplexy. J Med Assoc Ga 1958; 47:75.

115. Zervas NT, Mendelson G. Treatment of acute haemorrhage of pituitary tumours. Lancet 1975;1:604.

116. Chen S-T, Chen S-D, Ryu S-J, et al. Pituitary apoplexy with intracerebral hemorrhage simulating rupture of an anterior cerebral artery aneurysm. Surg Neurol 1988;29:322.

117. Challa VR, Richards F II, Davis CH II. Intracentricular hemorrhage from pituitary apoplexy. Surg Neurol 1981;16:360.

118. Clark JDA, Freer CEL, Wheatley T. Case report: pituitary apoplexy: an unusual cause of stroke. Clin Radiol 1987;38:75.

119. Itoyama Y, Goto S, Miura M, et al. Intracranial arterial vasospasm associated with pituitary apoplexy after head trauma: case report. Neurol Med Chir (Tokyo) 1990;30:350.

120. Lewin IG, Mohan J, Norman PF, et al. Pituitary apoplexy. BMJ 1988;297:1526.

121. Slaven ML, Budabin M. Pituitary apoplexy associated with cardiac surgery. Am J Ophthalmol 1984;98:291.

122. Walton JN. Subarachnoid haemorrhage of unusual aetiology. Neurology 1953;3:517.

123. Post MJ, David NJ, Glaser JS, et al. Pituitary apoplexy: diagnosis by computed tomography. Radiology 1980;134:665.

124. Armstrong MR, Douek M, Schellinger D, et al. Regression of pituitary macroadenoma after pituitary apoplexy: CT and MR studies. J Comput Assist Tomogr 1991;15:832.

125. Gomori J, Grossman RI, Goldberg H, et al. Intracranial hematomas: imaging by high-field MR. Radiology 1985;157:87.

126. Ostrov SG, Quencer RM, Hoffman JC, et al. Hemorrhage within pituitary adenomas: how often associated with pituitary apoplexy syndrome? AJR Am J Roentgenol 1989;153:153.

127. Veldhuis JD, Hammond JM. Endocrine function after spontaneous infarction of the human pituitary: report, review and reappraisal. Endocr Rev 1980;1:100.

128. Bjerre P, Lindholm J, Videbaek H. The spontaneous course of pituitary adenomas and occurrence of an empty sella in untreated acromegaly. J Clin Endocrinol Metab 1986;6:287.

129. Krueger EG, Unger SM, Roswit B. Hemorrhage into pituitary adenoma with spontaneous recovery an reossification of the sella turcica. Neurology 1960;10:691.

130. Majchrak H, Wencel T, Dragan T, et al. Acute hemorrhage into pituitary adenoma with SAH and anterior cerebral artery occlusion: case report. J Neurosurg 1983;58:771.

131. Taylor AL, Finster JL, Raskin P, et al. Pituitary apoplexy in acromegaly. J Clin Endocrinol Metab 1968;28:1784.

132. Bjerre P, Gyldensted C, Riishede J, et al. The empty sella and pituitary adenomas: a theory on the causal relationship. Acta Neurol Scand 1982;66:82.

133. Bjerre P, Lindholm J. Pituitary apoplexy with sterile meningitis. Acta Neurol Scand 1986;74:304.

134. Coxon RV. A case of haemorrhage into a pituitary tumour stimulating rupture of an intracranial aneurysm. Guys Hosp Rep 1943;92: 89.

135. Domingue JN, Wing SD, Wilson CB. Coexisting pituitary adenomas and partially empty sellas. J Neurosurg 1978;48:23.

136. Jellinek EH. Empty sella syndrome and pituitary apoplexy (letter). Lancet 1988;1:1053.

137. Jones NS, Finer N. Pituitary infarction and development of the empty sella syndrome after gastrointestinal haemorrhage. BMJ 1984;289:661.

138. Montalban J, Sumulla J, Fernandez JL, et al. Empty sella syndrome and pituitary apoplexy (letter). Lancet 1988;1:774.

139. Sadun AA. Acromegaly after pituitary apoplexy (letter). JAMA 1987;257:2034.

140. Tsementzis SA, Loizou LA. Pituitary apoplexy. Neurochirurgia (Stuttg) 1986;29:90.

141. Werner PL, Shalt JH, Kukreja SC, et al. Recurrence of acromegaly after pituitary apoplexy. JAMA 1982;247:2816.

142. Shenkin HA. Relief of amblyopia in pituitary apoplexy by prompt surgical intervention. JAMA 1955;17:1622.

143. Yuanxiu L. Blindness due to sellar region tumor-caused apoplexy: visual field investigation helps the diagnosis. Ophthalmologica 1980;181:203.

144. Kalyanaraman UP. Clinically asymptomatic pituitary adenoma manifesting as pituitary apoplexy and fatal third-ventricular hemorrhage. Hum Pathol 1982;13:1141.

145. Patel DV, Shields MC. Intraventricular hemorrhage in pituitary apoplexy: case report. J Comput Assist Tomogr 1979;3:829.

146. Cardoso ER, Peterson EW. Pituitary apoplexy and vasospasm. Surg Neurol 1983;20:391.

147. Kosary IZ, Braham J, Tadmor R, et al. Trans-sphenoidal surgical approach in pituitary apoplexy. Neurochirurgia (Stuttg) 1976;19:55.

148. Reutens DC, Edis RH. Pituitary apoplexy presenting as aseptic meningitis without visual loss and ophthalmoplegia. Aust N Z J Med 1990;20:590.

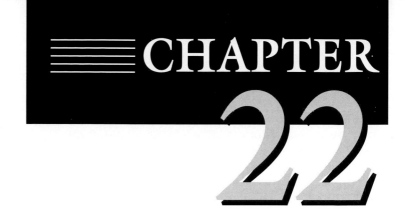

CHAPTER 22

Craniopharyngiomas

Ugur Türe and Ali F. Krisht

INTRODUCTION

Craniopharyngiomas account for 2.5 to 4.0% of all brain tumors (1). They are considered benign tumors and are thought to arise from squamous cell rests that are located along the pituitary stalk. This is why most of these tumors are adherent to the pituitary stalk and commonly present with diabetes insipidus (DI). If they arise from the proximal portion of the pituitary stalk, they are capable of infiltrating the region of the tuber cinereum and into the hypothalamic region. Craniopharyngiomas commonly compress the optic chiasm and result in visual deficits. They may grow to giant sizes, with significant suprasellar extension causing compression of the foramina of Monroe, resulting in secondary hydrocephalus.

Although craniopharyngiomas can become symptomatic at any age, they are commonly seen in children between 5 and 15 years of age. Matson (2) reported that craniopharyngiomas account for 9% of nonglial tumors in children. Several other series (3–14) found no significant predilection for a particular age, and the occurrence of craniopharyngiomas was the same in both sexes.

Although considered benign in nature, the anatomic location of craniopharyngiomas and their proximity to complex neural and vascular structures of the suprasellar and parasellar region renders their surgical removal hazardous, which could be associated with significant morbidity. However, advances in pharmacoendocrinology and refine-ments in microsurgical techniques have had a significantly positive impact on the management of craniopharyngiomas (15–29). Their total excision is possible in 70% of cases. Postoperative morbidity and long-term outcome have significantly improved with the availability of adequate hormonal replacement therapy. In this chapter, we discuss the pathophysiologic features, clinical presentation, diagnosis, and different aspects of the management of craniopharyngiomas and their outcome.

PATHOPHYSIOLOGIC FEATURES AND ORIGIN

In 1899, Mott and Barnett (30) were the first to suggest that craniopharyngiomas arise from the lining cells of Rathke's pouch. The histologic features of these tumors were later characterized by Erdheim (31) in 1904, who postulated that these tumors probably arise from embryonic squamous cell rests that originate from the incomplete involution of the hypophyseal–pharyngeal duct. This was later supported by findings that craniopharyngiomas can arise along the path of development of Rathke's pouch, from the pharyngeal wall all the way to the floor of the sella as well as within and above the sellar level (32). The accepted hypothesis that craniopharyngiomas have an embryologic background does not fully explain the variable behavior of these tumors. Evidence against this hypothesis comes from studies that showed the presence of cell rests resembling tissue of the hypophyseal duct in only 3% of neonates (33). In addition, there is no proof of neoplastic transformation of these rests. Results of several studies (34, 35) suggest the presence of differences in the histologic pattern seen in craniopharyngiomas in adults and in children. They suggest that these differences could be related to differences in their origin, with childhood craniopharyngiomas being related to embryonic rest cells and the adult variant of craniopharyngiomas being related to metaplasia of pituitary cells.

The histopathologic features in most craniopharyngiomas are characteristic. They have a central network of epithelial cells and an external layer of high columnar epithelium with variable amounts of polygonal cells. The epithelial cellular layers are supported by connective tissue stroma of mesodermal origin. They are usually associated with keratinlike material that is thought to be a result of liquefaction secondary to regressive changes in the epithelial cell layer (31). Degeneration of the central stroma may lead to formation of cysts. The cyst wall may be thin and membranous or thick and hard. Calcification is common in craniopharyngiomas. Cysts are encountered in up to 50% of craniopharyngiomas occurring in adults and in most of those occurring in children (11).

Craniopharyngiomas can induce a severe reaction of astrogliosis in the surrounding brain tissue that is particularly significant around the papillary tumor projections within the hypothalamus. The presence of this glial reaction around the tumor has been the subject of difference in opinion among surgeons regarding its role in surgical resection. Some authors suggest that the presence of this layer predisposes to hypothalamic damage during surgical resection when traction is applied on the craniopharyngioma tissue. Other authors suggest that the peritumor glial reaction provides a "glial envelope," which can help dissect the craniopharyngioma from the surrounding brain safely (36, 37). Although some craniopharyngiomas have a more aggressive course, there is no evidence of malignant degeneration at the histopathologic level. Liszozak et al. (38) reported on anaplastic changes seen on microscopy of what was considered to be aggressive craniopharyngiomas. The tendency of the aggressive craniopharyngiomas to produce cysts has been suggested by results of tissue culture studies done by Cobb and Wright (39). A detailed account of the pathologic aspects of craniopharyngiomas is given in Chapter 7.

ANATOMY AND LOCALIZATION

Craniopharyngiomas are thought to arise from different levels of the pituitary stalk. This is reflected in the differences in their growth pattern. Those arising from the distal portion of the pituitary stalk tend to grow within the sella turcica (Fig. 22.1). Those arising from the pituitary stalk are typically midline in location and grow within the intraarachnoid space. These craniopharyngiomas are usually lo-

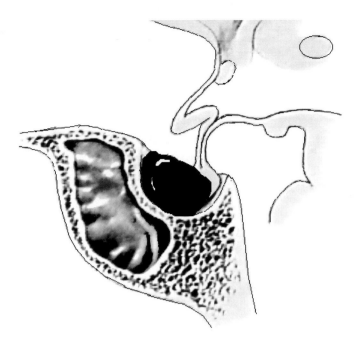

Figure 22.1. Diagram showing the location of a tumor arising from the distal portion of the pituitary stalk and contained within the sella.

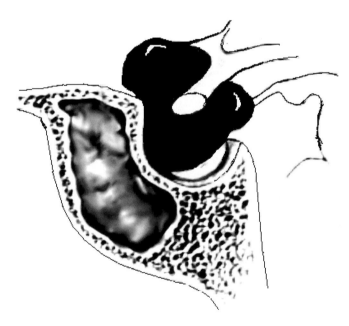

Figure 22.2. Tumor arising from the middle portion of the pituitary stalk and compressing the pituitary gland and filling the suprasellar region with compression of the optic apparatus.

cated in the suprasellar compartment, or they extend superiorly into the third ventricular region (Fig. 22.2). Those arising from the proximal portion of the pituitary stalk may grow predominantly within the third ventricular region, impinging on the foramina of Monroe and causing secondary hydrocephalus (Fig. 22.3). Remarkable individual variations are seen in the consistency of these tumors. They can be predominantly solid or predominantly cystic and

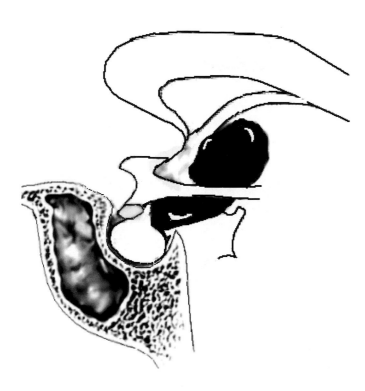

Figure 22.3. Diagram showing a tumor arising from the proximal portion of the pituitary stalk and extending behind the optic chiasm into the third ventricular region. Notice the bulging lamina terminalis.

enlarge to a giant size. They can also be mixed with solid areas of calcification. Their location in relationship to the optic apparatus depends on the location of the optic chiasm as well as the tumor size. When the chiasm is prefixed in position, the craniopharyngiomas tend to fill the entire suprasellar region, and the optic apparatus is pushed anteriorly and superiorly in this case. In postfixed chiasms, the tumor grows within the suprasellar region and between the two optic nerves, which are usually pushed laterally.

Although craniopharyngiomas grow in an expansile fashion, they tend to become adherent to the major arteries of the anterior circulation and their branches. This tendency limits the safe total resection of these tumors and forces the surgeon to leave tumor behind in some cases (8–10). Carmel et al. (3–7) reviewed the incompletely removed craniopharyngiomas and found that attachment to major arteries of the Circle of Willis is a more common cause for their subtotal resection compared with their adherence to the hypothalamus or the optic apparatus. It was suggested that the tumor may induce a mesenchymal reaction in the vessel wall, resulting in tougher and more adherent attachment to the blood vessels than the attachment seen with proliferation in the reactive hypothalamic tissue (3–7). The blood supply of craniopharyngiomas is thought to be derived from small vertebral feeders of the anterior Circle of Willis (35). When they are located within the sella, craniopharyngiomas derive their blood supply from small branches arising from the cavernous sinus portion of the

internal carotid artery. They rarely recruit blood supply from the posterior circulation unless the blood supply to the third ventricular and hypothalamic region is used by the tumor (3–7).

CLINICAL PRESENTATION

Growth failure occurs in 93% of children diagnosed with craniopharyngiomas. In adults, a history of decreased sexual drive was reported in 88% of men, and menstrual cycle irregularities were reported in 82% of women (2). Because craniopharyngiomas grow as extra-axial tumors, they may achieve a large size before they become symptomatic. Adding to the delay of their diagnosis is the fact that children often tolerate a significant degree of visual loss before they exhibit behavioral changes that can arouse the suspicion of their parents or teachers (3–7). In adults, the above-mentioned presenting symptoms could be caused by several other unrelated factors, which contributes to the delay in their diagnosis. In addition, when visual impairment occurs, macular vision is usually spared, similar to the case of pituitary adenomas, and this further adds to the delay in diagnosis. In the series of Carmel et al. (3–7), 80% of the adult patients complained of visual loss by the time they presented. Headaches are common in patients with craniopharyngiomas, and they are encountered in more than 50% of the patients. In adults, large tumors may present with psychiatric symptoms or cognitive deficits especially related to a memory loss. In such patients, hypersomnia, depression, apathy, and incontinence may be seen. Kahn and co-workers (34) reported that 3 of the 12 patients with mental changes presented with symptoms characteristic of Korsakoff's syndrome.

Endocrinopathies are common, but they are commonly missed in patients with craniopharyngiomas. More than half of the younger patients present with short stature, and most have a growth rate that is less than the expected average for their age. Hyperprolactinemia caused by stalk compression or direct compression of the hypothalamus is not infrequent. Patients with hyperprolactinemia typically present with galactorrhea and amenorrhea. Hypothalamic compression may occasionally lead to precocious puberty owing to loss of the hypothalamic inhibition exerted on the gonadotropin-releasing hormones in the preadolescent phase. Precocious puberty may not fully manifest if hypopituitarism develops secondary to compression of the pituitary gland. DI is more commonly seen in the preoperative period than the case with pituitary adenomas and other parasellar tumors. DI is also a more common occurrence in the postoperative period.

DIAGNOSIS
Endocrinologic Evaluation

A thorough endocrinologic evaluation is indicated in all patients with craniopharyngiomas. This evaluation should include the basic hormonal studies evaluating the anterior pituitary functions (levels of morning serum cortisol, 17-hydroxy corticosteroid, urinary free cortisol, growth hormone, prolactin, T4, luteinizing hormone, follicle-stimulating hormone, testosterone in men and estradiol in women, thyroid-stimulating hormone, and adrenocorticotropic hormone). Evaluation of blood electrolytes, including serum and urine osmolalities, is done to rule out DI. If there is a high suspicion of DI, then a 12-hour water deprivation test is indicated.

Ophthalmologic Evaluation

After obtaining a detailed history of the current illness, both a complete neurologic examination and a neuro-ophthalmologic evaluation are essential in all patients. Yasargil et al. (12–14) indicated that serious and destructive effects on the optic pathways occur in two-thirds of patients with craniopharyngiomas. Those destructive effects were more pronounced in children. The ophthalmologic evaluation is also essential for postoperative follow-up in case of recurrence and/or progression of the tumor.

Radiologic Evaluation

The introduction of computed tomography and magnetic resonance imaging has contributed significantly to the management of craniopharyngiomas and other lesions located in the sellar and parasellar regions (40). Calcification is best seen on computed tomographic images. Cystic components of the tumor have a low density on computed tomographic scans similar to cerebrospinal fluid density (Fig. 22.4). Magnetic resonance imaging allows a better

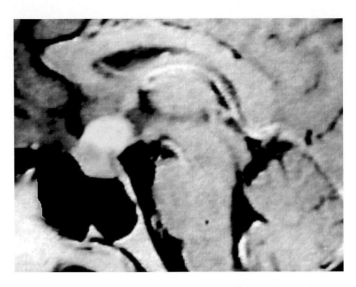

Figure 22.5. Sagittal T1-weighted magnetic resonance image showing a tumor arising from the pituitary fossa with suprasellar extension. The suprasellar component is predominantly cystic, and it is shown as hyperintense on the T1-weighted images.

delineation of the different densities within craniopharyngiomas. The sagittal and coronal reconstructions help provide information regarding tumor size, site, and consistency and its relationship to the surrounding structures (Fig. 22.5). Although magnetic resonance imaging provides significant radiologic details, it continues to fail in defining the degree of adherence or adhesiveness between the normal brain tissue and the pathologic craniopharyngioma tissue (41). Further refinement in neuroimaging that can help in such a task will provide beneficial information that can further help with the surgical planning, especially in determining the more appropriate surgical approach in different cases. Magnetic resonance angiography is recommended to identify the exact location of the blood vessels in the vicinity of the tumor and their relationship to the tumor. A detailed account of the radiologic features of craniopharyngiomas is given in Chapter 8.

SURGICAL MANAGEMENT

Depending on the location and size of the tumor, different surgical approaches can be used for craniopharyngiomas. The decision-making plan is based on the criteria of tumor size and location. Intrasellar tumors with no suprasellar extensions are best approached through the transnasal–transsphenoidal route (42–46). The detailed account of this approach is described in Chapter 26. Larger tumors with suprasellar extensions or smaller tumors located in the suprasellar region are approached using the pterional–transsylvian approach. A detailed account of the pterional–transsylvian approach is given in Chapter 27. Tumors located in the suprasellar compartment with significant extension into the third ventricular region are approached with the plan of a combined pterional and

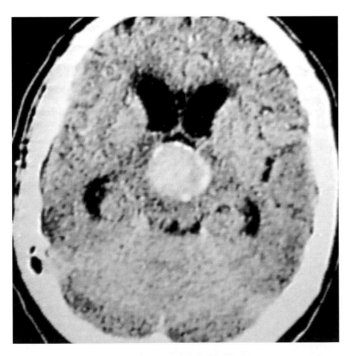

Figure 22.4. Axial computed tomographic scan of a large suprasellar craniopharyngioma with evidence of calcification and obstruction of the foramina of Monroe leading to secondary hydrocephalus.

transcallosal–transventricular approach as described by Ya-sargil et al. (12–14). If the tumor is purely intraventricular, the transcallosal–transventricular route is sufficient.

Pterional Approach

The pterional approach provides wide-angle access to the suprasellar region using the natural planes along the sphenoid wing. It carries the advantage of accessing the basal cistern for immediate drainage of spinal fluid and brain relaxation and avoidance of brain retraction. We recommend using an extended pterional approach with a medial burr hole located at the midline frontal region (Fig. 22.6). This extends the craniotomy medially and provides a wider angle to move the surgical microscope from the lateral transsylvian position to the most medial subfrontal position. The extended pterional approach adds the advantage of accessing the tumor through different anatomic windows, such as the space between the optic nerves, the opticocarotid space, and the space between the carotid artery and the oculomotor nerve.

After dissecting the arachnoid of the basal cisterns and opening the sylvian fissure (described in Chapter 27), the internal carotid artery bifurcation is identified and the A1 segment of the anterior cerebral artery is visualized in its proximal portion and its relationship to the tumor is defined. Cystic components of the tumor are first drained to decompress the tumor and release the pressure on the stretched optic nerves. If the tumor is solid in consistency,

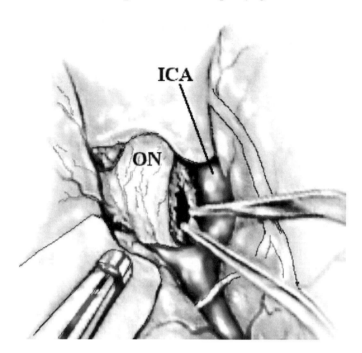

Figure 22.7.   Diagram showing tumor removal using the opticocarotid space. Notice the wide angle of exposure after opening the sylvian fissure and showing the carotid bifurcation. *ON*, optic nerve; *ICA*, internal carotid artery.

drilling of the optic canal and cutting the overlying dural fibrous band (falciform ligament) allows immediate decompression of the nerve and provides more room for its mobilization until the bulk of the tumor is excised. The tumor is then approached through the above-mentioned windows starting between the optic nerves, with attention to preserve the blood supply of the chiasm. Tumor removal is done with the suction and the pituitary rongeurs. Occasionally, the ultrasonic aspirator is needed. In hard and calcified tumors, the tumor should be broken into smaller fragments and removed in pieces to avoid inadvertent injury of the crossing small perforators supplying blood to the pituitary stalk and the chiasm. Further removal of the tumor can be done through the opticocarotid window (Fig. 22.7). Attention should be given while using this window to several small and stretched branches arising from the medial wall of the carotid artery and supplying the optic chiasm and hypothalamus. Prior debulking of the tumor will improve blood flow in these vessels and help identify them. These are the same branches that belong to the superior hypophyseal artery complex and provide blood supply to the optic chiasm, optic nerve, and pituitary stalk (47). The preservation of these vessels is essential to prevent postoperative ischemic visual deficits.

A third window that can be used is the window of the lamina terminalis. It is usually stretched and enlarged by the tumor and can safely be opened to remove the posterior portion of the tumor impinging on the hypothalamus and the third ventricular floor. The tumor capsule should carefully be dissected. It is usually attached to the surrounding

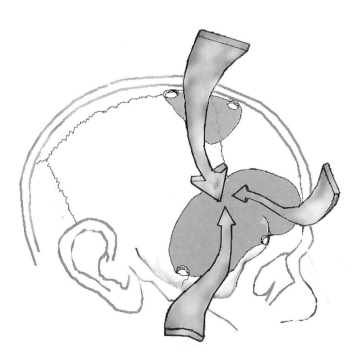

Figure 22.6.   Diagram showing the extended pterional craniotomy. The *inferior arrows* indicate the subfrontal and pterional transsylvian routes used to access the tumor in the suprasellar region. The *superiorly located arrow* shows the transcallosal-transforaminal route that is occasionally used to access tumors with third ventricular extensions.

gliotic brain in the hypothalamic region. If the tumor is adherent to the brain tissue, no heroic attempts should be tried, and the rest of the tumor may need to be removed through a different approach, such as the trans-callosal–transventricular one. In some cases, the pituitary stalk can be visualized and saved. Should this task prove difficult, there is no advantage to trying to save the stalk and leave residual tumor at the risk of a higher chance of recurrence.

Transcallosal-Transforaminal Approach

The addition of the transcallosal–transforaminal approach is used in tumors with significant intraventricular extension (48–52). When this approach is planned as part of a combined approach with a pterional–transsylvian one, a bicoronal or a curvilinear incision extending beyond the midline is used (53). A triangular-shaped craniotomy is done with two burr holes along the midline at the level of the coronal suture. The posterior midline burr hole is made behind the coronal suture, and the anterior midline burr hole is made 3 to 5 cm anterior to the coronal suture (Fig. 22.6). After opening the dura, the interhemispheric fissure is dissected under the microscope and magnification. The pericallosal arteries are identified as well as the corpus callosum. Cotton balls are applied to the most anterior and posterior aspects of the established interhemispheric space, and the corpus callosum is divided longitudinally at the level of the coronal suture (Fig. 22.8). After entry into the lateral ventricular cavity, the tumor is dissected through the

enlarged foramen of Monroe. The septum pellucidum can be opened to approach the tumor from the contralateral foramen of Monroe. Retraction of the forniceal system is avoided. The tumor is then debulked beginning at its central portion and moving, in a stepwise fashion, outward. This allows better identification of the surrounding capsule, which can be dissected from the surrounding adherent gliotic brain layer. The dissection of the capsule is done in an outward-to-inward fashion to avoid lateral diversion of the dissection, which may lead to injury of the lateral ventricular wall and hypothalamus. Occasionally, removal of the tumor leads to the interpeduncular fossa, in which visualization of the basilar artery and its branches is important to avoid their injury.

When the tumor is located purely in the third ventricular compartment, the transcallosal–transforaminal approach is usually sufficient. In tumors involving the suprasellar region and extending into the ventricular cavity, the combined approach is used, starting with the pterional one. Starting with the pterional approach has the advantage of achieving brain relaxation by opening the basal cisterns and also rendering the inferior portion of the tumor mobile after dissecting it from the optic apparatus and the anterior cerebral artery complex and its branches. The transcallosal approach is then used to complete the tumor resection. The tumor bed is reinspected again through the pterional approach for any residual tumor in the retrochiasmatic space. Hemostasis is then established, and the wound is closed afterward (14).

Results of several reports indicate that subtotal or partial resection of craniopharyngiomas is never a satisfactory treatment and leads to a high recurrence rate over time (3–7, 36, 37). Subtotal removal alone led to recurrence-free survival in less than 10% of patients reported by Sung and coworkers (11) during a 10-year period. Occasionally, craniopharyngiomas exhibit no significant growth after partial resection, with long-term symptom-free survival (53). Although no growth of partially resected craniopharyngiomas has been encountered, it is by no means the norm with these tumors. The greatest majority of subtotally removed tumors recur within 3 years of resection. High correlation is seen between the extent of resection and tumor-free survival time.

Total removal of craniopharyngiomas is possible in up to 70% of patients (2–14, 36, 37, 54–56). These series reported excellent results, with zero mortalities in some series (13). The mortality rates in large series have been reported to be between 5 and 10% (2). The opinion regarding the extent of resection continues to be a source of controversy. It is divided between recommendations for aggressive attempts at total removal and recommendations of subtotal resection followed by other treatment modalities such as radiation, topical chemotherapy, and cyst aspiration.

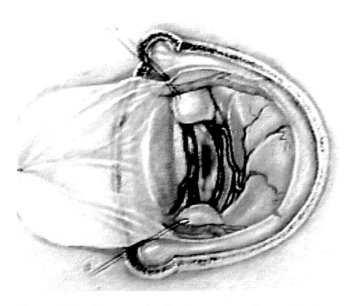

Figure 22.8. Diagram showing the exposure through the transcallosal approach with the window in the corpus callosum made at the level of the coronal suture between the anterior cerebral artery branches.

OTHER TREATMENT MODALITIES

Radiation Therapy

Craniopharyngiomas are considered radiosensitive tumors. Results of early reports by Carpenter and coworkers (57) indicated significant improvement in outcome after radiation therapy of craniopharyngioma cases. There was good control of tumor growth, especially in terms of cyst formation. They suggested a role for radiation therapy in damaging the lining epithelium of craniopharyngioma that was doubted by other authors (8–10). Later reports showed good outcomes after subtotal tumor removal and irradiation (58–62). As a result, several studies afterward indicated the beneficial effects of radiation therapy in increasing survival and prolonging the recurrence-free interval (11, 54, 58–60, 63). Some of the studies showed that the survival rates of patients treated with surgery and radiotherapy were better than those of patients treated with surgery alone, with a significant improvement in the recurrence-free survival interval (11). The term "radical subtotal removal" was introduced in a study by Baskin and Wilson (64) in 1986 in which the patients were radiated after subtotal aggressive resection of tumor. They reported a 91% remission rate and a low operative mortality of 3%. It has become clear that a more radical surgical removal prior to radiation contributes to longer survival and higher recurrence-free rates. This was further reinforced by results of a study done by Shapiro and coworkers (65) in which they showed the benefit of radical subtotal removal followed by radiation therapy to be superior to simple biopsy or cyst drainage followed by radiation.

Intracystic Radiation Therapy

The radioisotopes most commonly installed in the cystic portions of craniopharyngiomas are potassium-32, colloidal gold-198, and colloidal yttrium-91 (66–68). The protocols using intracystic radioisotopes necessitate accurate assessment of the cyst volume to calculate the amount of the radioactive substance to be injected into the cyst. Radiotherapists have different opinions about the amount of the radioactive substance needed for treatment of such cysts. This is complicated by the fact that different cysts may have different wall thicknesses that may cause variable penetration of the radiation into the surrounding brain tissue. Some studies suggested that delivering 2000 rad to the cyst wall would be adequate (16, 69). As more experience was gained with intracystic radiotherapy, the indications to its applications have become more defined. Intracystic radiotherapy is thought to be beneficial in large-volume cystic components of tumors but not in solid tumors or tumors with calcified walls (69). Disagreement exists regarding the method of delivery and installation of the radioisotopes, with proponents of the stereotactic techniques and proponents of direct placement of catheters in the cyst cavity. Although some centers use intracystic isotope therapy as the primary treatment of craniopharyngiomas, the availability of other more effective and safe treatment modalities suggests that their use should be restricted to large-volume recurrent cysts that are considered inoperable.

It is of interest to mention that several reports suggested using cyst aspiration as a temporary treatment in young children until an age is reached at which radiation therapy can be given safely. This is done by inserting an Ommaya reservoir connected through a burr hole to the cystic portion of the tumor. Interval aspiration of the cyst is guided by radiologic studies and clinical symptoms. Radiation is later given as mentioned above.

LONG-TERM OUTCOME

The introduction of magnetic resonance imaging and the recent advances in microsurgical techniques have had a significant favorable impact on the outcome of patients with craniopharyngiomas. The chances of achieving radical resection of these tumors is best in the primary occasion of surgery. Yasargil et al. reported good outcomes in 82% of adults and 75% of children who had a primary radical surgical resection and more than an average of 12.8 years follow-up (13). If the radical surgery was secondarily done after a previous subtotal resection, the rate of tumor control and good outcome decreased to 38.5% in adults and 3.6% in children. The overall good results achieved from radical surgical resection in both the primary and secondary radical surgical operations were 70.3%. The recurrence rate in the primarily operated group was 9.8% in children and 10.0% in adults, with an overall 10.0% recurrence rate (12–14). Compared with other reports in which subtotal resection was combined with radiation therapy, the results of radical surgery alone were better. Patients treated primarily with radiation have a 25% recurrence rate, and those treated with a combined partial surgical resection and radiation have a 26% recurrence rate (59, 60, 70). Other studies indicated the same points of higher recurrence rate when partial resection combined with radiotherapy was compared with radical total resection (70).

In tumors with such complexity, the optimum treatment is best provided by an experienced team of coworkers. Surgery of craniopharyngiomas should be done by surgeons experienced with lesions in the sellar, parasellar, and suprasellar areas so that results as good as 70 to 80% rates of radical surgical resection can be achieved. In the same sitting, those 20 to 30% left with residual tumors are handled by an experienced team of radiation oncologists providing a comprehensive plan that can be individualized to the best of each case.

REFERENCES

1. Kernohan JW. Tumors of congenital origin. In: Minckler J, ed. Pathology of the Nervous System. New York: McGraw-Hill, 1971:1927–1937.
2. Matson DD, Crigler JF Jr. Management of craniopharyngioma in childhood. J Neurosurg 1969;30:377–390.
3. Carmel PW. Tumours of the third ventricle. Acta Neurochir (Wien) 1985;75:136–146.
4. Carmel PW. Craniopharyngiomas. In: Wilkins RH, Rengachary SS, eds. Neurosurgery. New York: McGraw-Hill, 1996:1389–1400.
5. Carmel PW. Radical removal of craniopharyngioma, 1971–1991. In: Broggi G, ed. Craniopharyngioma: Surgical Treatment. New York: Springer-Verlag, 1995.
6. Carmel PW. Transcranial approaches for craniopharyngioma. In: Apuzzo M, ed. Brain Surgery: Complication Avoidance and Management. New York: Churchhill Livingstone, 1992:339–354.
7. Carmel PW, Autunes JL, Chang CH. Craniopharyngiomas in children. Neurosurgery 1982;11:382–389.
8. Hoffman HJ. Comment on paper by Patterson RH Jr, Danylevitch A. Neurosurgery 1980;7:116–117.
9. Hoffman HJ, da Silva M. Craniopharyngioma. In: Little JR, Awad IA, eds. Re-operative Neurosurgery. Baltimore: Williams & Wilkins, 1992:95–104.
10. Hoffman HJ, da Silva M, Humphreys RP, et al. Aggressive surgical management of craniopharyngiomas in children. J Neurosurg 1992;76:47–52.
11. Sung DI, Chang CH, Harisiadis L, et al. Treatment results of craniopharyngiomas. Cancer 1981;47:847–852.
12. Yasargil MG. Microneurosurgery. Stuttgart: Georg Thieme Verlag, 1996;IVB:29–68, 205–223, 313–338.
13. Yasargil MG, Curcic M, Kiss M, et al. Total removal of craniopharyngiomas: approaches and long term results in 144 patients. J Neurosurg 1990;73:3–11.
14. Yasargil MG, Ture U, Roth P. Combined approaches. In: Apuzzo MLC, ed. Surgery of Third Ventricle. 2nd ed. Baltimore: Williams & Wilkins, 1998.
15. Al-Mefty O, Hassounah M, Weaver P, et al. Microsurgery for giant craniopharyngiomas in children. Neurosurgery 1985;17585–595.
16. Antunes JL, Muraszku K, Quest DO, et al. Surgical strategies in the management of tumours of the anterior third ventricle. In: Brock M, ed. Modern Neurosurgery. Berlin: Springer-Verlag, 1982.
17. Apuzzo MLJ, Chikovani OK, Gott PS, et al. Trancallosal interfornical approaches for lesions affecting the third ventricle: surgical considerations and consequences. Neurosurgery 1982;10:547–554.
18. Apuzzo MLJ, Levy ML, Tung H. Surgical strategies and technical methodologies in optimal management of craniopharyngioma and masses affecting the third ventricle chamber. Acta Neurochir Suppl (Wien) 1991;53:77–88.
19. Apuzzo MLJ, Litofsky NS. Surgery in and around the anterior third ventricle. In: Apuzzo MLJ, ed. Brain Surgery. New York: Churchill Livingstone, 1993;1:541–579.
20. Banna M. Review article craniopharyngioma: based on 160 cases. Br J Radiol 1976;49:206–223.
21. Banna M. Craniopharyngioma in adults. Surg Neurol 1973;1:202–204.
22. Banna M, Hoare RD, Stanley P, et al. Craniopharyngioma in children. J Pediatr 1973;83:781–785.
23. Choux M, Lena G, Genitori L. Craniopharyngioma in children. Neurochirurgie 1991;37:1–174.
24. Dandy WE. Benign tumors in the third ventricle of the brain: diagnosis and treatment. Springfield, IL: Charles C. Thomas, 1933.
25. Dandy WE. Diagnosis, localization, and removal of tumors of the third ventricle. Bull Johns Hopkins Hosp 1922;33:188–189.
26. Garcia-Uria J. Surgical experience with craniopharyngioma in adults. Surg Neurol 1978;9:11–14.
27. Konovalov AN. Technique and strategies of direct surgical management of craniopharyngioma. In: Apuzzo MLJ, ed. Surgery of the Third Ventricle. Baltimore: Williams & Wilkins, 1987:542–553.
28. Symon L, Sprich W. Radical excision of craniopharyngioma: results in 20 patients. J Neurosurg 1985;62:174–181.
29. Symon L, Pell MF, Habib AH. Radical excision of craniopharyngioma by the temporal route: a review of fifty patients. Br J Neurosurg 1991;5:539–549.
30. Mott FW, Barnett JOW. Three cases of tumor of the third ventricle. Arch Neurol (London) 1899;1:417–440.
31. Erdheim J. Ueber Hypophysengangsgeshwulste and Hirncholesteatome. Sitzungsber Akad Wiss (Wien) 1904;113:537–726.
32. Podoshin I, Rolan L, Altman NM, et al. "Pharyngeal" craniopharyngioma. J Laryngol Otol 1970;84:93–99.
33. Goldberg GM, Eshbaugh DE. Squamous cell rests of the pituitary gland as related to the origin of craniopharyngiomas: a study of their presence in the newborn and infants up to age four. Arch Pathol Lab Med 1960;70:293–299.
34. Kahn EA, Gosch HH, Seeger JF, et al. Forty-five years experience with the craniopharyngiomas. Surg Neurol 1973;1:5–12.
35. Petito CK, De Girolami U, Earle KM. Craniopharyngiomas: a clinical and pathological review. Cancer 1976;37:1944–1952.
36. Sweet WH. Craniopharyngiomas (with a note on Rathke's cleft cysts). In: Schmidek HH, ed. Operative Neurosurgical Techniques. Orlando: Grune & Stratton, 1988:349.
37. Sweet WH. Craniopharyngiomas: a summary of recent data. In: Schmidek HH, Sweet WH (eds): Operative Neurosurgical Techniques. Philadelphia: WB Saunders, 1995;1:381–389.
38. Liszozak T, Richardson EP, Phillips JP, et al. Morphological, biochemical, ultrastructural, tissue culture and clinical observations of typical and aggressive craniopharyngiomas. Acta Neuropathol (Berlin) 1978;43:191–203.
39. Cobb JP, Wright JC. Studies on a craniopharyngioma in tissue culture: growth characteristics and alterations produced following exposure to two radiomimetic agents. J Neuropathol Exp Neurol 1959;18:563–568.
40. Naidich TP, Pinto RS, Kushner MJ, et al. Evaluation of sellar and parasellar masses by computed tomography. Radiology 1976;120:91–99.
41. Pusey E, Kortman KE, Flannigan BD, et al. MR of craniopharyngiomas: tumor delineation and characterization. AJNR Am J Neuroradiol 1987;8:439–444.
42. Laws ER. Transsphenoidal microsurgery in the management of craniopharyngioma. J Neurosurg 1980;52:661–666.
43. Laws ER. Transsphenoidal removal of craniopharyngioma. Pediatr Neurosurg 1994;21(suppl 1):57–63.
44. Ciric IS, Cozzens JW. Craniopharyngiomas: transsphenoidal method of approach: for the virtuose only? Clin Neurosurg 1980;27:169–187.
45. Fahlbusch R, Honegger J, Buchfelder M. Transsphenoidal microsurgery for craniopharyngioma. In: Schmidek HH, Sweet WH, eds. Operative Neurosurgical Techniques. Philadelphia: WB Saunders, 1995;1:371–379.
46. Honegger J, Buchfelder M, Fahlbusch R, et al. Transsphenoidal microsurgery for craniopharyngioma. Surg Neurol 1992;37:189–196.
47. Krisht AF, Barrow DL, Barnett D, et al. The microsurgical anatomy of the superior hypophyseal artery. Neurosurgery 1994;35:899–903.
48. Kjos BO, Brant-Zawadzki M, Kucharezyk W, et al. Cystic intracranial lesions: magnetic resonance imaging. Radiology 1985;155:363–369.
49. Long DM, Chou SN. Transcallosal removal of craniopharyngiomas within the third ventricle. J Neurosurg 1973;39:563–567.
50. Shucart WA, Stein BM. Transcallosal approach to the anterior ventricular system. Neurosurgery 1978;3:339–343.
51. Shucart W. Anterior transcallosal and transcortical approaches. In Apuzzo MLJ, ed. Surgery of the Third Ventricle. Baltimore: Williams & Wilkins, 1987:303–325.
52. Woiciechowsky C, Vogel S, Lehmann R, et al. Transcallosal removal of lesions affecting the third ventricle: an anatomic and clinical study. Neurosurgery 1995;36:117–123.
53. Bartlett JR. Craniopharyngiomas: an analysis of some aspects of symptomatology, radiology and histology. Brain 1971;94:725–732.
54. Hoff JT, Patterson RH Jr. Craniopharyngiomas in children and adults. J Neurosurg 1972;36:2922–2932.
55. Samii M, Bini W. Surgical treatment of craniopharyngioma. Zentralbl Neurochir 1991;52:17–23.

56. Samii M, Samii A. Surgical management of craniopharyngiomas in childhood: a rational approach to treatment. J Neurosurg 1979;50:617–623.

57. Carpenter RC, Chamberlin GW, Frazier CH. The treatment of hypophyseal stalk tumors by evacuation and irradiation. AJR Am J Roentgenol 1937;38:162–177.

58. Kramer S. Craniopharyngioma: the best treatment is conservative surgery and postoperative radiation therapy. In: Morley TP, ed. Current Controversies in Neurosurgery. Philadelphia: WB Saunders, 1976:336–343.

59. Kramer S, McKissock W, Concannon JP. Craniopharyngiomas: treatment by combined surgery and radiation therapy. J Neurosurg 1961;18:217–226.

60. Kramer S, Southard M, Mansfield CM. Radiotherapy in the management of craniopharyngiomas: further experiences and late results. AJR Am J Roentgenol 1968;103:44–52.

61. Fischer EG, Welch K, Shillito J, et al. Craniopharyngiomas in children: long-term effects of conservative surgical procedures combined with radiation therapy. J Neurosurg 1990;73: 534–540.

62. Laws ER. Conservative surgery and radiation for childhood craniopharyngiomas. J Neurosurg 1991;74:1025–1026.

63. Richmond IL, Wara WM, Wilson CB. Role of radiation therapy in management of craniopharyngiomas in children. Neurosurgery 1980;6:513–517.

64. Baskin DS, Wilson CB. Surgical management of craniopharyngiomas: a review of 74 cases. J Neurosurg 1986;65:22–27.

65. Shapiro K, Till K, Grant DN. Craniopharyngiomas in childhood: a rational approach to treatment. J Neurosurg 1979;50:617–623.

66. van den Berge JH, Blaauw G, Breeman WAP, et al. Intracavitary brachytherapy of cystic craniopharyngiomas. J Neurosurg 1992;77: 545–550.

67. Kodama T, Matsukado Y, Uemura S. Intracapsular irradiation therapy of craniopharyngiomas with radioactive gold: indication and follow-up results. Neurol Med Chir (Tokyo) 1981;21:49–58.

68. Kobayashi T, Kageyama N, Ohara K. Internal irradiation for cystic craniopharyngioma. J Neurosurg 1981;55:896–903.

69. Julow J, Lanyi F, Hajda M, et al. The radiotherapy of cystic craniopharyngioma with intracystic instillation of 90 Y silicate colloid. Acta Neurochir 1985;74:94–99.

70. Rajan B, Ashley S, Gorman C, et al. Craniopharyngioma: long-term results following limited surgery and radiotherapy. Radiother Oncol 1993;26:1–10.

Pediatric Pituitary Tumors

*Frederick A. Boop, Charles Teo,
and Kate Pihoker*

EPIDEMIOLOGY AND INCIDENCE

Although the suprasellar region is the second most common site for intracranial tumors during childhood, the finding of a pituitary adenoma in a child is distinctly uncommon. Even in large pediatric referral centers, less than five pediatric pituitary tumors per year can be expected, with most of those occurring in postpubertal children. In the series of Haddad et al. (1), only 2.8% of the pituitary tumors seen at their institution had symptomatic onset before 17 years of age. Given this, familiarity with the presentation of pituitary adenomas in children is critical if they are to be diagnosed and treated before the ravages of the disease are allowed to run their course. By way of review, note that incidental lesions of the pituitary gland are common. In the autopsy study of Teramoto et al. (2), of 1000 pituitary glands studied, 18% were found to harbor one or more lesions. Rathke's cleft cysts were the most common centrally located lesions, and adenomas were the most common eccentric lesions (2). Given this, the authors note that incidental lesions may not require treatment. This chapter concerns those pituitary adenomas that are symptomatic.

Symptomatic pituitary tumors account for no more than 1 to 2% of all childhood brain tumors (3). Hoffman (4) reviewed the experience at the Hospital for Sick Children in Toronto and found that during a 25-year period, 1.2% of their supratentorial tumors were pituitary adenomas. Gold (5) reviewed the epidemiologic features of these tumors and estimated an annual incidence of 0.1 per million. As with adult pituitary tumors, childhood pituitary tumors seem to be more common in females than in males, with the ratio varying depending on which hormones they secrete. In the largest reported series of childhood pituitary adenomas, Mindermann and Wilson (6) report female: male ratios of 4.5:1 for prolactinomas, but a 1:2 male predominance for growth hormone (GH)–secreting tumors. This male predominance for GH tumors was not reproduced, however, in the study by Partington et al. (3).

Reported series of pediatric pituitary tumors differ also in their definition of "pediatric." In some series, this includes children undergoing surgery before 16 or 18 years of age. Others include patients up to 20 years old. Still others include adults whose symptoms began historically in childhood. Despite these inconsistencies, results of all studies suggest that pituitary tumors rarely occur in children prior to puberty.

PATHOPHYSIOLOGY

Given the compact and complex anatomy of the suprasellar region, the presentation of the child with a pitui-

315

tary adenoma is related to its secretory status and its proximity to the pituitary gland, the optic chiasm, the third ventricle, and the hypothalamus. Tumors that are hormonally active will typically present as microadenomas because of the clinical manifestations of the hormonal excess. Tumors that are hormonally inactive will present with symptoms of mass effect, and tumors that hemorrhage will present with an abrupt, severe headache, mental status changes, or sudden visual deterioration (pituitary apoplexy).

The most common functional pituitary adenoma of childhood in the large series published by Mindermann and Wilson (6) is the prolactinoma. Note, however, that most of the children with this tumor were either pubertal or postpubertal. The most common presenting symptom was amenorrhea, occurring in 25% of the females. In 80% of them, primary amenorrhea was the initial diagnosis. Males tended to present later and had statistically larger tumors and higher prolactin (PRL) levels at the time of diagnosis.

In the prepubescent group of Mindermann and Wilson's study (6), the most common pituitary tumor was the adrenocorticotropic hormone (ACTH)–secreting tumor. This was the most common pituitary tumor of childhood in the study by Partington et al. (3), accounting for 44.4% of cases. Most of these tumors presented in childhood with typical symptoms of Cushing's disease: truncal obesity, increased facial soft tissue deposition, growth delay, and headache. In the study by Partington et al. (3), six children presented with Nelson's syndrome. Five of the six were prepubertal at the time of diagnosis.

In both of these large series, the third most common functional pituitary tumor of childhood was the GH-secreting adenoma. Even so, GH-secreting adenomas are exceedingly rare prior to puberty. Among these patients, 58.4% presented with accelerated growth or gigantism. Gigantism has been reported in association with these tumors in children as young as 2½ years of age (7). In postpubertal children whose growth plates have reached maturity, gigantism does not occur. In such patients, the typical appearance of acromegalic features is expected and was seen in one-third of the patients with GH-secreting tumors in the series of Mindermann and Wilson (6).

On rare occasions, children with pituitary tumors may present with precocious puberty. In one instance, this was associated with a prolactinoma that also secreted luteinizing hormone (LH) (8). Equally relegated to case reports is the thyroid-stimulating hormone–secreting adenoma that presents as multinodular toxic goiter (Graves' disease) (9).

The Mayo Clinic Group has pointed out that one of the most striking features of pediatric pituitary adenomas is the large proportion of them that are plurihormonal. In the study by Scheithauer et al. (10), 10% of pediatric pituitary tumors secreted more than one hormone, with 50% of GH-secreting adenomas being plurihormonal. Partington et al. (3) pointed out that this is significantly more common than that of adult pituitary tumors.

Finally, there is ongoing debate in the neurosurgical literature as to whether pituitary tumors in children are more biologically aggressive than in adults (11). This is refuted by Dyer et al.'s study (12), which documents a 13% incidence of invasiveness for pediatric pituitary tumors compared with a 35% incidence for adult pituitary tumors and suggests that the increased incidence of invasion in the adult tumors is related to the duration of the disease rather than to the biology of the neoplasm. Mindermann and Wilson's review (6) documents no correlation between invasiveness and recurrence. The likelihood of recurrence has been reviewed by Fisher et al. (11), whose limited data suggest that children with pituitary adenomas require more frequent radiographic and biochemical follow-up than do adults. In his series, most recurrences were noted less than 2 years following initial surgery. In Mindermann and Wilson's series (6), ACTH-secreting adenomas had the highest likelihood of recurrence at 17%. The review by Kane et al. (13) documents a 65% long-term cure rate with surgery alone; therefore, the preponderance of evidence suggests that pediatric pituitary tumors are no more aggressive than their adult counterparts.

HORMONAL AND METABOLIC CHANGES ASSOCIATED WITH PEDIATRIC PITUITARY TUMORS

Tumors of the pituitary gland can produce hormonal changes by interfering with the normal regulation of pituitary hormone secretion, as is also seen with craniopharyngiomas, or by secreting pituitary hormones themselves. Tumor location, tumor size, and patient age affect clinical manifestations, including associated endocrinopathies.

GH deficiency is the most common endocrine abnormality observed in children with pituitary tumors. Diabetes insipidus (DI) is the second most common endocrinopathy observed in association with pituitary lesions, resulting from tumor infiltration of the pituitary stalk or from mass effect causing inadequate secretion of antidiuretic hormone. Rarely, the syndrome of inappropriate antidiuretic hormone secretion (SIADH) is observed on presentation.

Central hypothyroidism is another endocrinopathy that may be present at the time of tumor diagnosis. Often its signs and symptoms are subtle, and it is diagnosed only through measurement of the child's serum thyroxine concentration. Of note is the occasional occurrence of a pituitary tumor in association with primary hypothyroidism. This has been observed in children as well as adults. Along with classic features of hypothyroidism (e.g., lethargy, dry skin, weight gain, and poor linear growth), children or adolescents may present with galactorrhea, headaches, and irregular menses (14, 15).

In adolescents with pituitary tumors, puberty is often delayed or arrested because of decreased gonadotropin levels and/or increased PRL levels. Females can have primary or secondary amenorrhea. Hyperprolactinemia can occur, producing galactorrhea and contributing to suppression of gonadotropin levels. Precocious puberty (development before age 8 years in girls and before age 9 years in boys), caused by loss of the central nervous system inhibition of gonadotropin-releasing hormone (GnRH) and gonadotropin secretion, is less frequently observed in association with pediatric pituitary tumors. The presentation of precocious puberty arises much more often in tumors above the sellar region, such as hypothalamic hamartomas. These tumors may actually produce GnRH, with subsequent central precocious puberty (Fig. 23.1).

Weight gain may be observed in children with large pituitary tumors or other suprasellar masses causing compression of neural structures. In the study by Sklar (16), 25% of children with craniopharyngiomas were found to be obese at presentation. Contributing factors can include pituitary dysfunction (central hypothyroidism or GH defi-

ciency) as well as hypothalamic dysfunction, which may produce inanition, decrease in metabolic rate, and appetite disturbances such as hyperphagia. Children with large lesions extending into the anterior hypothalamus may present with a diencephalic syndrome—with emaciation, alert appearance, hyperkinesis, and vomiting; more commonly, the diencephalic syndrome is associated with hypothalamic gliomas.

Most pituitary adenomas in children will be associated with more than one endocrine aberration, including hypersecretion of at least one pituitary hormone as well as some degree of hypopituitarism. Many tumors will produce growth arrest or a slowing of the growth velocity secondary to decreased GH secretion. The exception would be those tumors secreting GH and producing gigantism, which, although the third most common functional pituitary tumor in childhood, is nonetheless rare.

CLINICAL MANIFESTATIONS OF PEDIATRIC PITUITARY TUMORS

Signs and symptoms observed in children and adolescents with pituitary tumors may include endocrine manifestations, visual changes, headaches, symptoms of increased intracranial pressure, seizures, poor short-term memory, or behavioral changes. The type and size of the tumor and the age of the child all play a role in the clinical manifestations.

Short stature or decline in growth velocity is a common feature in most children with pituitary lesions. This is mainly attributable to GH deficiency but can also be a consequence of cortisol excess, hypothyroidism, or DI. Depending on the age of the child, delayed puberty or hypogonadism may be observed. Galactorrhea may occur with hyperprolactinemia, which may be caused by PRL secretion by the tumor itself or by disinhibition of the pituitary stalk.

Visual disturbances are often the presenting signs in children with pituitary tumors because of the pituitary gland's proximity to the optic chiasm. Decreased visual acuity, visual field defects, or even blindness may be noted on presentation. The insidious progression of visual loss is such that the visual disturbances are generally noted only late in the course, either because of the child's inability to see the chalkboard at school or because the child must sit close to the television at home to see the picture. Visual fields and visual acuity must be documented on presentation and at follow-up.

In pediatric pituitary adenomas, the specific hormones secreted by the tumor determine the clinical manifestations. These are usually microadenomas. Cushing's disease results from corticotroph adenomas producing excess ACTH. Cushing's syndrome causes obesity, growth arrest, pubertal arrest, striae, hypertension, and virilization. In children older than 7 years, ACTH-producing pituitary adenomas are the primary cause of Cushing's syndrome. The major difference in presentation of Cushing's disease in children versus adults is that growth arrest is a key feature,

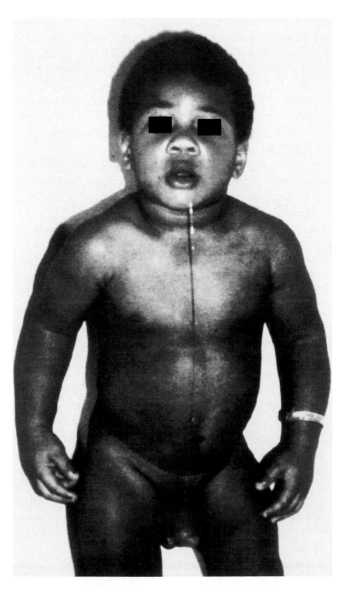

Figure 23.1. A 7-month-old male who presented with rapid growth and precocious puberty secondary to a hypothalamic hamartoma. The child was managed with medical therapy for his precocious puberty, and follow-up MRI scans revealed no change in lesion size.

and the obesity may be more generalized than truncal, with less evidence of muscle wasting. As in adults with ACTH-secreting adenomas, glucose intolerance and hypokalemia can also be seen in children.

PRL-secreting adenomas produce galactorrhea, delayed growth, and hypogonadism. Depending on the age of the patient, puberty may be delayed, and females may have either primary or secondary amenorrhea (17).

In prepubertal children, pediatric GH-secreting tumors produce gigantism. Children present with tall stature, large hands and feet, and prognathism. Glucose intolerance and sleep apnea may also be observed (18).

Symptoms of increased intracranial pressure, such as headache and vomiting, are reported in most children (80%) with *suprasellar* tumors, but papilledema is observed only in approximately 50% (19). Children with suprasellar tumors may also have a decline in school performance owing to memory problems, processing difficulties, or inanition (20). Similarly, emotional and behavioral problems may occur. These problems are attributable to alterations in the hypothalamus or other areas of the limbic system such as the septal nuclei. Children may have decreased motivation, increased aggression, emotional lability, or depression. The presence of such symptoms at diagnosis should be documented. With large tumors, anosmia may also be observed on presentation.

DIAGNOSTIC WORKUP IN PATIENTS WITH PITUITARY TUMORS IN THE PEDIATRIC GROUP

Endocrine

From an academic standpoint, pituitary function should be fully assessed on presentation. However, often it is not practical to perform dynamic testing of the pituitary axis. The most important aspects of pituitary function to determine preoperatively include the absence or presence of DI, thyroid status, and adrenal status. If the child is taking high-dose glucocorticoids at the time of evaluation, adrenal function cannot be assessed, and it must be assessed postoperatively.

DI classically produces polydipsia, polyuria, and nocturia. Careful questioning can often elucidate the magnitude of fluid intake and output. Children with an intact thirst mechanism and access to fluids can present with normal serum chemistries but dilute urine. Refer to Chapter 6 for a detailed account of diagnosis and workup of DI.

Thyroid function is determined simply by obtaining a serum sample for measuring thyroxine or free thyroxine. A thyroid-stimulating hormone measurement is not helpful in the assessment of central hypothyroidism, but levels will be significantly elevated in pituitary hyperplasia secondary to severe primary hypothyroidism. Theoretically, thyrotropin-releasing hormone stimulation can be used to distinguish between secondary (pituitary) and tertiary (hypothalamic) hypothyroidism. In clinical practice, this test is rarely necessary.

Adrenal function can be assessed by obtaining a morning cortisol measurement (8:00 AM). Symptoms of adrenal insufficiency include anorexia, weight loss, and lethargy. Provocative testing of the hypothalamic–pituitary–adrenal axis is used to document adrenal insufficiency (see Chapter 13 for a detailed account of diagnosis of Cushing's disease).

Other initial assessment should document growth and pubertal status. Height, weight, and Tanner stage should be noted. Screening tests to assess GH status include serum concentration of insulinlike growth factor-1 (IGF-1) or IGF binding protein-3 (IGFBP-3), which are GH-dependent proteins that are stable in the circulation. Concentrations of IGF-1 and IGFBP-3 can be obtained from a random serum sample. Also, a radiograph for bone age should be obtained to assess skeletal maturation. Provocative testing of GH with arginine, L-dopa, clonidine, or insulin may also be performed. If insulin-induced hypoglycemia is used as a test of GH status, cortisol status can also be assessed. In older children or those with any signs of pubertal development, LH, follicle-stimulating hormone, and PRL measurements should be obtained. The gonadotropin response to GnRH can be performed in conjunction with other provocative testing to evaluate the hypothalamic–pituitary–gonadal axis.

A serum PRL concentration should be obtained in all patients with pituitary tumors. Mild to moderate elevation of PRL level suggests disruption of the hypothalamic–pituitary axis. A PRL level greater than 200 μg/L (> 200 ng/mL) indicates a PRL-secreting adenoma, or prolactinoma.

For pituitary tumors producing ACTH and Cushing's syndrome, diagnostic studies must document hypercortisolism and ACTH dependence (21–24) (see Chapter 13). In almost all pediatric cases of ACTH-dependent Cushing's syndrome, the lesion is in the pituitary gland. There are rare case reports of ectopic ACTH in children with bronchial carcinoids, paragangliomas, or neuroblastomas (25).

Although GH-secreting tumors are the third most common tumors following PRL- and ACTH-secreting tumors, GH-secreting tumors are rare, particularly prior to puberty. Thus, the presentation of gigantism secondary to pituitary GH-secreting tumors is unusual. The diagnosis can be confirmed by obtaining elevated basal GH and IGF-1 or IGFBP-3 concentrations. With GH-secreting adenomas, GH fails to suppress in response to a glucose load, administered as a glucose tolerance test, so that glucose tolerance can be assessed simultaneously. Paradoxical increases in GH levels are often seen when thyrotropin-releasing hormone and GnRH are administered (18, 24).

Pituitary adenomas are a feature of multiple endocrine neoplasia type 1, along with tumors of the parathyroids and pancreatic islet cells. Most of the pituitary tumors associated with multiple endocrine neoplasia type 1 are prolactinomas or nonfunctioning tumors, but approximately 20%

secrete GH. This is an autosomal-dominant condition. If multiple endocrine neoplasia is suspected, chromosome 11 should be examined for the abnormal RET (REarranged during Transfection) oncogene. In addition, measurement of calcitonin, glucose, insulin, pancreatic polypeptide, potassium, gastrin, and glucagon levels should be performed to evaluate for associated tumors of the parathyroid glands and pancreatic islet cells (24, 26).

Radiology

The radiologic evaluation of the child with suspected sellar tumors is paramount. Many times, simple skull radiographs can make the diagnosis. The sphenoid sinus generally does not become fully pneumatized until 1 year of age. Thereafter, three radiographic types have been described. The preconchal type is that of infancy, in which the sinus has not developed. The conchal type is incompletely pneumatized and will require drilling through a thickened sellar floor in the event of a transsphenoidal approach. The fully pneumatized type has only a thin sellar floor that can be easily accessed through an osteotomy. Skull radiographs also allow assessment of the sphenoid septum. In the presence of a meningioma, one will typically see hyperostosis of the tuberculum sellae. The presence of suprasellar calcifications may suggest a craniopharyngioma. Erosion or expansion of the sella also suggests the presence of a chronic mass effect.

Computed tomography (CT) offers much better bony definition than plain skull radiographs. Coronal images give detailed anatomy of the skull base and nasal sinuses and is important in planning the transphenoidal approach. CT is also the study of choice for following residual calcifications in the patient who has had a craniopharyngioma resected, as these calcifications may not be detected by magnetic resonance imaging (MRI) (27).

MRI is certainly the test of choice in evaluating pituitary tumors. With the increasing prevalence of MRI imaging for headaches and associated symptoms, an increasing number of incidental pituitary lesions are being detected. It should be remembered that up to 20% of the normal population harbors a pituitary abnormality, such that the mere presence of a radiographic abnormality does not dictate the need for surgery. Furthermore, a physiologic enlargement of the gland will typically occur at puberty and can mimic a pituitary tumor.

The evaluation of the pituitary gland by MRI should normally include high-resolution thin section T1 and T2 images with and without gadolinium enhancement. Normally the anterior pituitary is isointense on T1 images, whereas the posterior pituitary is hyperintense. This characteristic signal is no longer attributed to fat within the neurohypophysis but is believed to be caused by the presence of neurosecretory vesicles (28). Thus, the loss of this hyperintensity accompanying the finding of a thickened infundibulum may suggest infiltration by a germinoma, an eosinophilic granuloma, or an inflammatory process such as

sarcoidosis. The presence of a spherical hypointense mass in the suprasellar region may suggest a Rathke's cleft cyst or may be caused by the flow void created by an aneurysm. If the question of a vascular abnormality is raised, magnetic resonance angiography or a formal angiogram may be needed prior to surgery.

Recognition of the characteristic pattern of enhancement following gadolinium enhancement is crucial to the correct interpretation of this study. Normally, a pituitary adenoma is not particularly vascular relative to the normal gland. As such, the normal gland will enhance immediately following the injection of contrast, whereas the tumor will appear relatively hypointense; however, after 20 to 30 minutes, the tumor will retain contrast, whereas the contrast will already be cleared from the normal gland. Therefore, a delayed study following the administration of contrast will demonstrate an enhancing tumor and a hypointense anterior pituitary gland. Given this variability, it is no wonder that MRI scanning for pituitary tumors carries a 20% false-positive and 20% false-negative rate (28).

Visual Examination

As mentioned earlier, one of the most important components in the evaluation of sellar lesions is the visual examination, which should include formal visual field testing in children old enough to cooperate. Visual examination should also include acuity testing and a dilated funduscopic examination. Often the detection of visual disturbances in children with chiasmal compression or infiltration will only become apparent to the family when the children are virtually blind. The classic picture of the bitemporal field defect must be documented and followed throughout the course of treatment. The visual fields are also a simple and reliable means of following up the patient postoperatively and are recommended at routine intervals in children with optic nerve gliomas or other processes that may potentially compress the chiasm. The finding of hypoplastic optic nerves may suggest a congenital process such as a craniopharyngioma. The finding of optic atrophy will suggest a slowly progressive process rather than a rapidly growing tumor. The finding of papilledema may accompany clinical symptoms of raised intracranial pressure and suggest ventricular obstruction and secondary hydrocephalus (29).

DIFFERENTIAL DIAGNOSIS

A current and concise review of suprasellar and sellar tumors in the pediatric age group is offered by Rutka et al. (30). The suprasellar region is second to the posterior fossa as the most common anatomic location of brain tumors in childhood. Given the complex developmental anatomy of this region, it is of little surprise.

One of the most important differentiating points in the child being evaluated for a possible pituitary tumor is that of physiologic hypertrophy of the normal gland. The pitui-

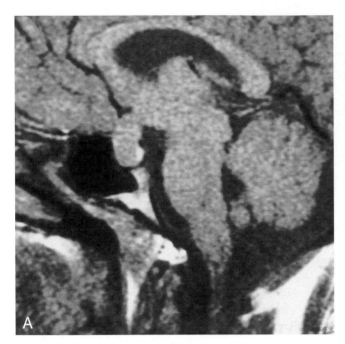
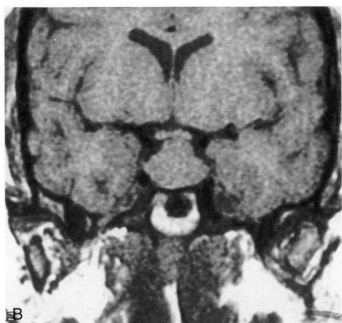

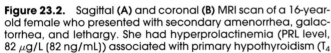

Figure 23.2.   Sagittal **(A)** and coronal **(B)** MRI scan of a 16-year-old female who presented with secondary amenorrhea, galactorrhea, and lethargy. She had hyperprolactinemia (PRL level, 82 μg/L (82 ng/mL)) associated with primary hypothyroidism (T₄ level, 32 nmol/L (2.5 μg/dL); thyroid-stimulating hormone level, 408 μIU/L (408 μIU/mL)). An MRI scan reveals significant pituitary hyperplasia, which resolved with thyroxine replacement therapy.

tary gland will normally enlarge at the time of puberty and, in the presence of headaches or delayed menarche, may raise the question of tumor versus normal gland. The anterior pituitary may also undergo physiologic enlargement secondary to end organ failure, as in the cases of primary hypothyroidism and hypogonadism (31). In such cases, the MRI demonstrates a full sella with bulging of the diaphragma sella but no discrete tumorous masses. One must rely on hormonal studies and follow-up MRIs to differentiate physiologic enlargement of the normal gland (hyperplasia) from neoplasia (Fig. 23.2A, B).

Craniopharyngiomas are the most common nonglial tumors of the suprasellar region, comprising 5 to 10% of all pediatric brain tumors (30). Approximately 70% of pediatric craniopharyngiomas arise within the sella. The remainder are suprasellar. In children with craniopharyngiomas, 40% present with growth arrest or short stature and 25% present with DI (19). Although less than half of children with craniopharyngiomas will have clinically apparent endocrine dysfunction, on testing, almost all will have some degree of hypopituitarism. Patients may also present with visual loss or symptoms of raised intracranial pressure secondary to ventricular obstruction. These tumors may be cystic or solid or may have components of both. They generally contain intratumoral calcifications that can be seen easily on CT scan.

Rathke's cleft cysts are also epithelial cystic tumors of the suprasellar region that are being seen more commonly now that MRI imaging is more prevalent. These lesions were found as the most common incidental lesion of the pituitary gland in the autopsy study by Teramoto et al. (2). They occur most frequently in the midline. Rathke's cleft cysts are filled with mucoid material and usually do not contain calcifications. Children with Rathke's cleft cysts may also present with hypopituitarism or DI. Because these cysts are often an incidental finding, the indications for surgery are documented visual disturbances or hypopituitarism (32). DI itself is not an indication for surgery (33) (Fig. 23.3A–D).

Hypothalamic/chiasmic gliomas most commonly occur in children younger than 10 years of age. They are usually low-grade glial neoplasms that can remain quiescent for years or that can undergo malignant degeneration and progress rapidly. In infancy, these patients may present with macrocephaly, roving nystagmus, or symptoms related to obstructive hydrocephalus. Older children may present with a diencephalic syndrome of weight loss, irritability, and decreased vision. The diagnostic procedure of choice is MRI, with many of these tumors being amenable to surgical debulking (30).

Suprasellar germ cell tumors account for a small percentage of suprasellar tumors in any pediatric series. Unlike these tumors of the pineal location, which are more common in males, those in the suprasellar region seem to have a female preponderance. They may present with the classic triad of DI, visual disturbance, and panhypopituitarism. Certainly, DI in the presence of a suprasellar tumor should raise the suggestion of germinoma. These tumors may also contain histologically mixed lesions, including embryonal carcinoma, choriocarcinoma, and teratoma. There are no characteristic radiographic features that will definitively characterize these lesion. At times, serum or cerebrospinal fluid beta human chorionic gonadotropin, α-fetoprotein, or carcinoembryonic antigen may help in characterizing these tumors.

Other rarely seen lesions included in the differential diagnosis of suprasellar pediatric tumors include hamartomas, meningiomas, cavernous hemangiomas, lymphomas, teratomas, aneurysms, arachnoid cysts, intrasellar mucocele, metastatic tumors, and inflammatory masses such as pseudotumor or hypophysitis.

MEDICAL MANAGEMENT OF PEDIATRIC PITUITARY TUMORS

The most common pituitary tumor in postpubertal children and the second most common overall is the prolactinoma. Although data are limited, it seems that these tumors in childhood respond at least as well to bromocriptine therapy as do adult prolactinomas. In the review by Tyson

et al. (34), all five patients given bromocriptine for these tumors had a dramatic response, with mean tumor shrinkage of 70% and resolution of biochemical abnormalities or visual field deficits in all cases. Kamel et al. (17) reported two additional cases of children with prolactinomas who were able to normalize their growth rates and have normal pubertal development following the institution of bromocriptine therapy. Tyson et al. (34) offer the position that bromocriptine therapy is preferable to surgery or radiation for prolactinomas; however, these authors do not address side effects of this medication or the fact that these children may require long-term treatment. These factors must be weighed against the fact that, in experienced hands, the mortality rate for transsphenoidal surgery now approaches zero (6), as does the need for hormonal replacement therapy following removal of microadenomas (12). In the authors' experience, children and their parents eventually tire of medical management and opt for surgical intervention.

Octreotide is a commercially available somatostatin analog that can be used to treat GH-secreting adenomas; however, at the moment, it is only available in parenteral form

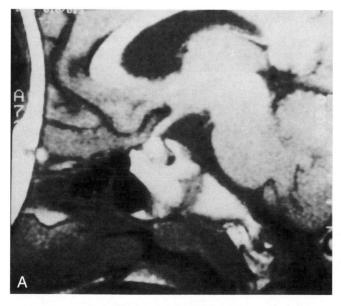

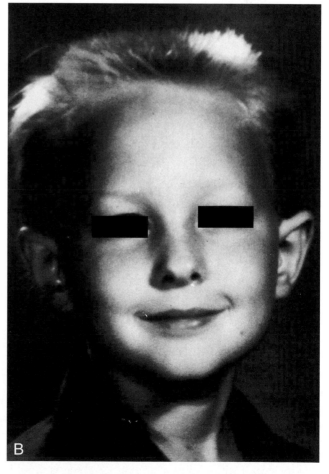

Figure 23.3. **A.** Sagittal T1-weighted MRI of a 13-year-old male with a Rathke's cleft cyst who presented with DI. **B–D.** These images reflect progression of changes in physical appearance. Although he appeared cushingoid, hypercortisolism was not de- monstrable at diagnosis. Surgery was performed 18 months after initial presentation, when growth and pubertal arrest were observed, with documented GH and gonadotropin deficiencies.

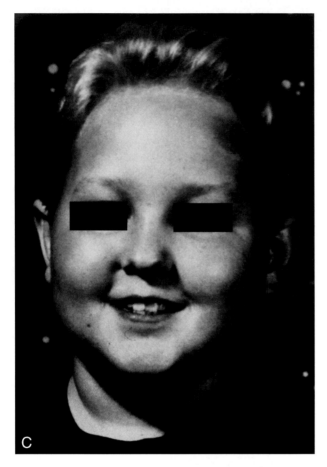

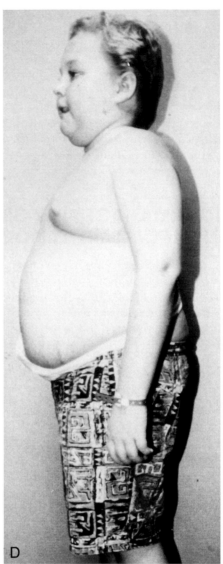

Figure 23.3.   *(continued)*

and treatment involves daily injections of the drug. As such, it is not practical for use in children.

SURGICAL MANAGEMENT

Preoperative Evaluation

The initial medical assessment of the pediatric patient diagnosed with a pituitary tumor includes a careful history and physical examination for signs and symptoms of endocrine dysfunction and baseline laboratory studies. The review of systems should include questions about polydipsia, polyuria, and nocturia and changes in appetite, behavior, or activity level. Height, weight, and pubertal status should be documented. Laboratory studies needed prior to surgery include serum thyroxine, electrolytes, urine specific gravity or osmolality, and a morning cortisol. Additional baseline studies need to be obtained for comparison in fol-

low-up, including a radiograph documenting skeletal maturation and IGF-1. In patients close to puberty or with evidence of pubertal development, LH and follicle-stimulating hormone, testosterone or estradiol, and prolactin levels should be measured. Children with DI should have the DI controlled and fluid and electrolyte imbalances corrected prior to surgery. Those with low cortisol levels should be covered with stress doses of glucocorticoids prior to surgery, and those with laboratory evidence of hypothyroidism should have this corrected before undergoing a general anesthetic unless an emergency, such as apoplexy, is encountered.

Indications for Surgery

The indication for surgery in children with a pituitary adenoma is no different than for adults. In patients with PRL-secreting microadenomas, and macroadenomas with no neurologic deficit, a trial of bromocriptine therapy is warranted. Bromocriptine may also be used for patients with macroadenomas who have neurologic deficit, but these patients require close neurologic, radiologic, and biochemical follow-up. Operative treatment for PRL-secreting adenomas is offered to those who show no response to medical therapy, those who are intolerant of the side effects of bromocriptine therapy, or those with progressive neurologic deficit. For patients with ACTH- or GH-secreting adenomas, the prognosis is excellent following transsphenoidal exploration and resection. For the rare patient presenting with headache alone or the child who is noted to have a pituitary adenoma as an incidental finding on an MRI scan done for other reasons, careful follow-up is best. With high-resolution MRI and sensitive endocrine testing, these lesions can be followed up until definitive symptoms or progression is documented.

Surgery

The surgical management of pituitary adenomas in childhood is little different than for adults. Occasionally, large tumors may require craniotomy for definitive resection, but most of these tumors can be dealt with through a transsphenoidal approach (35, 36). Examples of tumors requiring craniotomy include most craniopharyngiomas and large macroadenomas that extend into the middle cranial fossa. In approaching these tumors, it is important to plan for both the classic pterional as well as the subfrontal approach in case an intradural or extradural transethmoid extension is required to gain access to a deep sella. Although most tumors can be removed via a standard pterional craniotomy, the authors use the cranio-orbitozygomatic approach, coupled with wide opening of the sylvian fissure, to allow resection of suprasellar tumors with minimal brain retraction.

In performing transsphenoidal surgery in children, several factors should be kept in mind. First, the midface of the child is smaller than that of the adult such that a smaller speculum is often required. Second, in the rare child who presents before 8 years of age, if a sublabial approach is used, one must take care not to damage tooth buds of the secondary teeth. Finally, in younger children, the sinuses may not be well developed and should always be assessed by CT scan prior to surgery. In the surgical series of Dyer et al. (12), 17% of children required drilling of a conchal type, or incompletely pneumatized, sphenoid sinus. In no case did this pose a limitation to the surgical procedure (12).

The future of pituitary surgery will be transnasal, endoscope-assisted surgery. As better optics and microsurgical instruments are developed, this procedure is the natural progression of endoscopic sinus surgery (Fig. 23.4A–D). Rodziewicz et al. (37) have reported 10 cases in which the endoscopic guidance proved feasible and offer advice on their technique. The advantages of the endoscopic transnasal procedure in children are that it does not require fracture or removal of any facial bones, it is not hampered by a small nasal opening, and the potential complications of the translabial approach (septal perforation, saddle deformity, etc.) are lessened. In a recent report of 55 cases treated in this fashion by Jho and Carrau (38), the postoperative results were as good as those with standard transsphenoidal surgery.

Ram et al. (39) reported the intraoperative use of ultrasound to assist with identification of the microadenoma and verify the extent of resection. In this series, 23 of 28 pituitary tumors could be visualized by ultrasound, including 13 of 18 microadenomas (82% sensitivity) (39).

POSTOPERATIVE MANAGEMENT

In the immediate postoperative period, the most frequent acute endocrine disorders are DI and SIADH. For diagnosis and management of these disorders, both fluid intake and output need to be closely followed (see Chapters 6 and 26).

Cortisol deficiency is another endocrinopathy that may occur acutely in the immediate postoperative period. In clinical practice, management decisions regarding glucocorticoid treatment are often based on the presence of apparent remaining pituitary gland and morning cortisol concentrations. In children in whom these factors are inconclusive, maintenance glucocorticoids are often administered for 4 to 6 weeks, allowing the child to recover prior to further assessment (see Chapters 13, 14, and 26).

In the postoperative period, in patients who are taking high doses of glucocorticoids, serum glucose and urine glucose levels should be followed up because hyperglycemia secondary to stress and insulin resistance is commonly observed. This can require treatment with insulin. Careful consideration should be given to fluid status because glycosuria may exaggerate fluid losses.

Because all or part of the pituitary gland may have been removed during surgery, thyroid function should be reassessed postoperatively by obtaining a serum thyroxine or free thyroxine measurement approximately 1 to 2 weeks after surgery.

In patients with secretory pituitary adenomas, the particular hormone being secreted by the tumor may serve as a tumor marker; thus, the efficacy of surgical treatment can be determined by measuring the hormone(s) of note postoperatively. For Cushing's disease, serum cortisol level is measured 24 hours after perioperative glucocorticoid treatment is discontinued. An undetectable cortisol level is consistent with surgical cure. These patients need to receive "stress doses" of glucocorticoids in the event of an acute illness or trauma because they may have some suppression of the hypothalamic–pituitary–adrenal axis for several months. For those children or adolescents with GH- and/or PRL-secreting tumors, GH and PRL levels should be measured postoperatively, along with IGF-1 levels. These patients are frequently not cured by surgery, and medical

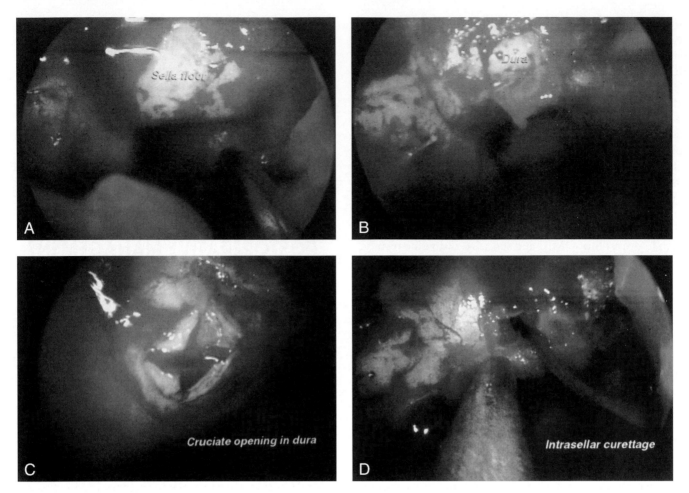

Figure 23.4. **A.** Endoscopic view of the sella during a transnasal approach. **B.** Removal of the sellar floor during a transnasal endoscopic pituitary tumor resection. **C.** Opening of the dura with endoscopic visualization. **D.** Removal of pituitary tumor by curettage with endoscopic visualization.

therapy is often added postoperatively. Dopamine agonists such as bromcriptine are used. Medical therapy may be needed for years. If medical therapy does not suppress GH and/or PRL or is not tolerated, then pituitary radiation may be required. Hypopituitarism often develops as a consequence of pituitary radiation.

Long-term Follow-up

Long-term management of pediatric patients with pituitary tumors should include endocrine consultation every 3 to 6 months. Height, weight, and pubertal status should be followed. Review of systems should be performed. In particular, questions related to possible hypothyroidism or adrenal insufficiency should be asked. Appetite should be assessed. Endocrine investigation includes thyroid hormone measurement every 6 to 12 months and skeletal age assessment approximately every year until growth is complete. GH deficiency is common and is documented with provocative tests such as clonidine, arginine, or L-dopa stimulation. With children in whom hypopituitarism is

highly suspected and in whom there is a history of seizures, insulin-induced hypoglycemia is not recommended as a test of GH status. Growth itself is not necessarily an indicator of GH status because many children, particularly those gaining weight rapidly, will demonstrate normal or even supranormal height velocities in the 6 to 12 months following surgery (40). These rapidly growing children are often observed to have high serum concentrations of insulin and IGF-1. Pubertal status must be followed closely because it can be early or delayed following pituitary surgery. Along with Tanner staging and skeletal maturation, LH, follicle-stimulating hormone, estradiol (females), testosterone (males), and PRL levels should be assessed when there is abnormal pubertal maturation. GnRH can be given to assess the pituitary–gonadal axis. When hypogonadotropic hypogonadism is present, treatment with testosterone (males) and estrogens/progesterone (females) is indicated. This is almost invariably the case in adolescents with craniopharyngiomas who present with delayed or arrested pubertal development (41). Particularly in children in whom these gonadal steroids are being used to induce and simulate normal puberty, visits to a pediatric endocrinologist every 3 to 6 months are recommended.

Adrenal insufficiency is treated with daily maintenance glucocorticoids, such as hydrocortisone or prednisone. The dose is tailored to the patient's needs. These children and their families need education and periodic review regarding the indications for stress doses of glucocorticoids. Patients should wear a Medic-Alert bracelet identifying their adrenal insufficiency.

DI can be transient, associated with a triphasic response (acute DI followed by SIADH, then DI that may be permanent), or permanent. Fluid intake and output, the presence of nocturia, and desmopressin acetate (DDAVP) doses should be discussed. Serum electrolytes should be assessed periodically.

A major morbidity of children with hypothalamic dysfunction, particularly with craniopharyngiomas, is obesity, occurring in approximately 50% of these patients (41). These children often have hyperphagia. They tend to have abnormal linear growth as well as rapid weight gain. In children in whom vision has been affected, improvement is usually observed (53%), but occasionally it worsens (25%) (41). Regular testing of visual fields and acuity must be done, particularly in patients with worsening vision. Other morbidities observed in children and adolescents after suprasellar tumors, particularly craniopharyngiomas, include behavioral, sleep, and academic difficulties.

Pituitary or hypothalamic dysfunction after surgery may produce substantial morbidity in the pediatric patient with a pituitary tumor. These problems can be numerous, complex, slowly evolving, and difficult to understand for the patients and their families. Early and regular consultation with a team including a pediatric endocrinologist, an ophthalmologist, and a neuropsychologist is helpful for anticipation, identification, and management of these problems.

TREATMENT OF RECURRENT OR RESIDUAL TUMOR

It is important to distinguish between tumor persistence and recurrence. Recurrence of tumor after cure is reserved for those children who had complete resection at the time of surgery, who had no postoperative imaging evidence of residual disease, and whose biochemical tumor markers returned to normal following surgery. Most larger series demonstrate that, in experienced hands, one may anticipate a 65 to 70% long-term cure rate with surgery alone. Recurrences are related to the type of hormonal secretion and to initial tumor size. In the review by Kane et al. (13), 70% of patients harboring microadenomas were free of disease following surgery, with a 25% recurrence rate (13). In contrast, only 33% of patients with macroadenomas were free of disease after surgery, and 4 (33%) of 11 had recurrence. In Mindermann and Wilson's study (6), ACTH- and GH-secreting adenomas both had a 17% recurrence rate. In Dyer et al.'s study (12), only 12% of patients with GH-secreting adenomas were cured by surgery, whereas 67% of PRL-secreting adenomas were cured. Partington et al. (3) documented a 25% long-term recurrence rate for ACTH-secreting tumors, and they believe that this recurrence rate is probably similar to that of the adult population.

For persistent or recurrent tumors, standard treatment options include reoperation, medical therapy, or radiotherapy. Reoperation for local recurrence is the treatment of choice for most tumors (6). In experienced hands, the complication rate for reoperative transsphenoidal surgery is still low. In children with persistently elevated levels of GH or ACTH, reoperation is crucial because the 5-year mortality for these diseases is higher in children than in adults. If reoperation does not cure the disease, then complete hypophysectomy, either surgically or by stereotactic radioablation, is recommended.

For large invasive prolactinomas, bromocriptine therapy is clearly effective and may help avoid the need for reoperation. For other tumor types, stereotactic radiosurgery is the standard of treatment if the tumor cannot be safely resected and is separated from the optic chiasm by several millimeters. The difficulty with radiotherapy for pediatric pituitary tumors is the high long-term incidence of panhypopituitarism that can be anticipated. Using conventional therapy, hypothalamic damage has also been reported, leading to memory problems, personality change, and visual loss (42, 43). Hoffman has also noted the development of moyamoya disease in several children who underwent conventional radiotherapy for suprasellar neoplasms (30). These side effects are clearly lessened using stereotactic radiosurgical techniques. Nonetheless, radiotherapy should be reserved only for those in whom both surgical and medical therapy have failed (1).

REFERENCES

1. Haddad SF, VanGilder JC, Menezes AH. Pediatric pituitary tumors. Neurosurgery 1991;29(4):509–514.
2. Teramoto A, Hirakawa K, Sanno N, et al. Incidental pituitary lesions in 1,000 unselected autopsy specimens. Radiology 1994;193:161–164.
3. Partington MD, Davis DH, Laws ER, et al. Pituitary adenomas in childhood and adolescence. J Neurosurg 1994;80:209–216.
4. Hoffman HJ. Pituitary adenomas. In: American Association of Neurological Surgeons, eds. Pediatric Neurosurgery: Surgery of the Developing Nervous System. New York: Grune & Stratton, 1982:493–499.
5. Gold EB. Epidemiology of pituitary adenomas. Epidemiol Rev 1981;3:163–183.
6. Mindermann T, Wilson CB. Pediatric pituitary adenomas. Neurosurgery 1995;36(2):259–269.
7. Gelber SJ, Heffez DS, Donohoue PA. Pituitary gigantism caused

by growth hormone excess from infancy. J Pediatr 1992;120:931–934.

8. Fabbiano M, Ceiscuolo T, Perone L, et al. Sexual precocity in a boy due to hypersecretion of LH and prolactin by a pituitary adenoma. Acta Endocrinol 1983;102:167–172.

9. Avramides A, Karapiperis A, Triantafyllidou E, et al. TSH-secreting pituitary macroadenoma in an 11-year-old girl. Acta Paediatr 1992;81:1058–1060.

10. Scheithauer BW, Horvath E, Kovacs K, et al. Plurihormonal pituitary adenomas. Semin Diagn Pathol 1986;3:69–82.

11. Fisher BJ, Gaspar LE, Stitt LW, et al. Pituitary adenoma in adolescents: a biologically more aggressive disease? Radiology 1994;192:869–872.

12. Dyer EH, Civit T, Visot A, et al. Transsphenoidal surgery for pituitary adenomas in children. Neurosurgery 1994;34(2):207–212.

13. Kane LA, Leinung MC, Scheithauer BW, et al. Pituitary adenomas in childhood and adolescence. J Clin Endocrinol Metab 1994;79:1135–1140.

14. Adams C, Dean HJ, Israels SJ, et al. Primary hypothyroidism with intracranial hypertension and pituitary hyperplasia. Pediatr Neurol 1994;10:166–168.

15. Williams RS, Williams JP, Davis MR, et al. Primary hypothyroidism with pituitary hyperplasia and basal ganglia calcifications. Clin Imaging 1990;14:330–332.

16. Sklar CA. Craniopharyngioma: endocrine abnormalities at presentation. Pediatr Neurosurg 1994;21(suppl 1):18–20.

17. Kamel N, Uysal AR, Cesur V, et al. Normal growth and pubertal development during bromocryptine therapy in two patients with prolactinoma. Endocr J 1995;42:581–586.

18. Lu PW, Silink M, Johnston I, et al. Pituitary gigantism. Arch Dis Child 1992;67:1039–1041.

19. Post KD, McCormick PC, Bello JA. Differential diagnosis of pituitary tumors. Endocrinol Metab Clin North Am 1987;16:609–643.

20. Shiminski-Maher T. Patient/family preparation and education for complications and late sequelae of craniopharyngiomas. Pediatr Neurosurg 1994;21(suppl 1):114–119.

21. Bickler SW, McMahon TJ, Campbell JR, et al. Preoperative diagnostic evaluation of children with Cushing's syndrome. J Pediatr Surg 1994;29:671–676.

22. Weber A, Trainer PJ, Grossman AB, et al. Investigation, management and therapeutic outcome in 12 cases of childhood and adolescent Cushing's syndrome. Clin Endocrinol 1995;43:19–28.

23. Mamelak AN, Dowd CF, Tyrrell JB, et al. Venous angiography is needed to interpret inferior petrosal sinus and cavernous sinus sampling data for lateralizing adrenocorticotropin-secreting adenomas. J Clin Endocrinol Metab 1996;81(2):475–481.

24. Magiokou MA, Mastorakos G, Oldfield EH, et al. Cushing's syndrome in children and adolescents. N Engl J Med 1994;331:629–636.

25. Oldfield EH, Doppman JL, Nieman LK, et al. Petrosal sinus sampling with and without corticotropin-releasing hormone for the dif-ferential diagnosis of Cushing's syndrome. N Engl J Med 1991;325:897–905.

26. Berezin M, Karasik A. Familial prolactinoma. Clin Endocrinol 1995;42:483–486.

27. Bonneville JF, Cattin F. The role of magnetic resonance imaging in the diagnosis of endocrine tumours of the sellar region in children. Horm Res 1995;43:151–153.

28. Kalifa G, Adamsbaum C, Carel JC, et al. Diagnosis of Cushing's disease in children: a challenge for the radiologist. Pediatr Radiol 1994;24:547–549.

29. Brodsky MC, Baker RS, Jamed LM. Optic atrophy in children. In: Pediatric Neuro-Ophthalmology. New York: Springer Verlag, 1996:125–163.

30. Rutka JT, Hoffman HJ, Drake JM, et al. Suprasellar and sellar tumors in childhood and adolescence. Pediatr Neuro-Oncol 1992;3(4):803–820.

31. Dadachanji MC, Bharucha NE, Jhankaria BG. Pituitary hyperplasia mimicking pituitary tumor. Surg Neurol 1994;42:397–399.

32. Rao GP, Blyth CPJ, Jeffreys RV. Ophthalmic manifestations of Rathke's cleft cysts. Am J Ophthalmol 1995;119:86–91.

33. Eguchi K, Uozumi T, Arita K, et al. Pituitary function in patients with Rathke's cleft cyst: significance of surgical management. Endocr J 1994;41(5):535–540.

34. Tyson D, Reggiardo D, Sklar C, et al. Prolactin-secreting macroadenomas in adolescents. AJDC 1993;147:1057–1061.

35. Laws ER, Scheithauer BW, Groover RV. Pituitary tumors in childhood and adolescence. Prog Exp Tumor Res 1987;30:359–361.

36. Tindall GT, Barrow DL. Disorders of the Pituitary. St. Louis: CV Mosby, 1986.

37. Rodziewicz GS, Kelley RT, Kellman RM, et al. Transnasal endoscopic surgery of the pituitary gland: technical note. Neurosurgery 1996;39(1):189–192.

38. Jho HD, Carrau RL. Endoscopic transphenoidal surgery in 55 patients. Presented at the annual meeting of the AANS. Denver, April 14, 1997.

39. Ram Z, Shawker TH, Bradford MH, et al. Intraoperative ultrasound-directed resection of pituitary tumors. J Neurosurg 1995;83:225–230.

40. Schoenle EJ, Zapf J, Prader A, et al. Replacement of GH in normally growing GH-deficient patients operated for craniopharyngioma. J Clin Endocrinol Metab 1995;80:374–378.

41. Curtis J, Daneman D, Hoffman HJ, et al. The endocrine outcome after surgical removal of craniopharyngiomas. Pediatr Neurosurg 1994;21(suppl 1):24–27.

42. Littley MD, Shalet SM, Beardwell EG. Radiation injury to the nervous system. In: Gutin PH, ed. Radiation and the Hypothalamic Pituitary Axis. New York: Raven Press, 1991:303–324.

43. Scott RM, Hetelekidis S, Barnes PD, et al. Surgery, radiation and combination therapy in the treatment of childhood craniopharyngioma: a 20 year experience. Pediatr Neurosurg 1994;21(suppl 1):75–81.

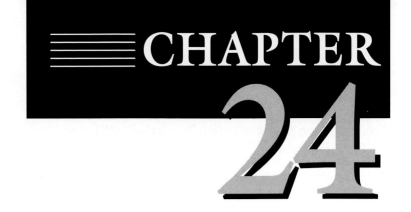

CHAPTER 24

Nonadenomatous Lesions of the Pituitary

William T. Couldwell and Martin H. Weiss

INTRODUCTION

Included in the differential diagnosis of mass lesions other than pituitary adenomas that can affect pituitary or visual function are a variety of tumors or benign cystic lesions in the region of the midline skull base. Many of these may be differentiated from primary pituitary lesions based on clinical history, physical examination, endocrinologic evaluation, and radiographic appearance. In most cases, such information is sufficient to establish the diagnosis; but, in some instances, histologic evaluation is required. Medical and surgical therapy is then individualized based on the underlying pathologic findings.

BENIGN PITUITARY CYSTS

The differential diagnosis of intrasellar and suprasellar cystic lesions includes a variety of neoplastic and nonneoplastic pathologic lesions. Although pituitary adenomas may contain cystic components and represent the most common cystic lesions of the pituitary, other tumoral causes include cystic craniopharyngiomas and the more uncommon suprasellar epidermoid cyst. Benign pituitary cysts

represent a disparate pathologic group of entities that often require histologic evaluation to differentiate. Benign pituitary cysts are a common autopsy finding and may occasionally become large enough to be symptomatic. Such nonneoplastic intrasellar cysts include Rathke's cleft cysts; less common cystic lesions in this region include arachnoid cysts, pars intermedia cysts, mucoceles, and parasitic (usually cysticercal) cysts (1–5).

Statistically, most cystic lesions other than cystic pituitary adenomas are believed to consist of remnants of Rathke's pouch (Rathke's cleft cysts; 2–8). Rathke's pouch is a transient embryologic structure (present in the third or fourth week of embryonic life) that represents an outgrowth of stomodeum and elongates to form the craniopharyngeal duct. The craniopharyngeal duct is the route by which the adenohypophysis ascends from the pharynx to its final location in the pituitary fossa. With further development of the pouch wall to form the anterior lobe of the pituitary, pars tuberalis, and pars intermedia, the residual lumen is reduced to a cleft, which usually regresses. It is hypothesized that persistence and enlargement of the cleft results in a symptomatic Rathke's cleft cyst. The cyst is characteristically lined by a single layer of cuboidal or columnar epithelium and is hypothesized to increase in size by the accumulation of mucus secreted by the cyst wall cells.

Although symptomatic Rathke's cleft cysts are uncommon, small, asymptomatic Rathke's cleft cysts are not infrequently seen on magnetic resonance imaging (MRI) and computed tomographic (CT) scans, and autopsy incidence of 2 to 26% has been reported (3, 5, 9–11). In the recent study reported by Oka et al. (12), most symptomatic Rathke's cleft cysts did not demonstrate enlargement of the sella. These authors suggested that this may be a distinguishing characteristic of these cysts that could help to differentiate such benign cysts from a cystic pituitary adenoma. One postulated theory for this difference may be that because the Rathke's cleft cyst is soft in consistency and usually originates in the central region of the pituitary gland, it easily extends to the suprasellar area through the cleft of the diaphragma sellae. Occasionally, Rathke's cleft cysts enlarge sufficiently to produce various clinical symptoms from compression of the pituitary gland, optic chiasm, or hypothalamus. Of 19 patients with symptomatic Rathke's cleft cysts recently reported, 11% presented with panhypopituitarism, 16% presented with amenorrhea/galactorrhea, 21% presented with diabetes insipidus (DI), and 47% presented with visual disturbance (13).

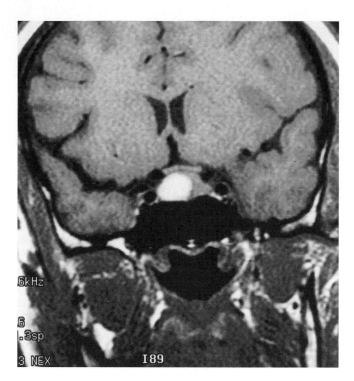

Figure 24.1. Rathke's cleft cyst.

Radiologic Evaluation

Radiologically, Rathke's cleft cysts are variable in their imaging features, and differentiation from craniopharyngiomas and cystic pituitary adenomas may be difficult. As noted above, the sella turcica is usually not enlarged in Rathke's cleft cysts, which may help distinguish these cysts from cystic pituitary adenomas radiographically; however, differentiating Rathke's cleft cysts from craniopharyngiomas may be difficult.

Results of most reports indicate that Rathke's cleft cysts are associated with high signal intensity on T1-weighted MRIs (Fig. 24.1). Proposed mechanisms for this high intensity include the presence of mucinous fluid (14), mucopolysaccharide within the fluid (15), and hemosiderin pigment (16) to produce this appearance. Surgical resection of the wall of large cysts has demonstrated deposition of hemosiderin pigment. The mechanism for this hemosiderin deposition is not clearly known, but it has been suggested that perhaps large cysts tend to bleed and that repetitive hemorrhage is associated with enlargement (12). Neovascularity within the granulation tissue surrounding the lesion may be the source of such hemorrhage.

Contrast enhancement on MRI or CT images has been reported to occur in approximately half of all cases. The contrast enhancement is hypothesized to occur secondary to pericystic granulation tissue (17); the granulation tissue may be induced by the mucous secreted by the goblet cells of the cyst wall.

Therapy

Because most Rathke's cleft cysts are asymptomatic, and hypodense lesions may be noted within the pituitary gland

on modern imaging studies in approximately 20% of patients without symptoms, only those patients with endocrinologic or neurologic compromise should be considered for surgical exploration. In most patients, treatment by simple transsphenoidal drainage is usually effective (1, 18, 19). The Rathke's cleft cyst should be treated by wide opening of the cyst wall and evacuation of the contents. Biopsy of the cyst wall confirms the benign nature of the cyst. Although transsphenoidal drainage is the surgical approach of choice, in a few instances craniotomy may be necessary for drainage, including when specific contraindications to transsphenoidal surgery are present ("kissing" carotid arteries at the level of the sphenoid bone, limiting the operative width available) and when a pure suprasellar cyst is clearly out of reach even to an extended transsphenoidal approach (18). In the recent series of patients reported by Egushi et al. (13), 69% of patients postoperatively demonstrated some improvement in pituitary function after 3 months. Amenorrhea and/or galactorrhea improved in all patients presenting with this problem, and visual disturbance improved in 89% of patients. However, DI and panhypopituitarism failed to improve in any patient. Thus, these authors concluded that surgical treatment is recommended even when the patient has only mild symptoms or signs, including pituitary dysfunction, to prevent irreversible panhypopituitarism.

The recent report of a delayed chiasmal syndrome after drainage of a symptomatic Rathke's cleft cyst (20) puts forth the possibility that delayed deficits may occur from tethering of the chiasm by the cyst wall after drainage.

EMPTY SELLA SYNDROME

Although not neoplastic, this entity can be mistaken for an intrasellar cystic mass on radiographic imaging. Empty sella syndrome results from a herniation of the arachnoid and subarachnoid space of the suprasellar cistern through an incompetent diaphragma sellae to occupy a significant volume within the sella. Developmental or degenerative incompetence of the diaphragma is necessary but not always sufficient to produce the empty sella syndrome. Various authors have demonstrated that although the diaphragma usually encircles the infundibulum closely, diaphragma defects may be present in 22 to 77% of patients (21–23).

The term "empty sella" was first applied to an anatomic finding described from autopsy studies by Busch in 1951 (22). He described a series of cases in which the pituitary gland was flattened inferiorly and posteriorly within the sella, together with an incompetent diaphragma sellae and a large infundibular foramen. Later, Kaufmann (23) recognized that the empty sella was a manifestation of an enlarged intrasellar expansion of the subarachnoid space. Since these seminal reports, the syndrome has been further categorized into primary empty sella syndrome, in which the enlargement of the subarachnoid space is not related to previous treatment, and secondary empty sella syndrome, in which the findings are related to previous treatment for a pituitary tumor.

Primary Empty Sella Syndrome

The cause of primary empty sella syndrome may be multifactorial. Predisposing factors include the presence of an incompetent diaphragma sellae, increased intracranial pressure (24–26), benign pituitary cysts (27), pituitary tumors (28), suprasellar tumors (29, 30), arachnoid cysts (31), and infarction or hemorrhage within the sella, resulting in some ablation of its contents. Although the presence of an incompetent diaphragma sella is permissive to the development of empty sella syndrome, it may not be sufficient in that although a significant percentage of individuals possess an incompetent diaphragma sellae as stated above, only 5.1 to 6.7% of autopsy cases reveal an empty sella (21–23).

Elevated intracranial pressure resulting from disparate causes may be associated with an increased incidence of empty sella syndrome. Increased intracranial pressure from brain tumors, hydrocephalus, sarcoidosis, Chiari malformations, and pseudotumor cerebri have been implicated. Benign intracranial hypertension (pseudotumor cerebri) disproportionately affects obese females, strikingly similar epidemiologic factors to those affected with empty sella syndrome, and may reflect a partial causality of the empty sella (32, 33).

Arachnoid cysts (31) or benign pituitary cysts of the pars intermedia (22) have been hypothesized to be involved in the genesis of disease in some patients with empty sella syndrome. Rupture of the pituitary cyst superiorly would provide a mechanism for the development of a communication with the subarachnoid space above.

Destruction or shrinkage of intrasellar contents (either normal or pathologic) has also been suggested as another mechanism for development of the empty sella. Patients with a history of previous pituitary apoplexy (34), Sheehan's syndrome (35), and treated primary hypothyroidism all share the feature of presenting increased space within the sella into which the suprasellar arachnoid may herniate.

Secondary Empty Sella Syndrome

Secondary empty sella syndrome may occur from herniation of arachnoid and subarachnoid space into the sella through an incompetent diaphragma sellae into a vacant sella following removal or shrinkage of intrasellar contents by surgery, radiation therapy, or medical therapy (24, 29, 36–39). Most commonly, secondary empty sella syndrome occurs after surgical resection or after successful medical or radiation therapy of a pituitary adenoma. Secondary empty sella syndrome affects both sexes equally and presents most commonly with visual field deterioration several weeks to years after therapy. The pattern of visual loss is not characteristic and may be the result of several factors, including herniation of the chiasm into the sella, scarring of the chiasm, or interruption of blood supply to the optic apparatus resulting from previous therapy. The visual loss may be worse and may progress more quickly than with primary empty sella syndrome (39).

Clinical Features

Review of contemporary series suggests that fewer than one-third of individuals with radiographic presence of an empty sella develop symptoms from the condition (40). Of patients with primary empty sella syndrome, more than 80% are women and more than 75% are obese. The most common ages of presentation are from 30 to 59 years (80% of patients). Neurologic presenting symptoms and signs include headaches (in up to 80% of cases reported), dizziness, seizures, impairment of balance, and rhinorrhea. Ophthalmologic complaints, which include decreased visual acuity and visual field loss, are less common (approximately 10% of patients) (37, 41). Occasionally, the patient may manifest an associated compressive endocrinopathy (26, 37, 42, 43). Endocrine symptoms leading to diagnosis of sellar pathology include amenorrhea/galactorrhea and loss of libido.

In contrast to the low frequency of endocrinologic symptoms and signs with adult empty sella syndrome, in the rare childhood presentation, endocrinologic abnormalities are present in 45 to 75% of patients (36, 44, 45). Craniofacial abnormalities and visual complaints are present in about one-third of patients. Headaches and nonspecific neurologic complaints are much less frequent than in adult patients.

Radiologic Evaluation

Plain roentgenograms usually reveal an enlarged sella, which still retains a "closed" configuration in that the posterior clinoids are not usually eroded (23, 46–48). In some patients, enlargement of the sella is associated with erosion of the sella, with posterior displacement of the dorsum sellae. The primary empty sella syndrome has been suggested to be responsible for up to 25% of enlarged sellae seen on lateral skull radiograms (49). On contemporary coronal CT scan, the empty sella appears as a low-density abnormality of the sella, often with erosion of the sellar floor (27, 37, 40, 50) (Fig. 24.2). The normal pituitary gland and infundibulum is usually displaced posteriorly and inferiorly, visualized well with intravenous contrast (50, 51).

The previous use of cisternography with CT for diagnosis has largely been supplanted by the use of present-generation MRI. On MRI, the empty sella appears isointense with cerebrospinal fluid (CSF) (T1 hypointensity and T2 hyperintensity), with the infundibular stalk traversing the sellar cavity. As with CT, the pituitary stalk and the compressed gland may be visualized and displaced posteriorly. The study of MRI signal characteristics is a useful method to differentiate an empty sella from a cystic pituitary mass; furthermore, in cystic tumors or in cases of cystic degeneration of the pituitary, the infundibular stalk cannot be identified below the top of the mass (52).

Therapy

Most patients with empty sella syndrome require no treatment. Endocrinopathy associated with primary empty sella syndrome is usually mild and may not require replacement therapy (53), and a conservative period of observation is warranted. The radiographic appearance, endocrinopathy, or visual deficit does not demonstrate progression in many cases. Conservative treatment requires rigorous endocrinologic and ophthalmologic follow-up. The associated obesity and hypertension so commonly seen with this disorder require only medical treatment. In the few cases in which progressive endocrinologic abnormalities occur, surgical intervention is warranted.

Progressive visual deterioration secondary to chiasmal stretching (54) (Fig. 24.2) also requires surgical intervention. This indication for surgery is more commonly encountered in patients with secondary empty sella syndrome. Although intradural chiasmapexy has been advocated by some authors, an extradural transsphenoidal approach has been proven to offer better results (55–58). The extradural transsphenoidal approach is performed by placing fat and fascia extradurally between the sellar floor and the dura, which avoids an intradural dissection. An interesting alternative approach advocated by Mortara and Norrell (59) is to perform a lamina terminalis otomy to vent the CSF pulsations from the third ventricle, which presumably incites the downward displacement of the median eminence and chiasm. Attempted lysis of chiasmal adhesions may result in deterioration of vision and in general is a fruitless endeavor.

CSF rhinorrhea associated with primary or secondary empty sella syndrome requires surgical intervention (58, 60, 61). As with other causes of nontraumatic CSF leak, the leak rarely ceases spontaneously. If the leak is clearly emanating from the sella, then transsphenoidal repair with fascial and fat packing is indicated (60). If increased intracranial pressure underlies the CSF leak, then measures to alleviate the increased pressure must be undertaken. CSF shunting, or tumor mass removal, should be performed as part of the overall management, and the possibility of developing a pneumocephalus after placement of a shunt must be recognized (62). For this reason, most authors advocate closure of the leak before shunting to avoid this complication.

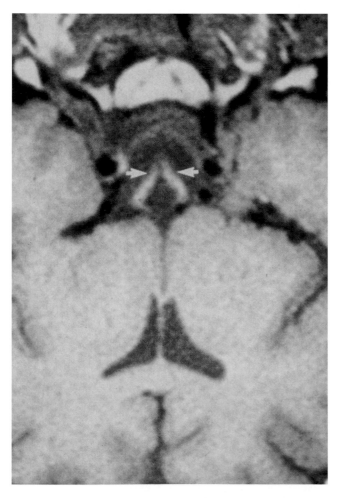

Figure 24.2. Empty sella syndrome. A 52-year-old female with progressive visual loss 8 months after transsphenoidal resection of a nonfunctional pituitary macroadenoma. Note the prolapse of the optic chiasm (*arrows*) into the sella region. This patient was successfully treated by the transsphenoidal approach with extradural chiasmapexy.

LYMPHOCYTIC HYPOPHYSITIS

The anterior pituitary gland is subject to inflammatory disorders. Originally, this "lymphocytic" or "granulomatous" hypophysitis was described most frequently in postpartum women (63–71), but more recently it has been recognized in men and in women without recent pregnancy (72–74). Lymphocytic hypophysitis may present with endocrine dysfunction and a diffuse mass, which may mimic a nonfunctional pituitary tumor.

A rare and presumably autoimmune disorder, lymphocytic hypophysitis is characterized by an extensive infiltration of the anterior pituitary with lymphocytes and plasma cells. The pathophysiologic process begins as an acute inflammatory process with diffuse enlargement of the gland (71, 75, 76). Cytotoxic lymphocytes are noted to be infiltrating the secretory cells. A preponderance of T cells over B lymphocytes exists, and T4 cells outnumber T8 cells in a ratio of 2:1 (77, 78). With continued inflammation the normal pituitary architecture becomes difficult to recognize and with progressive inflammation may ultimately progress to diffuse interstitial fibrosis and gland atrophy (70, 79). The neurohypophysis does not seem to be primarily involved with the process. The rarity of the disorder and the lack of specific radiologic or endocrinologic features have made it difficult to diagnose without a tissue biopsy.

Lymphocytic hypophysitis has been commonly noted to be associated with other autoimmune processes, strongly suggesting a common etiologic mechanism. Reported associated autoimmune diseases include thyroiditis, adrenalitis, pancreatitis, parathyroiditis, and pernicious anemia (80–82). The inciting antigen has not been identified. However, an interesting hypothesis has been put forth by Vanneste and Kamphorst (76), who noted that previous or concurrent meningitis may be an inciting etiologic factor.

Clinical Features

Lymphocytic hypophysitis should be considered in the differential diagnosis of a pituitary mass or pituitary dysfunction presenting in relation to pregnancy (63, 67–69, 83). Most reported cases have occurred in women (approximately 75% of parous women with the disorder presented within 1 year of parturition). However, results of an increasing number of reports show that lymphocytic hypophysitis is occurring in nulliparous women and men (72–74, 84, 85). Most commonly, presentation includes pituitary insufficiency, headaches, and visual field defects.

Hormonal abnormalities encountered may cover a spectrum from single hormonal insufficiency to panhypopituitarism. The most frequent presenting endocrinologic abnormality is adrenal insufficiency, with associated symptoms of nausea, vomiting, hypotension, fatigue, and anorexia. Less common presentations in the female include amenorrhea and galactorrhea. Although the presentation is usually one of anterior pituitary dysfunction, rare cases

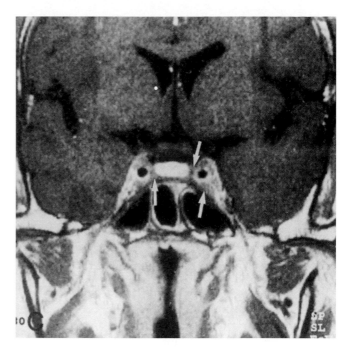

Figure 24.3.   Lymphocytic hypophysitis.

have been reported of a prominent presentation with DI (86) or clinical cavernous cranial nerve involvement (84, 87). The endocrinopathy is transient in a few reported cases, indicating that not all cases of lymphocytic hypophysitis lead to permanent hypopituitarism.

With adenohypophyseal enlargement, the patient may present with headaches or visual compromise. Both visual field and acuity deficits have been reported (88).

Radiologic Evaluation

The sella may be uniformly enlarged. Erosion of the dorsum sellae has been noted without erosion of the floor of the sella, presumably because of the short course of the disease. No strict characteristic features of the appearance of the mass exist to differentiate the lesion from a pituitary adenoma (64, 89) (Fig. 24.3). The lesion is generally homogeneous in appearance on MRI and either hypointense or isointense with brain parenchyma. The hypophysitis usually intensely enhances with gadolinium contrast on MRI (66, 90) and iodinated contrast on CT (66). When present, intense enhancement of the dura adjacent to the pituitary mass and thickening and enhancement of the pituitary stalk may suggest the diagnosis.

Therapy

Because of the rarity of the disease, lymphocytic hypophysitis has seldom been diagnosed preoperatively, and no controlled trials of therapy have been reported. In cases with evolving symptomatic chiasmal compression, transsphenoidal surgery for establishing the diagnosis and for decompression is warranted. The pituitary gland may be uniformly involved with the process; decompression should then be undertaken laterally to preserve the midline infundibulum and pituitary stalk, the posterior gland, and the portal hypophyseal system. Also, it is imperative to identify early any pituitary insufficiency to enable immediate replacement therapy, especially hypothyroidism and hypoadrenalism.

Some authors have suggested steroid therapy for suspected lymphocytic hypophysitis to decrease the immune response and the inflammation (91). In patients with suspected lymphocytic hypophysitis and a pituitary mass, a trial of steroids may be therapeutic, but the results reported to date have been variable. In some patients, the size of the gland has been reported to diminish with chronic steroid therapy, and pituitary dysfunction may recover in such cases (91, 92). However, Stelmach and O'Day (88) described a woman presenting in the third trimester of pregnancy with a rapidly evolving bitemporal hemianopia and reduced visual acuity caused by a 2-cm suprasellar mass. A short course of high-dose steroids, which was initiated to promote fetal lung maturity, produced marked resolution of the field loss. However, as the steroid level was reduced, the visual field loss recurred, which prompted a surgical exploration in which lymphocytic hypophysitis was diagnosed and a partial resection of the adenohypophysitis was undertaken. In another pregnant patient diagnosed with lymphocytic hypophysitis and treated with corticosteroids, no effect was noted either in decreasing the size of the mass or on the progressive visual loss (93). The patient subsequently underwent a partial hypophysectomy for decompression of the visual apparatus and confirmation of the diagnosis. Taken together, short-term efficacy of steroids in this disorder is unpredictable, and conservative treatment with steroids should be considered only in those patients in whom vision is not threatened (94).

PITUITARY AND SELLAR METASTASES

Either the pituitary gland directly or the sellar region may become involved with metastatic tumor spread.

A variety of tumors have been reported to metastasize to the pituitary gland itself (95), including carcinoid tumor (96); pancreatic endocrine tumor (97); rhabdomyosarcoma (98); and gastric (99), renal cell (100), breast (101–103), endometrial (100), prostate (104), lung (102), and bladder (105) carcinomas. Although clinical symptomatic metastasis represents a rare event (106,107), autopsy series indicate that metastases to the pituitary gland are not rare (108,109). In the series by Takakura et al. (110), metastases to the pituitary were present in 6% of all patients with cancer and in 20% of patients dying of breast cancer.

Extrapituitary metastases to the sellar region are uncommon, most being secondary to bony metastases of the skull base. A variety of other tumors occur in the sphenoid bone and clivus, including bony tumors and direct spread of nasopharyngeal or sphenoid sinus carcinoma, lymphoma, or plasmacytoma. Mechanisms of metastatic tumor spread to the skull base in this area include venous routes, for example, the paravertebral venous plexus, which anastomoses with the venous drainage at the base of the skull (111). During a Valsalva maneuver, blood flow is reversed through the inferior vena cava into the vertebral veins, and access to the skull base is achieved. If metastatic cells pass through dural veins, subdural seeding is possible; contiguous spread through Virchow-Robin spaces allows intracerebral metastases to occur. Direct arterial spread may occur to the region of the posterior pituitary, usually in those instances in which metastatic spread to the lungs has already occurred (the "multistep" metastatic hypothesis).

Clinical Features

When metastases do occur to the pituitary gland, the presenting symptoms are often those of progressive panhypopituitarism, DI, or visual loss. Malignancy of the pituitary fossa may mimic nonfunctional pituitary tumors clinically. Neurologic manifestations include both visual loss and cavernous cranial neuropathies; rapidly progressive visual loss, extraocular movement palsies, and facial sensory loss may help distinguish the presentation of metastatic tumor from a benign adenoma. A corollary of this is that when a pathologist evaluates an alleged "nonfunctional" adenoma, metastases should be included in the differential diagnosis.

Radiologic Evaluation

In purely pituitary metastases, the lesion may be located intrasellar or a combination of intrasellar and suprasellar (Fig. 24.4). The pituitary fossa is usually normal in these cases, attesting to the shorter latency of tumor growth than with primary pituitary tumors (112). All metastatic tumors that affect the skull base have certain MRI features in common. T1-weighted sequences typically demonstrate low-signal tumor tissue replacing the normally bright marrow fat. On T2-weighted sequences, the tumor is usually hyperintense with marrow.

Therapy

Therapy of the metastatic tumor is predicated on the primary tumor histologic features and the extent of disease elsewhere. Surgical intervention may be necessary to establish the diagnosis in many cases in which underlying carcinoma has not been diagnosed and to alleviate visual compromise from tumor mass (98, 104). Adjunctive systemic chemotherapy or local radiotherapy may then be indicated as directed by the underlying histologic features of the tumor.

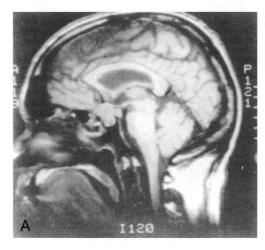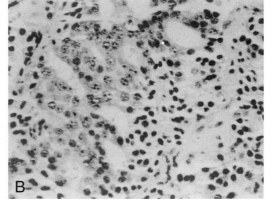

Figure 24.4. Metastatic lesions of the sella. This 61-year-old male presented with a 2-month history of increasing bifrontal headaches and peripheral visual loss. Ophthalmologic evaluation revealed a marked bitemporal hemianopia, and MRI revealed a large sellar mass with suprasellar extension **(A)**. Results of endocrinologic evaluation were normal. In the face of relentlessly progressive visual loss and questionable pituitary patho-logic features, a transsphenoidal craniotomy was performed. A firm, rubbery lesion was encountered within the parenchyma of the pituitary extending into the suprasellar cistern. Pathologic evaluation revealed adenocarcinoma compatible with a prostate primary **(B)**. (Reprinted with permission from Couldwell WT, Weiss MH. Pituitary parenchymal metastasis from adenocarcinoma of the prostate. J Neurosurg 1989;71:139.)

SUPRASELLAR GERMINOMAS

Germinomas are tumors of germ cell derivation that occur primarily in adolescents and young adults. Germ cell tumors account for 0.5 to 2% of all primary intracranial tumors but are more prevalent in Japan, constituting 2.1 to 4.5% of intracranial tumors in that country (113, 114). Within the cranium, germinomas are located most commonly in the region of the pineal gland; in the suprasellar–retrochiasmal region; within the third ventricle, interpeduncular, or quadrigeminal plate regions; or within the pituitary fossa. No sex preference has been noted in suprasellar germinomas, in contrast to the male predominance noted with tumors of the pineal region. These tumors are not encapsulated, and they infiltrate so extensively that complete surgical excision is not possible without producing extensive neurologic deficits.

Clinical Features and Radiologic Evaluation

Patients with suprasellar tumors most commonly present with DI (95% of patients), visual difficulties (including optic atrophy), or endocrinopathy (115). If tumor infiltrates into the region of the hypothalamus, the patient may develop signs of autonomic dysfunction, including changes in heart rate, blood pressure, temperature, and gastric motility. Pituitary insufficiency may be pituitary or hypothalamic in origin. Less commonly, the tumor may present by causing increased intracranial pressure with hydrocephalus

(third ventricular extension) or from associated symptoms such as Parinaud's syndrome from germinoma located in the region of the pineal gland.

Diagnosis is usually made by MRI, in which the tumors intensely enhance with gadolinium contrast (116). CSF may be informative in patients suspected of harboring a suprasellar germinoma. The spinal fluid almost always shows a pleocytosis and elevated protein content, especially if tumor is noted to involve the ependyma of the ventricular system. CSF studies should include assays for α-fetoprotein, placental alkaline phosphatase, and human chorionic gonadotropin, which may individually or all be secreted by the tumor. High levels of any of these markers may obviate the need for diagnostic surgery (117, 118).

Therapy

Therapy usually consists of surgical biopsy or partial removal for verification of histologic features. Germinomas have been demonstrated to be exquisitely sensitive to radiation therapy (119, 120). More recently, chemotherapeutic regimens including cisplatin have been used with success (121). Chemotherapy alone or in combination with radiation therapy has been reported to be an effective alternative for the treatment of suprasellar germ cell tumors of all types. Chemotherapy used alone has been advocated to avoid the deleterious long-term effects of high-dose radiation therapy on the developing nervous system in young children. Long-term survival without radiation therapy or chemotherapy is not likely.

REFERENCES

Benign Pituitary Cysts

1. Baskin DS, Wilson CB. Transsphenoidal treatment of non-neoplastic intrasellar cysts: a report of 38 cases. J Neurosurg 1984;60:8–13.
2. Berry RG, Schlezinger NS. Rathke-cleft cysts. Arch Neurol 1959;1:48–58.
3. Bysoumi ML. Rathke's cleft and it cyst. Edinburgh Med J 1948;55:745–749.
4. Fager CA, Carter H. Intrasellar epithelial cysts. J Neurosurg 1966;24:77–81.
5. McGrath P. Cysts of sellar and pharyngeal hypophyses. Pathology 1971;3:123–131.
6. Fairburn B, Larkin IM. A cyst of Rathke's cleft. J Neurosurg 1964;21:223–225.
7. Kucharczyk W, Peck WW, Kelly WM, et al. Rathke cleft cysts: CT, MR imaging, and pathological features. Radiology 1987;165:491–495.
8. Rasmussen AT. Ciliated epithelium and mucous secreting cells in the human hypophysis. Anat Rec 1929;41:273–283.
9. Rottenberg GT, Chong WK, Powell M, et al. Cyst formation of the craniopharyngeal duct. Clin Radiol 1994;49:126–129.
10. Shanklin WM. On the presence of cysts in the human pituitary. Anat Rec 1949;104:379–407.
11. Shanklin WM. The incidence and distribution of cilia in the human pituitary with a description of microfollicular cysts derived from Rathke's cleft. Acta Anat (Basel) 1951;11:361–382.
12. Oka H, Kawano N, Suwa T, et al. Radiological study of symptomatic Rathke's cleft cysts. Neurosurgery 1994;35:632–637.
13. Eguchi K, Uozumi T, Arita K, et al. Pituitary function in patients with Rathke's cleft cyst: significance of surgical management. Endocrinol J 1994;41:535–540.
14. Maggio WW, Cail WS, Brookeman JR, et al. Rathke's cleft cyst: computed tomographic and magnetic resonance imaging appearances. Neurosurgery 1987;21:60–62.
15. Nemoto Y, Inoue Y, Fukuda T, et al. MR appearance of Rathke's cleft cysts. Neuroradiology 1988;30:155–159.
16. Wagle VG, Nelson D, Rossi A, et al. Magnetic resonance imaging of symptomatic Rathke's cleft cyst: report of a case. Neurosurgery 1989;24:276–278.
17. Okamoto S, Handa H, Yamashita J, et al. Computed tomography in intra- and suprasellar epithelial cysts (symptomatic Rathke's cleft cysts). AJNR Am J Neuroradiol 1985;6:515–519.
18. Couldwell WT, Weiss MH. Transnasal transsphenoidal approach. In: Apuzzo MLJ, ed. Surgery of the Third Ventricle. 2nd ed. Baltimore: Williams & Wilkins, 1996.
19. Voelker JL, Campbell RL, Rossi A, et al. Clinical, radiographic and pathological features of symptomatic Rathke's cleft cysts. J Neurosurg 1991;74:535–544.
20. Fischer EG, DeGirolami U, Suojanen JN. Reversible visual deficit following debulking of a Rathke's cleft cyst: a tethered chiasm? J Neurosurg 1994;81:459–462.

Empty Sella Syndrome

21. Bergland RM, Ray BS, Torack RM. Anatomical variations in the pituitary gland and adjacent structures in 225 human autopsy cases. J Neurosurg 1968;28:93–99.
22. Busch W. Die Morphologie des Sella Turcica und ihre Beziehungen zur hypophyse. Virchows Arch 1951;320:437–458.
23. Kaufman B. The "empty" sella turcica: a manifestation of the intrasellar subarachnoid space. Radiology 1968;90:931–941.
24. Berke JP, Buxton LF, Kokmen E. The "empty" sella. Neurology 1975;25:1137–1143.
25. Kaye AH, Tress BM, Brownbill D, et al. Intracranial pressure in patients with the empty sella syndrome without benign intracranial hypertension. J Neurol Neurosurg Psychiatry 1982;45:209–216.
26. Lee WM, Adams JE. The empty sella syndrome. J Neurosurg 1968;28:351–356.
27. Schumacher M, Gilsbach J. A new variety of "empty sella" with cystic intrasellar dilatation of the recessus infundibuli. Br J Radiol 1979;52:862–864.
28. Dominique JN, Wing SD, Wilson CB. Coexisting pituitary adenomas and partially empty sellas. J Neurosurg 1978;48:23–28.
29. Hoyt WF, Baghdassarian SA. Optic glioma of childhood: natural history and rationale for conservative management. Br J Ophthalmol 1973;53:793.
30. Iraci G, Gerosa M, et al. Gliomas of the optic nerve and chiasm. Childs Brain 1981;8:326.
31. Friedmann G, Marguth F. Intrasellläre liquorzysten. Zentralbl Neurochir 1961;21:33–41.
32. De Paepe L, Abs R, Verlooy J, et al. Benign intracranial hypertension as a cause of transient partial pituitary deficiency. J Neurol Sci 1993;114:152–155.
33. Foley KM, Posner JB. Does pseudotumor cerebri cause the empty sella syndrome? Neurology 1975;25:565–569.
34. Login I Santen RJ. Empty sella syndrome: sequelae of spontaneous remission of acromegaly. Arch Intern Med 1975;135:1519–1521.
35. Fleckman AM, Schubart D, Caceres E, et al. Empty sella of normal size in Sheehan's syndrome. Am J Med 1983;75:585–591.
36. Costigan DC, Daneman D, Harwood-Nash D, et al. The "empty sella" in childhood. Clin Pediatr (Phila) 1984;23:437–440.
37. Gallardo E, Schacter D, Caceres E, et al. The empty sella: results of treatment in 76 successive cases and high frequency of endocrine and neurological disturbances. Clin Endocrinol (Oxf) 1992;37:529–533.
38. Matson DD, Crigler JF Jr. Management of craniopharyngioma in childhood. J Neurosurg 1977;30:377.
39. Sapiazante R, deDivitis E, Stella L, et al. The empty sella. Surg Neurol 1981;16:418–426.
40. Ferreri AJ, Garrido SA, Markarian MG, et al. Relationship between the development of diaphragma sellae and the morphology of the sella turcica and its contents. Surg Radiol Anat 1992;14:233–239.
41. Buckman MT, Husain M, Carlow TJ, et al. Primary empty sella syndrome with visual field defects. Am J Med 1976;61:124–128.
42. Brismar K, Efendíc S. Pituitary function in the empty sella syndrome. Neuroendocrinology 1981;32:70–77.
43. Buchfelder M, Brockmeier S, Pichl J, et al. Results of dynamic endocrine testing of hypothalamic pituitary function in patients with a primary "empty" sella syndrome. Horm Metab Res 1989;21:573–576.
44. Nass R, Engel M, Stoner E, et al. Empty sella syndrome in childhood. Pediatr Neurol 1986;2:224–229.
45. Wilkinson IA, Duck SC, Gager WE, et al. Empty sella syndrome: occurrence in childhood. Am J Dis Child 1982;136:245–247.
46. Gabriele OF. The empty sella syndrome. Am J Roentgenol 1968;104:168–170.
47. Kaufman B, Chamberlin WB Jr. The ubiquitous "empty" sella turcica. Acta Radiol Diagn (Stockh) 1972;13:413–425.
48. Sage MR, Chan ESR, Reilly PL. The clinical and radiological features of the empty sella syndrome. Clin Radiol 1980;31:513–519.
49. Weisberg LA, Zimmerman EA, Frantz AG. Diagnosis and evaluation of patients with an enlarged sella turcica. Am J Med 1976;61:590–596.
50. Haughton VM, Rosenbaum AE, et al. Recognizing the empty sella by CT: the infundibulum sign. Am J Roentgenol 1981;136:293.
51. Hoffman J, Barrow DL. Radiological evaluation of pituitary lesions. In: Barrow DL, Selman WR, eds. Neuroendocrinology. Baltimore: Williams & Wilkins, 1992:237–257.
52. Connolly ES, Carmel PW. Empty sella syndrome. In: Wilkins RH, Rengachary SS, eds. Neurosurgery. 2nd ed. New York: McGraw-Hill, 1996:1367–1373.
53. Pompili A, Calsova F, Appetecchia M. Evolution of primary empty sella syndrome. Lancet 1990;336:1249.
54. Bursztyn EM, Lavyne MH, Aisen M. Empty sella syndrome with intrasellar herniation of the optic chiasm. Am J Neuroradiol 1983;4:167–168.

55. Hamlyn PJ, Baer R, Ashfar F. Transsphenoidal chiasmopexy for long standing visual failures in the secondary empty sella syndrome. Br J Neurosurg 1988;2:277–279.
56. Hudgins WR, Raney LA, Young SW, et al. Failure of intrasellar muscle implants to prevent recurrent downward migration of the optic chiasm. Neurosurgery 1981;8:231–232.
57. Welch K, Stears JC. Chiasmapexy for the correction of traction on the optic nerves and chiasm associated with their descent into an empty sella: case report. J Neurosurg 1971;35:760–764.
58. Weiss MH, Kaufman B, Richards DE. Cerebrospinal fluid rhinorrhea from an empty sella: transsphenoidal obliteration of the fistula: technical note. J Neurosurg 1973;39:674–676.
59. Mortara R, Norell H. Consequences of a deficient sellar diaphragm. J Neurosurg 1970;32:565–573.
60. Couldwell WT, Weiss MH. Cerebrospinal fluid fistulae. In: Apuzzo MLJ, ed. Brain Surgery: Complication Avoidance and Management. 1992:2329–2343.
61. Garcia-Uria J, Carrillo R, Serrano P, et al. Empty sella and rhinorrhea: a report of eight treated cases. J Neurosurg 1979;50:466–471.
62. Ikeda K, Nakano M, Tani E. Tension pneumocephalus complicating ventriculoperitoneal shunt for cerebrospinal fluid rhinorrhea: case report. J Neurol Neurosurg Psychiatry 1978;41:319–322.

Lymphocytic Hypophysitis

63. Asa SL, Bilbao JM, Kovacs K, et al. Lymphocytic hypophysitis of pregnancy resulting in hypopituitarism: a distinct clinicopathological entity. Ann Intern Med 1981;95:166–171.
64. Baskin DS, Townsend JJ, Wilson CB. Lymphocytic adenohypophysitis of pregnancy simulating a pituitary adenoma: a distinct pathological entity. J Neurosurg 1982;56:148–153.
65. Holck S, Laursen H. Prolactinoma coexistent with granulomatous hypophysitis. Acta Neuropathol (Berl) 1983;61:253–257.
66. Levine SN, Benzel EC, Fowler MR, et al. Lymphocytic adenohypophysitis: clinical, radiological, and magnetic resonance imaging characterization. Neurosurgery 1988;22:937–941.
67. Molitch ME, Hedley-White T. Case records of the Massachusetts General Hospital, Case 5–1985: a 33-year-old woman with a question of pituitary tumor. N Engl J Med 1985;312:297–305.
68. Naik RG, Ammini A, Shah P, et al. Lymphocytic hypophysitis. Case report. J Neurosurg 1994;80:925–927.
69. Patel MC, Guneratne N, Haq N, et al. Peripartum hypopituitarism and lymphocytic hypophysitis. QJM 1995;88:571–580.
70. Sautner D, Saeger W, Ludecke DK, et al. Hypophysitis in surgical and autopsy specimens. Acta Neuropathol (Berl) 1995;90:637–644.
71. Thodou E, Asa SL, Kontogeorgos G, et al. Clinical case seminar: lymphocytic hypophysitis: clinicopathological findings. J Clin Endocrinol Metab 1995;80:2302–2311.
72. Hartmann I, Tallen G, Graf KJ, et al. Lymphocytic hypophysitis simulating a pituitary adenoma in a nonpregnant woman. Clin Neuropathol 1996;15:234–239.
73. Lee JH, Laws ER Jr, Guthrie BL, et al. Lymphocytic hypophysitis: occurrence in two men. Neurosurgery 1994;34:159–162.
74. McCutcheon IE, Oldfield EH. Lymphocytic adenohypophysitis presenting as infertility: case report. J Neurosurg 1991;74:821–826.
75. Mayfield RK, Levine JH, Gordon L, et al. Lymphoid adenohypophysitis presenting as a pituitary tumor. Am J Med 1980;69:619–623.
76. Vanneste JAL, Kamphorst W. Lymphocytic hypophysitis. Surg Neurol 1987;28:145–149.
77. Jensen MD, Hardwerger BS, Scheithauer BW, et al. Lymphoid hypophysitis with isolated corticotropin deficiency. Ann Intern Med 1986;105:200–203.
78. Parent AD, Cruse JM, Smith EE, et al. Lymphocytic hypophysitis: autoimmune reaction? Adv Biosci 1988;69:465–469.
79. Nishioka H, Ito H, Miki T, et al. A case of lymphocytic hypophysitis with massive fibrosis and the role of surgical intervention. Surg Neurol 1994;42:74–78.
80. Gleason TH, Stebbins PL, Shanahan MF. Lymphoid hypophysitis in a patient with hypoglycemic episodes. Arch Pathol Lab Med 1978;102:46–48.
81. Lack EE. Lymphoid "hypophysitis" with end organ insufficiency. Arch Pathol Lab Med 1975;99:215–219.
82. Sobrinho-Simtes M, Brandno A, Paiva ME, et al. Lymphoid hypophysitis in a patient with lymphoid thyroiditis, lymphoid adrenalitis, and idiopathic retroperitoneal fibrosis. Arch Pathol Lab Med 1985;109:230–233.
83. Abe T, Matsumoto K, Sanno N, et al. Lymphocytic hypophysitis: case report. Neurosurgery 1995;36:1016–1019.
84. Nussbaum CE, Okawara SH, Jacobs LS. Lymphocytic hypophysitis with involvement of the cavernous sinus and hypothalamus. Neurosurgery 1991;28:440–444.
85. Pestell RG, Best JD, Alford FP. Lymphocytic hypophysitis: the clinical spectrum of the disorder and evidence for an autoimmune pathogenesis. Clin Endocrinol Oxf 1990;33:457–466.
86. Koshiyama H, Sato H, Yorita S, et al. Lymphocytic hypophysitis presenting with diabetes insipidus: case report and literature review. Endocrinol J 1994;41:93–97.
87. Supler ML, Mickle JP. Lymphocytic hypophysitis: report of a case in a man with cavernous sinus involvement. Surg Neurol 1992;37:472–476.
88. Stelmach M, O'Day J. Rapid change in visual fields associated with suprasellar lymphocytic hypophysitis. J Clin Neuroophthalmol 1991;11:19–24.
89. Hungerford GD, Biggs PJ, Levine JH, et al. Lymphoid adenohypophysitis with radiologic and clinical findings resembling a pituitary tumor. Am J Neuroradiol 1982;3:444–446.
90. Ahmadi J, Myers GS, Segall HD, et al. Lymphocytic adenohypophysitis: contrast-enhanced MRI imaging in five cases. Radiology 1995;195:30–34.
91. Bitton RN, Slavin M, Decker RE, et al. The course of lymphocytic hypophysitis. Surg Neurol 1991;37:71.
92. Beressi N, Cohen R, Beressi JP, et al. Pseudotumoral lymphocytic hypophysitis successfully treated by corticosteroid alone: first case report. Neurosurgery 1994;35:505–508.
93. Reusch JE, Kleinschmidt-DeMasters BK, Lillehei KO, et al. Preoperative diagnosis of lymphocytic hypophysitis unresponsive to short course dexamethasone: case report. Neurosurgery 1992;30:268–272.
94. Prasad A, Madan VS, Sethi PK, et al. Lymphocytic hypophysitis: can open exploration of the sella be avoided? Br J Neurosurg 1991;5:639–642.

Pituitary and Sellar Metastases

95. Sioutos P, Yen V, Arbit E. Pituitary gland metastases. Ann Surg Oncol 1996;3:94–99.
96. Rossi ML, Bevan JS, Fleming KA, et al. Pituitary metastasis from malignant bronchial carcinoid. Tumori 1988;74:101–105.
97. Genka S, Soeda H, Takahashi M, et al. Acromegaly, diabetes insipidus, and visual loss caused by metastatic growth hormone-releasing hormone-producing malignant pancreatic endocrine tumor in the pituitary gland. J Neurosurg 1995;83:719–723.
98. Jalalah S, Kovacs K, Horvath E, et al. Rhabdomyosarcoma in the region of the sella turcica. Acta Neurochir (Wien) 1988;88:142.
99. van-Seters AP, Bots GT, van-Dulken H, et al. Metastasis of an occult gastric carcinoma suggesting growth of a prolactinoma during bromocriptine therapy: a case report with a review of the literature. Neurosurgery 1985;16:813–817.
100. McCormick PC, Post KD, Kandji AD, et al. Metastatic carcinoma to the pituitary gland. Br J Neurosurg 1989;3:71–79.
101. Chaudhuri R, Twelves C, Cos TC, et al. MRI in diabetes insipidus due to metastatic breast carcinoma. Clin Radiol 1992;46:184–188.
102. Juneau P, Schoene WC, Black P. Malignant tumors of the pituitary gland. Arch Neurol 1992;49:555–558.
103. Mayr NA, Yuh WTC, Muhonen MG, et al. Pituitary metastases: MR findings. J Comput Assist Tomogr 1993;17:432–437.
104. Couldwell WT, Weiss MH. Pituitary parenchymal metastasis from adenocarcinoma of the prostate. J Neurosurg 1989;71:138.
105. Kawamura J, Tsukamoto K, Yamakawa K, et al. Diabetes insipidus due to pituitary metastasis from bladder cancer. Urol Int 1991;46:217–220.
106. Branch CL Jr, Laws ER Jr. Metastatic tumors of the sella turcica masquerading as primary pituitary tumors. J Clin Endocrinol Metab 1987;65:469–474.
107. Ruelle A, Palladino M, Andrioli GC. Pituitary metastases as presenting lesions of malignancy. J Neurosurg Sci 1992;36:51–54.
108. Kovacs K. Metastatic cancer of the pituitary gland. Oncology 1973;27:533–542.

109. Nelson PB, Robinson AG, Martinez AJ. Metastatic tumor of the pituitary gland. Neurosurgery 1987;21:941–944.

110. Takakura K, Sano K, Hojo S, et al. Metastatic Tumors of the Central Nervous System. Tokyo: Igaku-Shoin, 1982.

111. Batson OV. The function of the vertebral veins and their role in the spread of metastases. Ann Surg 1940;112:138–149.

112. Schubiger O, Haller D. Metastases to the pituitary-hypothalamic axis: an MR study of 7 symptomatic patients. Neuroradiology 1992;34:131–134.

Suprasellar Germinomas

113. Jellinger K. Primary intracranial germ cell tumors. Acta Neuropathol (Berl) 1973;25:291–306.

114. Walsh JW. Suprasellar germinomas. In: Wilkins RH, Rengachary SS, eds. Neurosurgery. 2nd ed. New York: McGraw-Hill, 1996: 1407–1410.

115. Buchfelder M, Fahlbusch R, Walther M, et al. Endocrine disturbances in suprasellar germinomas. Acta Endocrinol (Copnh) 1989; 120:337–342.

116. Fujisawa I, Asato R, Okumura R, et al. Magnetic resonance imaging of neurohypophyseal germinomas. Cancer 1991;68: 1009–1014.

117. Allen JC, Nisselbaum J, Wepstien F, et al. Alphafetoprotein and human chorionic gonadotropin determination in cerebrospinal fluid: an aid to the diagnosis and management of intracranial germ-cell tumors. J Neurosurg 1979;51:368–374.

118. Shinoda J, Miwa Y, Sakai N, et al. Immunohistochemical study of placental alkaline phosphatase in primary intracranial germ-cell tumors. J Neurosurg 1985;63:733–739.

119. Jenkin RDT, Simpson WJK, Keen CW. Pineal and suprasellar germinomas: results of radiation treatment. J Neurosurg 1978;48: 99–107.

120. Sung DI, Harisliadis L, Chang CH. Midline pineal tumors and suprasellar germinomas: highly curable by irradiation. Radiology 1978;128:745–751.

121. Patel SR, Buckner JC, Smithson WA, et al. Cisplatin-based chemotherapy in primary central nervous system germ cell tumors. J Neurooncol 1992;12:47–52.

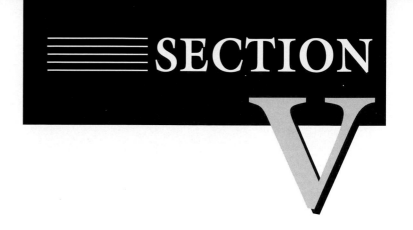

SECTION V

Surgery of Pituitary Lesions

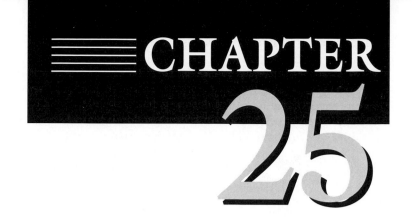

Pituitary Tumors: Anesthetic Considerations

Ghaleb A. Ghani

INTRODUCTION

Surgery on the pituitary gland through the transsphenoidal approach presents the anesthesiologist with particular problems. The anesthesiologist shares the airway with the surgeon. The pathologic features in the pituitary gland can have major impact on the anesthetic management. The patient is prone to particular complications in the perioperative period.

PREOPERATIVE EVALUATION

Most patients are currently evaluated as outpatients a few days before surgery. A thorough medical history is taken. The anesthesiologist will have the advantage of the endocrinologist's evaluation and the results of the different hormonal levels. The list of patient medications is reviewed. Special attention is given to thyroid and steroid replacement therapy, including the dosages. Patients receiving bromocriptine are asked about symptoms of gastroparesis (possible increased risk of aspiration), vomiting, and orthostatic hypotension—known side effects of the drug (1). Occasionally, medications are discontinued during the en-docrine evaluation. These drugs need to be restarted as soon as the workup is completed. This is especially important for thyroid replacement therapy. Patients with acromegaly need a special evaluation for airway changes. Patients are asked about snoring, restless sleep, and somnolence in the day time, which are symptoms of sleep apnea caused by the airway changes. Cardiovascular system evaluation includes history of exercise tolerance and angina. Blood pressure is measured. The electrocardiogram is examined for conduction defects, ischemia, and ventricular hypertrophy. Physical examination should include cardiac auscultation for heart murmurs caused by the aortic or mitral valve dysfunction. Patient's hands should be examined for collateral circulation to the fingers from the ulnar artery. This is done by performing the Allen's test (2). If the result of the Allen's test is abnormal, and an arterial line is planned, then an alternate site such as the dorsalis pedis or brachial artery should be used instead of the radial artery. The patient is instructed to have nothing by mouth after midnight before the day of surgery, except medications. Patients who are obese, who are receiving bromocriptine, or who have symptoms of gastroesophageal reflux are given a histamine H_2 receptors blocker and antacid at bedtime the night before surgery. These medications, along with any antihypertensive drugs, beta-blockers, and thyroid replacement, are also taken the morning of surgery with a few sips of water. If an awake endotracheal intubation is planned, then the patient should be prepared mentally and physically. An explanation is given to the patient of the need for and the various steps of the procedure. Also, a "drying agent," e.g., 0.2 mg of glycopyrrolate, is ordered to be given intramuscularly 30 minutes to 1 hour before the intubation procedure starts.

TRANSSPHENOIDAL PROCEDURES

Anesthetic Management

Intraoperative monitors include the standard American Society of Anesthesiologists monitors (noninvasive blood pressure, electrocardiogram, pulse oximeter, end-tidal carbon dioxide, temperature, and esophageal stethoscope). Invasive monitors are dictated by the diagnosis, the patient's general health, and the concurrent diseases. An arterial line is used in patients with acromegaly, Cushing's disease, labile blood pressure, pulmonary disease, or coronary artery disease. An arterial line is also recommended if there is a need for frequent blood sampling for glucose measurement or arterial blood gases. Extra invasive monitors like central venous pressure or pulmonary artery catheter are dictated by the presence of other concomitant diseases. This will also depend on the anesthesiologist's judgment. Newfield et al. (3) reported the occurrence of venous air embolism in 3 of 31 consecutive patients who underwent transsphenoidal operations. They recommended the use of precordial Doppler and a right atrial catheter during this procedure. However, they placed their patients in a semisitting position with the head tilted up about 40°. We position our patients flat with minimal head elevation. In this position, the risk of venous air embolism is minimal, and our experience supports this view. We monitor our patients with end-tidal carbon dioxide and end-tidal nitrogen. We believe that the routine use of precordial Doppler and the right atrial catheter is not needed. Occasionally, a central venous pressure line is necessary for good venous access, e.g., in patients who are obese or who have Cushing's disease and whose peripheral veins are difficult to cannulate. Because the anesthesiologist will have access to the left arm, the intravenous access and arterial line should be inserted in the left arm if possible. This will make drug infusion and blood sampling easier and faster. The anesthesiologist will also be able to evaluate the lines for proper function during the procedure. Insertion of a Foley catheter used to be our practice, but we have discontinued it in the past few years. If the patient is unable to urinate in the postoperative period, a Foley catheter is inserted then.

Because of the technical difficulties, we do not use visual evoked response during pituitary surgery. This view is shared by others (4). Also, there is a concern that direct pressure on the eye globe can cause corneal abrasion or blindness (5). However, patients should be evaluated for visual acuity and extraocular eye movements as soon as they emerge from anesthesia. This evaluation should be repeated in the postanesthesia care unit. Visual loss or extraocular eye movement deficit can be caused by hematoma in the pituitary bed (6–9). In that case, the patient may need to be taken back to surgery for evacuation of the hematoma (6, 8).

The agent chosen for induction is not critical. One can choose thiopental sodium (Pentothal), etomidate, or propofol and adjust the dose according to the individual patient. Propofol is a better choice as an induction agent for patients with hyperactive airway diseases such as asthma or a long-standing history of smoking. Conversely, etomidate causes less cardiovascular depression, making it the preferable agent for induction in high-risk patients. These induction agents are generally used in combination with a short-acting narcotic such as fentanyl or sufentanil. The choice of muscle relaxants will depend on the status of the airway, heart rate, blood pressure, and liver and renal functions.

The airway is not easily accessible to the anesthesiologist once the procedure is started. The endotracheal tube (ETT) has to be inserted orally and not nasally. Because of the way the head and neck are positioned and the anesthesia circuit is arranged, a regular (polyvinyl chloride) ETT may get kinked in the pharynx or at the corner of the mouth. The use of a reinforced ETT will avoid this problem.

The ETT is positioned in the left corner of the mouth. Because the surgeon makes the incision under the upper lip, the upper lip cannot be used to fix the ETT. Instead, the tube is taped to the left side of the face and to the submandibular area in a transverse fashion (Fig. 25.1). An oral airway is not inserted during the procedure because it interferes with the surgery. An esophageal stethoscope, however, is inserted and is taped to the side of the ETT. In patients with a thick beard, the ETT can be wired to one of the left upper premolar teeth. If this option is used,

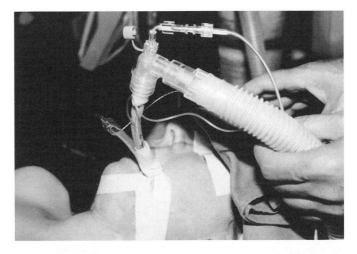

Figure 25.1. The ETT is placed in the left corner of the mouth, fixed with tape over the left side of the face and the submandibular area. No tape is put on the upper lip. An esophageal stethoscope is inserted along the ETT.

one should remember to cut the wire at the end of the procedure, while the patient is still in a suitable level of anesthesia. If a reinforced ETT is used, then the anesthesiologist must insert an oral airway after the procedure is completed but before the patient is awakened from anesthesia to prevent the patient from biting on the tube. If the patient bites on the reinforced tube, it will collapse. Once this happens, most brands of reinforced tubes will not reexpand, causing an airway obstruction. An ophthalmic ointment is placed in the conjunctival sacs and the eyes are taped shut. After the ETT is secured, the operating room table is turned around about 45° to the right.

In patients with large (10 mm or more) tumors, a catheter or a needle is inserted into the subarachnoid space in the lumbar area. This is done after induction of anesthesia. If a needle is used, a special mattress that has a cutout that allows the needle to protrude undisturbed when the patient is supine, will be necessary (10). If this option is chosen, efforts should be made during positioning of the patient to be sure that the needle is not against the edge of the mattress. The catheter or needle is connected to a drainage system. After verification of free flow of cerebrospinal fluid (CSF), the drainage control is turned to the "off" position.

Before the three-points head holder is applied by the surgeon, efforts need to be made to minimize the hypertensive and cardiac response to this stimulating step. This can be done by deepening the anesthetic with inhalational or intravenous agents or by giving a vasoactive drug like nitroglycerine or esmolol. Also, the sites of the head holder in the scalp can be infiltrated with a local anesthetic before applying the pins. The head is positioned in flexion of the neck, extension of the head, and rotation to the right. The anesthesiologist should guard the ETT during this process to prevent accidental extubation. After the final position, auscultation of the chest is done to exclude endobronchial intubation. A folded sheet is put on the patient's chest and the ETT and anesthesia circuit is allowed to rest on that sheet. This is done to minimize the risk of accidental extubation of the trachea by the surgeon's manipulations. The anesthesia circuit is anchored over the sheet with tape originating from the patient's right shoulder (Fig. 25.2).

The arrangement of the different teams is shown in Figure 25.3. We generally do not use fluoroscopy. The right arm is tucked securely on the operating room table, and the left arm is secured on an arm board. The arm board is adjusted to allow the surgeon to have access to the left lower quadrant of the abdomen to harvest a piece of fat. Occasionally, a lateral radiograph of the skull is needed to assist the surgeon in getting "reoriented." The anesthesiologist should accommodate the radiology technician during this process. Of more importance, vigilance is heightened during this process to prevent or discover an interruption of the monitors or disconnections in the anesthesia circuit and the ETT.

Some advocate insertion of a pharyngeal pack so blood does not gravitate into the stomach and cause postoperative nausea and vomiting (10). We believe that this is not neces-

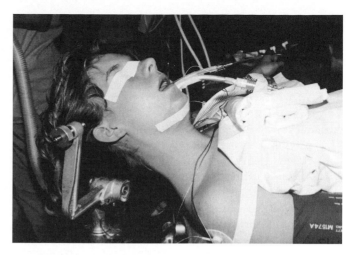

Figure 25.2. The patient is positioned for the procedure using the head holder. No oral airway is in place. The ETT connector and the anesthesia circuit rest on a sheet placed on the patient's chest. The circuit is anchored with adhesive tape originating from the patient's right shoulder. The right arm is tucked securely on the operating room bed.

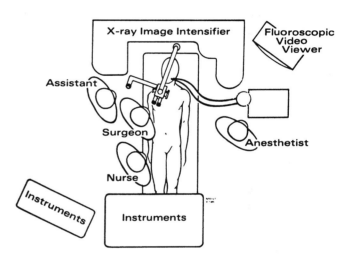

Figure 25.3. Operating room arrangement for transsphenoidal pituitary procedures showing the location of the team members and equipment. (Reprinted with permission from the Mayo Foundation from Black S, Cucchiara R. Clinical Neuroanesthesia. In: Cucchiara RF, Mitchenfelder JD, eds. New York: Churchill Livingstone, 1990:304.)

sary and therefore do not practice it. Frequently the surgeon applies cotton applicators, soaked with 4% cocaine, to the nasal mucosa for the vasoconstrictive effect. In patients with severe coronary artery disease or history of dysrhythmias, cocaine should not be used. An alternate vasoconstriction agent, e.g., oxymetazoline hydrochloride (Afrin), can be used instead.

General anesthesia is maintained with an inhalational agent. A muscle relaxant is frequently used. Use of the muscle relaxant is not necessary if a high concentration of the inhalational agent is used and tolerated by the patient. If the inhalational agent concentration is low, then the use of a muscle relaxant becomes necessary to eliminate the risk of the patient's movement. Addition of a short-acting narcotic, like fentanyl, is highly desirable in our view. The big advantage of the use of narcotics is the smooth emergence. When narcotics are used, patients generally tolerate the ETT well, without straining or bucking on emergence. This view is shared by others (10). Ventilation is controlled mechanically to maintain normocarbia or mild hypocarbia.

The volume of intravenous fluids needed include the fluid deficit, maintenance and blood loss replacement. Because the surgical field is small, the "third space" loss and evaporation of fluids is minimal. This fact should be kept in mind when one estimates the fluids requirements. The sella turcica is bordered by the cavernous sinuses and internal carotid arteries. Injury to these structures, although rare, can cause a large amount of blood loss. Therefore, one has to secure good venous access in advance if the need for rapid fluid transfusion arises. However, in our experience, the need for blood transfusion in transsphenoidal procedures is extremely rare. It is common to have episodes of hypertension and tachycardia during the procedure. The cause of these episodes is thought to be secondary to the surgical stimulation and/or the use of epinephrine or cocaine by the surgeon. These episodes are transient and can be treated by deepening the anesthetic level or a bolus of vasoactive drug like nitroglycerine or esmolol. Abou-Madi et al. (11) reported significant reduction in the hypertensive and tachycardic response during the nasal dissection by infiltrating the upper gingiva, nasal mucosa, nasal septum, and floor of the nose with 1% lidocaine with 1/200,000 epinephrine. Caution needs to be exercised with the use of local anesthetics because if they are injected into the cribriform plate and subarachnoid space, a total spinal anesthesia may occur (12).

If a lumbar subarachnoid catheter or needle was inserted, the surgeon may ask the anesthesiologist to drain a certain volume of CSF. This is done generally by gravity and not by active aspiration. The surgeon may need to increase the CSF pressure to secure complete resection of the tumor. Some centers inject air for that purpose (13). We inject normal saline. One must use *preservative-free* solution. The injection of air or saline should be done under strict sterile conditions. If air is injected then nitrous oxide (N_2O) should be eliminated from the anesthetic mixture, otherwise the injected air will increase in size by diffusion of N_2O to the air space. An alternative is to inject a filtered $N_2O–O_2$ mixture withdrawn from the inspired gas line. If this is done, then N_2O does not need to be discontinued. Injection of $N_2O–O_2$ mixture instead of air may be necessary if N_2O, narcotics, relaxant technique is being used.

Because of the potential loss of adrenocorticotropic hormone, glucocorticoid therapy is necessary. Our method is to give 100 mg of hydrocortisone intravenously at the beginning of the procedure. This is repeated every 8 hours in the postoperative period. Patients with a history of elevated blood glucose level secondary to diabetes mellitus, Cushing's disease, or acromegaly will need intraoperative moni-

toring of blood glucose level. If hyperglycemia is diagnosed, then insulin administration may be required. The guidelines for insulin administration are outlined in a recent review (14).

Occasionally the surgeon requests a Valsalva maneuver. The object of this is to check for hemostasis, to look for a CSF leak, or to bring the tumor into the sella. The maneuver is done manually with the bag in the circuit. If the patient is not deeply anesthetized, the Valsalva maneuver may cause the patient to buck secondary to the stretch reflex. It is preferable to take measures to prevent this. A dose of intravenous lidocaine or an intravenous agent like thiopental sodium or propofol will be adequate.

After the adenoma is excised, closure of the wound takes a short time. This point should be kept in mind for adjusting the anesthetic drugs. In the process of closing the surgical wound, the surgeon will insert bilateral nasopharyngeal airways of the appropriate size. These nasal airways help in maintaining the airway patent after extubation. This is important if the upper airway is compromised, such as in the acromegalic patient (15). The nasal airways can also be used to suction blood from the pharynx, both before and after extubation. Because the patient's head is fixed with the three-points head holder, an appropriate level of anesthesia should be maintained until the head holder is removed. Efforts are made to minimize the risk of coughing and bucking during the process of removal of the head holder. Lidocaine, 1.5 mg/kg given intravenously, is effective for that purpose.

Once the head holder is removed, the anesthesiologist has access to the patient's airway. The muscle relaxant is reversed. An oral airway is inserted and blood in the pharynx is suctioned. N_2 and other inhalational agents are turned off. When the patient is breathing adequately and is responsive to commands, the ETT is removed. It is not uncommon for the systemic blood pressure to be elevated at this stage. If this increase is excessive, especially if there are electrocardiographic changes of myocardial ischemia, the hypertension should be treated. The drug of choice depends on the patient's history. If the patient is known to be hypertensive, then labetalol is a good choice, especially if the hypertension is accompanied by an increase in the heart rate, as is usually the case. Patients with no history of hypertension are better treated with a short-acting agent like nitroglycerine. Esmolol can be added to the nitroglycerine if the heart rate is elevated. One has to keep in mind that hypertension at this stage can be caused by pain. If that is the case, then an analgesic (e.g., fentanyl) should be given. Analgesics at this stage should be given in small increments. If the dose is excessive, the patient may develop upper airway obstruction and hypoventilation. Before the analgesic drug is given, the anesthesiologist should be certain that the patient is not suffering from hypoxia or hypercarbia.

If a needle was inserted in the lumbar spinal canal, then that needle is removed before the patient awakens from anesthesia. If, conversely, a catheter was used, then one has the option of either taking the catheter out or leaving it in place to drain CSF. That decision is made by the surgeon. The deciding factors are the size of the tumor, the size of the ventricles preoperatively, and the possibility of developing CSF rhinorrhea.

Acromegaly

Acromegaly is the result of excessive secretion of growth hormone in the adults. Clinical manifestations include hyperhidrosis, headache, visual disturbances, amenorrhea, impotence, diabetes mellitus, and carpal tunnel syndrome (1).

Using the Allen's test, Campkin (16) reported an impaired ulnar artery circulation, to one or both hands, in 5 of 10 patients with acromegaly. He cautioned against inserting an intra-arterial catheter in the radial artery in these patients. Instead he used the dorsalis pedis artery. Our experience, however, doesn't resemble that of Campkin. We use the radial artery for the intra-arterial catheter. We had no ischemic problems to the fingers in more than 100 patients with acromegaly.

Two other aspects of the disease are important to the anesthesiologist: the airway changes and cardiovascular manifestations. The airway changes in acromegalic patients are listed in Table 25.1.

After a thorough evaluation of the airway, a decision has to be made between "awake" fiberoptic intubation or intubation conventionally (general anesthesia, muscle relaxant, and rigid laryngoscopy). Because the changes in the larynx and pharynx cannot be fully evaluated before induction of anesthesia, we believe that awake fiberoptic intubation should be the first choice to secure the insertion of the ETT. The conventional method is reserved for mild degrees of the disease, especially if combined with favorable airway anatomy or the patient's refusal of awake intubation. An advantage of fiberoptic intubation, besides securing the airway under a controlled environment, is avoiding trauma to the airway, which may predispose the patient to postoperative airway problems.

A blind nasal intubation is not an option because the *nasal* ETT will interfere with the surgical approach. *Asleep* fiberoptic intubation is not recommended because of the difficulty in visualizing the laryngeal structures secondary to anatomic changes in the airway and loss of muscle tone under general anesthesia and muscle relaxation. If one chooses to perform the intubation under general anesthesia, it is recommended to use succinylcholine for muscle relaxation. This will facilitate awakening the patient if endotracheal intubation was unsuccessful. Although tracheostomy has been suggested in acromegalic patients (17, 18, 26), experience in the fiberoptic technique in the last decade or so made the need for tracheostomy unnecessary (19, 27, 28).

Cardiovascular manifestations in acromegaly include systemic hypertension (29), cardiomegaly, accelerated coronary artery disease, aortic and mitral valve disease (30), cardiomyopathy, conduction defects (31–33), congestive

Table 25.1. *Airway Changes in Acromegaly*

Prognathism
Spreading of lower teeth
Thickened lips
Enlarged tongue (17)
Large nose, hypertrophy of nasal turbinates (18)
Hypertrophy of the soft palate and tonsils and pharyngeal mucosa (18)
Hypertrophy of laryngeal structures (epiglottis, aryepiglottic folds, ventricular folds, and vocal cords) (17, 19)
Fixation of vocal cords (20, 21)
Narrowing of the glottis (17, 21)
Calcification and ossification of the laryngeal cartilages (22)
Narrowing of the cricoid width (23)
Decreased range of motion in the cricoarytenoid joints
Enlarged larynx externally
Recurrent laryngeal nerve palsy (24)
Hoarsness and coarseness of voice (24)

The implications of these changes are as follows:
Tendency to have a sleep apnea (1, 25).
Difficult mask fit, which may make positive-pressure ventilation, with the mask, difficult. There may be a need for a larger face mask.
Airway obstruction after induction of general anesthesia. Maintaining the airway patent, with the use of oral airway and jaw thrust, may be difficult if not impossible.
Visualization of the laryngeal structures, by the rigid laryngoscope, may be difficult or not possible (17, 26).
Because of the glottis narrowing, there is a need to choose an endotracheal tube smaller than the standard size for patients of the same sex, size, and age.
Patient may have the tendency to have postoperative airway obstruction (22). This necessitates caution in the use of anesthetic agents, especially narcotics and hypnotics, and the need to keep the endotracheal tube in place until the patient is responsive to commands. Trauma to the airway, on induction, should be avoided.

How to secure the airway in the acromegalic patient will depend on:
The extent of airway changes by the disease.
The presence or absence of other features known to make endotracheal intubation difficult.
The skills and preferences of the anesthesiologist.
The patient's psychological status.

heart failure (29, 30, 33), and arrythmias. Most arrhythmias are supraventricular, and their presence warrants a search for hyperthyroidism (29). Patients with long-standing sleep apnea may develop pulmonary hypertension and right heart failure. The implications of these manifestations are as follows:

1. The patient may need preoperative evaluation by the cardiologist. These changes are quantitated but, more important, the patient's condition should be optimized.

2. Intraoperatively, the patient will need more invasive monitors: an intra-arterial catheter is usually needed. The need to insert a central venous pressure or pulmonary artery catheter will be dictated by the

patient's condition and the anesthesiologist's judgment.

3. The patient's response to painful stimuli, anesthetics, and vasoactive drugs tends to be exaggerated. Extra efforts should be made to predict and minimize these responses by proper selection of drugs, the doses and timing of giving the drugs in relation to various steps of the procedure.

4. Postoperatively, the patient may need to be taken care of in the intensive care unit.

Cushing's Disease

This disease is caused by adrenocorticotropic hormone–secreting adenomas. Clinical features include truncal obesity, short neck with buffalo hump, hirsutism, acne, plethora, hypertension, diabetes mellitus, mental disturbances, menstrual or libido disorders, myopathy, and osteoporosis (4). Sleep apnea exists in one-third of the patients. Excessive daytime drowsiness and snoring are frequent complaints (34). Left ventricular hypertrophy is often seen and is thought to be caused by hypertension. Echocardiographic studies indicate that the left ventricular hypertrophy may be accompanied by asymmetric septal hypertrophy, which may resolve following treatment (35). Patients frequently complain of symptoms of gastroesophageal reflux. Hypokalemic alkalosis secondary to excess mineralocorticoids may be present. Easy bruisability makes the skin susceptible to injury. Because of this and the osteoporosis, patients should be handled gently during transportation. Tape on the skin should be removed carefully.

Patients are at increased risk of infection because of the immunosuppressive effect of glucocorticoids (36–38). Extra attention therefore should be given to the aseptic technique. Patients with Cushing's disease tend to bleed excessively. One, however, has to be careful with fluid transfusion because these patients have fluid retention and hypertension. Postoperatively, patients who are cured will require maintenance of glucocorticoid therapy (39).

Anesthetic management differs in the following:

1. Use of H_2 blockers and antacids in the perioperative period is encouraged.

2. Because of the obesity and the frequent symptoms of gastroesophageal reflux, rapid sequence induction may be necessary to minimize the risk of aspiration.

3. Airway management with the mask and endotracheal intubation is generally harder than usual. However, the need for awake fiberoptic intubation is rare.

4. Venous access may be difficult, therefore central venous access may be necessary.

5. A direct arterial line is highly desirable because of the need to monitor the blood glucose level and arterial blood gases. Direct blood pressure monitoring will make the management of the labile blood pressure easier.

6. The hypertensive response to painful stimuli tends to be excessive. Effort, therefore, should be made to minimize these responses.

Prolactinomas

Prolactin-secreting adenomas represent approximately 40% of pituitary tumors (39). These tumors cause galactorrhea, amenorrhea, and infertility in females and impotence in males. By the time the diagnosis is made, these adenomas tend to be larger in males than in females. Patients with prolactinomas tend to be young and in good health. Invasive monitors are generally not indicated unless the patient has another concurrent disease.

Pituitary Apoplexy

Pituitary apoplexy, an acute clinical syndrome, results from pituitary hemorrhage or infarction. It is characterized by headache, vomiting, ocular paresis, visual loss, photophobia, facial pain or numbness, and decreased level of consciousness. Sixty-two percent of patients reported having previous endocrine symptoms (40). The procedure is frequently done on an urgent basis to prevent visual loss. Replacement of corticosteroid will be necessary. Maneuvers like hyperventilation, the use of mannitol, and CSF drainage may be necessary to improve the surgical access (40–42). Postoperatively most patients will need steroid and thyroid replacement therapy.

Bifrontal Craniotomy

For large tumors that extend outside the sella, the surgical approach may require frontal craniotomy. The anesthetic management is beyond the scope of this chapter but will follow the basic principles of neuroanesthesia. CSF drainage from the lumbar spinal canal is highly recommended. Measures to relax the brain—osmotic diuretics, hyperventilation, proper use of anesthetic drugs, and proper positioning of the head and neck—are applied. Monitors should include an arterial line and a Foley catheter. A supplemental dose of glucocorticoids is necessary. Patients have a higher incidence of developing diabetes insipidus (DI). The diagnosis of DI is complicated by the fact that these patients frequently receive mannitol. From our experience, when DI develops, it starts a few hours after the start of the surgical dissection. The polyuria starts after the diuresis caused by mannitol therapy has tapered off. Once the diagnosis of DI is made, our treatment of choice is aqueous vasopressin (5 to 10 units subcutaneously). Postoperatively, the patient is admitted to the neurointensive care unit.

CSF Rhinorrhea

Occasionally, a patient with CSF rhinorrhea will need surgical repair of the CSF leak. The anesthetic implications of this procedure are as follows:

1. Patients may have pneumocephalus (43); therefore, N_2O should not be used in the anesthetic mixture, otherwise the pneumocephalus will increase in size.

2. Positive-pressure ventilation with the mask *theoretically* can cause bacteria in the nasopharynx to be pushed into the subarachnoid space. Therefore, positive-pressure ventilation before endotracheal intubation is not encouraged. The anesthetic technique of choice in this circumstance is rapid sequence induction.

3. Insertion of a lumbar CSF catheter is necessary to drain CSF postoperatively. This will decrease the intracranial pressure and allow the surgical repair to heal.

4. The surgeon may need the anesthesiologist's help to localize the site of the CSF leak by Valsalva maneuver.

5. On emergence from anesthesia, extra efforts are taken by the anesthesiologist to prevent coughing and bucking. Adding short-acting narcotics (e.g., fentanyl or sufentanil) to the anesthetic drugs will aid this goal. Lidocaine, 1.5 mg/kg intravenously, is also given at this stage for the same purpose.

Postanesthesia Care Unit

Patients stay in the postanesthesia care unit for 1 to 2 hours, during which time they are closely monitored and given humidified O_2. Hypertension and/or tachycardia are treated with the appropriate drugs. Analgesia is provided by increments of analgesics such as hydromorphone hydrochloride (Dilaudid), morphine, or fentanyl. Nausea is treated with either droperidol or ondansetron. The patient is instructed not to blow his or her nose and not to cough vigorously. Level of consciousness is monitored. Visual acuity and extraocular eye movements are tested frequently. Any deficit in these should be discussed with the surgeon immediately. New deficit or deterioration may require exploration of the surgical site (7, 8). The patient's urine output is monitored for the possibility of development of DI.

Postoperative Care

Most patients will be discharged from the postanesthesia care unit to a regular hospital bed. Rarely, an intensive care unit is needed when the patient is unstable, needs invasive monitors, or needs infusions of vasoactive drugs.

Postoperatively, mouth breathing or breathing through the nasopharyngeal airways causes the patient to complain of dry mouth. Therefore, humidified oxygen therapy is provided in the postoperative period. Urine output is monitored for the possibility of developing DI. Extraocular eye movement, visual acuity, and level of consciousness are checked periodically.

Diabetes Insipidus

DI is characterized by excretion of a large volume of diluted urine. DI can be neurogenic or nephrogenic (44, 45). Neurogenic DI is caused by diminished or absent antidiuretic hormone release. Although DI can be caused by other entities, e.g., head trauma or carcinomatous metastases to the pituitary gland, this discussion focuses on pituitary surgery.

DI may be present in the preoperative period. It may not be evident in the patient with panhypopituitarism until replacement of steroid therapy is started (46) because glucocorticoids and probably mineralocorticoids are necessary to facilitate the renal excretion of the water load (46). This condition should be known to the anesthesiologist in the preoperative period.

The onset, severity, and clinical course of DI depends on the location and degree of injury to the posterior pituitary, stalk, or hypothalamus. In patients with prolactinomas, the incidence of DI is 60%, but in most patients it is transient (47). It is permanent in only 3% (47). However, in patients with craniopharyngiomas, the incidence of DI is higher. Seckl et al. (48) reported the development of DI in eight of nine children operated on for craniopharyngioma. Two children died within 48 hours of surgery. In the other six children, the DI was permanent.

Intraoperatively, DI is seen more with frontal craniotomy than transsphenoidal procedures. The difference in the incidence could be caused by the extent of the tumor, surgical approach, and duration of the procedure. After transsphenoid procedure, it is rare for the DI to be seen in the immediate postoperative period. Most commonly, it starts in the first postoperative day (45). The first presenting symptom is high urine output. If the urine output is not replaced, hypovolemia and cardiovascular instability will result. The urine is diluted, and the result is increasing serum sodium levels. If the patient is awake he or she will complain of thirst, and intake of oral fluids will be high.

The differential diagnosis of DI includes:

1. Hyperglycemia and glucosuria.
2. Excessive intravenous fluids administration in the perioperative period (45).
3. Excessive water intake (primary polydipsia).
4. Use of diuretics.
5. A preexisting renal condition (nephrogenic DI) (44).
6. Corticosteroid deficiency (49).

Management of the patient with possible DI starts with:

1. Review of the patient's history for the possibility of nephrogenic DI.
2. Review of the patient's records for fluids (intravenous and/or oral) intake and urine output.
3. Measurement of plasma sodium level, osmotic pressure, and glucose level.
4. Testing of the urine for specific gravity, sodium level, osmotic pressure, and presence of glucose.

One has to keep in mind the possibility of:

1. Diuretics given unintentionally.

2. Inaccurate record keeping.

3. Increased urine output, which could be caused by elimination of retained fluids caused by the pituitary adenomas. This was observed in patients with suprasellar extension and in prolactin-secreting tumors (50).

The diagnosis of DI is made if the plasma sodium level exceeds 143 to 145 mmol/L with continuing diuresis of hypotonic urine (osmotic pressure below 200 mOsm and specific gravity below 1.005) (51). If the diagnosis of DI is not clear, then the physician could slow the rate of intravenous fluids for 1 to 2 hours. If the high urine output continues, the diagnosis of DI is confirmed. Caution should be exercised to avoid hypovolemia and dehydration. Once the diagnosis of DI is made, treatment consists of fluid replacement and vasopressin therapy. The type of intravenous fluids and the rate depends on the level of hypernatremia and the fluid balance. Fluids used are hypotonic solutions (one-half or one-quarter normal saline). Hypernatremia, especially of chronic nature, should be corrected slowly, at the rate of 1 mOsmol every hour. Brain edema can result if chronic hypernatremia is corrected too fast.

Vasopressin therapy of choice, in the immediate postoperative period, is aqueous vasopressin, 5 to 20 units given subcutaneously. This can be repeated every 4 to 6 hours. Most of the DI is transient. If DI proved to be permanent, then vasopressin tannate-in-oil can be used, 5 to 10 IU intramuscularly every 24 to 48 hours. Intranasal desmopressin, 1-desamino-8-d arginine vasopressin (DDAVP), cannot be used during the immediate postoperative period because of the nasal packs. Fluid balance needs to be observed once the vasopressin is given. Overzealous treatment of DI with vasopressin can cause fluid overload and a clinical state similar to the syndrome of inappropriate antidiuretic hormone secretion.

Vasopressin should be used with caution in pregnant women and patients with coronary artery disease because of the oxytocic and coronary artery constriction properties of the drug (52).

In patients with coronary artery disease, nitroglycerin can be added to minimize the risk of myocardial ischemia. Nikolic and Singh (53) cautioned against the use of vasopressin in combination with cimetidine. He described a patient who, under this circumstance, developed bradyarrhythmia and atrioventricular block requiring insertion of a pacemaker.

REFERENCES

1. Melmed S. Acromegaly. N Engl J Med 1990;322:966–977.
2. Allen EV. Thromboangitis obliterans: methods of diagnosis of chronic occlusive arterial lesions distal to wrist with illustrative cases. Am J Med Sci 1929;178:237–244.
3. Newfield P, Albin MS, Chestnut JS, et al. Air embolism during transsphenoidal pituitary operations. Neurosurgery 1978;2:39–42.
4. Matjasko J. Perioperative management of patients with pituitary tumors. Semin Anesthesia 1984;3:155–167.
5. Grundy BL. Monitoring of sensory evoked potentials during neurosurgical operation: methods and applications. Neurosurgery 1982;11:556–575.
6. Black PM, Zervas NT, Candia GL. Incidence and management of complications of transsphenoidal operation of pituitary adenomas. Neurosurgery 1987;20:920–924.
7. Wilson CB, Dempsey LC. Transsphenoidal microsurgical removal of 250 pituitary adenomas. J Neurosurg 1978;48:13–22.
8. Barrow DL, Tindall GT. Loss of vision after transsphenoidal surgery. Neurosurgery 1990;27:60–68.
9. Zervas NT. Surgical results in pituitary adenomas: results of an international survey. In: Black PMCL, Zervas NT, Ridgway EC Jr, et al., eds. Secretory Tumors of the Pituitary Gland. New York: Raven, 1984:377–385.
10. Messick JM, Laws ER, Abboud CF. Anesthesia for trans-sphenoidal surgery of the hypophyseal region. Anesth Analg 1978;57:206–215.
11. Abou-Madi M, Trop D, Barnes J. Aetiology and control of cardiovascular reactions during trans-sphenoidal resection of pituitary microadenomas. Can Anaesth Soc J 1980;27:491–495.
12. Jill JN, Gershon NI, Gargiulo PO. Total spinal blockade during local anesthesia of the nasal passages. Anesthesiology 1983;59:144.
13. Spaziante R, DeDivitus E. Forced subarachnoid air in transphenoidal excision of pituitary tumors (pumping technique). J Neurosurg 1989;71:864–867.
14. Hirsh IB, McGill JB, Cryer PE, et al. Perioperative management of surgical patients with diabetes mellitus. Anesthesiology 1991;74:346–359.
15. Signgelyn FJ, Scholtes JL. Airway obstruction in acromegaly: a method of prevention. Anaesth Intensive Care 1988;16:491–492.
16. Campkin TV. Radial artery cannulation: potential hazard in patients with acromegaly. Anaesthesia 1980;35:1008–1009.
17. Kitahata LM. Airway difficulties associated with anesthesia in acromegaly. Br J Anaesth 1971;43:1187–1189.
18. Southwick JP, Katz J. Unusual airway difficulty in the acromegalic patient: indications for tracheostomy. Anesthesiology 1979;51:72–73.
19. Ovassipian A, Doka JC, Rosma DE. Acromegaly: use of fiberoptic laryngoscopy to avoid tacheostomy. Anesthesiology 1981;54:429–430.
20. Grotting JK, Pemberton JDEJ. Fixation of the vocal cords in acromegaly. Arch Otolaryngol 1950;52:608–617.
21. Bhatia ML, Misra SC, Prakash J. Laryngeal manifestations in acromegaly. J Laryngol Otol 1966;80:412–417.
22. Edge WG, Whitwam JG. Chondro-calcinosis and difficult intubation in acromegaly. Anaesthesia 1981;36:677–680.
23. Hassan SZ, Matz GJ, Lawrence AM, et al. Laryngeal stenosis in acromegaly: a possible cause of airway difficulties associated with anesthesia. Anesth Analg 1976;55:57–60.
24. Siegler J. Acromegaly associated with laryngeal obstruction. J Laryngol 1952;66:620–621.
25. Perks WH, Harrocks PM, Cooper RA, et al. Sleep apnea in acromegaly. BMJ 1980;280:894–897.
26. Burn, James MB. Airway difficulties associated with anaesthesia in acromegaly. Br J Anaesth 1972;44:412–414.
27. Messick JM, Cucchiara RF, Faust RJ. Airway management in patients with acromegaly. Anesthesiology 1982;56:157.
28. Venus B. Acromegalic patient: indications for fiberoptic bronchoscopy but not tracheostomy. Anesthesiology 1980;52:100.
29. McGuffin WL, Sherman BM, Roth J, et al. Acromegaly and cardiovascular disorders. Ann Intern Med 1974;81:11–18.
30. Lie JT, Grossman SJ. Pathology of the heart in acromegaly: anatomic findings in 27 autopsied patients. Am Heart J 1989;100:41–52.

31. Aloia JF, Field RA. The heart and the endocrine system in cardiac and vascular diseases. Conn HL, Horowitz O, eds. Philadelphia: Lea and Febiger, 1971;2:1252–1261.

32. Rabinowitz D, Spr SP, Bledsoe T. The pituitary gland. In: Harvey AM, ed. The Principles and Practices. 18th ed. New York: Appleton-Century-Crofts, 1972:839–840.

33. Pepine CJ, Aloia J. Heart muscle disease in acromegaly. Am J Med 1970;48:530–534.

34. Shirley JE, Schteingart DE, Rajiv T. Sleep architecture and sleep apnea in patients with Cushing's disease. Sleep 1992;15:514.

35. Sugihara N, eShimizu M, Kila Y. Cardiac characteristics and postoperative courses in Cushing's syndrome. Am J Cardiol 1992;69:1475.

36. Enquist A, Backer OG, Jarnum S. Incidence of postoperative complications in patients subjected to surgery under steroid cover. Acta Chir Scand 1974;140:343.

37. Dale DC, Fauci AS, Wolff SM. Alternate-day prednisone: leukocyte kinetics and susceptibility to infections. N Engl J Med 1974;291:1154.

38. Winstone NE, Brook BN. Effects of steroid treatment on patients undergoing operation. Lancet 1961;1:973.

39. Flier JS, Underhill LH. Diagnosis and management of hormone-secreting pituitary adenomas. N Engl J Med 1991;324:822–831.

40. Bills DC, Meyer FB, Laws ER, et al. A retrospective analysis of pituitary apoplexy. Neurosurgery 1993;33:602–609.

41. Bonicki W, Zaluska AK, Koszewski W. Pituitary apoplexy: endocrine surgical and oncological emergency: incidence, clinical course and treatment with reference to 799 cases of pituitary adenomas. Acta Neurochir (Wien) 1993;120:118.

42. Gaillarad RC. Pituitary gland emergencies. Baillieres Clin Endocrinol Metab 1992;6:57.

43. Shields CB, Valdes-Rodriguez AG. Tension pneumocephalus after transphenoidal hypophysectomy: case report. Neurosurgery 1982;11:687–689.

44. Roizen MF. Diseases of the endocrine system. In: Katz B, Beumof JL, Kadis LB, eds. Anesthesia and Uncommon Diseases. 3rd ed. Philadelphia: WB Saunders, 1990:265.

45. Shucart WA, Jackson I. Management of diabetes insipidus in neurosurgical patients. J Neurosurg 1976;44:65–71.

46. Green H, Harrington AR, Valtin H. On the role of antidiuretic hormone in the inhibition of acute water diuresis in adrenal insufficiency and the effects of gluco and mineralocorticoids in reversing the inhibition. J Clin Invest 1970;49:1724–1736.

47. Faria MA, Tindall GT. Transsphenoidal microsurgery for prolactin-secreting pituitary adenomas. J Neurosurg 1982;56:33–43.

48. Seckl JR, Dunger DB, Lightman SL. Neurohypophyseal peptide function during early postoperative diabetes insipidus. Brain 1987;110:737–746.

49. Davis BB, Bloom ME, Field JB, et al. Hyponatremia in pituitary insufficiency. Metabolism 1969;18:821–832.

50. Hans P, Stevenaert A, Albert A. Study of hypotonic polyuria after transsphenoidal pituitary adenomectomy. Intensive Care Med 1986;12:95–99.

51. Verbalis JG, Robinson AG, Moses AM. Postoperative and posttraumatic diabetes insipidus. In: Czernichow P, Robinson AG, eds. Diabetes Insipidus in Man. Basel: Karger, 1985:256.

52. Corliss RJ, McKenna DH, Sialers S, et al. Systemic and coronary hemodynamic effects of vasopressin. Am J Med Sci 1968;256:293.

53. Nikolic G, Singh JB. Cimetidine, vasopresin and chronotropic incompetence. Med J Aust 1982;2:435.

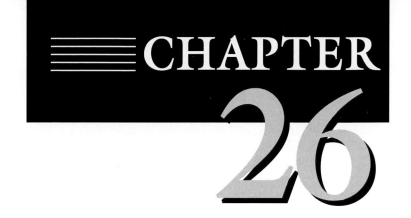

CHAPTER 26

Transsphenoidal Surgery: Operative Techniques

C. Michael Cawley and George T. Tindall

INTRODUCTION

A host of neoplastic and nonneoplastic lesions may arise from the pituitary gland or its neighboring structures. These lesions are manifest clinically by either hypersecretion or hyposecretion of one or more of the pituitary gland's products or by compression of nearby anatomic structures causing specific neurologic deficits. After nearly a century of refinement and rediscovery, the transsphenoidal approach has evolved as the preferred route for removal of most sellar lesions.

First described in 1907 by Schloffer, the technique was refined in the early twentieth century (1–3). Cushing developed the sublabial transseptal technique for accessing the pituitary fossa via the sphenoid sinus (1). He used this approach extensively and with relatively good results but later abandoned it in favor of a transcranial procedure. Cushing's decision led to the disappearance of the procedure from the American surgical scene for almost 50 years.

However, a few Europeans—most notably Hirsch (4) and Dott (5)—continued to perform a large number of transsphenoidal procedures, with excellent results. Out of their experience, and with the advent of new microsurgical techniques, Guiot in France (6) and Hardy in Canada (7)

further refined the operation and repopularized the technique in the United States. With a morbidity of less than 2% and a mortality rate of less than 0.5%, the procedure today stands as one of the most effective operative procedures performed by neurosurgeons.

INDICATIONS FOR SURGERY

Adenomas of the adenohypophysis are by far the most common lesions found in the region of the sella, accounting for one third of sellar and juxtasellar lesions in large series. Other neoplastic lesions arising from the pituitary include craniopharyngiomas (9% in adults, 50% in children), pituitary carcinomas, and sarcomas. Neighboring tumors not of pituitary origin include hypothalamic and optic apparatus gliomas (11%) and meningiomas (10%). Nonneoplastic lesions that affect pituitary structure and function include aneurysms (most often of the anterior communicating complex [7%]), arachnoid cysts (2%), Rathke's cleft cysts (2%), hamartomas (2%), and the special case of the "empty sella" syndrome (3%). Various inflammatory disorders may also affect the pituitary, such as sarcoidosis, histiocytosis X, and lymphocytic hypophysitis (8, 9).

Extra Glandular Lesions

The clinical presentation of these lesions varies to some degree among each disorder; however, most will become clinically apparent because of either local mass effect or systemic endocrinopathy. Most lesions not arising from the gland will present with mass effect and the attendant focal neurologic deficits. Occasionally, extra glandular lesions will also present with an endocrinopathy—most often hypopituitarism caused by mass effect hindering the function of the gland. Any lesion that threatens vision should be treated, and surgical decompression is the safest and most efficacious option for extra glandular sellar masses. Should these lesions present only with endocrinologic compromise, the risks of surgery must be weighed against those of daily hormone replacement.

Glandular Lesions

For most intrinsic pituitary lesions (most often adenomas), the decision regarding surgical versus medical therapy depends on several factors such as patient preference, tumor type, and tumor invasion. As with extra glandular lesions, intrinsic lesions (most often adenomas) may present with mass effects or endocrine derangements that often produce one of the following characteristic clinical syndromes.

Amenorrhea-Galactorrhea

Prolactin-secreting adenomas are one of the most common lesions in the sella and are responsible for the amenorrhea-galactorrhea syndrome. Like other adenomas, these masses may grow to compress the optic apparatus overlying the sella and result in visual field defects (usually bitemporal hemianopia). A serum prolactin level of at least 150 μg/ L ($\geq$ 150 ng/mL) usually indicates the presence of a prolactinoma; provocative tests are not necessary. In the patient who exhibits symptoms of hyperprolactinemia yet has a serum prolactin level of 150 μg/L (150 ng/mL), the "stalk effect" must be considered. Stalk effect results from the loss of normal dopaminergic inhibition of the prolactin-secreting lactotrophs. These inhibitory influences originate in the hypothalamus and descend to the adenohypophysis via the portal system. Compression of the stalk by a sellar mass results in a failure of these inhibitory factors to reach the adenohypophysis. Thus, any mass in or around the sella that interferes with prolactin inhibitory factors will result in an elevation of the serum prolactin level usually in the range of 60 to 100 μg/L (60 to 100 ng/mL). Such lesions are often referred to as "pseudoprolactinomas."

For those patients with documented prolactinomas, both surgery and medical therapy with dopamine agonists such as bromocriptine or pergolide are effective therapeutic options. Therapy with these drugs will reliably decrease serum prolactin levels and usually shrink the tumor. However, this therapy is lifelong: if the medication is stopped, the tumor will regrow. Therefore, in those patients who do not wish to undergo lifelong drug therapy, or in those who cannot tolerate the side effects of dopamine agonist therapy, surgery is an appropriate option.

In those patients with extremely high serum prolactin levels (e.g., > 750 μg/L [> 750 ng/mL]), surgery is unlikely to result in a cure. In these special cases, the high levels of hormone indicate that the tumor has probably spread beyond the confines of the sella, most likely into the cavernous sinuses, and that surgical resection alone will not be successful. Medical therapy and/or radiotherapy should be considered as either a primary or an adjunct treatment option in this situation.

Cushing's Disease

Patients with clinical stigmata of hypercortisolism are referred to as having "Cushing's syndrome." When hypercortisolism has a pituitary origin it is referred to as "Cushing's disease." Spontaneous, noniatrogenic hypercortisolism may occur as a result of a pituitary adenomas or an ectopic adrenocorticotropic hormone (ACTH)–producing lesion (usually a pulmonary tumor). A battery of endocrinologic tests, including measurements of morning serum cortisol, 24-hour urine free cortisol, and peripheral and inferior petrosal sinus ACTH levels may be used along with radiologic studies of the sella, adrenals, and common sites of tumors elaborating "ectopic ACTH" are performed to ascertain the cause of an elevated serum cortisol level. A pituitary source accounts for 60 to 65% of all cases of noniatrogenic hypercortisolism.

The serious clinical manifestations of ACTH-secreting adenomas are caused solely by a functional endocrinopathy and not by mass effects because these tumors are usually microadenomas. Surgery is the mainstay in the treatment of this disorder. The antifungal agent ketoconazole has been used with some success as a medical therapy for Cushing's disease. However, though surgical excision may be difficult because of problems identifying these small tumors on radiographic examination and at surgery, adequate surgical extirpation is superior to partial control with medical therapy. Repeat surgery for further tumor removal or partial hypophysectomy is also indicated should a first transsphenoidal procedure fail to cure the disease.

Acromegaly

Growth hormone (GH)–secreting adenomas account for between 20 and 30% of all pituitary adenomas. The clinical consequences of excessive GH secretion include acromegaly in adults and gigantism in prepubertal children. The serious adverse effects of this disease in terms of health and longevity are discussed elsewhere. The clinical picture of patients harboring GH-secreting tumors is usually obvious; confirmatory tests include failure of suppression of the serum GH level to less than 88 pmol/L (< 2 ng/mL) after oral glucose challenge and elevation of the insulinlike growth factor-1 (somatomedin C) level. Most GH-secreting adenomas will have reached a size large enough to be identified on magnetic resonance imaging (MRI).

A few of these tumors will respond to dopamine agonist therapy; however, more recently the somatostatin analog octreotide has been used with greater success in both non-surgical and presurgical treatment. The treatment of choice remains surgical excision via the transsphenoidal route. Immediate and permanent lowering of serum GH levels to below 88 pmol/L (< 2 ng/mL) followed by sustained normalization of serum somatomedin C levels herald a cure.

Nonfunctional Adenomas

Nonfunctional adenomas comprise most pituitary adenomas. These lesions are not associated with any clinically recognizable endocrinopathy. They exert their clinical effects via local compression of the pituitary gland, hypothalamic pathways, or neighboring central nervous system structures. Most often patients harboring such tumors will present with either hypopituitarism or symptoms and signs referable to compression of the optic apparatus or other cranial nerves. Amenorrhea-galactorrhea may also occur because of elevation of prolactin levels as a result of the stalk effect. Rarely, neurologic dysfunction may result from compression of the third ventricle and subsequent hydrocephalus. The treatment of such lesions is surgical because they threaten sensitive neurologic structures and are poorly responsive to administration of pharmacologic agents useful for functional adenomas.

Pituitary Apoplexy

This syndrome is most often seen in the puerperal period or in those patients already harboring pituitary tumors. The acute onset of severe headache, diminished visual acuity, hypotension, or shock; alterations in consciousness; and, in some cases, death are the result of hemorrhage into the gland itself or into a preexisting tumor. A few patients will recover spontaneously without surgical intervention; however, most cases require emergent evacuation of the hematoma to save vision and cranial nerve function. Appropriate hormone replacement—most importantly hydrocortisone—therapy is mandatory and can lead to immediate and dramatic clinical improvement.

CONTRAINDICATIONS TO SURGERY

Relatively few contraindications to the transsphenoidal approach to the pituitary exist. The procedure requires general anesthesia and is tolerated well by most patients. Proper corticosteroid coverage in the perioperative period as described below will decrease the likelihood of adverse effects resulting from manipulation of the normal gland during tumor removal.

Major active medical problems that would prohibit the elective use of general anesthesia may contraindicate transsphenoidal surgery. Active sinus infection is also a relative contraindication to elective surgery, although the rate of either central nervous system or general wound infection following transsphenoidal surgery is extremely low. Serious endocrinopathies such as unstable Cushing's disease or incompletely controlled hyperthyroidism may lead to perioperative hemodynamic derangements and thus are also contraindications to surgery.

PREOPERATIVE PREPARATIONS

After clinical, radiologic, and endocrinologic studies have established the diagnosis, several preparative tests are required to later gauge the success of the procedure and to ensure that the patient is in optimum condition to undergo a major operation. As mentioned above, control of any preexisting medical problems is mandatory. Of special concern is the adequate control of hypercortisolism, hyperthyroidism, and diabetes. In addition to diagnostic endocrine testing, baseline measurement of prolactin, free thyroxine, luteinizing hormone, follicle-stimulating hormone, and serum sodium levels and urine output (to assess antidiuretic hormone activity) should be performed in all patients. Additional preoperative testing including chest radiography, electrocardiography, and hematologic profiling is performed, as with any other surgery, based on the patient's age and medical condition. Baseline formal visual field testing should be done if results of clinical examination or historical information suggest field defects or if the mass lesion impinges significantly on the optic apparatus. Automated testing is preferred because it allows for more reliable repeat examinations.

On the day of surgery, stress doses of hydrocortisone are administered. Hydrocortisone should be given in divided dosages of 300 mg on the day of surgery and gradually reduced by 50 to 100 mg each day thereafter until it can be discontinued. Broad spectrum antibiotics (nafcillin or vancomycin, 1 g intravenously) that cover normal upper respiratory and skin flora and that have good central nervous system penetration are given at least 30 minutes prior to incision (10, 11).

OPERATIVE TECHNIQUE
General Considerations

The patient is placed supine with both arms tucked at the side. After induction of anesthesia and endotracheal intubation, the authors place the patient in a three-point Mayfield head holder with two prongs on the left temporal convexity perpendicular to the coronal plane and the third over the right temporal convexity. The patient's head is then tilted laterally toward the left shoulder. Prior to setting the head position, a final adjustment bringing the head

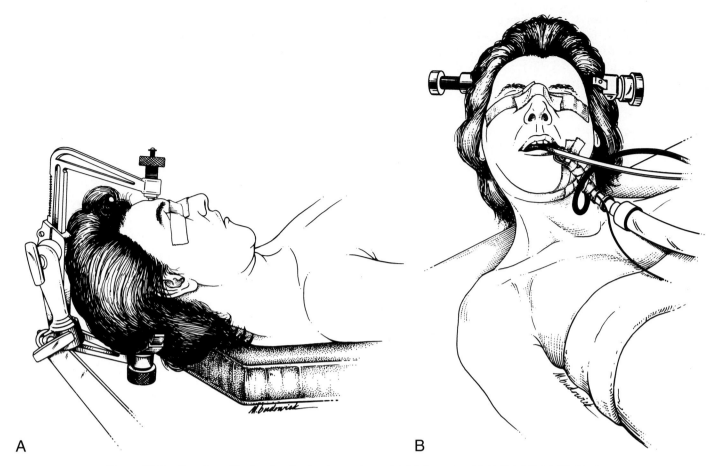

A   B

Figure 26.1.   Head positioning for the transnasal or sublabial approach to the sphenoid sinus.

straight up above the level of the heart and extending the head about the occipital cervical junction allows for both minimal venous congestion and an optimal line-of-sight for the surgeon (Fig. 26.1, *A* and *B*). Should the use of C-arm fluoroscopy be anticipated, care should be taken to avoid obscuring the lateral sellar profile during placement of the radiopaque head holder. Alternatively, the Mayfield may be placed in an anteroposterior orientation or may be replaced with a horseshoe head rest (9, 10).

Pneumatic compression devices or elastic wraps are placed on the lower extremities. The use of an indwelling bladder catheter is optional. The patient's left lower abdomen is prepared for fat graft harvest and is kept as a separate sterile surgical field throughout the case. The endotracheal tube is taped to the left of the midline, and a pharyngeal pack to prevent ingestion of blood may be used. At least 10 minutes prior to incision, the nostrils are packed with cotton pledgets soaked in 5% cocaine, oxymetazoline, or 0.5% lidocaine containing epinephrine 1:200,000; this will allow shrinkage of the turbinates and will optimize hemostasis during initial exposure. No subcutaneous lidocaine injection is performed for a transnasal–transsphenoidal approach; however, if the approach is sublabial, lidocaine with

epinephrine may be injected along the upper gingiva and into the inferior portion of the nasal septum. An aseptic aqueous solution such as povidone-iodine (Betadine) is swabbed around the nose, nostrils, and upper lip.

The use of intraoperative subarachnoid spinal catheters is considered in patients in whom there is significant suprasellar tumor extension. In these cases, infusion of a few milliliters of preservative-free normal saline will increase the cerebrospinal fluid (CSF) pressure and force the diaphragma sellae—and any suprasellar tumor—down into the operative field in the sella. Likewise, drainage of several milliliters of CSF may allow further manipulation of a bulky tumor. When indicated, the authors use a small silastic lumbar drainage catheter inserted via a Tuohy needle into the lumbar subarachnoid space. Alternatively, a spinal needle may be placed and taped into position attached to a drainage bag. In this last case, a split mattress must be used on the operating table to facilitate positioning (11).

Some surgeons use intraoperative C-arm fluoroscopy to guide the surgical approach to the sphenoid sinus and sella and to monitor the position of instruments in and above the sella. The authors prefer to use such assistance only in selected cases, such as in those patients whose preoperative radiographs reveal a sphenoid sinus abnormality or in reoperations in which the nasal anatomy may be obscured.

The Transnasal-Transseptal Approach

Four different surgical approaches to the sphenoid sinus have been described. Most modern surgeons use either the transnasal or the sublabial route to access the sphenoid sinus. The transantral and transmaxillary approaches, which will not be discussed here, are rarely required and are usually accomplished with the assistance of an otolaryngolo-gist. During the past 10 years, the authors' preference has become the transnasal approach. Advantages of this approach include the lack of a gingival incision and greater facility in initiating a plane of dissection between the septal cartilage and nasal mucosa.

Once the patient has been prepared as outlined above, a 1- to 2-cm incision is made with either a #15 blade or a monopolar electrocautery in the columella at the junction of the skin and nasal mucosa, usually on the patient's right side (Fig. 26.2, A–D). A suture may be passed through the inferomedial columella to help in traction of the nostril.

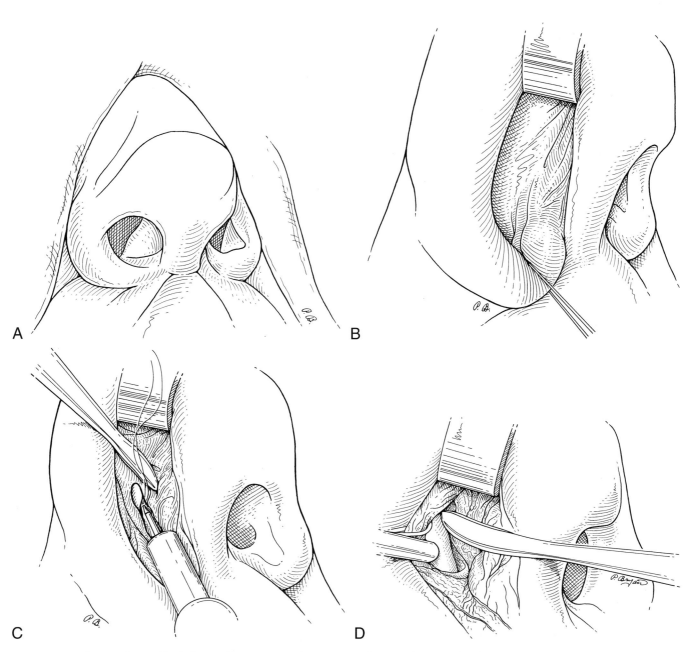

A   B

C   D

Figure 26.2. The initial incision and establishment of the submucosal plane along the contralateral cartilaginous septum for the transnasal approach.

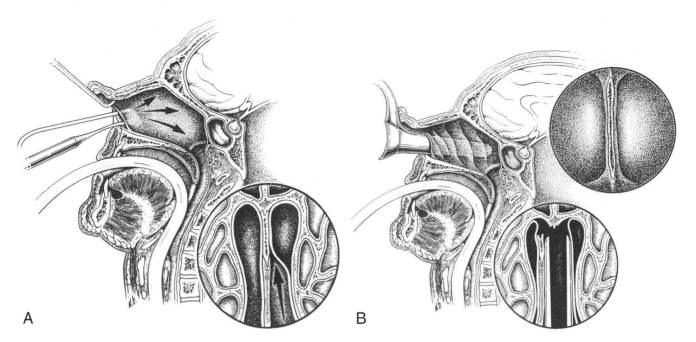

Figure 26.3. The progressive submucosal dissection along the cartilaginous and bony septum, exposing the sphenoid crest.

A dissector is used to enter the subperichondral plane. This plane is dissected across the anterior aspect of the cartilaginous septum, and then posteriorly and inferiorly along the left side of the quadrangular cartilage. With progressively larger nasal speculums, the mucosa is dissected off the cartilaginous septum until its junction with the perpendicular plate of the ethmoid bone is encountered (Fig. 26.3A). At this point, the operation proceeds, as described below, in a similar fashion to the other sphenoid approaches.

The Sublabial-Transseptal Approach

This approach is the one initially devised by Cushing and later repopularized by Guiot and Hardy. Its advantages include a wider opening for the nasal speculum, obviating the need for a cosmetically evident alar relaxing incision, which may be required in those patients with small nostrils in whom the transnasal approach is attempted. Once the upper lip is everted with a pair of skin hooks, a bilateral incision is made in the mucosa just above the vestibule from the canine fossa to the maxillary bone. Subperiosteal dissection elevates the mucosa to the pyriform apertures that are then enlarged with rongeurs, allowing access to the nasal floor at the inferomedial aspect of the junction of the cartilaginous septum with the anterior vomer. Unilateral or bilateral mucosal dissection is carried out posteriorly along the vomer to its junction with the perpendicular plate of the ethmoid bone. Elevation proceeds superiorly to the junction of the bony vomer with the quadrangular plate. At this point, care must be taken to maintain the correct dissection plane because the mucosa is often quite adherent at the junction of the vomer and the cartilaginous septum.

Sphenoid Sinus and Sella Access

Once the perpendicular plate of the ethmoid is encountered, the authors prefer to continue a unilateral subperiosteal mucosal elevation along the left side of the plate until the rostrum of the sphenoid is evident. At this point, a larger nasal speculum is introduced and with gentle force is directed to the patient's right, and the root of the plate is fractured from the rostrum (Fig. 26.3B). This maneuver displaces the entire septum—bony and cartilaginous—away from the midline, allowing bilateral visualization of the rostrum of the sphenoid sinus. Because none of the bony septum is actually removed, there is little risk of postoperative saddle-nose deformity. In addition, should later reconstruction of the sellar floor be required, a ready site for bone harvest is available.

Further elevation of mucosa away from each side of the sphenoid rostrum will reveal the so-called "keel of the boat," composed of the sphenoid rostrum and the midline remnant of the displaced perpendicular plate of the ethmoid bone (i.e., the sphenoid crest). Both superiorly and inferiorly the rostrum will taper, as would the bottom of a boat seen from below. Toward the rostral end of the surgical field the paired sphenoid ostia should also become evident. At this point, the large bivalve Cushing-Landolt speculum is then inserted and gently opened. The operating microscope is brought into the field.

Enlargement of the sphenoid ostia with microrongeurs is followed by complete removal of the sphenoid rostrum with either continued rongeuring or the use of a high-speed drill (Fig. 26.4A). Once the anterior wall of the sinus is opened, the sphenoid mucosa is exenterated and the sphenoid septa are removed. The sellar floor is identified.

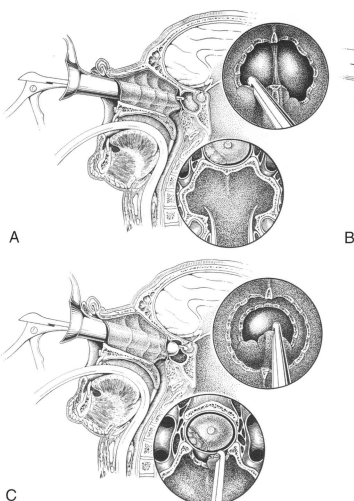

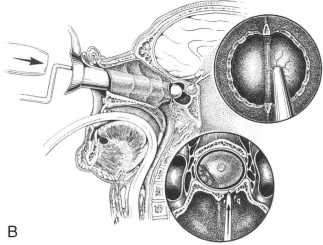

Figure 26.4. Entry into the sphenoid sinus and removal of the floor of the sella.

The authors prefer to use a high-speed drill to remove this small plate of bone, although microchisels and small variable-angle rongeurs may also be adequate (Fig. 26.4, *B* and *C*). Care should be taken because the sellar floor is often thinned because of expansion of the underlying tumor. Resection of the sellar floor should continue in a circumferential pattern until one notices a change in the color of the underlying dura. The bluish tint of the dura will identify the lateral cavernous sinuses and the superior intercavernous or circular sinus. Inferiorly, bone removal should continue until the ledge of the sellar floor merges into the clivus. Prior to opening the dura, meticulous attention to hemostasis and adequate lateral exposure is mandatory. In some cases, C-arm fluoroscopy may be used to confirm correct positioning prior to a dural incision.

Tumor Removal

Macroadenomas

A #11 blade is used to create a linear durotomy. With a small-angled dissector, a plane is developed between the gland and tumor and the inner aspect of the dura. Small-angled microscissors are used to further open the dura in a stellate fashion (Fig. 26.5, *A* and *B*). With larger tumors, the intracranial pressure will often push the tumor into the operative field, facilitating removal. Four-quadrant curettage with various Hardy ring curettes allows further tumor resection from both the lateral, superior, and inferior recesses. Identification of the normal gland is essential (Fig. 26.5*C*). Usually located posterosuperiorly to the tumor, the normal gland will appear reddish-orange in color and is of a firm consistency. Most adenomas, on the other hand, are grayish in color and are much more friable. Should the tumor/gland interface not be apparent, a Hardy spoon dissector may be used to meticulously develop a plane. This is essential if total tumor removal and sparing of the gland is to be achieved.

Once the bulk of a large pituitary tumor is removed, the diaphragma sella will descend into the pituitary fossa. Care should be taken to identify the dura and not create a dural rent. Such herniation of the diaphragma into the sella allows closer inspection for any residual tumor. In fact, if the diaphragma does not descend, there is likely residual tumor superior to the sella. In some instances, *infusion* of a few millimeters of preservative-free saline into an indwelling

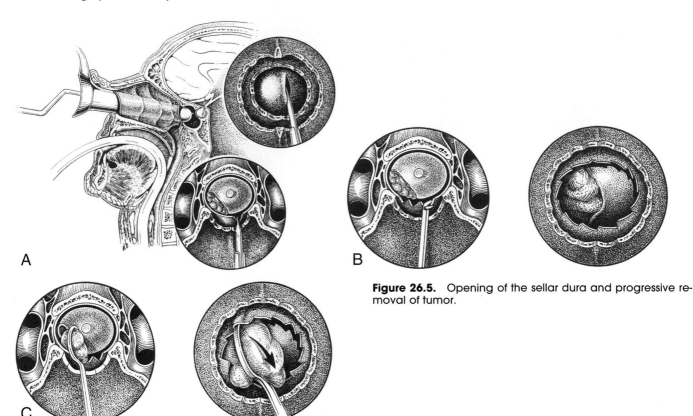

Figure 26.5. Opening of the sellar dura and progressive removal of tumor.

lumbar subarachnoid catheter may force the diaphragma and any occult tumor into the surgical field. Likewise, should the diaphragma prolapse to an excessive degree, *removal* of several millimeters of CSF may allow it to ascend and clear the operative field. In this manner, even significant suprasellar tumor extensions may be completely removed via transsphenoidal surgery. In those cases in which copious suprasellar tumor remains despite such maneuvers, either a staged procedure—allowing the suprasellar contents to descend over time and reoperating transsphenoidally in 2 to 3 weeks—or a later transcranial approach should be considered.

Microadenomas

Most microadenomas are obvious once the dura is adequately opened. Some microadenomas, especially in patients with Cushing's disease, may be either so small or so situated within the normal pituitary gland that locating and removing them may prove difficult. Correlation of the surgical view with MRI findings is imperative if the microadenoma is to be located without undue damage to the normal gland. If the tumor is not visible on opening of the dura, a transverse incision is made in the gland. Blunt dissection of the lateral wings of the pituitary will usually result in herniation of the adenoma out of the transverse incision. Development of a tumor/gland interface is of paramount importance. All abnormal tissue is removed with ring curettes and cup biopsy forceps. Frequent frozen section ex-

amination of biopsy specimens assists in complete tumor removal and sparing of the normal gland. Those patients harboring an ACTH-secreting adenoma often have no abnormal mass apparent on MRI or at surgery. In these cases, the results of preoperative inferior petrosal sinus sampling will assist the surgeon in lateralizing the source of aberrant ACTH production (12). If a tumor is not found, a hemihypophysectomy may be performed on the side lateralized by inferior petrosal sinus sampling.

Sellar Cysts

The most commonly encountered sellar cysts are Rathke's cleft and arachnoid cysts. The former is an epithelial-lined pouch resulting from persistence of a remnant of the primitive stomodeum between the anterior and intermediate lobes of the pituitary gland. Most Rathke's cleft cysts can be managed with surgical excision via the transsphenoidal route. Once the cyst is encountered, the readily accessible portions of its wall should be resected and sent for frozen pathologic diagnosis. The cyst contents are then drained. Total removal of the cyst wall is not recommended if this requires extensive dissection around the hypothalamus, optic apparatus, or intracranial vessels. Unlike craniopharyngiomas, even after only partial resection of the cyst wall, recurrence is rare. Arachnoid cysts are treated in a similar manner, requiring only fenestration and drainage of the cyst into the sphenoid sinus. One potential drawback of the transsphenoidal approach in the treatment of these cysts is that fenestration into the subarachnoid space may be difficult. In fact, surgery for arachnoid cysts carries up to a 28.6% complication rate in one series (13). These complications included both persistent CSF rhinorrhea and meningitis.

Craniopharyngiomas

These tumors may be purely intrasellar, suprasellar, or both. They may lead to acute or chronic hydrocephalus, visual impairment, or neuroendocrine derangements. The transsphenoidal approach for resection of such tumors is indicated if the tumor is predominantly intrasellar and beneath the diaphragma sella. In most of these cases, the sella will be significantly expanded by tumor, facilitating exposure. Those tumors with moderate suprasellar extension but a smoothly delineated midline upper border may also be amenable to transsphenoidal resection. For those tumors with more extensive suprasellar extension, or in those patients with a small sella, transcranial routes should be considered.

The surgical technique in approaching these tumors is similar to that for adenomas. However, a wide opening of the sphenoid sinus, the sellar floor, and the dura is important if a total excision is to be accomplished. Although the capsule will be closely adherent to surrounding structures, every attempt should be made to develop a subdural, extracapsular plane and to remove the lesion in toto without violating the cystic sac. All safe attempts should be made to remove the capsule completely to reduce the incidence of recurrence. The pituitary gland itself is usually displaced anterosuperiorly in those tumors arising from the sella and often must be sharply dissected away from the tumor capsule. Likewise, the capsule may also be adherent to the diaphragma sella or the pituitary stalk. In this situation, total tumor excision may require resection of some of the tumor-infiltrated dura with a consequent intraoperative CSF leak.

CLOSURE

Once the resection of a sellar tumor has been completed, meticulous hemostasis must be achieved. Gently packing the resection site with adipose tissue is usually sufficient. Once the tumor bed is dry, absolute alcohol may be instilled to further sterilize the tumor bed in an attempt to achieve total eradication of abnormal cells. This step is contraindicated in the presence of a dural tear.

Autologous fat graft harvested from the abdomen is used to gently pack the intrasellar tumor resection site. The authors do not routinely reconstruct the sellar floor, although a small piece of pressed Avitene may act as a scaffold for the intrasellar fat packing. In those cases in which reconstruction of the sellar floor is desired, a piece of the perpendicular plate of the ethmoid bone may be used. The sphenoid sinus is also packed with fat, and the nasal speculum

is removed. The bony and cartilaginous nasal septum is then repositioned in the midline.

The columellar incision used in the transnasal approach is closed loosely with a running 3–0 catgut suture; the sublabial incision is closed with interrupted simple 3–0 catgut suture. The authors use well-lubricated, soft, curved latex nasal airway tubes as nostril packs, which are placed posteriorly into the nasopharynx and must be inserted with care to avoid penetration onto any mucosal tears. An endotracheal suction catheter may be placed down each tube to act as a guide in placement and to evacuate any blood in the nasopharynx that might be ingested. The airway tubes are loosely secured to the cartilaginous septum by means of a single 2–0 silk suture placed through the external aspect of each tube and the columella. On the morning of postoperative day 1, the packs are removed. The patient is instructed to refrain from blowing his or her nose and to apply only light dabbing pressure to the nostrils.

POSTOPERATIVE CARE AND FOLLOW-UP

As noted, corticosteroid support is tapered from 100 mg twice a day on postoperative day 1 to 20 mg every morning and 10 mg every night for the first 4 postoperative days. If the patient's morning serum cortisol level is low after the previous night's dosage has been held, maintenance doses of 20 mg in the morning and 10 mg at night are prescribed until the first postoperative office visit at 1 month. Perioperative antibiotic therapy (nafcillin, 1 g every 8 hours, or vancomycin, 1 g every 12 hours) is continued for a total of three doses postoperatively. Nasal decongestants such as pseudoephedrine are prescribed on a request basis to help alleviate the feeling of nasal fullness. After discharge from the hospital, the patient is seen again at 1 month and at 6 months and thereafter at 1-year intervals. During the first clinic visit after surgery, postoperative testing of the endocrine axes is carried out and repeated periodically if any derangement persists. Follow-up MRI with gadolinium is performed at 3 months postoperatively and then at yearly intervals for 3 years. If any visual field defects were present preoperatively, visual fields should be evaluated 2 to 3 months following surgery.

COMPLICATIONS AND THEIR MANAGEMENT
Intraoperative

Complications may be encountered intraoperatively. During the approach to the sella, the surgeon must be sure that on removing the sellar floor, the bony floor of the frontal fossa or the clivus are not inadvertently penetrated. The use of intraoperative fluoroscopy (C-arm) or intraoperative skull radiographs should allow precise localization and thus prevent this complication (Fig. 26.6).

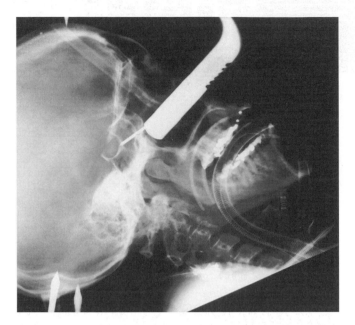

Figure 26.6. Lateral intraoperative skull radiograph demonstrating correct localization at the floor of the sella.

During removal of the sellar floor and lateral exposure of the sellar dura, copious venous bleeding may occur owing to entrance into the cavernous sinus. This bleeding is usually controlled with Surgicel, Avitene, or cotton-pledget packing. In some cases, elevation of the head of the bed may assist in the control of more vigorous hemorrhage. In this situation, the surgeon should refrain from overzealous packing to avoid compression palsies of the cranial nerves traversing the sinus. Also, the intracavernous carotid artery may rarely be damaged. Injury to this vessel is usually the result of overly aggressive dissection of laterally extending tumor. Gentle probing of the lateral recesses of the pituitary fossa and the cavernous sinuses with a blunt ring curette are usually safe, but if preoperative images suggest encasement of the carotid artery with tumor, aggressive attempts to follow tumor laterally into the cavernous sinuses should not be performed. Once a carotid injury is suspected, the site of hemorrhage is packed off, and, after the operation is completed, an angiogram is performed to assess the extent of the injury. Another well-described catastrophic vascular injury is that of the small perforating arteries supplying the optic apparatus, resulting in blindness. These perforators may be compromised during aggressive removal of an adherent capsule from underneath the optic chiasm.

The most common intraoperative complication associated with transsphenoidal pituitary surgery is an iatrogenic CSF leak (13). This is usually the result of disruption of the diaphragma sella. In some cases, the tumor itself will have invaded the dura; thus, in the course of tumor resection, a dural tear cannot be avoided. Should a tear be encountered, tumor evacuation should proceed. On closure, some authors advocate the placement of a fascial graft over the tear. In our experience, adipose tissue placed over the tear usually suffices. Large leaks may require the use of fibrin glue to obtain a tight seal.

Postoperative

Postoperative complications of transsphenoidal surgery are usually caused by endocrine derangements. As noted above, proper corticosteroid coverage is imperative in the perioperative period. Hypocortisolism is usually manifest by anorexia, nausea, weakness, and postural hypotension. To prevent this situation, hydrocortisone is continued after surgery and is tapered to physiologic doses of 20 to 30 mg daily after the fifth postoperative day. Discontinuation of corticosteroid therapy follows documentation of recovery of the hypothalamic–pituitary–adrenal axis with a morning serum cortisol level of at least 275 nmol/L ($\geq$ 10 μg/dL) after withholding hydrocortisone therapy for 24 hours.

Urine output should be monitored closely to promptly diagnose diabetes insipidus. This condition is seen transiently in approximately 20 to 25% of patients undergoing transsphenoidal pituitary surgery. In 1 to 2% of patients it may persist for months or permanently. Diabetes insipidus results from the disruption of the outflow of antidiuretic hormone and should be suspected when the patient's urinary output exceeds fluid intake by 300 mL/h. In this setting, a serum sodium level higher than 145 mmol/L (> 145 mEq) or a urine specific gravity less than 1.005 confirms the diagnosis (8). In the acute postoperative period, diabetes insipidus is best managed by allowing the patient free access to water and by using aqueous vasopressin, 5 units subcutaneously every 4 to 6 hours as needed. More long-term urine-concentrating defects are treated with intranasal desmopressin acetate.

Other postoperative complications include the rare development of sinusitis, wound infection, or meningitis. These should be treated in a routine manner. Long-term cosmetic deformities of the nose, including septal perforation and saddle-nose deformity, may be avoided by meticulous dissection and maintenance of both the bony and cartilaginous nasal septum. CSF leakage may become apparent postoperatively. If a significant leak occurs in the acute postoperative period, placement of a lumbar spinal fluid drain is performed. Drainage for 72 hours usually allows most leaks to seal. In those cases in which CSF rhinorrhea comes to the clinician's attention in a delayed fashion, simple lumbar drainage may not be adequate in sealing a well-established fistula. In these cases, diagnostic studies such as cisternography and therapeutic measures such as repeat operation may be required.

REFERENCES

1. Cushing H. Surgical experiences with pituitary disorders. JAMA 1914;63:1515.
2. Kanavel AB. The removal of tumors of the pituitary body by an infranasal route: a proposed operation with a description of technique. JAMA 1909;53:1704.
3. Schloffer H. Zur frage der operationen an der hypophyse. Beitr Klin Chir 1906;50:767.
4. Hirsch O. Eine neue methode der endonaasalen operation von hypophysentumoren. Wien Med Wochenschr 1909;59:636.
5. Dott NM, Bailey P. A consideration of the hypophyseal adenomata. Br J Surg 1925;13:314.
6. Guiot G, Thibaut B. L'extirpation des adenomes hypophysaries par voie transsphenoidale. Neurochirurgia (Stuttg) 1959;1:133.
7. Hardy J, Wigser SM. Transsphenoidal surgery of pituitary fossa tumors with televised radiofluoroscopic control. J Neurosurg 1965;23:612.
8. Cawley CM, Tindall GT. Pituitary and neighboring tumors. In: Hurst JW, ed. Medicine for the Practicing Physician. Stamford, CT: Appleton & Lange, 1996:540.
9. Laws ER. Transsphenoidal approach to pituitary tumors. In: Schmidek HH, Sweet WH, eds. Operative Neurosurgical Techniques. Philadelphia: WB Saunders, 1996:283.
10. Rabb CH, Couldwell WT, Weiss MH. Pituitary tumors: anatomy and surgical approach. In: Tindall CT, Cooper PR, Barrow DL, eds. The Practice of Neurosurgery. Baltimore: Williams & Wilkins, 1996:1121.
11. Tindall GR, Barrow DL. Tumors of the sellar and parasellar area in adults. In: Youmans JR, ed. Neurological Surgery. Philadelphia: WB Saunders, 1990:3447.
12. Zovickian J, Oldfield EH, Doppman JL, et al. Usefulness of inferior petrosal sinus venous endocrine markers in Cushing's disease. J Neurosurg 1988;68:205.
13. Black PMCL, Zervas NT, Candia GL. Incidence and management of complications of transsphenoidal operation for pituitary tumors. Neurosurgery 1987;29(6):920.

CHAPTER 27

The Pterional Approach

Ali F. Krisht

INTRODUCTION

The best approach to any intracranial lesion is the approach that achieves maximal exposure with minimal manipulation or retraction to the brain tissue. For lesions in the suprasellar area and the inferior third ventricular region, the ideal approach is the pterional craniotomy, with its conveniently located natural planes and spaces at the level of the skull base. The sphenoid ridge provides a plane with ideal access to the suprasellar region along the anterior frontotemporal junction. This natural plane can further be widened by drilling the sphenoid ridge along its medial extension to the level of the superior orbital fissure and by flattening the orbital roof as well.

The pterional approach evolved as a result of several of its variations that were previously used. Dandy (1, 2) used a frontotemporal craniotomy but without removing the sphenoid ridge. He used a larger craniotomy with frontal lobe retraction to approach aneurysms of the anterior circle of Willis. Yasargil (3, 4) was the first to describe the pterional approach in detail, and he popularized its use for lesions of the anterior circle of Willis and the suprasellar region. He carefully described the steps of the bony exposure and the drilling of the sphenoid ridge, followed by the

opening of the sylvian fissure and the basal arachnoid. This allows the entire frontal lobe to fall backward with gravity and leads to minimal or no retraction of the brain itself. The addition of magnification, improved lighting, and the stereoscopic binocular vision provided by the operating microscope leads to visualization of a large field of the undersurface of the brain in the supra and parasellar region and easier access to the inferior third ventricular space. The addition of a mobile microscope allows maximal use of the "keyhole" concept of exposure, which leads to more exposure and a lesser need for brain retraction.

CLINICAL EVALUATION

Patients with lesions involving the inferior third ventricular region and the suprasellar area should undergo thorough clinical and endocrinologic evaluation. In addition to a detailed history of the current illness and a complete neurologic examination, a neuro-ophthalmologic evaluation is performed on all patients. A complete endocrinologic evaluation is done, evaluating both anterior and posterior lobe pituitary function. This evaluation should include at least levels of AM serum cortisol, urinary free cortisol, growth hormone, prolactin, T4, luteinizing hormone, follicle-stimulating hormone, and testosterone levels in men and estradiol levels in women. Serum and urine osmolalities are also evaluated both prior to and after a 12-hour water deprivation test when diabetes insipidus (DI) is considered (5).

DIAGNOSTIC EVALUATION

A variety of pathologic lesions involve the inferior third ventricular region (Table 27.1), including primary lesions such as craniopharyngiomas or lesions arising in the vicinity and secondarily involving the inferior third ventricular portion such as pituitary adenomas and meningiomas (5–7).

Recent advances in neuroradiologic studies have improved our ability to visualize the detailed anatomy of lesions located in the suprasellar and inferior third ventricular region. These modern imaging techniques, including computed tomography and magnetic resonance imaging (MRI), have an important role in preoperative evaluation and surgical planning. They provide information regarding tumor consistency and vascularity and its relationship to the surrounding neural elements. The sagittal and coronal MRI images are especially helpful in showing the extent of suprasellar extension of these tumors and whether the third ventricular wall is infiltrated or only compressed. This information is important in planning the surgical approach and in the decision making of whether the tumor can be removed totally through the pterional approach or whether an additional and/or combined approach is needed.

Conventional cerebral angiography is helpful in defining the relationship of the vascular structures and their distorted anatomy in the vicinity of the tumor. However, the recently introduced magnetic resonance angiography is a less invasive modality that may replace cerebral angiography. Figure 27.1 shows MRIs of a variety of lesions that may involve the suprasellar and inferior third ventricular region, approached through the pterional approach.

PREOPERATIVE CONSIDERATIONS

Surgical Decision Making

Tumors arising in the suprasellar and inferior third ventricular region have different growth patterns depending on several factors, the most important of which is the exact location from which the tumor arises. Tumors such as pituitary adenomas and craniopharyngiomas arise from the intrasellar compartment and extend superiorly to the suprasellar region. Craniopharyngiomas may also arise from the middle part of the pituitary stalk in the suprasellar region and grow superiorly, extending into the third ventricular compartment. Some craniopharyngiomas, juvenile pilocytic gliomas, and others may be more restricted to the third ventricular region with possible impingement on suprasellar neural and vascular structures. The consistency of these tumors can be variable. Some tumors are solid, others are cystic, and some are mixed. The cystic components may compose the bulk of these tumors. Calcification is commonly seen with craniopharyngiomas and may increase the difficulty of their surgical removal. The size of the tumor and its location in relationship to the optic chiasm decides the pattern of deformity in the optic apparatus. If the chiasm is prefixed, the tumor growth in the suprasellar compartment pushes the optic apparatus anteriorly and superiorly, flattening the optic nerves. With postfixed chiasms, the tumor growth is more anterior between the optic nerves. There can still be a posterior suprasellar extension of the tumor into the inferior third ventricular region.

This information is important in the preoperative surgical decision making. The surgical approach is decided on based on the location and the size of the tumor. In general, tumors growing within the sella that have no suprasellar extension should be approached through the transnasal–transsphenoidal route. Large intrasellar tumors with suprasellar extensions are best approached through the pterional–transsylvian route. Tumors located in the suprasellar compartment with a significant suprasellar extension into the third ventricular compartment are still approached through the pterional–transsylvian route as part of or in combination with another approach, such as the transcallosal–transventricular approach.

Anesthetic Considerations

All patients are treated with parenteral hydrocortisol in the immediate preoperative period. Hydrocortisol can be replaced with dexamethasone (Decadron) to help decrease postoperative brain swelling. Patients are given antibiotics (nafcillin or vancomycin) and prophylactic anticonvulsant therapy (Dilantin).

Anesthesia is usually induced with thiopental and muscle relaxants. Maintenance anesthesia is usually done using a combination of nitrous oxide, a narcotic, and a muscle relaxant. The use of inhalation anesthetics is minimized, especially when dealing with large tumors and possible increase in the intracranial pressure. In the immediate preoperative phase, patients are given 20 to 40 mg of furosemide (Lasix) to help achieve better brain relaxation. Furosemide can be supplemented with 1 g/1 kg of body weight of mannitol bolus if needed. We attempt to avoid hypotension, especially in elderly patients who are likely to have diffuse ath-

Table 27.1. *Lesions That Can Be Approached Through the Pterional Approach*

Common	Uncommon
Aneurysm	Dermoid
Craniopharyngioma	Epidermoid
Pituitary adenoma	Lipoma
Meningioma	Rathke's pouch cyst
Metastatic tumor	Choristoma
Germinoma	Paraganglioma
Optic nerve glioma	Gangliocytoma
Hypothalamic glioma	Abscess or infectious cyst
Arachnoid cyst	Yolk sac tumor

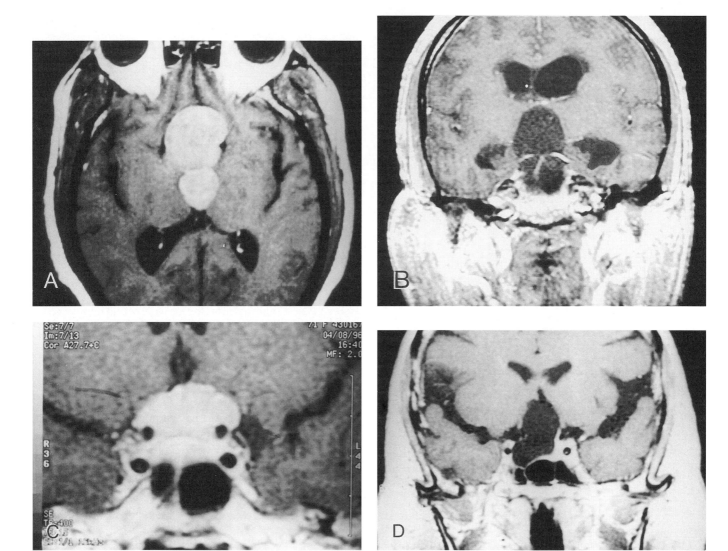

Figure 27.1. **A.** Axial T1-weighted gadolinium-enhanced MRI of giant invasive pituitary adenoma extending into the third ventricular region. **B.** Coronal T1-weighted MRI of large cystic craniopharyngioma extending into the third ventricular region. **C.** Coronal T1-weighted gadolinium-enhanced MRI of tuberculum sellae meningioma. **D.** Coronal T1-weighted MRI of suprasellar arachnoid cyst.

erosclerotic disease and are more prone to develop cerebral infarctions and ischemia when hypotensive. In these patients, we even tend to avoid diuretic use to keep them well hydrated. This is usually affordable taking into consideration that most patients in this age group have some degree of cerebral atrophy, and as soon as the spinal fluid pathways are opened, a good brain relaxation is easily achieved. The carbon dioxide pressure level is kept from 30 to 32 mm Hg. This extent of hyperventilation and opening of the basal cisterns is always enough to achieve adequate brain relaxation.

OPERATIVE APPROACH

Head Position

The patient is put in the supine position and the head is slightly tilted (20 to 30°) opposite the side in which the

incision will be made. A right-sided craniotomy is usually preferred for lesions along the midline as well as right-sided lesions. This is most comfortable approach knowing that most surgeons are right-handed. The neck is elevated above the chest and the head is dropped backward in a hyperextended position to allow the frontal lobes to fall with gravity. This will help minimize the need for frontal lobe retraction. The head is fixed in place with a three-point fixation device such as the Mayfield–Kees head holder. The position brings the malar eminence to the most superior point of the field, and the sphenoid ridge assumes a vertical direction to the plane of the operating field (Fig. 27.2). Care must be taken to avoid extreme positions that may lead to compression of the trachea, jugular veins, and carotid and vertebral arteries. In overweight and obese patients, the venous drainage may well be compromised, especially if the neck is short; for this reason, the patient's trunk is put

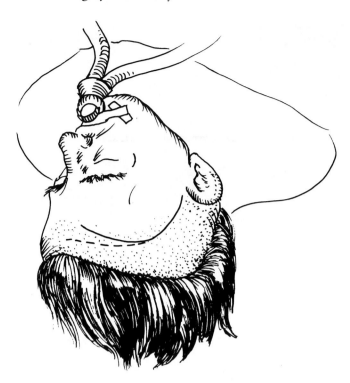

Figure 27.2.   Head position for the pterional approach.

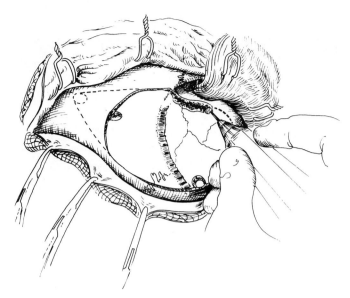

Figure 27.3.   Figure indicates the location of burr holes used for the pterional approach. The *dotted line* indicates the modified medial extension of the pterional flap.

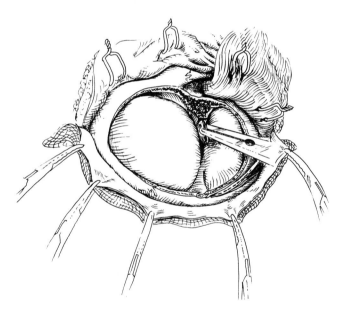

Figure 27.4.   The pterional bone window and the removal of the sphenoid wing.

in a 30° elevation. This elevation will enhance the venous outflow of the intracranial cavity and allow better relaxation of the brain.

Surgical Technique

The skin incision begins at a point 1 cm anterior to the tragus of the ear and follows a curvilinear line behind the hairline to reach the midsagittal plane. The skin flap is reflected anteroinferiorly, and the superficial temporal fascia is dissected behind the zygomatic arch to identify and preserve the frontalis branch of cranial nerve VII. We also preserve the pericranium and reflect it for possible further use as a dural graft. The temporalis muscle is then cut at its insertion, leaving a small cuff of fascia along the superior temporal line for suturing it back in place at the end of the procedure.

The standard position of the burr holes are indicated in Figure 27.3. For tumors located in the suprasellar region with significant suprasellar extension, we modify the pterional craniotomy to extend more medially and inferiorly just above the medial aspect of the superior orbital ridge. This extension allows a more medial subfrontal approach, especially for tumors arising between the optic nerves in case of a postfixed chiasm. After the bone flap is made, dural tack up stitches are applied for epidural hemostasis. The sphenoid ridge is then drilled along its medial extension as far as the lateral aspect of the superior orbital fissure (Fig. 27.4). During this maneuver the meningeo-orbital artery is coagulated and cut. The dura is then opened in a

U-shaped fashion above the sylvian fissure (Fig. 27.5). The opening may be extended medially when the craniotomy is modified and extended to the medial subfrontal region. The dura is reflected anteriorly, and, if needed, relaxing incisions are made on its posterior aspect. The surgical microscope is introduced to the field at this stage, and any further dissection is done under magnification.

After opening the dura, the priority is for achieving brain relaxation to minimize retraction and achieve maximal exposure. The chiasmatic cistern region is approached by

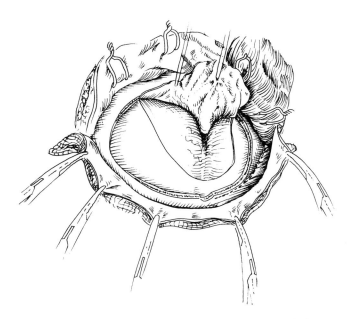

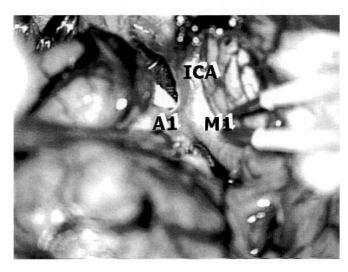

Figure 27.7. Intraoperative photograph of the internal carotid artery (*ICA*) bifurcation after splitting the sylvian fissure. *A1*, proximal anterior cerebral artery; *M1*, proximal middle cerebral artery.

Figure 27.5. The dura opened and reflected anteriorly over the sylvian fissure.

gentle retraction of the frontal lobe with the microsuction, and then both the chiasmatic and the carotid cisterns are opened to allow spinal fluid drainage and brain relaxation. Patience at this step will achieve a much more relaxed brain that will be easier to manage with minimal or no retraction, especially when considering the long hours needed for the excision of some tumors in this region (Fig. 27.6). After adequate brain relaxation is achieved, attention is shifted to the sylvian fissure. We advocate using the transsylvian approach to the suprasellar and inferior third ventricular region for many reasons. Dissecting the sylvian fissure helps in visualizing the carotid bifurcation and the course of the

anterior cerebral artery, which could be significantly distorted; thus, help avoid its injury. Opening the sylvian fissure allows the disengagement of the temporal from the frontal lobes and allows the frontal lobe to fall backward with gravity without the need for retraction. In addition, the transsylvian–pterional approach, with its modified medial extension, allows more than a 90° angle of exposure, extending from the sylvian fissure to the anterior midline plane.

The microdissection of the sylvian fissure is started by opening the arachnoid on the frontal (or medial) side of the superficial middle cerebral veins overlying the sylvian fissure. The dissection is extended first into the depth of the fissure along one of the M2 branches of the middle cerebral artery until the M1 segment is identified. The M1 segment is followed along its course toward the carotid artery bifurcation. The fissure is split in a deep to superficial direction and progressing proximally until the bifurcation is reached. This will lead, as mentioned above, to better visualization of the proximal M1 and A1 segments and their relationship to the tumor (Fig. 27.7).

In attacking lesions in this area, attention is first directed to the extent of tension that is applied by the tumor to the stretched optic apparatus, and an immediate attempt to relax this tension by shrinking the tumor is made. Cystic components are drained first to decrease the tumor size. If the tumor is solid in consistency and the optic nerve is stretched, the optic canal is first drilled and the overlying fibrous dural band (falciforme dural fold) is cut. This will decompress and relax the nerve, allowing it to be more tolerant to manipulation during the tumor removal phase. The tumor can then be approached through one of several windows. Through the modified medial extension of the pterional approach, the medial subfrontal approach is used

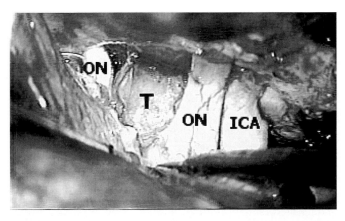

Figure 27.6. Intraoperative photograph of the suprasellar and chiasmatic region. Notice the excellent visualization of the tumor and optic apparatus after dissecting the basal arachnoid and using minimal retraction with the microsuction and the bipolar. *T*, tumor; *ON*, optic nerve; *ICA*, internal carotid artery.

to approach tumors between the optic nerves. The overlying stretched arachnoid is coagulated and cut distal to the chiasm to avoid injury to its blood supply. The tumor is then debulked using the suction and the pituitary rongeur with gentle traction on the tumor itself. The ultrasonic aspirator can be used occasionally. If the tumor is calcified and hard to remove, the large calcific pieces are broken into small fragments and removed with a pituitary rongeur.

The tumors can also be approached through the opticocarotid window. Attention should be given through this approach to the several small branches arising from the medial wall of the carotid artery and supplying the inferior aspect of the optic chiasm. These small branches may be stretched and hard to visualize until the tumor is debulked. They belong to the superior hypophyseal artery complex, which supplies the optic chiasm, the pituitary stalk, and the optic nerves, and their preservation is essential to prevent postoperative ischemic visual deficits (8). The third window that can be used is the lamina terminalis. When the lamina terminalis is stretched and enlarged by the tumor, it can safely be opened and the tumor removed without significant risk of injury to the hypothalamus. It is important to preserve the plane between the tumor, or its capsule, and the surrounding gliotic brain layer. If the tumor has a giant superior extension with a significant intraventricular component, an attempt to complete surgical removal may be risky, and residual tumor is left to be removed using another approach, such as the transcallosal–transventricular approach. In the case of small suprasellar tumors, the pituitary stalk can usually be identified, and an attempt should be made to preserve both its anatomic continuity and its blood supply (Fig. 27.8). In larger tumors this becomes more difficult, and preserving the pituitary stalk has no advantage if it risks leaving significant residual tumor behind, especially in the case of craniopharyngiomas.

On concluding the tumor resection phase, the retrochiasmatic and interpeduncular spaces are inspected for any residual tumor, and complete hemostasis is established. The wound is then closed in layers in a routine fashion.

POSTOPERATIVE CARE

After a short stay in the recovery room, patients are kept in the intensive care unit for a night or two. They are kept on fluid restrictions for the first 48 hours after surgery (< 750 to 1000 mL/24 hr). Accurate intake and output records are kept to watch for DI. If the urine output is greater that 250 cc/hr for 2 hours or greater than 500 cc/hr in 1 hour, DI is suspected and serum sodium level and osmolality are obtained in addition to a urine specific gravity. If the sodium level is greater than 142 mmol/L and the urine specific gravity is less

than 10.10, vasopressin (Pitressin) or desmopressin acetate (DDAVP) is administered parenterally, and the dose is repeated every 6 or 12 hours as needed. If the DI is suspected to be permanent, desmopressin acetate nasal spray is started, and, for convenience, it is usually given at bedtime. Steroids are continued in the postoperative period and are tapered to a maintenance dose of 20 mg in the AM and 10 mg in the PM in adults. The need for hormonal replacement therapy is determined by reevaluating the pituitary gland functions in the first or second week after discharge. We usually obtain an AM cortisol level and T4 levels during the first week after discharge. The rest of the anterior pituitary hormone functions can be assessed at a later stage within the 30-day postoperative period. Patients with an uncomplicated postoperative course are discharged within 5 to 7 days of the surgery day.

COMPLICATIONS

The most common complications associated with the pterional approach are not different than those encountered with other intracranial neurosurgical procedures. As mentioned above, DI is common when surgical manipulation occurs around the pituitary stalk region. This is most commonly encountered with surgery of craniopharyngiomas. Hypopituitarism usually occurs preoperatively because of large lesions compressing the pituitary gland, but it can also be encountered in the postoperative period as a possible complication of the surgical procedure. Hypopituitarism is most commonly seen after the transcranial approach to pituitary adenomas. With experience, the surgeon should be able to recognize the normal pituitary tissue and avoid the complete resection of the pituitary gland. Leaving a small portion of the gland is usually enough to maintain adequate hormonal production without the need for replacement therapy.

Loss of vision is not uncommon after surgery through the pterional approach. Vision loss is most commonly encountered when dealing with lesions in the suprasellar area. The most common cause of visual loss is the disruption of the blood supply to the optic chiasm or the optic nerves. This is usually the case even though the anatomic continuity of those structures is preserved. The visual loss is more pronounced in patients who had a prolonged preoperative course with a significant preoperative visual loss. In general, patients who had recent decrease in their vision tend to improve faster. A detailed understanding of the microvascular anatomy of the optic nerves and optic chiasms as well as meticulous microdissection techniques are the most important factors that can help avoid postoperative worsening of vision. Postoperative coma and autonomic dysfunction are infrequent postoperative complications that may occur as a result of hypothalamic injury (9). They are rarely encountered when one or unilateral hypothalamic injury oc-

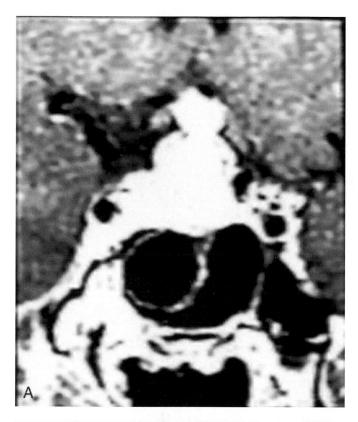

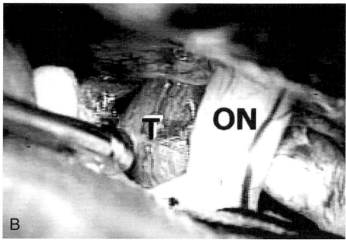

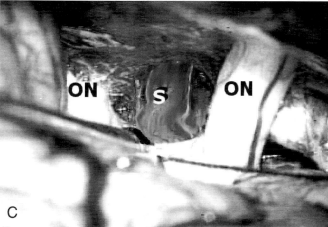

Figure 27.8. **A.** MRI of a pituitary adenoma with a dumbbell shape and that can best be removed through a cranial approach. **B.** Intraoperative photograph of the tumor (*T*) and the stretched optic nerve (*ON*) through a right pterional approach. **C.** Intraoperative photograph after tumor removal showing decompression of the optic apparatus (*ON*, optic nerves) and preservation of the pituitary stalk (*S*), which pushed anteriorly and to the left side in this case.

curs. Coma and autonomic dysfunction are more commonly seen when both sides of the hypothalamus are significantly injured. This can best be avoided by applying the traction against the tumor and not the surrounding brain during dissection. Another important step is to avoid violation of the capsule or pseudocapsule of the tumor and inadvertent entry into the surrounding brain tissue. It is of utmost importance to have good experience with the deformed and pathologic anatomy encountered with tumors involving the suprasellar and inferior third ventricular region.

CONCLUSION

The pterional approach, with its conveniently located natural planes, provides an ideal approach to lesions involving the suprasellar area and inferior third ventricular region. When combined with opening the basal cisterns and spinal fluid drainage, maximal brain relaxation is achieved, and, as a result, minimal use of brain retraction is needed. The modified medial extension of the pterional craniotomy provides an additional anterior subfrontal approach that can be used to safely access the tumor extension between the optic nerves as well as the superior extension into the inferior third ventricular region. It is a time-honored approach that should be mastered by every practicing neurosurgeon.

REFERENCES

1. Dandy WE. Intracranial Arterial Aneurysms. New York: Havner Publishing, 1969:103–132. (Fascimile of the 1944 edition reprinted by arrangement with Corness University Press.)
2. Dandy WE. Surgery of the Brain (A Monograph From Lewis Practice of Surgery). Hagerstown, MD: WF Prior, 1945; 12:405.
3. Yasargil MG, Fox JL. The microsurgical approach to intracranial aneurysms. Surg Neurol 1975;3:7–14.
4. Yasargil MG. Microneurosurgery, Volume II. Stuttgart: George Thieme Verlag, 1984.
5. Daughaday WH. The adenohypophysis. In: Williams RH, ed. Textbook of Endocrinology. 5th ed. Philadelphia: WB Saunders, 1974: 31–79.
6. Rhoton AL, Yamamoto I, Peace DA. Microsurgery of the third ventricle: part 2. Neurosurgery 1981;8:357–373.
7. Symon L. Microsurgery of the hypothalamus with special reference to craniopharyngioma. Neurosurg Rev 1983;6:43–49.
8. Krisht AF, Barrow DL, Barnett D, et al. The microsurgical anatomy of the superior hypophyseal artery. Neurosurgery 1994;35(5): 899–903.
9. Plum F, Van Uitert R. Neuroendocrine diseases and disorders of the hypothalamus. In: Reichlin S, Balderssarini RJ, Martin JB, eds. The Hypothalamus. New York: Raven Press, 1978:415–473.

Combined Pterional and Transsphenoidal Approach to Pituitary Tumors

Nelson M. Oyesiku, Cargill H. Alleyne Jr, and George T. Tindall

INTRODUCTION

The surgical approaches to pituitary adenomas have undergone considerable refinement during the past century. In 1889, Horsley (1) first removed the pituitary gland using a subtemporal approach, and subsequently he performed nine such procedures to remove pituitary tumors. Caton and Paul (2), in 1893, used a lateral subtemporal approach combined with orbital exenteration to explore the sella. Krause (3), in 1900, recommended a subfrontal approach to the pituitary. The birth of the transsphenoidal approach began with publications by Scholffer and by von Eiselsberg in 1907, and later by Hockenegg and Kosher (4). Their radical transnasal procedures were later refined by Kanavel, Hirsch, and others (4). Cushing preferentially used the intracranial approach after concluding that the recurrence rate with the transsphenoidal route was too high (5). The transsphenoidal route regained popularity after it was reevaluated by Guiot (6) and later by Hardy and Wigser (7) using the operating microscope and the image intensifier.

Today the transsphenoidal approach remains the preferred approach to most sellar lesions, especially pituitary adenomas. However, there remains a small subgroup of lesions that is more optimally approached by a combined transsphenoidal and pterional technique. Although these procedures may be staged (8–10), this chapter describes the indications and technique of the simultaneous combined approach. This approach has been previously described by Barrow et al. (11) and Loyo et al. (12).

INDICATIONS AND ADVANTAGES OF THE COMBINED APPROACH

The transsphenoidal approach is successfully employed not only for lesions confined to the sella, but also for large lesions with significant extrasellar extension if the extension remains central and the configuration of the tumor is symmetric. In these cases, the usual scenario of tumor evolution is a progressive enlargement of the tumor with gradual

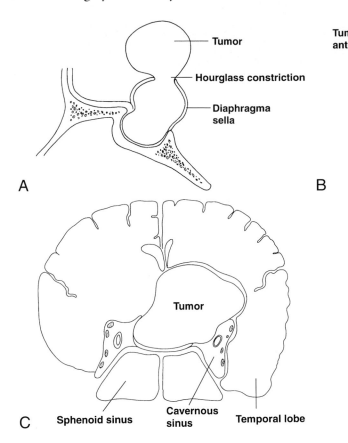

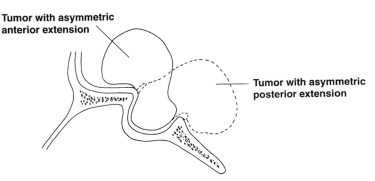

Figure 28.1. Configurations of tumors that benefit from the combined approach. **(A)** Hourglass constriction and tumors with asymmetric suprasellar extension in the **(B)** sagittal plane and **(C)** coronal plane.

stretching of the diaphragma sellae above. If, however, the diaphragma sellae is partially incompetent around the pituitary stalk, the tumor can extend through this hiatus and then expand asymmetrically in the suprasellar region. The resulting tumor configuration is then usually "dumbbell" with an "hourglass" constriction (Fig. 28.1A). An approach to this tumor by either the transsphenoidal or the transcranial route alone would obviously not accomplish the task of safe and complete decompression of the sellar and suprasellar compartments. It is in these cases that a combined approach could prove invaluable. Other tumor configurations that lend themselves well to this technique include tumors with asymmetric suprasellar extension in the sagittal plane (either in the anterior or posterior fossa) (Fig. 28.1B) and those with asymmetric suprasellar extension in the coronal plane (into the middle fossa) (Fig. 28.1C).

About 5 to 7.5% of large pituitary tumors may be fibrous (13, 14). Many tumors of this consistency are difficult or impossible to successfully remove by the transsphenoidal route because the extensive suprasellar component may not descend even if the sella has been effectively decompressed. Snow et al. suggest that fibrous tumors tend to appear isointense to brain on magnetic resonance images (15), and as many as 70% of tumors that are isointense on T2-weighted magnetic resonance images are firm (16). Although a transsphenoidal extracapsular approach has been described for firm, fibrous adenomas (17), this is not uni-

formly effective; in these cases, a combined approach might be more appropriate.

One disadvantage of the transsphenoidal approach is the inability to directly visualize the optic nerves and their blood supply from the inferior plexus of vessels from the superior hypophyseal artery. In fact, worsening of visual acuity and visual fields as a result of damage to the blood supply to the optic nerves or direct injury has been noted after transsphenoidal surgery in 0 to 11% of patients (18–23). Risk factors for visual complications include the size of the tumor (macroadenomas) or its configuration ("bottleneck" or dumbbell-shaped tumors), existing visual impairment, previous surgery, and radiation therapy. Therefore, patients with bicompartmental lesions and any of these risk factors may be better served by a combined approach.

Another situation in which the combined approach may be considered over the transcranial approach alone is when a prefixed chiasm is present in a patient with a tumor occupying the suprasellar region with extension into the sella. In this case, the operative exposure between the chiasm and the tuberculum sellae is limited, and visualization of the intrasellar portion of the tumor is suboptimal. An alternative method would be to drill off the tuberculum sellae, as described by Rand (24).

If total tumor removal can be achieved by this combined, simultaneous approach, then postoperative radiation therapy may be averted. Another advantage cited by

Loyo et al. (12) is the ability to divide the pituitary stalk early in the procedure if it is invaded by tumor. Thus, injury to the hypothalamus is avoided when traction is applied from below.

TECHNIQUE

Preparation

Two separate operative fields are prepared and maintained throughout the procedure. To facilitate this, two operating microscopes and two sets of operating room personnel (surgeon and scrub nurse) are needed (Fig 28.2). After the induction of general anesthesia, the patient's head is fixed in a Mayfield head holder. The Mayfield may be oriented in an anteroposterior direction or in a transverse direction far enough posteriorly so that it would not preclude an intraoperative lateral skull film if this should be needed later. The head is positioned with the head flexed to about 20° and tilted and rotated to the patient's left or right depending on the side on which the craniotomy approach will be made. The frontotemporal scalp is shaved, prepared, and sterilely draped as for a craniotomy. The nose is prepared with povidone-iodine solution and draped as for a transsphenoidal approach. The left lower quadrant of the abdomen is also prepared for harvesting a fat graft that will be used in the transsphenoidal portion of the operation. The set of sterile instruments used for the fat harvest and for the craniotomy is kept separate from the set of transsphenoidal instruments. A sterile drape is hung between two poles and placed just above the eyebrows to partition the two operative fields. Typically, the transsphenoidal surgeon stands and the transcranial surgeon sits.

Endonasal Transsphenoidal Approach

The details of this exposure are well described in Chapter 26.

Once the sphenoid sinus anterior wall is exposed, the rest of the procedure is performed with an operating microscope equipped with a 300-mm objective lens and 12.5× oculars. The sinus is opened with an osteotome or a Kerrison rongeur placed in the laterally located sphenoid ostia. The sinus opening is enlarged so that the most lateral aspect of the sella is visualized. If necessary, the location of the sellar floor can be confirmed with an intraoperative lateral skull film obtained with a metallic instrument placed at the expected position of the sella. The anterior wall of the sella is opened with an osteotome and a mallet. The opening is enlarged with a Kerrison rongeur laterally to the cavernous sinus, inferiorly to the sellar floor, and superiorly to the intercavernous sinus. A vertical incision is made in the dura with a No. 11 bayonet-handled scalpel. A wide elliptical durotomy is then performed with an angled microscissors. A large tumor will be readily apparent and is removed. A thin, flattened pituitary gland can often be identified posterosuperiorly and spared.

Pterional Approach

The pterional approach to the suprasellar region is performed simultaneously with the transsphenoidal approach. The details of the pterional approach are well described in Chapter 27.

With the suprasellar region exposed, the tumor should be easily visualized. The optic chiasm and nerves are dissected free of tumor, and any tumor that has extended to the frontal, temporal, and retrochiasmatic regions is excised. The suprasellar portion of tumor is then delivered inferiorly to the transsphenoidal surgeon by gently using a microdissector or spatula. The transcranial surgeon takes care not to devascularize the inferior aspect of the optic nerves and protects the chiasm under direct vision while the transsphenoidal surgeon removes the tumor delivered from above.

Closure

When the tumor has been completely removed, a small piece of adipose tissue previously harvested from the abdomen is placed in the sella and sphenoid sinus. If there is a cerebrospinal fluid leak, the sella can be sealed with a combination of fibrin glue and fat and a spinal drain can be left in place. After ensuring that the cerebrospinal fluid leak has sealed, the speculum is withdrawn, the septum is manually replaced in the midline, and the nasal mucosa is closed with 3–0 chromic interrupted sutures. Nasal airways (trumpets) are placed in each nostril to reapproximate the nasal mucosa and to facilitate nasal breathing. These trumpets are removed on the first postoperative day. The pterional opening is closed in the routine fashion. The retractors are removed and the dura is closed with 3–0 Vicryl sutures. The bone flap is replaced and anchored with 2–0 Nurulon sutures or rigid cranial fixation plates and screws, and the temporalis fascia is closed with 2–0 Vicryl sutures. The galea and skin are closed in layers.

COMPLICATIONS

Potential complications are identical to those encountered in either the transsphenoidal or the pterional approach and include cerebrospinal fluid leak, infection, mucosal tears, carotid injury, visual deficits, and hypothalamic injury. The fear of increased infection rates from simultaneous exposure of the intracranial and sphenoid sinus cavities seems unfounded (11).

The combined, simultaneous transsphenoidal and pterional approach described in this chapter need not be used for most pituitary tumors; however, for the treatment of a small subgroup of large asymmetric compartmentalized tumors, the combined approach may be the treatment of choice.

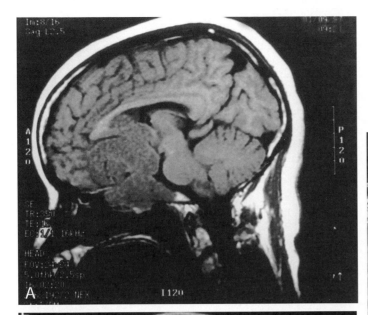

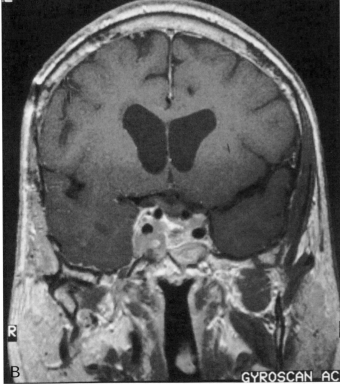

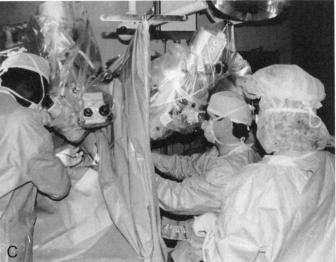

Figure 28.2. C. Intraoperative picture of the two surgical teams operating at the same time.

Figure 28.2. Sagittal preoperative (**A**) and coronal postoperative (**B**) T1-weighted MRI. There has been a near total resection of the tumor. Pituitary function was unchanged from preoperatively. Vision improved completely.

REFERENCES

1. Horsley V. On the technique of operations on the central nervous system. Br Med J 1889;2:411–423.
2. Caton R, Paul FT. Notes of a case of acromegaly treated by operation. Br Med J 1893;2:1421–1423.
3. Krause F. Surgery of the Brain and Spinal Cord. Vol 1, translated by Haubold HA. New York: Rebman, 1912:117–120; Vol 2, translated by Thorek M. 792–802.
4. Davey LM. Early historical aspects of the pituitary gland. In: Goodrich I, Lee KJ, eds. The Pituitary. Amsterdam: Elsevier Science Publishers, 1987.
5. Henderson WR. The pituitary adenomata: a follow-up study of the surgical results in 338 cases (Dr. Harvey Cushing's series). Br J Surg 1939;26:811–921.
6. Guiot G. Transsphenoidal approach in surgical treatment of pituitary adenomas: general principles and indications in nonfunctioning adenomas. In: Kohler PO, Ross GT, eds. Diagnosis and Treatment of Pituitary Tumors. Amsterdam: Excerpta Medica, 1973:159.
7. Hardy J, Wigser WR. Transsphenoidal surgery of pituitary fossa tumors with televised radiofluoroscopic control. J Neurosurg 1965;23:612–619.
8. Bynke O, Hillman J. Role of transsphenoidal operation in the management of pituitary adenomas with suprasellar extension. Acta Neurochir (Wien) 1989;100:50–55.
9. Takakura K, Teramoto A. Management of huge pituitary adenomas. Acta Neurochir (Suppl) 1996;65:13–15.
10. Kobayashi T, Nakane T, Kageyama N. Combined transsphenoidal and intracranial surgery for craniopharyngioma. Prog Exp Tumor Res 1987;30:341–349.
11. Barrow DL, Tindall GT, Tindall SC. Combined simultaneous transsphenoidal transcranial operative approach to selected sellar tumors. Perspect Neurol Surg 1992;3:49–57.
12. Loyo M, Kleriga E, Mateos H, et al. Combined supra-infrasellar approach for large pituitary tumors. Neurosurgery 1984;14:485–488.
13. Laws ER. Comment. Neurosurgery 1984;14:488.
14. Wilson CB. Neurosurgical management of large and invasive pituitary tumors. In: Tindall GT, Collins WF, eds. Clinical management of pituitary disorders. New York: Raven Press, 1979:335–342.
15. Snow RB, Lavyne MH, Lee BCP, et al. Craniotomy versus transsphenoidal excision of large pituitary tumors: the usefulness of magnetic resonance imaging in guiding the operative approach. Neurosurgery 1986;19:59–64.
16. Patterson RH. The role of transcranial surgery in the management of pituitary adenoma. Acta Neurochir (Suppl) 1996;65:16–17.
17. Hashymoto N, Handa H, Yamagami T. Transsphenoidal extracapsular approach to pituitary tumors. J Neurosurg 1986;64:16–20.
18. Trautmann JC, Laws ER Jr. Visual status after transsphenoidal surgery at the Mayo Clinic. Am J Ophthalmol 1983;96:200–208.
19. Cohen AR, Cooper PR, Kupersmith MJ, et al. Visual recovery after transsphenoidal removal of pituitary adenomas. Neurosurgery 1985;17:446–452.
20. Sullivan LJ, O'Day J. Visual outcomes of pituitary adenoma surgery: St. Vincent's Hospital 1968–1987. J Clin Neuro-ophthalmol 1991;II(4):262–267.
21. Harris PE, Afshar F, Coates P, et al. The effects of transsphenoidal surgery on endocrine function and visual fields in patients with functionless pituitary tumors. QJM 1989;71:417–427.
22. Ebersold MJ, Quast LM, Laws ER Jr, et al. Long-term results of nonfunctioning pituitary adenomas. J Neurosurg 1986;64:713–719.
23. Barrow DL, Tindall GT. Loss of vision after transsphenoidal surgery. Neurosurgery 1990;27:60–68.
24. Rand RW. Transfrontal transsphenoidal craniotomy in pituitary and related tumors. In: Rand RW, ed. Microsurgery. 3rd ed. St. Louis: CV Mosby, 1984.

CHAPTER 29

Skull Base Approaches for Giant Invasive Pituitary Tumors

Michael J. Harrison and Ossama Al-Mefty

INTRODUCTION

Although pituitary tumors are entities commonly managed by neurosurgeons, giant invasive pituitary tumors are infrequently encountered. The overwhelming majority of pituitary adenomas may be managed by transsphenoidal surgery, and Wilson (1, 2) estimates that less than 1% of his patients were not suitable for a transsphenoidal approach. Data from our institution reveal only 35 patients in whom cavernous sinus exploration was performed for giant invasive pituitary tumors during the past 15 years (A Krisht, O Al-Mefty, unpublished data, 1997). Yet, to exclude these lesions from discussion based on infrequency eliminates a facet of the disease process and restricts our understanding of pituitary adenomas.

Ambiguity still abounds even over the terminology of "giant" or "massive" in regards to pituitary tumors (2–6), and various authors have proposed schemata to classify "giant" tumors. Jefferson was the first to introduce the term "giant," but he did not qualify the requisite dimensions (7). Symon et al. (6) defined giant pitui-

tary adenomas as lesions that extend more than 40 mm from the midline jugum sphenoidale in any direction or within 6 mm of the foramen of Monro. Wilson (1) categorized lesions that grossly displace the third ventricle as giant. This implies extension of 30 mm or more above the tuberculum sellae and is in accordance with the classification of Mohr et al. (5), with certain subtle differences. We concur with the classification of Wilson and Mohr (Table 29.1) but will additionally confine our discussion to lesions with extension into the cavernous sinus and/or sphenoid sinus.

RATIONALE AND INDICATIONS FOR RESECTION OF GIANT INVASIVE PITUITARY ADENOMAS

Pituitary adenomas invading the cavernous sinus have long been viewed by neurosurgeons as unresectable and thus incurable. Control was only thought possible if the lesion was completely responsive to radiation therapy (1,

Table 29.1. *Classification of Pituitary Adenomas Based on Size*

Extension
  Suprasellar extension
    O: None
    A: Occupies cistern
    B: Recesses of 3rd ventricle obliterated
    C: 3rd ventricle grossly displaced
  Parasellar extension
    D: Intracranial (intradural)[a]
    E: Into or beneath cavernous sinus (extradural)

Site of adenoma
  Floor of the sella turcica intact
    I: Sella normal or focally expanded; tumor < 10 mm
    II: Sella enlarged; tumor ≥ 10 mm
  Sphenoid
    I: Localized perforation of sellar floor
    II: Diffuse destruction of sellar floor
  Distant spread
    V: Spread via cerebrospinal fluid or bloodborne

[a] *Designate anterior (1), middle (2), or posterior (3) fossa.*

8). However, with the evolution of skull base techniques and improved microanatomic knowledge, surgical exploration of the cavernous sinus has become commonplace, and these lesions, which were once believed to be incurable, are now amenable to aggressive surgical resection (9–14). A common feature of pituitary tumors that allows for aggressive resection is the consistency of the tumor. Most pituitary adenomas are soft, friable lesions that can be readily removed with gentle curettage and suction. Fewer than 5% of pituitary adenomas will contain extensive connective tissue, rendering them tough and unamenable to suction extirpation (1). Adenomas tend not to invade the carotid artery or cranial nerves and may be removed from the cavernous sinus while preserving the artery and nerves. In fact, pituitary adenomas are more readily resected from the cavernous sinus than lesions such as meningiomas, and the attendant morbidity pertaining to cranial nerve dysfunction is much lower (12). Yet, still one must ask in what circumstances should giant invasive adenomas be subjected to radical surgical attack.

Some lesions will have solely suprasellar extension without involvement of the parasellar region. These tumors lend themselves to transsphenoidal resection in all but exceptional cases in which the tumor is firm and fibrous or in which there is an hourglass configuration with a narrow waist created by the diaphragma sella. In this unusual situation, the tumor will not collapse and the optic chiasm cannot be adequately decompressed via the transsphenoidal route. A standard bifrontal or pterional craniotomy may be used to remove the tumor, as discussed elsewhere in this text, or a cranio-orbitozygomatic osteotomy (COZ) may be used, which we advocate and subsequently describe.

Certain adenomas display invasion of bone along with extension into the paranasal sinuses. For most patients, a standard transsphenoidal approach will allow for manage-

ment of these lesions. Addition of a maxillotomy can provide additional room if required. However, when cavernous sinus involvement is accompanied by invasion of the paranasal sinuses, a COZ can be tailored to allow for resection of the paranasal sinus component as well as the tumor in the cavernous sinus. By extending the COZ to the midline, the planum sphenoidale may be drilled to enter the ethmoid and sphenoid sinuses so that this component of the tumor is resected through what has been termed a "transbasal approach" (15). We disfavor the simultaneous transsphenoidal and transcranial resection of pituitary tumors as reported by some authors and believe that this will lead to a higher incidence of infection and cerebrospinal fluid (CSF) leak (16). By using standard skull base approaches, virtually all lesions can be resected through a single exposure; when this cannot be accomplished we would elect to use two different exposures separated in time.

Several situations are, in our opinion, indications for radical surgical resection of giant invasive pituitary adenomas. When a giant tumor with solely suprasellar extension is found during transsphenoidal surgery to be firm and fibrous, the optic chiasm often cannot be adequately decompressed from below. Some authors would advocate radiation therapy in this situation, but it is our belief that aggressive surgical decompression of the optic nerves prior to any contemplated radiation yields better long-term control and a lower incidence of postradiation effects on the optic apparatus. This position is supported by the literature (17, 18). Similarly, pituitary tumors can become so large that they present with symptoms of mass effect and increased intracranial pressure. Surgical resection to remove tumor and alleviate mass effect is mandated in this situation. Radiation therapy without surgical resection is less likely to succeed and is likely to make subsequent exploration more treacherous. If tumor has invaded the cavernous sinus or extended extracranially, an attempt at complete removal should be undertaken at the initial resection. The initial exploration is the best and often only true opportunity to effect a cure.

In rare situations, cavernous sinus invasion can lead to severe pain in the distribution of the trigeminal nerve. When this pain is debilitating and refractory to medical management, surgical attack of the lesion is warranted. Excellent pain control can be achieved with resection of the lesion, and, if needed, surgery may be supplemented with radiation therapy.

It is well established that secretory tumors such as those in Cushing's disease or acromegaly have dramatically shortened life expectancies when the endocrinopathy is not controlled. Radiation may be effective in helping to control the endocrine dysfunction, but if complete surgical resection can be accomplished then the need for radiation therapy, with its potential side effects, may be obviated or the effectiveness of radiation can be increased (17). With the exception of prolactinomas, we advocate aggressive surgi-

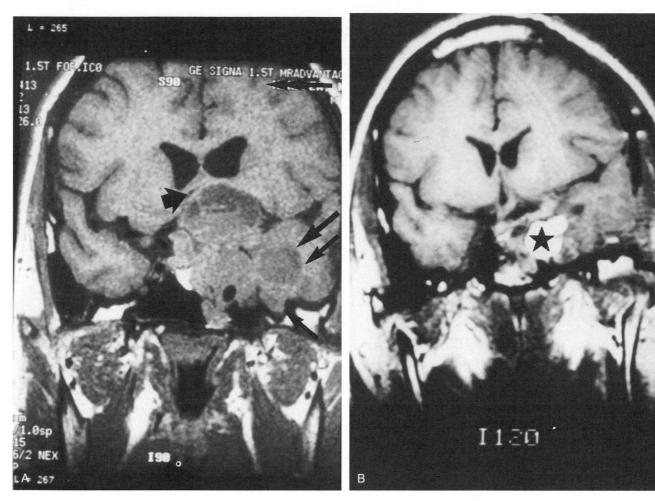

Figure 29.1. A 17-year-old male who presented to another institution with gigantism and was found to have a growth hormone–secreting pituitary adenoma. He underwent partial resection of the tumor without abatement of his endocrinopathy and then was referred to our institution for further therapy. **A.** A magnetic resonance image (MRI) in coronal section without contrast of the patient on arrival at our hospital. A large tumor is seen extending into the left cavernous sinus (*thin arrows*) and obliterating the third ventricle (*thick arrow*). **B.** A postoperative MRI with contrast in coronal section was obtained after surgical resection of the tumor (*COZ*). A normal third ventricle, infundibulum, and optic chiasm are seen. Fat was inserted at the time of surgery to avert a CSF leak and is clearly visualized (*star*). The growth hormone level normalized following the surgery.

cal resection of any endocrinologically active pituitary tumor regardless of the extent of invasion (Fig. 29.1).

Any tumor invading the cavernous sinus is likely to present with diplopia secondary to affectation of cranial nerves 3, 4, and/or 6. Once progressive cranial nerve dysfunction is established, a radical attack is mandated to maximize the potential for cranial nerve recovery. As mentioned previously, the potential for cranial nerve injury during cavernous sinus exploration for a pituitary adenoma is much less than with meningiomas of the cavernous sinus, and in fact the potential for cranial nerve preservation or recovery is greater. In our experience with cavernous sinus exploration for 35 giant invasive pituitary adenomas, no patient at long-term follow-up had worsening of their cranial neuropathy (A Krisht, O Al-Mefty, unpublished data, 1997).

One last situation in which resection of a pituitary adenoma is indicated is for tumor progression despite radiation therapy and/or bromocriptine administration. In centers in which skull base surgery is performed on a regular basis, it is not uncommon for a patient to be referred following a biopsy and radiation when the tumor is seen to progressively enlarge (Fig. 29.2). Since the introduction of bromocriptine, prolactinomas have been largely relegated to the category of nonsurgical disease regardless of size or degree of extension (7). The response to dopamine agonist therapy is normally rapid and dramatic (Fig. 29.3). However, rare situations occur in which a prolactinoma will progress despite optimal medical management with bromocriptine and similar medications, such as pergolide. When prolactinoma progression is clearly documented, then radical surgical resection including exploration of the cavernous sinus and paranasal sinuses is warranted. Once again, these lesions tend to be soft and suckable and do not possess a propensity to invade the cranial nerves or carotid artery. Radical resection followed, when indicated, by radiation and/or medical therapy can be rewarding.

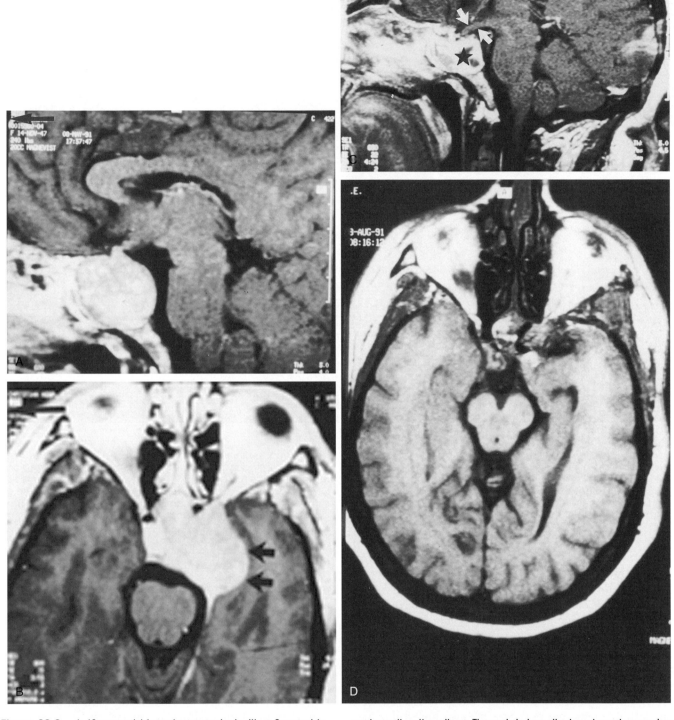

Figure 29.2. A 43-year-old female presented with a 2-year history of dizziness, headaches, and intermittent diplopia. The patient underwent a craniotomy and partial resection of her tumor at another institution, which resulted in a third nerve palsy. Subsequent to this, the tumor increased in size and the patient was referred to our institution for management. An MRI with gadolinium enhancement in sagittal section **(A)** revealed a bulbous lesion filling the sellar region, compressing the optic chiasm, and eroding the clivus. The axial view displays invasion and expansion of the cavernous sinus (*arrows*) by the tumor **(B)**. A COZ and complete microsurgical resection of the tumor was performed. Postoperative MRI examinations with contrast are shown. In the sagittal view **(C)**, the optic chiasm falls back into a normal position (*white arrows*) and the sellar is seen packed with fat (*star*). In the axial view **(D)**, complete resection of the tumor within the cavernous sinus is seen.

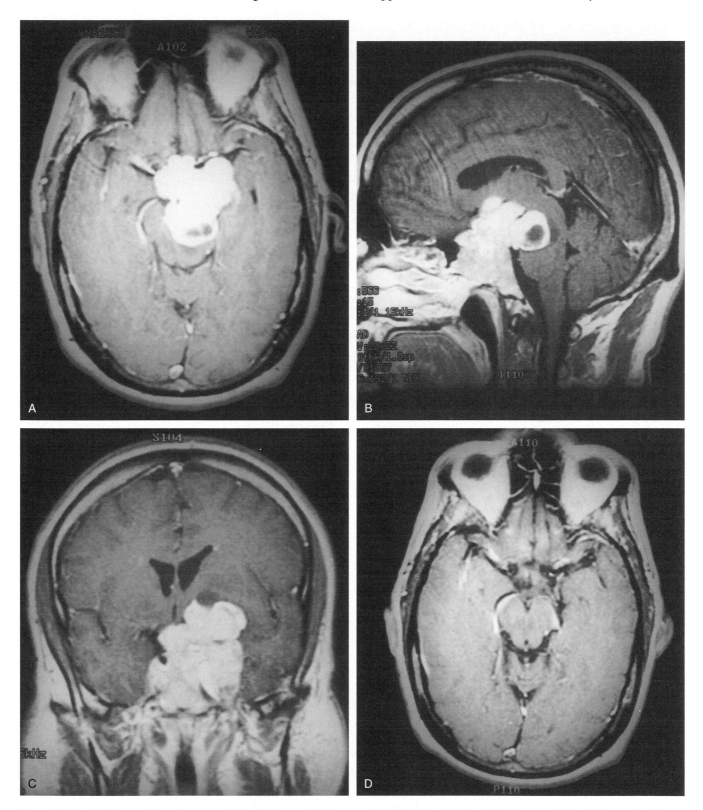

Figure 29.3. A 46-year-old male presented with loss of libido, headaches, and a subtle bitemporal hemianopia only detected with formal visual fields. Prolactin level was found to be greater than 20,000 µg/L (20,000 ng/mL). The patient was started on bromocriptine therapy and a repeat MRI and prolactin level were obtained 2 months later. The prolactin level was 46 µg/L (46 ng/mL) at this time, and the MRI examination revealed dramatic reduction in the tumor mass. Axial **(A)**, sagittal **(B)**, and coronal **(C)** images from the patient at presentation. Axial **(D)**, sagittal **(E)**, and coronal **(F)** views at 2-month follow-up. All images are gadolinium enhanced.

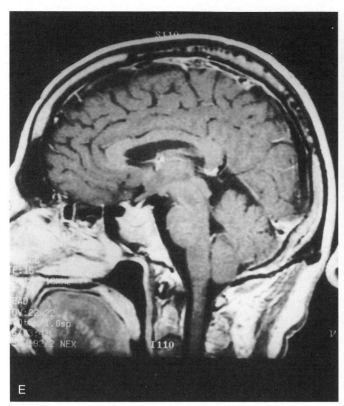
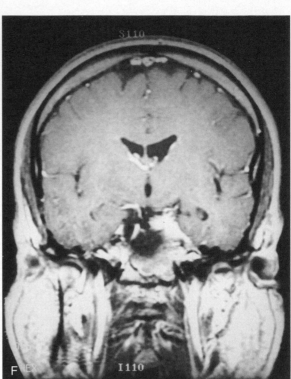

Figure 29.3. *(continued)*

SURGICAL APPROACHES FOR GIANT INVASIVE TUMORS

Once the indication for surgical resection of an invasive adenoma has been established, the surgical approach must be determined. The approach is selected based on the extension of each tumor and any extenuating circumstances of the individual patient. With extension into the paranasal sinuses and extensive invasion of the clivus, modifications of the transsphenoidal approach will be needed. When a craniotomy is appropriate, such as with cavernous sinus invasion with or without extension into the paranasal sinuses, the COZ approach can be tailored to address virtually any lesion.

The COZ Approach

The COZ approach is the approach we would use to resect most giant invasive pituitary adenomas. It provides access to midline structures, including the paranasal sinuses and clivus inferiorly, and allows the surgeon to direct the microscope superiorly to resect tumors from the third ventricle. When tumor extends laterally into the cavernous sinus, this approach renders superb exposure of the cavernous sinus and all adjacent structures. Most important, the COZ approach allows proximal and distal control of the cavernous carotid artery. By removing the orbital rim and roof in continuity with a fronto-temporal craniotomy and

performing a zygomatic osteotomy, excellent exposure of these lesions is obtained while minimizing the need for retraction (Fig. 29.4). If the tumor is larger with significant posterior extension into the incisura or inferiorly into the posterior fossa, removal of the petrous apex allows good exposure to the midclivus (9, 19, 20). The COZ approach provides several distinct advantages over the pterional approach: (*a*) it brings deep-seated lesions closer to the surgeon, providing the shortest possible distance for dissection; (*b*) it creates several potential corridors for attacking the lesion (subfrontal, transsylvian, and subtemporal); (*c*) avenues along the base of the skull intercept the vascular supply to the lesion at the onset of tumor resection, thus minimizing blood loss; (*d*) a single bone flap is created, thus minimizing the need for reconstruction and maximizing cosmetic results; and (*e*) brain retraction is minimized by the removal of this additional bone.

Two of the axioms of skull base surgery are that each approach must be tailored to the needs of the patient and that bone must be removed to avoid brain retraction. Removal of the orbital rim to access the pituitary gland was reported by McArthur (21) in 1912 and later by Frazier (22) in 1913. The supraorbital approach is best suited for midline suprasellar masses and can be used to follow pituitary tumors or craniopharyngiomas through the lamina terminalis into the third ventricle and can spare a patient a subsequent transcallosal approach in certain situations. If access to the sphenoid and ethmoid sinuses is desired, the

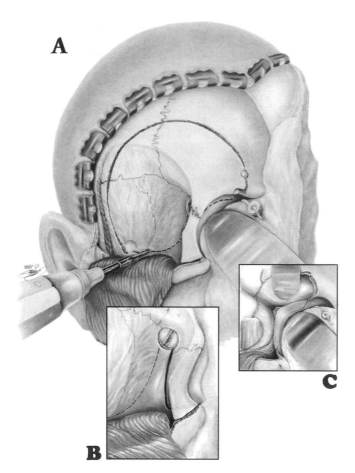

Figure 29.4. This illustration demonstrates some of the key points of the COZ. **A.** A bicoronal skin incision has been created allowing a large sheet of pericranium to be harvested extending posteriorly beneath the scalp almost to the occiput. This vascularized pericranium will be key in reconstructing the skull base and guarding against CSF leaks. An osteotomy through the zygomatic arch has been performed allowing the temporalis muscle to mobilize flush with the floor of the temporal fossa. The bone flap is created in a single piece to include the orbital roof, providing optimal cosmesis. **B.** The keyhole burr hole must be placed at the frontozygomatic suture in a fashion so that an opening is created into the orbit, frontal fossa, and middle fossa simultaneously. **C.** After the craniotomy is performed, including a large portion of the lateral wall and roof of the orbit, further bone may be removed extradurally into the superior orbital fissure and including the anterior clinoid. By maximizing bony removal, brain retraction can be minimized. (Reprinted with permission from Arnautovic K, Al-Mefty O, Angtuaco E. A combined microsurgical skull base and endovascular approach to giant and large paraclinoid aneurysms. Surg Neurol (In Press).)

anterior clinoid, tuberculum sellae, planum sphenoidale, and anterior cranial fossa can be removed with a high-speed drill to gain exposure of the air sinuses and down the clivus to the foramen magnum. The COZ can be extended to the opposite side to widen the exposure and to increase the degrees of freedom in which the microscope can be rotated (23–25).

The patient is positioned supine, and spinal drainage is used. The table is flexed such that the head and trunk are elevated 20 to 25°. The head is placed in three-point pin fixation and rotated 30 to 35° to the contralateral side and

extended such that the frontal lobes will fall away from the floor of the anterior cranial fossa with gravity. The head is maintained neutral and rotation is avoided to facilitate orientation of the surgeon.

A bicoronal skin incision extending from the zygoma of the operative side to the superior temporal line on the contralateral side is created. This incision is extended only through the galea aponeurotica, and great care is exercised to spare the pericranium. During this dissection, the superficial temporal artery is spared to maintain vascularity to the flap in the event that bypass graft is needed later during the procedure. The scalp flap is "peeled" down in a subgaleal plane until the fat pad is identified between the two outer layers of the temporalis fascia. Both outer layers of temporalis fascia are then incised down to muscle extending from the anterior aspect of the superior temporal line to the root of the zygoma. This is a modification of the technique described by Yasargil et al. (26) for the preservation of the frontalis branch of the facial nerve. The fat and fascia are retracted anteriorly over the frontal process of the zygoma with hooks. The scalp flap is then dissected and undermined posteriorly toward the occiput while sparing the pericranium. The pericranium is incised as far posteriorly as can be reached under the flap and dissected anteriorly onto the orbital rims, rendering a large, vascularized pericranial flap. This pericranium will be used at the conclusion of the procedure to repair any defect created in the skull base, and it is thus advantageous to harvest the largest, thickest pericranial flap possible. As the pericranium is dissected across the orbital rim, the supraorbital and supratrochlear branches of the trigeminal nerve will be encountered. They are usually contained within a bony foramen and must be dissected free and preserved with an osteotome or a high-speed drill to avoid an insensate forehead. The pericranial flap will be in continuity with the periorbita, dissection will turn beneath the orbital roof, and the periorbita will be freed from the orbit and preserved. During this phase of the surgery, care must be taken to avoid exerting pressure on the orbital contents and thus jeopardizing vision.

The zygomatic bone is then exposed with subperiosteal dissection to expose it from its root on the temporal bone, anteriorly onto the zygoma proper, and superiorly onto the frontal process of the zygoma along the lateral rim of the orbit. Osteotomies are then created posteriorly on the zygomatic arch just anterior to the temporomandibular joint and anteriorly adjacent to the coronoid process of the mandible. The cuts are made obliquely so that the zygoma can be anchored when it is plated in position at the end of the case. The zygoma is then reflected downward with the masseter still attached. The temporalis muscle is detached from its insertion along the superior temporal line and anteriorly down to the zygoma and then retracted posteriorly and inferiorly. The temporalis muscle is detached anteriorly beneath the frontal process of the zygoma and swept posteriorly to reveal the junction of the zygomatic, sphenoid, and frontal bones. In addition, the temporalis muscle is detached from the superior temporal line and dissected inferiorly such that the squamous part of the temporal bone and the greater wing of the sphenoid is widely exposed down to the infratemporal fossa. Three burr holes are then created. The first is placed at MacCarty's keyhole, providing access to the frontal fossa, middle fossa, and orbit (24). A second burr hole is created in the frontal bone behind the hairline and medial to the superior temporal line. This allows for the dura to be dissected free from the undersurface of the frontal bone without placing a burr hole on the forehead in a cosmetically displeasing location. The third burr hole is place just above the temporal root of the zygoma. An osteotomy is then created in the lateral rim of the orbit as far inferiorly as possible. This is done under direct visualization with either a B5 or a B1 bit on the Midas Rex drill (alternatively, a Gigli saw or a reciprocating saw may be used). The periorbita is protected during the osteotomy with a malleable brain retractor. The cut is extended into the infratemporal fossa, then turned 90° to join the orbital portion of the keyhole. A free frontotemporal bone flap is then created with a craniotome, and the craniotomy is extended into the orbit as close to midline as possible. Along the orbital rim at the midline, the frontal sinus will be entered and the footplate must be removed from the craniotome to produce osteotomies through both posterior and anterior tables of the frontal sinus to open the roof of the orbit. At this point the orbital roof is the only structure holding the free bone flap in place. This bone can be thick, however, and should never be fractured free. Although usually the roof can be fractured in an appropriate direction, it can skew posteriorly into the optic canal with resultant injury to the optic nerve. This cut across the roof of the orbit is produced with an osteotome and a mallet. The dura along the frontal floor and the periorbita are protected during this maneuver with malleable brain retractors. This creates a large, unilateral, frontotemporal craniotomy with an orbital osteotomy in combination with the zygomatic osteotomy that was previously performed. It should be emphasized that with the craniotomy, a generous portion of the temporal and sphenoid bone is included such that the temporal portion of the craniotomy is flush with the floor of the temporal fossa. As mentioned previously, this can be combined with a bifrontal craniotomy, if needed, for larger lesions.

The remaining roof and lateral wall of the orbit is then removed. This removal can be done piecemeal with a rongeur or alternatively resected in one piece with a high-speed drill such that it can be replated at the end of the case. If this orbital flap is replaced during closure, the possibility of enophthalmos and pulsatile exophthalmos is avoided. After the orbital roof is removed, the lesser wing of the sphenoid is resected with rongeurs and a drill to completely unroof the superior orbital fissure. This will lead into the anterior clinoid. The anterior clinoid can be partially or completely removed prior to the dural opening, but from this point onward the operating microscope should be used. When bone removal is performed prior to dural opening, lumbar drainage should be used to minimize brain retraction.

As previously mentioned, control of the internal carotid artery (ICA) proximal and distal to the cavernous sinus is of paramount importance for safe exploration of the cavernous sinus. Two stages are required for this. First, the proximal ICA can be controlled in the neck or in the petrous bone. Because extensive exploration of the middle fossa is required for any cavernous sinus surgery, we standardly control the proximal ICA in the petrous bone. Second, the subclinoid ICA must be exposed and controlled. The subclinoid segment of the carotid artery is exposed by resection of the remainder of the bony encasement of the superior orbital fissure, the anterior clinoid, and the optic canal and strut. This is accomplished with a high-speed diamond drill and can be done extradurally or following dural opening under direct visualization of the optic nerve and ICA. By removing the anterior clinoid and unroofing the optic canal, not only is the subclinoid ICA exposed, but the optic nerve is mobilized over a long segment, facilitating exposure during later tumor removal. If aerated anterior clinoid or ethmoid air cells are entered during drilling, care must be taken at closure to pack these with fat to avoid a CSF leak. The subclinoid carotid artery, once exposed, has exited the cavernous sinus through the distal carotid dural ring and lies extradurally prior to piercing the proximal ring and entering the subarachnoid space. The dura propria of the optic nerve is then opened, completing the mobilization of the optic nerve. This will provide greater visualization of the superior cavernous sinus and in most patients will expose the ophthalmic artery as it branches from the carotid artery.

To gain proximal control of the ICA, the intrapetrous portion of the artery is exposed in Glasscock's triangle (27–29). Following the initial craniotomy, bone should be removed by rongeur so that the opening is flush with the floor of the middle fossa. The microscope is brought into the field and the dura is elevated from the temporal bone beginning posteriorly over the root of the zygoma. Venous oozing may be encountered from the onset of the procedure and can be controlled in various fashions. Gel foam or bone wax can be employed, but recently we have found a paste of gel foam powder and thrombin to be excellent in this situation. A branch of the middle meningeal artery is identified in the dura, and as the dura is raised from the temporal floor, the branch is followed back to the foramen spinosum, where it enters the skull. The middle meningeal artery is coagulated and cut. The foramen spinosum lies just lateral and posterior to the foramen rotundum with the mandibular branch of the trigeminal nerve. Posterior and medial to V3, the greater and lesser superficial petrosal nerves are identified. The greater superficial petrosal nerve (GSPN) will run superficially and parallel to the intrapetrous carotid artery along its lateral border. Classically, it has been taught that the GSPN should be sectioned sharply at this point to avoid traction on the nerve, which can potentially result in a facial nerve palsy. If a long segment of artery is to be unroofed, section of the GSPN is probably prudent, but it will result in a dry eye that can be irritating to the patient and, when accompanied by a facial nerve or V1 deficit, may lead to exposure keratitis. Alternatively, the GSPN can be dissected free from the dura along the artery and preserved. We have encountered no difficulty in doing this, particularly when a Fogarty catheter is used to obtain proximal control, as described by Wascher et al. (30). In up to 40% of cases, the carotid will be only partially covered by bone or not at all. If bone is absent, the periosteum covering the artery will be exposed as the dura is elevated. When bone is present, the horizontal portion of the petrous canal over the ICA is unroofed with a high-speed diamond drill. Only a small opening needs to be created such that a number 2 French Fogarty arterial embolectomy catheter can be inserted into the bony canal extra-arterially. The catheter is threaded back toward the vertical segment of the petrous carotid about 1 cm so that if needed, the catheter can be inflated and occlude the carotid by compression within the bony canal. Only if a bypass is contemplated is extensive drilling and mobilization of the carotid required. If this is done it may be prudent to section the GSPN. If the horizontal segment of the petrous carotid is extensively drilled, the eustachian tube, which lies lateral to the artery and below the tensor tympani muscle, may be opened. If this occurs, the tube must be plugged with muscle or fat during closure to avert a CSF leak.

Once control of the ICA is obtained, surgical resection of the pituitary tumor is undertaken (Fig. 29.5). Initially the extracavernous portion of the tumor is removed using standard microsurgical technique. The cavernous sinus will only be entered after all other tumor is resected and the tumor is followed into the cavernous sinus. The corridor of entry into the cavernous sinus will be dictated by the tumor. There are numerous points of entry into the cavernous sinus that have been described as triangles, but in practice the overwhelming majority of cases will be approached through a superior or a lateral approach. Parkinson's triangle on the lateral wall of the cavernous sinus may also be exploited during a lateral approach and may be used in combination with superior entry into the cavernous sinus. Because of the growth pattern of pituitary adenomas with invasion from the medial wall of the cavernous sinus, superior entry tends to supply the best access to the pathologic lesion. Superior entry is obtained after removal of the anterior clinoid and mobilization of the optic nerve. The superior dural wall is opened along the carotid artery and the artery is followed proximally into the sinus. The structures within the cavernous sinus medial to the cavernous carotid artery are accessed well with this approach. The superior approach is carried out after the sylvian fissure is opened widely, and surgery is conducted primarily transsylvian and subfrontally.

If tumor resection is to be carried out through the lateral wall of the cavernous sinus, once again the sylvian fissure is widely split, and surgery may be conducted transsylvian or subtemporally contingent on anatomy. Different trian-

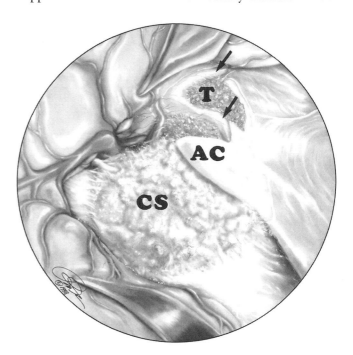

Figure 29.5. Once bony removal is completed, dura is opened and the sylvian fissure is opened widely. In this fashion, CSF is maximally removed, leading to greater relaxation of the brain with optimization of the operating space. In this figure, a pituitary tumor (*T*) is seen invading the cavernous sinus (*CS*, lateral wall of cavernous sinus), engulfing the carotid artery, and elevating and stretching the optic nerves (*arrows*) and chiasm. *AC*, anterior clinoid.

gles have been described by which the cavernous sinus is entered, but each surgical resection is somewhat different and the surgeon must modify his or her attack depending on the anatomic distortion produced by the tumor. After the cavernous sinus has been entered, tumor is removed by suction as the nerves and carotid artery are skeletonized and preserved (Fig. 29.6). Bleeding may be brisk, but where the sinus is filled by tumor, bleeding will be considerably less than where the sinus is not filled with tumor. A certain degree of bleeding from the tumor must be tolerated, but if copious, it must be controlled by packing with cellulose (Surgicel). When the bulk of the tumor is removed, venous bleeding will frequently increase dramatically as the cavernous sinus is reopened.

Once the cavernous sinus has been skeletonized and all tumor removed, fat is harvested from the abdomen or thigh and placed all around the nerves and the ICA. This is particularly important if the ethmoid or sphenoid sinuses are entered. When the paranasal sinuses are violated, they must be denuded of mucosa and packed thoroughly to avoid a postoperative CSF leak.

Closure must be meticulous to avoid a CSF leak, which is the bane of all skull base surgery. After fat is packed into all sinuses and between the cranial nerves and carotid artery, fascia harvested from the thigh or a portion of the pericranium is placed in the floor of the temporal fossa and tacked in position to reproduce the lateral wall of the

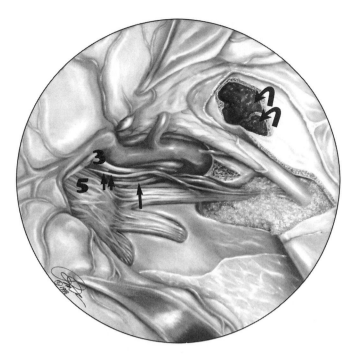

Figure 29.6. Following removal of the anterior clinoid and resection of the planum sphenoidale to enter the sphenoid sinus (*two curved arrows*), the falciform ligament tethering the optic nerve is cut. This maximizes the length and reduces tension on the optic nerve prior to resection of the tumor. All intradural tumor is removed first, and then tumor is resected from the sellar and sphenoid sinus. Next, attention is directed toward the tumor in the cavernous sinus. The lateral wall of the cavernous sinus is removed with identification of the third (3), fourth (*two straight arrows*), and fifth cranial nerves (5, gasserian ganglion). Tumor is "sucked" from around these nerves with gentle suction. The cranial nerve VI (*single straight arrow*) and intracavernous carotid artery will be the last to be identified during the dissection. If there is difficulty in identifying cranial nerve VI, its entrance into Dorello's canal should be sought and the nerve followed through the sinus from its entry. The arteries and nerves of the cavernous sinus are represented here following resection of tumor.

cavernous sinus. Dura is closed watertight even if a duraplasty must be performed. Last, the frontal sinus is obliterated and muscle and fat are packed into the frontonasal duct and the vascularized pericranium is tucked over the sinus and positioned over any skull base defect along the frontal floor, ethmoid sinuses, and sphenoid sinus.

Extended Transsphenoidal Approach

By combining a maxillotomy with a transsphenoidal approach, significantly wider exposure is gained to the skull base (13, 31). The addition of a maxillotomy allows the introduction of a drill through the opening for extensive removal of bone where tumor has invaded the paranasal sinuses and clivus. Lesions extending from the superior sellar region and caudally to the foramen magnum may be attacked through this approach. We have used this approach primarily for chordomas, but the exposure is well suited for any midline lesion. Emphasis must be placed on

midline because lateral dissection is limited, and this approach is ill suited for tumors in which most of the mass is intracranial or in which extensive cavernous sinus invasion is present. The COZ approach, as previously detailed, should be used for such lesions. This approach is ideal for lesions that have broken into the paranasal sinuses and invaded and extended down the clivus. Tumors that have significant midline extension into the third ventricle can be attacked with this approach, but the rationale for introducing the maxillotomy is to widen the exposure and allow drilling of the clivus. Anand et al. (10) previously described approaches that incorporated division of the hard palate, but we rarely use this technique for pituitary tumors. For lesions extending down the clivus below the foramen magnum, a palatal split may be necessary, but this would be exceptional with pituitary tumors. Splitting the palate is not necessary for pituitary adenomas because it adds to the morbidity of the procedure and, during closure, eliminates the buttress for packing fat and fascia against clival dura when repairing openings in the dura. The addition of a maxillotomy will create an increased risk of a postoperative CSF leak when the dura is opened.

The patient is positioned supine on the table, as with the standard transsphenoidal approach, and the head is kept mobile. This mobility can be exploited to the surgeon's advantage during drilling, when rotation of the head can enhance exposure. We use C-arm fluoroscopy for the approach, and in recent cases we have used frameless stereotactic guidance, which adds a measure of safety when drilling along the petrous carotid arteries. In addition, frameless stereotactic guidance delineates tumor margins, providing a greater chance for complete tumor extirpation. The addition of the maxillotomy requires little additional time compared with the standard transsphenoidal exposure, which is detailed elsewhere in this book.

A sublabial incision is created about 1 cm above the gingival mucosa in the standard fashion as when performing a transsphenoidal approach. The incision is extended about 4 cm further laterally on the intended side of the maxillotomy (Fig. 29.7). A subperiosteal dissection is performed to expose the nasal mucosa in the pyriformis opening, except dissection is carried out lateral to the pyriformis opening on the side of the maxillotomy. The subperiosteal dissection is extended up the frontal process of the maxilla just below the inferior aspect of the orbit. The limiting factor in this dissection is the infraorbital nerve, which marks the most superior aspect of the exposure at the infraorbital foramen. The nerve must be spared to avoid a numb cheek postoperatively (Fig. 29.8). The rostral–caudal extent of the dissection must be sufficient to accommodate the entire height of the self-retaining retractor blade. If the maxillotomy is insufficient to allow the self-retaining retractor blade to drop into the opening, no benefit is gained from this extra dissection. Dissection is carried out laterally about 3 to 4 cm, and this will determine the additional width obtained by this exposure. After the standard transsphenoidal exposure is performed in which the cartilaginous nasal septum is disarticulated from the hard palate and vomer, the nasal septum is swung contralateral to the side of the maxillotomy. We have found that when a tumor extends more to one side of the clivus that a maxillotomy on the contralateral side will provide superior exposure of the lesion. When a tumor extends more into the left cavernous sinus and clivus, a right maxillotomy will be performed. Thus, if a right maxillotomy is to be performed, the submucosal tunnel is created down the right side of the nasal septum, and the septum will be swung into the patients left nasal cavity. Prior to creating the maxillotomy, the mucosa is elevated along the lateral aspect of the pyriformis opening sufficiently to accommodate the opening in the maxilla. We have used an oscillating saw to create the maxillotomy on the anterior wall of the maxilla, but, alternatively, a B5 bit on the Midas Rex drill or a reciprocating saw can be used. The maxillotomy is created up to the infraorbital foramen and laterally about 3 to 4 cm or a sufficient distance to permit maximal opening of the self-retaining retractor (we use Hardy retractors). The maxillotomy will incorporate the medial and anterior wall of the maxilla. Following the maxillotomy, any bone that is left along the medial wall of the maxilla (lateral aspect of the pyriformis opening) should be removed with a rongeur. When the self-retaining retractor system is opened maximally, it will push mucosa into the opening in the maxilla created by the maxillotomy. This is what provides the additional width to the exposure (Fig. 29.9). Along the inferior aspect of the vomer, the mucosa must be elevated inferiorly along the clivus to gain maximal caudal exposure. If needed, part of the superior aspect of the hard palate can be removed with a high-speed drill to gain superior visualization inferiorly. In this fashion, exposure is gained of the entire bony clivus, from the superior aspect of the sella to the anterior lip of the foramen magnum. We have used frameless stereotactic guidance during drilling along the petrous carotid arteries and have found it to be helpful. The remainder of the approach is identical to that described for transsphenoidal exposure. After tumor resection, dural repair, and fat grafting are completed, the maxillotomy is repositioned with a microplating system. Postoperative swelling over the maxilla will be more prominent than with a simple transsphenoidal approach, but there is no difference in the long-term cosmetic outcome.

LONG-TERM OUTCOME

As previously noted, only 35 giant invasive pituitary adenomas have been managed at our institution during the past 15 years. Eisenberg et al. (unpublished data) recently analyzed 14 of these patients in detail, and their analysis provides the basis for the following discussion. Among these 14 pituitary adenomas, 5 secreted prolactin, 3 secreted growth hormone, and 6 were not hormonally active. The indications for craniotomy and cavernous sinus dissection were intracranial extension of tumor unresponsive to

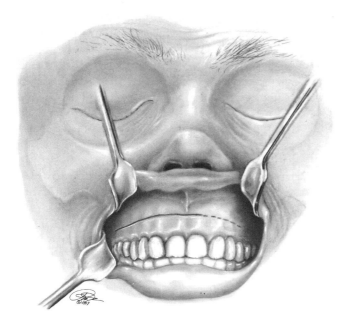

Figure 29.7. As with a standard transsphenoidal procedure, an incision is created below the upper lip about 1 cm above the gingival labial sulcus and is carried down to the periosteum of the maxilla. Illustrated in this figure is the greater lateral extension of the incision to the side of the intended maxillotomy.

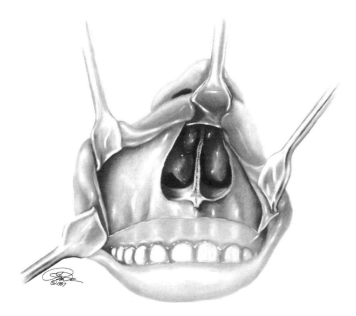

Figure 29.8. Mucosa is then elevated up the maxilla to the infraorbital foramen housing the infraorbital nerve. This will be the superior limit of the mucosal dissection. After the routine dissection, in which mucosa is elevated out of the floor of the pyriformis opening and along the nasal septum, the cartilaginous nasal septum is disarticulated from the hard palate and mobilized to the side contralateral to the intended maxillotomy. A maxillotomy is then created in the anterior and medial wall of the maxilla to remove an L-shaped piece of bone. The maxillotomy extends superiorly to but sparing the infraorbital nerve and laterally a sufficient distance to allow *complete* opening of the self-retaining nasal speculum. The dimensions of the maxillotomy provides the exact width gained for the exposure by this addition to standard transsphenoidal surgery.

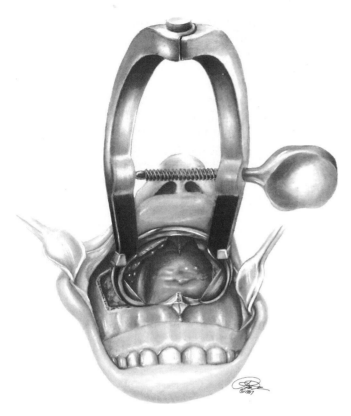

Figure 29.9. This illustration demonstrates the wide exposure of the clivus and parasellar region gained with the extended transsphenoidal approach. By sweeping mucosa into the maxillary sinus with the retractor blade, enough width is gained to allow comfortable manipulation of a drill and attack of tumor extending down the clivus.

transsphenoidal resection (6 cases), invasive growth hormone–secreting tumor (3 cases), ocular motor neuropathy (2 cases), CSF leak (2 cases), hemorrhage into the tumor bed following subtotal transsphenoidal resection (1 case),

and recurrent tumor following radiotherapy (1 case). Extraocular motor function was worsened by surgery in only 2 of the 14 patients. Of 10 patients with excellent extraocular motor function, 8 had excellent function postoperatively. No patient had improved extraocular function following surgery. Thus, once progression of diplopia is noted, surgery should be undertaken as soon as possible to preserve function. Complete tumor resection was obtained in 10 of the 14 patients, for a total resection rate of 71.4%. Incomplete resection was caused by extensive invasion into the sphenoid and both temporal bones. One of these patients had been referred after seven previous surgeries and radiation therapy. Two patients had recurrence following total resection (one prolactinoma and one nonfunctional). The patient with the prolactinoma is well controlled with bromocriptine therapy at 17-month follow-up. The patient with the recurrent nonfunctional tumor expired from disease progression despite three subsequent surgeries. Two patients with subtotal resection of their tumors had continued growth of residual adenoma (one prolactinoma and one nonfunctional). The patient with the prolactinoma is well controlled with bromocriptine therapy at 22-month follow-up. The patient with the nonfunctional adenoma has experienced progression of disease despite further surgery and radiation.

When analyzing the above data we noted that the outcome for giant pituitary tumors of the cavernous sinus is inferior to that for lesions such as trigeminal schwannomas in the same series but superior to data reported for meningiomas of the cavernous sinus (12). When appropriate indications for cavernous sinus exploration are present for pituitary tumors we remain enthusiastic about aggressive surgical resection. This enthusiasm is bolstered by data for giant invasive pituitary adenomas when aggressive resection is not undertaken. When giant pituitary tumors are treated with standard resection and radiation alone, long-term survival is less than 16% (17).

REFERENCES

1. Wilson CB. Neurosurgical management of large and invasive pituitary tumors. In: Tindall GT, Collins WF, eds. Clinical Management of Pituitary Disorders. New York: Raven Press, 1979:335–342.
2. Wilson CB. A decade of pituitary microsurgery: The Herbert Olivercrona Lecture. J Neurosurg 1984;61:814–833.
3. Guidetti B, Fraioli B, Cantore GP. Results of surgical management of 319 pituitary adenomas. Acta Neurochir (Wien) 1987;85:117–124.
4. Jefferson G. Extrasellar extension of pituitary adenomas. Proc R Soc Med 1940;33:433–458.
5. Mohr G, Hardy J, Comtois R, et al. Surgical management of giant pituitary adenomas. Can J Neurol Sci 1990;17:62–66.
6. Symon L, Jakubowski J, Kendall B. Surgical treatment of giant pituitary adenomas. J Neurol Neurosurg Psychiatry 1979;42:973–982.
7. King LW, Molitch ME, Gittinger JW Jr, et al. Cavernous sinus syndrome due to prolactinoma: resolution with bromocriptine. Surg Neurol 1983;19:280–284.
8. Ludecke DK. Invited commentary: value of transcavernous surgery in the treatment of pituitary adenomas. Eur J Endocrinol 1995;133:147–148.
9. Al-Mefty O, Smith RR. Clival and petroclival meningiomas. In: Al-

Mefty O, ed. Meningiomas. New York: Raven Press, 1991:517–553.
10. Anand VK, Harkey HL, Al-Mefty O. Open-door maxillotomy approach for lesions of the clivus. Skull Base Surg 1991;1:217–225.
11. Anson JA, Segal MN, Baldwin N, et al. Resection of giant invasive pituitary tumors through a transfacial approach: technical case report. Neurosurgery 1995;37:541–546.
12. DeMonte F, Smith H, Al-Mefty O. Outcome of aggressive removal of cavernous sinus meningiomas. J Neurosurg 1994;81:245–251.
13. Fraioli B, Esposito V, Santoro A, et al. Transmaxillosphenoidal approach to tumors invading the medial compartment of the cavernous sinus. J Neurosurg 1995;82:63–69.
14. Matsuno A, Sasaki T, Saito N, et al. Transcavernous surgery: an effective treatment for pituitary macroadenomas. Eur J Endocrinol 1995;133:156–165.
15. Arita N, Shintaro M, Sano M, et al. Surgical treatment of tumors in the anterior skull base using the transbasal approach. Neurosurgery 1989;24:379–384.
16. Loyo M, Kleriga E, Mateos H, et al. Combined supra-infrasellar approach for large pituitary tumors. Neurosurgery 1984;14:485–488.

17. Hashimoto N, Handa H, Yamashita J, et al. Long-term follow-up of large or invasive pituitary adenomas. Surg Neurol 1986;25: 49–54.
18. Hughes MN, Llamas KJ, Yelland ME, et al. Pituitary adenomas: long-term results for radiotherapy alone and post-operative radiotherapy. Int J Radiat Oncol Biol Phys 1993;27:1035–1043.
19. Al-Mefty O, Fox JL, Smith RR. Petrosal approach for petro-clival meningiomas. Neurosurgery 1988;22:510–517.
20. Haddad G, Al-Mefty O. Approaches to petroclival tumors. In: Wilkins RH, Rengachary SS, eds. Neurosurgery. 2nd ed. New York: McGraw-Hill, 1996:1695–1706.
21. McArthur LL. An aseptic surgical access to the pituitary body and its neighborhood. JAMA 1912;58:2009–2011.
22. Frazier CH. An approach to the hypophysis through the anterior cranial fossa. Ann Surg 1913;57:145–152.
23. Al-Mefty O. Clinoidal meningiomas. J Neurosurg 1990;73: 840–849.
24. Al-Mefty O, Smith RR. Tailoring the cranio-orbital approach. Kwio J Mws 1990;39(4):217–224.
25. Al-Mefty O. The cranio-orbital zygomatic approach for intracranial lesions. Contemp Neurosurg 1992;14:1–6.
26. Yasargil MG, Reichman MV, Kubik S. Preservation of the fronto-temporal branch of the facial nerve using the interfascial temporalis flap for pterional craniotomy: technical article. J Neurosurg 1987; 67:463–466.
27. Glasscock ME III, Miller GW, Drake FD, et al. Surgery of the skull base. Laryngoscope 1978;88:905–923.
28. Glasscock ME III. Exposure of the intra-petrous portion of the carotid artery. In: Hamberger CA, Wersall J, eds. Disorders of the Skull Base Region. Stockholm: Almqvist and Wiksell, 1969: 135–143.
29. Paullus WS, Pait TG, Rhoton AL Jr. Microsurgical exposure of the petrous portion of the carotid artery. J Neurosurg 1977;47: 713–726.
30. Wascher TM, Spetzler RF, Zabramski JM. Improved transdural exposure and temporary occlusion of the petrous internal carotid artery for cavernous sinus surgery: technical note. J Neurosurg 1993; 78:834–837.
31. Rabadan A, Conesa H. Transmaxillary-transnasal approach to the anterior clivus: a microsurgical anatomical model. Neurosurgery 1992;30:473–482.

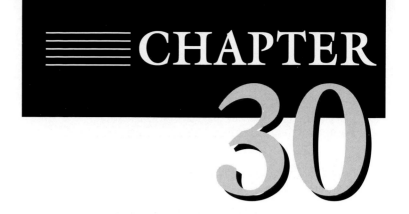

Endoscopic Surgery of Pituitary Adenomas

Hae-Dong Jho

INTRODUCTION

When Hirsh in Vienna reported transsphenoidal pituitary surgery in 1910, he adopted endonasal techniques using multiple staged operations, including resection of the middle turbinate and ethmoidectomy. Despite successful endonasal surgery in his first patient, he did not continue to use the endonasal route for transsphenoidal pituitary surgery. Instead, he changed his endonasal transsphenoidal techniques to a transseptal approach via a nasal hemitransfixion incision (1). The endonasal approach was revived by Griffith and Veerapen (2) in 1987. In their microscopic transsphenoidal pituitary surgeries, they placed a transsphenoidal retractor directly into the nasal cavity to reach the rostrum of the sphenoidal sinus. Cooke and Jones (3) in 1994 reported benign outcomes with the endonasal approach when they used it in their microscopic pituitary surgery with a transsphenoidal retractor. This endonasal route incorporating the natural nasal air pathway has been used for the endoscopic pituitary surgery described in this chapter. Use of an endoscope in replacement of the operating microscope as the visualizing tool eliminates the need for a transsphenoidal retractor or nasal speculum, which microscopic surgery requires.

Although the idea for use of an endoscope in pituitary surgery had once lingered in the past (4), it was never clinically substantiated in pituitary surgery until recently. Use of endoscopes became practical earlier in sinunasal surgery than in pituitary surgery. Since a sinunasal endoscope was adopted in paranasal sinus surgery with modern equipment, endoscopic sinus surgery has gradually replaced conventional invasive sinus surgery (5). Rhinologists have been able to operate on lesions involving the sphenoidal sinus with the endoscope as the sole visualizing tool. The sellar floor can be easily exposed when the surgeon visualizes the internal cavity of the sphenoid sinus. The angled lens of the endoscope enables the surgeon to look into anatomic corners that the operating microscope cannot. Panoramic visualization and close-up views of the important structures are additional advantages provided by the use of endoscopes. Encouraged by comparable surgical outcome and quick postoperative patient recovery obtained in sinunasal surgery by an endoscopic technique, the sinunasal endoscope was implemented in pituitary surgery.

The endoscopic pituitary surgery technique described here adopts an endonasal route through the natural nasal cavity without an additional ethmoidectomy or resection of the middle turbinate. Rigid sinunasal endoscopes that are 17 cm in length and 4 mm in diameter and have 0, 30, or 70° lenses are used. These endoscopes do not have working channels in the shaft. Surgical instruments are introduced through the same nostril next to the endoscope.

Different techniques in use of the endoscope in pituitary surgery as well as surgical anatomy, instruments, detailed surgical techniques, patient management, and advantages and disadvantages of endoscopic pituitary surgery are described in this chapter.

SURGICAL ANATOMY FOR ENDONASAL ENDOSCOPIC PITUITARY SURGERY

The endonasal endoscopic technique for pituitary surgery does not involve complicated anatomic structures in passage through the nasal cavity to reach the sella. Important neurovascular structures are located adjacent to the sella itself. The middle turbinate is easily visualized with a 0° endoscope when the patient's head is positioned horizontally and neutrally. Lateral to the middle turbinate is the ostium of the maxillary sinus. When the middle turbinate is pushed laterally, the sphenoid ostium is under direct endoscopic view. Fluoroscopic roentgenographic C-arm images of the lateral skull can visualize a surgical instrument placed to aim at the vertical dimension of the sella. At the rostrum of the sphenoid sinus inferior to the middle turbinate, the posterior septal artery arises from the sphenopalatine artery and crosses to reach the posterior portion of the nasal septum. When inferior exposure is required, the posterior septal artery has to be coagulated with a monopolar suction coagulator. The caudal end of the middle turbinate often leads to the floor level of the sella.

The nasal septum is easy to fracture from the rostrum of the sphenoid sinus at the midportion level. However, at the lower portion of the nasal septum, the septal insertion to the rostrum of the sphenoid sinus is sometimes difficult to fracture because of the thick bone of the vomer. Further inferior dissection at the rostrum of the sphenoid sinus will lead the surgeon to the middle or inferior clivus. Superior dissection leads to the ethmoid sinus, through which the anterior fossa base can be reached. When an anterior sphenoidotomy is performed, anatomic bony structures will then be under direct and clear endoscopic view. Clival indentation can be visualized then by looking midline and inferiorly. On either side of the clival indentation the carotid bony protuberances that lead up to the cavernous sinus can be noted. Superior to the clival indentation is the sella. At the 11 o'clock and 1 o'clock points superior to the sella are the optic protuberances. Between the optic protuberance and the cavernous sinus the opticocarotid recess is notable as a lateral indentation (Fig. 30.1A, B). When the sphenoid sinus septum is septated in a complex and multiple manner, the bony anatomy may not be as distinct as usual. In that case, fluoroscopic corroboration is useful for the surgeon's orientation leading to the sella.

When the bone covering the carotid protuberance and cavernous sinus is removed and the dura mater is opened, the carotid artery lateral to the clival indentation swings

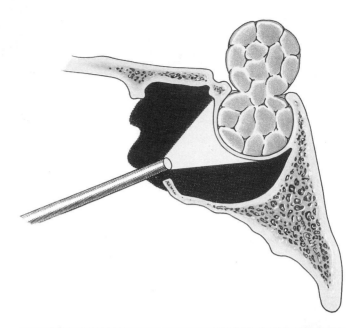

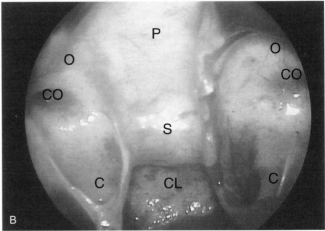

Figure 30.1. **A.** Schematic drawing demonstrates endoscopic exposure of the sellar region through the sphenoid sinus. **B.** The 0°-lens endoscope depicts the sella (*S*), clival indentation (*CL*), carotid artery bony protuberances (*C*), optic nerve bony protuberances (*O*), caroticooptic recesses (*CO*), and planum sphenoidale (*P*).

superiorly and makes an S-shaped serpentine turn in the cavernous sinus before it penetrates the inner dural ring reaching the subarachnoid space lateral to the optic nerve. Because the ophthalmic cranial nerves run along the lateral wall of the cavernous dura mater, the exposure of the carotid artery does not disclose the cranial nerves in the cavernous sinus. However, the abducens nerve runs lateral to the lower portion of the S-shaped carotid siphon from the Dorello's canal to the superior orbital fissure. Rostral to the sella, the optic nerves and the dura mater at the planum sphenoidale can be exposed by removal of the optic bony protuberance and the planum sphenoidale. The supradiaphragma area can easily be exposed by additional bone removal at the anterosuperior portion of the sella. A 30°

endoscope inserted into the sella visualizes the diaphragma sella and suprasellar structures nicely (Fig. 30.2*A, B*). When the pituitary gland is completely resected and the arachnoid membrane is opened, the optic nerves, optic chiasm, optic tract, inferior hypothalamus, anterior cerebral artery complex, and arteries of posterior circulation are under direct view of the 30° endoscope. When the clival bone is removed, an anterior view of the pons and midbrain will be under direct view of the 0° endoscope. Endoscopes with 30 and 70° lenses can visualize the further rostral parts of the brainstem in the posterior fossa. To operate under the 30 or 70° endoscope, surgical instruments have to be accordingly curved in shape.

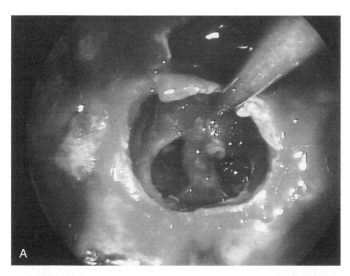

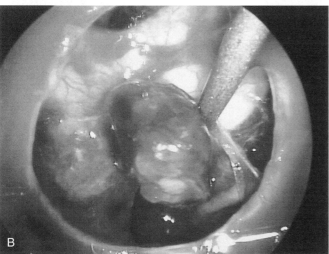

Figure 30.2. In a patient with a craniopharyngioma, the pituitary stalk was sectioned distally for complete tumor resection in addition to the excision of the tumor. The pituitary stalk is visualized at the center of the opening of the dura mater at the anterior wall of the sella and the edge of the diaphragma sella through a 0°-lens endoscope **(A)**. When the 30°-lens endoscope is introduced into the sella, the pituitary stalk at the center and the optic chiasm are directly visualized through the diaphragma sella **(B)**.

IMPLEMENTATION OF THE ENDOSCOPE IN PITUITARY SURGERY

The endoscope can be adopted in pituitary surgery either as the sole surgical tool for visualization (6–16) or as a supplemental tool to the operating microscope (17, 18). Conventional microscopic pituitary surgery has achieved good surgical outcome with minimal morbidity (19–21). To augment visibility into anatomic corners or into the suprasellar region, a 30°-angled endoscope can be used. Advantages of using the endoscope are its capability to visualize areas and to provide close-up views that the limited peripheral visualization of the operating microscope cannot. Although it has not been substantiated scientifically yet, a proximal endoscopic view at the tumor–pituitary interface may enable the surgeon to perform a more complete resection of the tumor. However, supplementary use of an endoscope during microscopic pituitary surgery is cumbersome for surgeons who are used to microscopic pituitary surgery. Setting up for the use of an endoscope may further crowd the operating room, which is already saturated with heavy equipment. Operating under an endoscope through the tunnel provided by transsphenoidal retractors is often a nerve-provoking experience for the surgeon who is not familiar with endoscopic techniques. Nevertheless, it may provide the surgeon with assurance of its usefulness with increase of his experience. When the surgeon's confidence in use of the endoscope increases, an endoscope can be used as the sole visualizing tool, replacing the operating microscope completely.

Another way to initiate use of the endoscope is to simply replace the operating microscope with the endoscope as the only visualizing tool. Although a few of the author's early patients were operated on under the operating microscope with supplementary use of the endoscope, the endoscopic techniques described in this chapter were developed using the endoscope alone. This endoscopic technique eliminates use of a transsphenoidal retractor or nasal speculum because the endoscope in application does not require much space when an endonasal route is used. If endoscopic techniques use a conventional transseptal route, the transsphenoidal retractor is required, and, subsequently, the patient's quick postoperative recovery will be compromised by nasal packing and the mucosal incision. In addition, use of the transsphenoidal retractor decreases the surgeon's operating space from a large natural nasal cavity to a narrow tubular cavity that the retractor provides. However, endoscopic pituitary surgery is technically demanding, and there certainly is a learning curve dependent on the surgeon's increasing experience. In our earlier patients, placement of telfa or Gel-film next to the middle turbinate was almost routine to minimize postoperative dripping of blood. A small piece of Gel-foam was also laid at the anterior wall of the sella. Lately, laying foreign materials in the sphenoid sinus or nasal cavity has not been required at all owing simply to the minimized mucosal trauma relative to the surgeon's increased experience. In our patients, postoperative nasal dripping of blood has been trivial. However, it should not be surprising because of the intrinsic learning curve of using an endoscope in pituitary surgery to hear a surgeon's frustration or complaints following his first few attempts. The endoscope is still simply a surgical tool. Its usefulness and benefit in pituitary surgery should be evaluated by surgeons who have experience in conventional microscopic pituitary surgery. Technical adroitness in handling a sinunasal endoscope alone should not be the justification for surgeons to attempt pituitary tumor surgery.

EQUIPMENT FOR ENDONASAL ENDOSCOPIC PITUITARY SURGERY

Endoscopes

Although ideally shaped endoscopes for pituitary surgery are not yet commercially available, the endoscopes used in our endonasal pituitary surgery are 4-mm-diameter and 17-cm-long rigid sinunasal endoscopes with 0, 30, and 70° lenses (Fig. 30.3). These endoscopes do not have built-in working channels or irrigation-suction ports. Surgical instruments are inserted parallel to and next to the endoscope through the same nostril. Use of an endoscope with a built-in working channel may enable the surgeon to perform a biopsy of a tumor or decompression of the optic system or of the pituitary gland with subtotal resection of a tumor; however, its use is not practical in performing delicate dissection to achieve total resection of tumor from

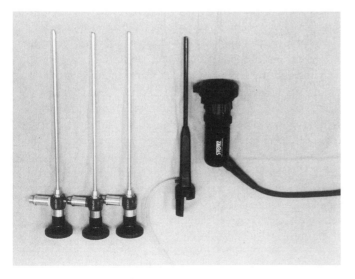

Figure 30.3. The endoscopes used in our endonasal pituitary surgery are 4-mm-diameter and 17-cm-long sinunasal endoscopes with 0-, 30-, and 70°-angled lenses. Although they are not ideal yet and not made for pituitary surgery or other neurosurgical use, they are suitable for endoscopic pituitary surgery.

the surrounding pituitary gland. Because a flexible endoscope reduces clarity of the image, only rigid endoscopes were used. Our operations were performed mostly with a 0° endoscope. The 30° endoscope was used for further investigation of the rostral area and for exploring the intrasellar cavity and suprasellar region.

Although it is not ideal for neurosurgical use and not specifically made for endonasal transsphenoidal surgery, the 4-mm-diameter endoscope with 17-cm length has proven suitable for endonasal transsphenoidal pituitary surgery. When endonasal endoscopic resection of a posterior fossa tumor was performed, this particular endoscope was marginally short in length. Although the 0° endoscope can be rotated in any direction without disturbing the surgeon's surgical orientation, an endoscope with an angled lens requires fixed positioning for surgical orientation. When the angled endoscope is fixed to the surgeon's anatomic orientation in the video monitor, its accompanying appendages often limit the surgeon's access to the nasal cavity. To improve the instrumental problems of the endoscope in its use for transsphenoidal surgery so that the surgeon can have unlimited access to the nostril around the endoscope shaft, the endoscope's appendages, such as the light source and video camera attachments, should enter the shaft either along the axis of the shaft or in a mildly angled fashion. In most of the currently available endoscopes, the light source enters the endoscope at a right angle. A longer endoscope may be an alternative answer for this problem. An endoscope with a 21- to 24-cm shaft length is better suited for endonasal pituitary surgery and provides ample operating space between the patient's face and the endoscopic appendages.

An endoscope with a 70° lens has been used occasionally to access a posterior view of a structure; however, maneuvering surgical instruments under the 70° endoscope requires a high level of endoscopic surgical skill. A surgeon needs to get used to the reversed mirror images of the 70° endoscope to operate under its visualization. We have not encountered a situation that requires a 70° endoscope during surgery for pituitary adenomas. We used a 70° endoscope in posterior fossa tumor resection and for exploration of the anterior fossa skull base. To operate under the 70° endoscope, surgical instruments need to be curved accordingly to be maneuvered to the surgical target.

We have used a 5-mm-diameter stereoscopic endoscope (3-D) in two patients. Although the depth perception with the 3-D video image was an advantage over the two-dimensional flat images, the spectacles worn for the 3-D endoscope increased the surgeon's visual fatigue. The benefit in computer technology providing virtual reality surgery remains to be proven in the future. The sharpness and clarity of endoscopic images in the video monitor are still inferior to that of direct microscopic visualization. When the improved technology of a high-definition monitor comes into practical use, the clarity of video images will certainly improve.

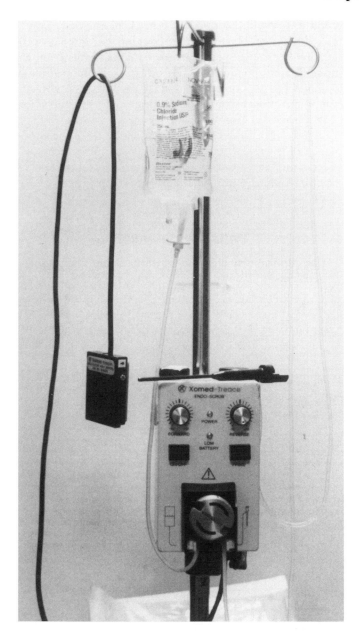

Figure 30.4. The endoscope lens cleansing device (Endo-scrub, Xomed-Treace, Bristol-Myers Squibb, Jacksonville, FL) is an indispensable tool for cleaning the lens without removing the endoscope from the surgical field. The power-driven irrigation-suction device cleanses the lens and is activated by the surgeon's foot pedal.

Endoscope Cleansing Device (Endoscrub)

Without a lens cleansing attachment, the value of the endoscope can be severely limited by inevitable fogging and bloodstaining of the lens. Although a defogging lubricant has been used to minimize these problems, its use only reduces fogging of the lens induced by temperature differences between room and body temperature. A recently introduced lens cleansing device (Endoscrub, Xomed-Treace, Bristol-Myers Squibb, Jacksonville, FL) has been an advance toward this goal (Fig. 30.4). Its function is similar to that of the windshield wiper in a car. A

thin tube is placed over the endoscope shaft and a power-driven irrigation-suction mechanism is activated to clean the lens by a foot pedal. This motorized irrigation-suction device cleans the lens by irrigation and removes water bubbles from the lens by reverse flow of suction. This lens cleansing device eliminates the cumbersome effort of wiping and cleaning the lens by frequently removing the endoscope from the surgical field. Although this device has not completely solved the problem of cleansing the lens yet, it has reduced the surgeon's unnecessary work load significantly. This device is essential for an uninterrupted endoscopic operation. A better lens cleansing system is yet to be devised in the future.

Rigid Endoscope Holder ("Genny" Holder)

During the nasal portion of the procedure, the endoscope is held in the surgeon's nondominant hand and a surgical instrument is held in the other hand. However, once the anterior sphenoidotomy is completed and the anterior wall of the sella is exposed, an endoscope holder is used to fix the endoscope. The endoscope holder will render steady video images as well as allowing the surgeon to use two hands freely. Our endoscope holder consists of a commercially available Greenberg retractor mounting system and a custom-made connecting device that was developed with the help of our operating room head nurse, "Genny." A Greenberg clamp with a jointed bar is mounted to a three-pin head fixator. The Genny holder is connected to the Greenberg bar. The Genny holder has two additional joints that can be tightened by a screw-shaped tightener. At the end of the holder, a small clamp with a plastic inner ring holds the endoscope tightly (Fig. 30.5). This endoscope holding clamp at the terminal of

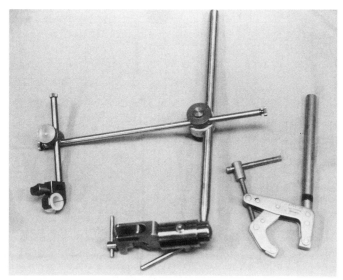

Figure 30.5. Our endoscope holder consists of a combination of a Greenberg retractor mounting system and our own custom-made distal joint (Genny holder). It will provide rigid fixation of the endoscope and allow the surgeon to use both hands freely.

the holding device is made small so that it provides the surgeon with the maximum available operating space around the endoscope shaft. Our endoscope holder renders rigid fixation of the endoscope. Current commercially available endoscope holders are either not rigid enough to hold the endoscope tightly or are so bulky at the endoscope holding terminal joint that it obliterates valuable operating space around the endoscope shaft near the nostril. This endoscope holder is another piece of essential equipment for endoscopic pituitary surgery in addition to the endoscopic lens cleansing device.

Fluoroscopic C-Arm

As with the conventional microscopic transsphenoidal technique, the fluoroscopic C-arm images are used to corroborate surgical anatomy, especially to determine the extent of the vertical dimension of the anterior sphenoidotomy and also the vertical dimension of the sella. Although the operations can be performed without use of fluoro-

scopic imaging in most patients, its use has helped to optimize the size of the anterior sphenoidotomy and has occasionally been indispensable in patients with complex multiseptated sphenoidal sinuses. If the endoscope holder is connected to computer-assisted frameless stereotactic equipment, fluoroscopic roentgenographic corroboration of the surgical anatomy may not be necessary. Stereotactic equipment can also be adopted independently of the endoscope holder, replacing the fluoroscopic C-arm. The cost-effectiveness and accuracy of computer-assisted stereotaxis may dictate future implementation of stereotaxis in endoscopic pituitary surgery.

Surgical Instruments

The surgical instruments used for endoscopic pituitary surgery are sinunasal surgery instruments for the nasal part of the operation and microscopic transsphenoidal instruments for the sellar part of the operation. In addition, various other microsurgical instruments are used for tumor

Figure 30.6. Surgical instruments used for our endoscopic pituitary surgery are those used for sinunasal surgery **(A)** and microscopic transsphenoidal surgery, and various other microsurgical instruments **(B)**.

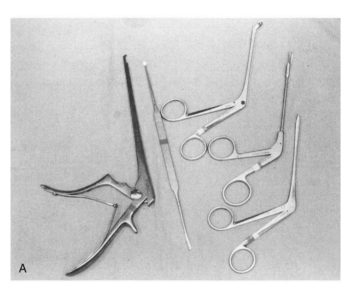

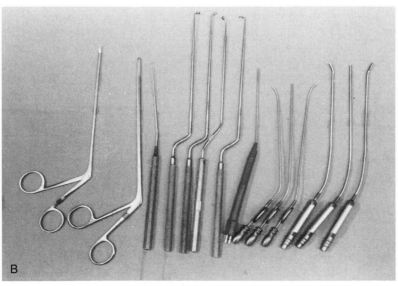

removal (Fig. 30.6*A, B*). The intranasal procedure is performed mostly with a number 7 French suction cannula, a number 8 suction monopolar coagulator, a Cottle elevator, a micropituitary rongeur, and a straight ethmoidal rongeur. In addition, variously angled ethmoidal rongeurs, ethmoidal scissors, transsphenoidal bipolar forceps, and a high-speed microsurgical drill are occasionally used. A number 8 French monopolar suction-coagulator is a valuable tool for bloodless dissection of the sphenoidal rostrum. Use of a suction-coagulator will minimize postoperative nasal blood dripping. The sellar procedure is performed using a small straight bone curette; Kerrison rongeurs with a 1- or 2-mm footplate; occasionally a high-speed microsurgical drill; left- and right-angled, single-bladed Kurze microscissors; variously angled pituitary ring curettes; a 45°-angled Jannetta microdissector; variously curved number 7 and number 5 suction cannulas; micropituitary rongeurs; and a single-bladed, bipolar coagulator. The single-bladed, bipolar coagulator has two electric cables to function as a bipolar coagulator with one cable at the core and the other at the shell. Most of the surgical instruments are made up of existing transsphenoidal instruments with some offhand modification and other microsurgical instruments. The ideal surgical instruments would be single-bladed, slender tools with the shape and mechanics similar to that of a micropituitary rongeur. Valuable tools for microdissection of a tumor are a 100-μm-diameter, 45°-angled, and bayoneted Jannetta microdissector and variously curved number 5 French suction cannulas. Recently introduced dural microclips enabled us to perform dural reconstruction using a fascial graft even after a wide opening of the skull base dura mater.

INDICATIONS FOR OPERATION

Although our endonasal endoscopic transsphenoidal technique has been used mostly in patients with pituitary adenomas, we have been expanding the implication of our technique to various other skull base lesions, such as anterior fossa skull base lesions, cavernous sinus lesions, various sellar and suprasellar lesions, and posterior fossa tumors. Generally speaking, surgical indications for endoscopic pituitary surgery are the same as those for conventional microscopic pituitary surgery. In addition, this endoscopic pituitary surgical technique enables direct access to a tumor located at the suprasellar region; therefore, a suprasellar tumor that used to require a transcranial approach may still be approachable by the endoscopic transsphenoidal technique. However, endoscopic access to tumors located at the middle fossa is still limited. The middle fossa can be reached lateral to the cavernous sinus. However, the cavernous sinus, intracranial carotid artery, and optic nerve system will hinder access to the middle fossa. Recently, the threshold of surgical indication has been reduced owing to minimal surgical risk and to the patients' quick surgical recovery, especially in the elderly population.

PREOPERATIVE PREPARATION

All of the patients underwent preoperative formal endocrine testing. Formal visual evaluation, including visual acuity and field testing, was also performed preoperatively. Preoperative magnetic resonance imaging (MRI) was obtained on every patient, and most had a preoperative computed tomographic (CT) scan. The exquisite delineation of the bony structures of the sinus, provided by thinly sliced axial and coronal CT scans, seemed to be valuable to assess bony anatomy in the sphenoid sinus and nasal cavity and its relationship to the sella floor, optic nerve canals, bony coverage over the cavernous sinuses, and carotid canals. CT scans have recently been obtained selectively only when an MRI scan suggests complicated anatomy in the sphenoidal sinus. However, the true value of CT scans has been under scrutiny.

The patients with preoperative hypopituitarism were treated in advance with hormonal replacement prior to operation. Most of our earlier patients were treated with perioperative "stress doses" of hydrocortisone. Recently, however, perioperative steroids have been avoided when an endocrine deficit was lacking preoperatively and not expected postoperatively. Prophylactic antibiotics, comprising 1 g of cefazolin or, occasionally, 1 g of vancomycin and 80 mg of gentamicin if the patient has an allergy to cefazolin, were administered intravenously as a single intraoperative dose. A topical clindamycin (600 mg in 500 cc of normal saline) solution was used as an irrigation solution through the suction-irrigation lens cleansing device to irrigate the nasal cavity and the sphenoid sinus throughout the procedure. Although Foley catheters were inserted in the operating suites in our earlier patients, its use has been recently selected only for patients who have a risk of developing diabetes insipidus. When a Foley catheter is inserted and the patient does not need a strict hourly intake and output measurement postoperatively, it is removed directly after surgery. The anesthesiologist is advised to restrict intraoperative intravenous fluid administration to less than 2000 cc to eliminate postoperative confusion between postoperative diuresis and possible diabetes insipidus.

OPERATIVE TECHNIQUE

Positioning and Intraoperative Preparation of a Patient

The positioning and preparation of patients is similar to that for conventional microscopic surgery (Fig. 30.7). General anesthesia is induced and maintained with orotracheal intubation. The patient is positioned supine, with the hips and the knees gently flexed. A pillow is placed under the knees. The torso is elevated about 20° to place the level of the head higher than that of the heart to possibly reduce the intracranial venous pressure. This elevation of the torso may eliminate unwanted venous bleeding around the cav-

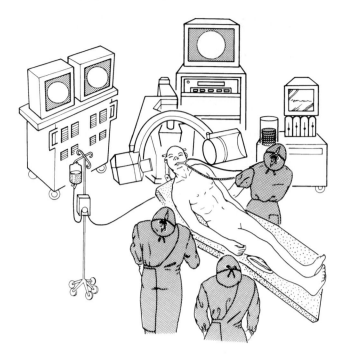

Figure 30.7. Schematic drawing demonstrates patient positioning and operating room arrangement. Fluoroscopic equipment (C-arm) is used as in conventional transsphenoidal surgery. The patient's torso is elevated about 20° to minimize sinus bleeding. The video monitor displaying the endoscopic image is placed to face the surgeon directly, and the C-arm monitor is placed at the left-hand side of the surgeon. An endoscope cleansing device is mounted to a pole holding a bottle of irrigation saline.

ernous sinuses. The elevation of the head and torso may increase risk of air embolism. However, we have not yet encountered a single case of intraoperative air embolism. A Doppler monitor is used to detect possible air embolism. The patient's head is tilted about 10° to the left and is extended gently to maintain the face to the horizontal plane. The operating table is rotated toward the surgeon about 10 to 20° to minimize the surgeon's discomfort during the operation. The head is fixed in this position using a three-pin head fixation system. Fluoroscopic equipment (C-arm) is applied to provide an intraoperative lateral image of the nasal cavity, sphenoid sinus, and sella turcica. The corneas are protected with ophthalmic ointment and the eyelids are closed with the coverage of soft vinyl adhesives. The oropharyngeal cavity is packed with a roll of gauze bandage to prevent possible aspiration of stagnant blood from the oropharynx at the end of surgery. The face, nasal cavity, and lower abdominal wall are then prepared with 5% povidone-iodine solution. Cotton patties, 1/2 × 3 in, soaked with a decongestant are placed into the nasal cavities. The patient, C-arm fluoroscope, and endoscopic/video camera equipment are draped aseptically. A lens cleansing irrigation-suction system (Endoscrub) is then assembled and attached to the endoscope. The endoscope is also connected to a closed circuit video system. The endoscope video monitor system provides a continuously moni-

tored view and allows video recording and hard copy filming of the surgery. An endoscope holding device is mounted to the head fixation system.

Surgical Technique

The side of the nasal cavity to be used is determined by the width of the nasal cavity and the laterality of the tumor. Preferably the wider side of the nasal cavity is used. It would be advisable to approach a laterally located microadenoma through the contralateral nostril because an endonasal approach is a few degrees off from the midline and would lead to the contralateral sella more easily. Still, the width of the nasal cavity is the main determining factor for which nostril is to be used. When disparity of the nasal cavities is minimal, a laterally located microadenoma is approached through the contralateral nostril. In most of our patients, the operation was performed through one nostril. In our experience with more than 80 patients, only 2 patients who had Cushing's disease required an approach using both nostrils. They had narrow nasal airways mostly caused by mucosal hypertrophy and congestion. This narrowness of the nasal cavities limited simultaneous passage of the endoscope and operating instruments through the same nostril. The endoscope was placed through one nostril and the surgical instruments were inserted through the other. A two-nostril technique will certainly increase surgical trauma to the nasal mucosa.

The decongestant-soaked patties placed earlier are then removed from the nasal cavities. Under endoscopic visualization, the mucosa over the rostrum of the sphenoid, middle turbinate, and posterior septum is infiltrated with a solution of lidocaine 1% with epinephrine 1/100,000. Recently, lidocaine infiltration has been eliminated because no additional nasal bleeding was encountered intraoperatively or postoperatively without the use of lidocaine with epinephrine. Although decongestant-soaked patties have been used continuously, the value of a decongestant is also questionable. The endoscope is held in the surgeon's nondominant hand while a surgical instrument is carried into the nasal cavity in the other hand. This freehanded endoscope holding technique is used until the anterior wall of the sella is exposed. With the 0° endoscope, the nasal cavities are inspected one at a time to determine which nostril is to be used. The patient's head is positioned in a way that the middle turbinate is visualized naturally at the center of the endoscopic view (Fig. 30.8). Two 1/2 × 3-in cotton patties are placed between the middle turbinate and the nasal septum. The middle turbinate is gently squeezed and pushed laterally under the coverage of cotton patties to access the sphenoethmoid recess and the sphenoid sinus ostium. The ipsilateral sphenoid ostium is identified (Fig. 30.9), and a trajectory to the sella is corroborated from time to time with fluoroscopic imaging. The mucosa at the anterior wall of the sphenoid sinus is then coagulated with a number 8 French suction-monopolar coagulator. The septal artery is coagulated and divided to prevent intraoper-

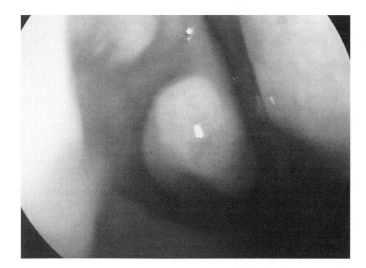

Figure 30.8. Under the 0° endoscope, the right-sided middle turbinate is exposed at the center of the surgical field. The middle turbinate is outfractured to access the ipsilateral sphenoid ostium.

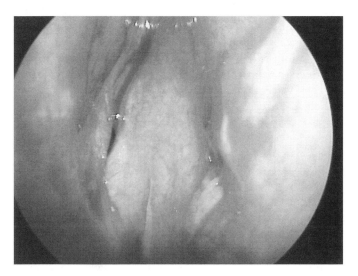

Figure 30.9. The right-sided sphenoid ostium is visible medial to the middle turbinate, which is displaced laterally.

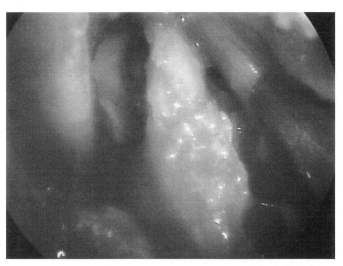

Figure 30.10. Bilateral sphenoid ostia are enlarged and the sphenoidal septum is exposed at the center.

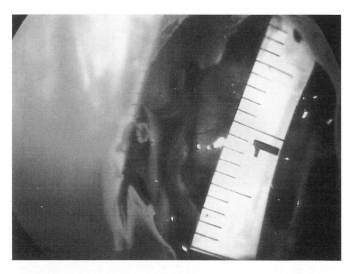

Figure 30.11. Anterior sphenoidotomy is performed about 1.5 × 2 cm in size.

the bone from the rostrum and the sphenoid septum are saved for the reconstruction of the sella. The anterior wall of the sella is exposed and confirmed again with fluoroscopic imaging. When a patient has a small sphenoid sinus, a high-speed microsurgical drill is used to make an adequate opening to reach the sella. Use of a drill under the endoscope is not difficult at all. When an anterior sphenoidotomy is finished, the 0° endoscope will provide a view of the clival indentation, the carotid protuberances, and the anterior wall of the sella (Fig. 30.12). If the 30° endoscope is applied, it depicts a further rostral panoramic view of the sphenoid sinus, including the floor of the planum sphenoidale, the optic and carotid protuberances, the caroticooptic recesses, and the anterior wall of the sella.

Once the anterior wall of the sella has been well exposed, the endoscope is mounted to the endoscope holding de-

ative and postoperative nasal bleeding. The nasal septum attached to the anterior wall of the sphenoid sinus is fractured and pushed away to the other side with the sharp edge of a Cottle elevator. Although the thick bone of the vomer is sometimes difficult to fracture away, the sharp end of the Cottle elevator helps to crack the vomer. The mucosa of the sphenoid rostrum is dissected and pushed away with attachment to the fractured nasal septum and vomer. The contralateral sphenoid ostium is identified by submucosal dissection of the contralateral sphenoid rostrum. The sphenoid rostrum between the ostia is enlarged by using Kerrison and ethmoid rongeurs (Fig. 30.10). The vertical dimension of the anterior sphenoidotomy is determined by fluoroscopic images. The sphenoidal septum is removed to expose the anterior wall of the sella (Fig. 30.11). Pieces of vice. The endoscope is placed superiorly in the nostril and nasal cavity as much as possible. This maneuver will stretch the nostril, allowing maximum operating space in the nasal cavity for the surgeon to be able to maneuver surgical instruments. A small hole is made with a small, sharp, straight bone curette at the anterior wall of the sella. If the bone is too thick to be penetrated with a curette, a high-speed microsurgical drill is used. Often a high-speed drill is required in patients with acromegaly or Cushing's disease caused by microadenomas. The remaining bone of the floor and anterior wall of the sella is removed with micro-Kerrison rongeurs (Fig. 30.13). The bone removal is made

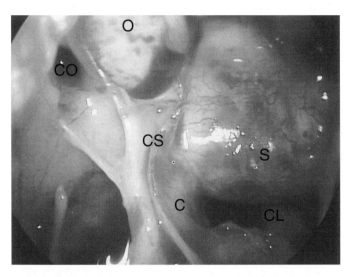

Figure 30.12. The sphenoid septum is removed and the anterior wall of the sella is exposed. In this patient, the septum is deviated to the right and inserted to the right carotid protuberance and anterior cavernous sinus area. The sella (*S*), clival indentation (*CL*), right carotid protuberance (*C*), bone covering the right anterior cavernous sinus (*CS*), right optic protuberance (*O*), and right caroticooptic recess (*CO*) are noticeable.

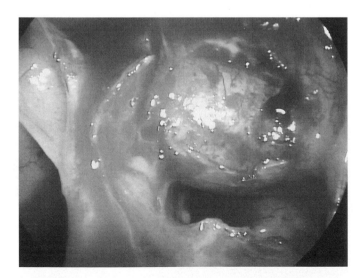

Figure 30.13. The anterior wall of the sella is removed from cavernous sinus to cavernous sinus and from the floor of the sella to the circular sinus at the top.

from cavernous sinus to cavernous sinus and from the floor of the sella to the circular sinus. For the removal of microadenomas, the opening of the anterior wall of the sella is performed adjacent to the tumor, exposing a little more than half of the sella. But the opening of the sella still has to be large enough to expose the margin of the normal pituitary tissue adjoining the tumor. The dura mater is exposed. Before making a dural incision, the dura mater is coagulated with a single-bladed bipolar or suction-monopolar coagulator. The dura mater is then opened horizontally with a 45°-angled Jannetta microdissector. The dural incision is enlarged with use of curved, single-bladed Kurze microscissors. If unexpected bleeding is encountered from the dural sinus during the dural incision, gentle packing with microcottonoids will control bleeding. Bipolar or suction-monopolar coagulation may occasionally be required for dural bleeding. A horizontal dural incision is made first, followed by a vertical incision. Often, the tumor tissue of microadenomas will spill out when the dura is opened. Precautionary measures are required so as not to lose a specimen through suctioning. A specimen is then removed with a micropituitary rongeur. Once a sufficient amount of specimen has been gathered for pathologic diagnosis, the rest of the tumor is removed, mostly using straight and variously curved number 5 or number 7 French suction cannulas in conjunction with simultaneous use of a pituitary curette. When a cavity is created by tumor removal, the endoscope is then advanced into the tumor cavity. This closeup endoscopic view will provide increased distinction between the tumor tissue and the normal pituitary gland. Often, the tumor tissue is grayish in color, which is in contrast to the normal pituitary gland. The normal pituitary gland is orange or pinkish orange in color. The posterior pituitary gland appears to be a glistening white color under the endoscope. The tumor is removed continuously using micropituitary rongeurs, suction cannulas, and pituitary curettes while preserving normal pituitary gland tissue as much as possible. When the tumor has been debulked, the tumor capsule is dissected from surrounding tissue with a microdissector or microscissors. For hormone-secreting adenomas, a thin layer of the normal pituitary gland tissue adjacent to tumor is shaved off to maximize the chance of cure (Fig. 30.14). Often the surgical maneuver requires two hands, with surgical instruments in each hand. When the tumor has been completely removed, the margin of the preserved pituitary gland will be exposed at the tumor resection site. At this point, repeated Valsalva maneuvers are performed to find leakage of cerebrospinal fluid (CSF). If either the tumor resection cavity is too large or CSF leakage is encountered, an abdominal free fat graft is placed at the tumor resection cavity (Fig. 30.15).

The removal of macroadenomas that are extended to the suprasellar region often requires the insertion of a 30° endoscope into the sella, which will provide a superior view toward the suprasellar portion of the tumor. When the 30° endoscope is rotated, it will show a lateral view toward the lateral wall of the sella and an inferior view toward the

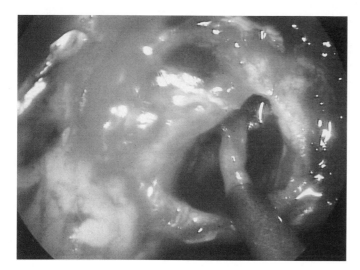

Figure 30.14. After removal of the tumor, a thin layer of the normal pituitary tissue is shaved off from the tumor resection cavity to achieve a better chance of cure in patients with hormone-secreting adenomas.

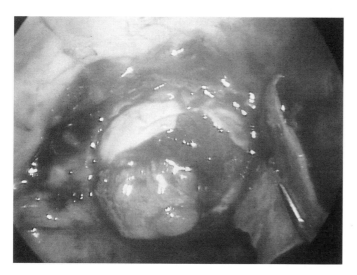

Figure 30.15. A small piece of abdominal fat graft is placed at the tumor resection cavity when the tumor resection cavity is too large or CSF leakage is encountered intraoperatively. A piece of bone is laid on the right inferior corner for bony reconstruction of the anterior wall of the sella.

floor of the sella, depending on the rotation of the angled endoscope. For removal of suprasellar tumors, the diaphragma sella is identified along the periphery of the tumor. The tumor is removed circumferentially along the edge of the diaphragma sella using a curved suction cannula. Anteriorly located tumor is removed first to delineate the anatomic dimension of the diaphragma sella. Once the anatomic orientation of the diaphragma sella has become certain to the surgeon, the tumor is removed further posteriorly along the edge of the diaphragma. The tumor removal is gradually advanced toward the center of the tumor close to the origin of the pituitary stalk. The arachnoid membrane will herniate down along the edge of the dia-

phragma sella when the tumor is trimmed out by suctioning. The tumor tissue is removed circumferentially at the periphery of the tumor, leaving the eye of the tumor at the center as the last piece of the tumor to be removed. Normal pituitary gland tissue is still preserved as much as possible. When all the tumor has been removed, the arachnoid membrane will then appear in view. The center of the flower-shaped arachnoid membrane will be the pituitary stalk. Rotating the 30° endoscope then permits inspection of the medial wall of the cavernous sinuses and the floor of the sella. Any residual tumor is thoroughly removed. When the arachnoid membrane is removed, the optic nerves and chiasm will be under direct visualization. However, if possible, the arachnoid membrane is kept intact to minimize the chance of CSF leakage. Even if the suprasellar portion of the tumor is large, it will gradually descend down along with brain pulsation. Sometimes the fibrotic nature of the tumor that frequently results from previous bromocriptine treatment gives the surgeon difficulty when removing the suprasellar portion of the tumor with conventional use of a pituitary curette and suctioning. If required, further rostral exposure by bone removal of the tuberculum sella and extended dural incision at the anterosuperior supradiaphragmatic dura and the anterior portion of the diaphragma sella will provide direct visualization of the suprasellar portion of the tumor. This wider exposure allows further microdissection of the tumor from the surrounding tissue under the direct visualization. The dura can be closed with dural microclips. No attempt is made to remove the intracavernous portion of the tumor. However, the cavernous sinus can be explored by opening the anterior and medial wall if it is required. The cavernous sinus has been entered for resection of other types of tumors.

After completion of the tumor removal, a 1- or 2-cm curvilinear skin incision is made along the inferior margin of the umbilicus to harvest a free fat graft. An appropriately sized portion of the free fat graft is placed in the sella. A watertight seal is confirmed by repeated Valsalva maneuvers. A gentle in and out motion of the fat graft will be observed on Valsalva maneuvers. If CSF leakage or extreme extrusion of the fat graft is noticed on Valsalva maneuvers, a new, proportionately adjusted, segment of the fat graft is placed. The fat graft is placed as a single piece if possible rather than as multiple small pieces to avoid dislodging a fragment. The anterior wall of the sella is reconstructed using a piece of bone saved during anterior sphenoidotomy (Fig. 30.16). When pieces of bone were not available because of previous transseptal pituitary surgery, the sphenoid sinus was packed with an absorbable gelatin sponge to provide further support to the fat graft in our earlier patients; in our later patients, a titanium mesh was placed for bony reconstruction (Fig. 30.17). The middle turbinate is placed back in its normal position. The abdominal incision is closed in subcuticular fashion. In our earlier patients, we used absorbable gelatin film at the middle meatus, allowing airflow at the level of the inferior meatus. If the middle meatus was too traumatized during the procedure, an ab-

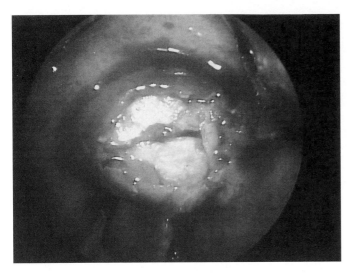

Figure 30.16. Three pieces of the bone are used for reconstruction of the anterior wall of the sella in this patient.

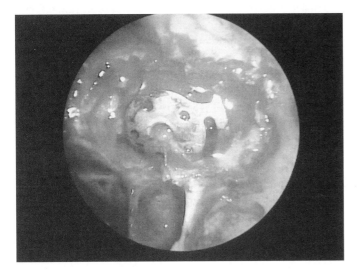

Figure 30.17. When sphenoidal bone is not available for sellar bone reconstruction because of previous transsphenoidal surgery, a small titanium mesh is placed for sellar reconstruction.

sorbable gelatin film roll was used to prevent possible adhesions near the ostium of the maxillary sinus. However, as mucosal trauma has become minimal with increased experience, no extra measure has been necessary in the nasal cavity. Besides bony reconstruction of the sella, nothing has been laid in the sphenoid sinus or nasal cavity in our more recent patients. This has minimized postoperative artifacts on MRI scans.

POSTOPERATIVE MANAGEMENT

In our earlier series, the patients were observed in a regular room overnight in the hospital. Recently, patients with microadenomas have been surgically treated on an outpa-

tient basis. Postoperative headache or discomfort is minimal. Most often, analgesics are not required at all postoperatively. A few drops of blood may drip postpharyngeally or through a nostril, which will dissipate over a few days. The patients are advised not to blow their nose for a month. Postoperatively, the patients were kept on a 5-day course of oral erythromycin. The most common problem in our earlier patients was postoperative diuresis. Postoperative diluted large-volume urination required differential diagnosis from diabetes insipidus and was a frequent cause of delays in early discharge from the hospital. Since intraoperative hydration was reduced to less than 2 L during the subsequent operations, postoperative diuresis has not been much of a problem. Once diabetes insipidus is diagnosed by urine specific gravity and serum electrolytes in conjunction with the classic symptoms of polyuria and polydipsia, desmopressin is used intravenously or intranasally. Among our first 50 patients, 2 developed temporary diabetes insipidus requiring one or two doses of desmopressin and 1 patient with a craniopharyngioma developed permanent diabetes insipidus that was expected preoperatively.

Perioperative stress doses of steroids were routinely used in our earlier patients but recently have not been used for patients who had normal preoperative endocrine function and minimal manipulation of the pituitary gland during an operation. For those patients, a morning cortisol level may be measured the day after the operation to confirm that it is higher than 414 nmol/L ($> 15\ \mu g/dL$). When stress doses of steroids are used, the patient is discharged with hydrocortisol treatment, 20 mg every morning and 10 mg every night. The patients with Cushing's disease were discharged with dexamethasone treatment, 2 mg twice a day. Postoperative dexamethasone therapy in patients with Cushing's disease enabled us to measure early postoperative 24-hour free urinary cortisol levels to determine completeness of the tumor resection. Patients with Cushing's disease often require prolonged steroid treatment over a few months to a year. An ordinary postoperative physiologic dosage of steroids in patients with Cushing's disease may cause an Addisonian crisis. Patients with Cushing's disease should be strongly advised not to skip taking postoperative steroids because the inadvertent skipping of steroids during the early postoperative period can be lethal. The nasal cavity is examined the following day prior to the patient being discharged. All patients underwent formal endocrine evaluation within a few weeks postoperatively. All patients obtained MRI scans of the brain 6 weeks postoperatively. Postoperative visual evaluations were performed only in patients who showed preoperative visual impairment or additional indications. Patients with microadenomas causing hyperprolactinemia, Cushing's disease, and acromegaly were followed up with interval endocrine testing. Patients with macroadenomas and hormone-nonsecreting adenomas are followed up with interval MRI scans of the brain thereafter.

SURGICAL OUTCOME

In our first 52 operations in 50 patients, 48 operations were performed endonasally. Among these 48 operations, 27 were performed with patients being discharged home the day following their operations. Eight operations required a two-night hospital stay and another eight operations required a three-night hospital stay following their operations because of postoperative diuresis that required differential diagnosis from diabetes insipidus. The remaining patients stayed longer because of CSF leakage and for social reasons.

Among eight patients with Cushing's disease, six had normal postoperative serum adrenocorticotropic hormone and normal 24-hour urinary free cortisol levels after one operation. The other two patients required reoperations for incomplete reduction of their cortisol levels after their first operation. After the second operation, one patient had a normal 24-hour urinary free cortisol with panhypopituitarism and another continued to have mildly increased cortisol levels for which stereotactic Gamma Knife surgery was rendered.

In 17 patients with prolactinomas, 5 had microadenomas, 9 had sellar macroadenomas, and 3 had macroadenomas involving the suprasellar region and cavernous sinus. Postoperatively, 10 patients had normalized prolactin levels, 4 had still mildly elevated prolactin levels, and 3 had residual tumors in the cavernous sinuses with increased prolactin levels. Four patients with mildly elevated prolactin levels were elected for observation with prolactin level checks at intervals. The two patients with residual cavernous sinus tumors were treated with stereotactic gamma-surgery and the other was treated with bromocriptine. Among the 19 patients with nonsecreting adenomas, 7 had sellar macroadenomas, 9 had macroadenomas involving the suprasellar region, and 3 had macroadenomas involving the suprasellar and cavernous sinus region. Sixteen patients had total resection and three had subtotal resection owing to tumor invasion into the cavernous sinus. One patient with residual tumor was treated with Gamma Knife surgery and another was treated with conventional fractionated radiation treatments. The third patient with residual tumor was elected for observation with sequential MRI scans because of his advanced age.

Six patients had a metastatic adenocarcinoma, germinoma, postcraniotomy CSF leak, posterior fossa chordoma, Rathke's cleft cyst, and craniopharyngioma, respectively. The patient with a metastatic adenocarcinoma was biopsied followed by radiation treatment. The patients with the germinoma and with the chordoma had subtotal resection followed by conventional radiation for germinoma and gamma-surgery for chordoma. The patient with a craniopharyngioma had total resection of the tumor with expected postoperative panhypopituitarism. The postcraniotomy CSF leak was repaired successfully.

COMPLICATIONS

Postoperative CSF leakage is a major possible complication in transsphenoidal surgery. In our first case of an endonasal endoscopic procedure, postoperative CSF leakage occurred in a patient with metastatic adenocarcinoma of the sella. The patient underwent an endonasal endoscopic biopsy. One bite of tumor tissue was procured with a pituitary rongeur in the sella. No fat graft was placed. The patient developed postoperative CSF leakage. The CSF leak was repaired with endonasal endoscopic placement of an abdominal fat graft. Another patient with a recurrent pituitary adenoma following a previous transsphenoidal operation developed a postoperative CSF leak. We were concerned about a possible CSF leak intraoperatively because of a wide defect of the bone and dura mater at the anterior wall and the floor of the sella from the previous operation. Surrounding supportive structures to hold an abdominal free fat graft were lacking. Pieces of bone were not available for bone reconstruction because of the previous transseptal approach. However, use of a titanium mesh could have prevented CSF leak in this patient. We had to be cautious with the packing of the fat graft into the sella so as not to cause optic compression. Despite the placement of a generously sized fat graft into the sella, the patient developed a postoperative CSF leak. The CSF leak was repaired with placement of a larger fat graft into the sella and sphenoid sinus on the second postoperative day. Recently, every effort was made to reconstruct the anterior bony wall of the sella in all patients with either the patient's own bone or titanium mesh. In cases of microadenoma, a fat graft was not placed. Although fibrin glue has not been used in our patients, the use of fibrin glue made out of the patient's own blood may facilitate a secure, watertight seal of the dural opening. Postoperative CSF leakage was another reason for prolonged patient hospitalization.

Most of our patients were able to be discharged the day following their operation mostly because they did not require obstructive nasal packing. Recently, patients with microadenomas were discharged from the hospital a few hours after their operations. As mentioned previously, the most common cause of delay in patient discharge in our series was postoperative diuresis requiring a differential diagnosis from diabetes insipidus. Judicious intraoperative fluid management has reduced the incidence of postoperative diuresis. Because late electrolyte imbalances can occur in delayed fashion so many days that patient's routine hospitalization for a certain number of days does not warrant avoidance of such a complication. However, the length of the patient's hospitalization should be individualized depending on the patient's endocrine and electrolyte conditions. Other complications that we encountered in our first 50 patients included temporary diabetes insipidus in 2 patients, expected permanent diabetes insipidus in a patient with a craniopharyngioma, worsening of anterior pituitary function in 6 patients, asymptomatic synechia of the nasal mucosa in 1 patient, and chronic sphenoid sinusitis in 1 patient. The chronic sphenoid sinusitis was noted during a routine postoperative visit in 6 weeks and was successively treated with 5-day antibiotics.

ADVANTAGES AND DISADVANTAGES OF THE ENDONASAL ENDOSCOPIC TECHNIQUE

Avoidance of postoperative nasal packing seems to be a significant advantage for quick recovery and early release from the hospital. The endoscopic approach through a natural endonasal route not requiring use of a retractor eliminates the need of any sort of postoperative nasal packing. Postoperative pain and discomfort is also minimal. The microscopic endonasal technique requires a retractor; however, our endoscopic endonasal technique does not. Quick postoperative recovery and short hospitalization in our group of patients was made possible by the selection of this natural endonasal route without use of a retractor. We have not yet encountered a patient who has had too narrow a nasal pathway to undergo this endonasal endoscopic technique. This endonasal technique does not require sublabial incision or nasal transfixion incision and subsequently minimizes the chance of dental, gingival, and sinunasal complications. Our endoscopic technique does not use ethmoidectomy or resection of the middle turbinate.

The main advantage of the endoscopic technique is that the 30°-angled lens can visualize the diaphragma sella and the suprasellar region directly. The optic system, hypothalamus, and intracranial vessels can be directly demonstrated with the angled endoscope after removal of the suprasellar portion of the tumor. By rotating the angled-lens endoscope, the corners of the sella and sphenoidal sinus can also be visualized directly. The endoscope can provide a panoramic view of the sphenoid sinus demonstrating the bony protuberance of the optic nerves and carotid arteries. Although risk of injury to the carotid artery, the optic system, and the hypothalamus is low with conventional microscopic transsphenoidal surgery, the capability of the endoscope to visualize those structures directly may further reduce incidence of such a rare catastrophe. An endoscopic close-up view at the juncture of tumor and pituitary gland tissue has seemed to be much clearer than the remote view provided by an operating microscope. Whether this endoscopic close-up view is going to contribute to better surgical outcome in pituitary adenoma surgery remains to be proven.

The disadvantages of endoscopic pituitary surgery compared with conventional microscopic surgery are monitor-provided two-dimensional flat images and reduced clarity and sharpness of the monitor picture. Therefore, endoscopic video images are still inferior to those of direct microscopic visualization. Another disadvantage will be the learning curve for neurosurgeons who are already well trained for conventional microscopic surgery. Despite a neurosurgeon's painstaking training in microsurgery, those who are not used to endoscopic surgical maneuvers will have to spend extra time getting used to new endoscopic surgical skills. Maneuvering surgical instruments during endoscopic endonasal transsphenoidal surgery is somewhat similar to how one would pick up food with one chopstick held parallel in each hand. One of the major concerns of microscopic pituitary surgeons has been the possibility of uncontrollable bleeding with limited exposure. As with microscopic pituitary surgery, significant bleeding has been encountered from the tumors with high vascularity. The endoscopic endonasal technique itself has not been a handicap in particular when dealing with this type of tumor. Venous sinus bleeding occasionally became cumbersome, but not a single case has needed to be aborted. Because of the intrinsic learning curve, the operation time for endoscopic surgery was initially longer than that for microscopic surgery. Once the surgeon becomes accustomed with this endoscopic technique, the operation time will become comparable or even shorter.

ACKNOWLEDGMENTS

The author thanks Arthur P. Nestler and Robin A. Coret for their assistance in the preparation of this manuscript.

REFERENCES

1. Landolt AM. History of transsphenoidal pituitary surgery. In: Landolt AM, Vance ML, Reilly PL, eds. Pituitary Adenomas. New York: Churchill Livingstone, 1996:307–314.
2. Griffith HB, Veerapen R. A direct transnasal approach to the sphenoid sinus: technical note. J Neurosurg 1987;66:140–142.
3. Cooke RS, Jones RAC. Experience with the direct transnasal transsphenoidal approach to the pituitary fossa. Br J Neurosurg 1994; 8:193–196.
4. Guiot G, Rougerie J, Fourestler A, et al. Une nouvelle technique endoscopique: exploration endoscopiques intracraniennes. La Presse Medicale 1963;71:1225–1228.
5. Stammberger H. Endoscopic endonasal surgery: concepts in treatment of recurring rhinosinusitis, part II: surgical technique. Otolaryngol Head Neck Surg 1986;94:147–156.
6. Carrau RL, Jho HD, Ko Y. Transnasal-transsphenoidal endoscopic surgery of the pituitary gland. Laryngoscope 1996;106:914–918.
7. Jankowski R, Auque J, Simon C, et al. Endoscopic pituitary tumor surgery. Laryngoscope 1992;102:198–202.
8. Jho HD. Endoscopic endonasal pituitary surgery: technical aspects. Contemp Neurosurg 1997;19(6):1–7.
9. Jho HD, Carrau RL, Ko Y. Endoscopic pituitary surgery. In: Wilkins RH, Rengachary SS, eds. Neurosurgical Operative Atlas. Baltimore: Williams & Wilkins, 1996;5(1):1–12.
10. Jho HD, Carrau RL. Endoscopy assisted transsphenoidal surgery for pituitary adenoma: technical note. Acta Neurochir (Wien) 1996; 138:1416–1425.
11. Jho HD, Carrau RL. Endoscopic endonasal transsphenoidal surgery: experience with 50 patients. J Neurosurg 1997;87:44–51.
12. Jho HD, Carrau RL, Mclaughlin ML, et al. Endoscopic transsphenoidal resection of a large chordoma in the posterior fossa. Acta Neurochir (Wien) 1997;139:343–348.

13. Jho HD, Carrau RL, Ko Y, et al. Endoscopic pituitary surgery: an early experience. Surg Neurol 1997;47:213–223.
14. Sethi DS, Pillay PK. Endoscopic management of lesions of the sella turcica. J Laryngol Otol 1995;109(10):956–962.
15. Shikani AH, Kelly JH. Endoscopic debulking of a pituitary tumor. Am J Otolaryngol 1993;14(4):254–256.
16. Wurster CF, Smith DE. The endoscopic approach to the pituitary gland (letter). Arch Otolaryngol Head Neck Surg 1994;120:674.
17. Gamea A, Fathi M, EL-Guindy A. The use of the rigid endoscope in trans-sphenoidal pituitary surgery. J Laryngol Otol 1994;108:19–22.
18. Helal MZ. Combined micro-endo trans-sphenoid excisions of pituitary macroadenomas. Eur Arch Otorhinolaryngol 1995;252(3):186–189.
19. Black PMcL, Zervas NT, Candia GL. Incidence and management of complications of transsphenoidal operation for pituitary adenomas. Neurosurgery 1987;20:920–924.
20. Hardy J. Trans-sphenoidal approach to the pituitary gland. In: Wilkins RH, Rengachary SS, eds. Neurosurgery. New York: McGraw-Hill, 1985:889–898.
21. Zervas NT. Surgical results in pituitary adenomas: results of international survey. In: Black PMCL, Zervas NT, Ridway EC Jr, et al., eds. Secretory Tumors of the Pituitary Gland. New York: Raven Press, 1984:377–385.

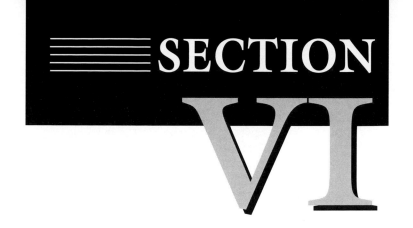

SECTION
VI

Radiation Therapy of
Pituitary Tumors

Radiation Therapy and Radiosurgery of Pituitary Tumors

Douglas Kondziolka, John C. Flickinger, and
L. Dade Lunsford

INTRODUCTION

The use of radiation to treat tumors of the pituitary gland has had a long history (1, 2). Improvements in radiation techniques and associated results occurred with the development of medical linear accelerator systems and improvements in brain imaging. More recently, stereotactic radiosurgery has been used to deliver single-session conformal irradiation to pituitary tumors of the sella or cavernous sinus region. Although the goals of both treatments include reduction and stabilization of the tumor mass, preservation or improvement in visual function (3, 4), and reduction in abnormal hormone secretion with preservation of neurologic function, the techniques and expectations of the two treatments differ greatly.

Radiation therapy (XRT) plays an important role as part of planned combined therapy (with partial resection) for pituitary macroadenomas as salvage therapy after failed surgical or medical therapy or as primary therapy in patients who are poor surgical candidates or who refuse surgery. The use of conventional XRT is rarely indicated for the treatment of pituitary microadenomas. Stereotactic radiosurgery has been used for the treatment of small-volume pituitary tumors (5–9), including both microadenomas and smaller macroadenomas that may involve the cavernous sinus region. Because of the high dose delivered to the tumor, the dose received by the optic nerve and chiasm to the tumor margin is important to limit visual complications. Radiosurgery must be used judiciously for tumors that directly compress the optic apparatus (10, 11).

It is important not to base modern treatment policies for pituitary tumors on studies from the pre-1970s era. Prior to the development of detailed hormone assays, petrosal sinus sampling, direct imaging, and improvements in transsphenoidal surgery, conclusions made regarding XRT are for the most part outdated. In this chapter, the techniques of conventional XRT (fractionated linear accelerator-based irradiation), the indications and results of this treatment for functional and nonfunctional tumors, and discussion of the technique and role of stereotactic radiosurgery for pituitary tumors are presented.

TECHNIQUE OF XRT
Dosimetry

Medical linear accelerators are almost always used to deliver fractionated pituitary XRT. Although cobalt teletherapy has been used successfully in the past, linear accelerator–based XRT is preferred because of sharper radiation field borders. X-ray energy beams of between 4 and 25 MV are appropriate for multiple-field (≥ 3) radiotherapy to the pituitary region. The use of a single set of right and left lateral fields is inappropriate because of the unnecessarily high delivery of radiation to the temporal lobes. To limit such parenchymal irradiation, a combination of three or four fields of arc rotations are used. The standard three-field technique employs the combination of right and left lateral fields with either an anterior field or a single anterior-cephalad oblique field. Arc rotations also have been used to limit radiation outside the treatment volume. The rationale of multiple static fields (instead of arcs) reflects the use of shaping blocks that are constructed for each field. Multileaf collimators with dynamic collimation may allow arc rotations to be constructed with adequate field shaping. This technology still requires evaluation.

Recently, relocatable stereotactic frames have been used to deliver more conformal fractionated XRT to the pituitary region. During each irradiation session during the course of treatment, a noninvasive frame is attached to the head to provide some degree of stereotactic guidance. In this fashion, irradiation outside the target volume is reduced.

Dose Selection

The optimum dose for fractionated XRT to a pituitary adenoma is somewhat controversial. One group reported high tumor control rates (78 versus 56%) using 40 to 50 Gy in 4 to 5 weeks versus 30 to 40 Gy in 3 to 4 weeks (3). Many authors have considered doses less than 45 Gy to be suboptimal and recommend treatment to 55 Gy. We reviewed results of fractionated XRT in 100 patients with pituitary macroadenomas treated at the University of Pittsburgh from 1964 to 1987 (12, 13). Tumor control rates at doses of 38 to 45 Gy were higher than those in 53 patients treated with between 46 and 65 Gy. Other groups also support the use of doses in the 45-Gy range (14–16). There is no evidence to suggest that different tumor types require different radiation doses. Currently, we limit total dose to no greater than 45 Gy using 1.8-Gy fractions. With this dose, we expect long-term tumor control in the range of 70 to 90% with less than or equal to 1% rates of optic neuropathy.

HORMONE-SECRETING PITUITARY TUMORS

Prolactinoma

Primary management strategies for prolactin (PRL)-secreting pituitary tumors include dopamine agonist therapy and microsurgical resection (17, 18). XRT plays a secondary role. Because of favorable results with medical therapy, radiotherapy is reserved for the treatment of PRL-secreting macroadenomas that do not favorably respond to medical management or surgery.

Results of some studies have shown that postoperative XRT in patients with prolactinoma reduces but rarely normalizes PRL levels; however, increased rates of normalization occur in the long term when XRT is combined with intermittent medical therapy (19, 20). Such incomplete normalization of PRL levels after XRT may be related to an undesired reduction in PRL-inhibiting hormone secretion. This reduction may also explain observed hyperprolactinemia that occurs following XRT of nonsecreting pituitary tumors (21). Rush et al. (20) compared the results of surgery, XRT, and dopamine agonist therapy alone with surgery and XRT for patients with PRL levels above 200 μg/L (> 200 ng/mL). Although significant PRL level reductions were noted in patients who received surgery and XRT, none of seven patients achieved normal values. However, in the groups that also had medical therapy, normal values were routinely achieved. Tsagarakis et al. (22) provided an update in a series of 36 patients with microprolactinomas and macroprolactinomas who had XRT and intermittent dopamine agonist therapy without surgery. They found that PRL levels fell to normal in 18 of 36 patients, with reductions in another 28%. They concluded that XRT produced a progressive fall in the serum PRL level in most patients and that pregnancy was safely undertaken early on in therapy because hypogonadism was a more delayed effect. In a recent report by Tsang et al. (23) from Toronto, patients with prolactinomas were less likely to achieve normalized hormone levels with XRT alone (25% at 10 years) compared with patients with acromegaly (46%) or Cushing's disease (53%). In their series, the incidence of permanent hypopituitarism requiring replacement included hypothyroidism (47%), adrenal insufficiency (47%), and hypogonadism (53%). They determined that pituitary irradiation was the specific causal factor of these problems in only 22, 10, and 10% of these syndromes, respectively.

Acromegaly

XRT has played an important role in the management of both primary and recurrent acromegaly (24, 25). Eastman et al. (26) reported in 1979 that doses of 40 to 50 Gy were associated with a 77% reduction in growth hormone (GH) levels 5 to 10 years after irradiation. The percentage of patients achieving levels less than 220 pmol/L (< 5 ng/mL) varied from 17% at 2 years to 60% at 10 years. This report demonstrated a progressive decline of GH secretion over years. Irrespective of the rate of reduction of GH secretion, the metabolic and anatomic features of acromegaly improved. This was an important finding because the medical manifestations of acromegaly can be life threatening.

Others have found that the pretreatment level of GH, as for prolactinoma, influences the results of therapy. Data from the University of California at San Francisco revealed that patients with fasting GH levels below 1980 pmol/L

(< 45 ng/mL) achieved postradiation fasting GH levels of less than 440 pmol/L (< 10 ng/mL) in 100% of patients by 3 years. This rate was only 71% for pre-XRT GH levels above 2200 pmol/L (> 50 ng/mL) (27, 28).

As increasingly stricter criteria for "endocrine cure" have been proposed, it has been more difficult to achieve fasting GH levels less than 88 pmol/L (< 2 ng/mL). Caruso et al. (24) found in 53 patients that such levels were achieved in 62% at 6 years. An additional study from the University of Hamburg compared results for the treatment of acromegaly using proton therapy (13 patients) versus conventional XRT (17 patients) (15). There was no significant difference in the rate of normal GH levels at 5 years between the two groups. Higher rates of pituitary insufficiency and oculomotor deficits were noted in the proton group in this small series. Tsang et al. (23) again found that XRT led to significant reductions in GH-secreting adenomas (< 440 pmol/L [< 10 ng/mL]), although this reduction often took more than 5 years. They found a 10-year tumor control rate of 60%, which increased toward 90% at 15 years.

Cushing's Disease

Until recently, few modern reports of the use of XRT for Cushing's disease were available. Early reports were published prior to the current refinements of transsphenoidal surgery and in an era when the absolute diagnosis of Cushing's disease versus Cushing's syndrome was uncertain. In general, older series reported remission rates in the range of 50 to 70% (30–34). Typical radiation doses varied from 40 to 50 Gy.

In a recent series, Estrada et al. (35) reported longer-term outcomes in 30 patients with persistent or recurrent Cushing's disease after prior transsphenoidal surgery. The mean radiation dose was 50 Gy. Twenty-five patients (83%) had clinical remission during median follow-up of 42 months. Hormonal remission began 6 to 60 months following XRT but in most cases occurred during the first 2 years. None of these 25 patients had a relapse of Cushing's disease after remission was achieved (35). They noted that 17 patients had GH deficiency after XRT, 10 had hypogonadism, 4 had hypothyroidism, and 1 had adrenal insufficiency.

Tsang et al. (23) reported remission rates of 53% at 10 years after pituitary irradiation (n = 25 patients). For recurrent tumors, they advocated repeat pituitary surgery and immediate postoperative XRT. They suggested that XRT be given consideration prior to bilateral adrenalectomy to prevent the development of Nelson's syndrome. No cases of Nelson's syndrome had been observed in their series after pituitary XRT.

Stereotactic radiosurgery has proven useful in patients with pituitary tumors causing Cushing's disease and is discussed below (9).

Nonsecreting Pituitary Tumors

Patients with nonsecreting pituitary tumors often present with symptoms of regional brain compression such as visual field deficits, cranial neuropathies, headache, or pituitary insufficiency. Complete surgical resection can be performed for tumors confined to the sellar and suprasellar region. When the cavernous sinus is involved, a complete microsurgical resection is often not possible without high risk. Fractionated XRT is an important primary adjuvant treatment to obtain growth control of nonsecreting pituitary tumors with reduction in recurrence rates to less than or equal to 25% (13, 14, 16, 36, 37). Although fractionated XRT has been used as sole management for such tumors, initial surgical resection provides the histologic diagnosis and decompression of the optic apparatus.

The need for extended follow-up beyond 10 years is important to address the effects of XRT. Several recurrences developed in both the University of Pittsburgh and the Royal Marsden series during the second decade, even with doses greater than 45 Gy (13, 14). The New York University group showed that tumor control rates following radiotherapy alone (sometimes with biopsy) were similar to those following subtotal resection and radiotherapy in 101 patients with 8-year follow-up (97% in both groups) (16). In the recent Royal Marsden series, the 20-year tumor control rates were 100% for 31 patients with intrasellar tumors, 92% for 180 patients with suprasellar tumors less than 2 cm in diameter, and 91% for 34 patients with suprasellar tumors greater than 2 cm in diameter (14).

Visual Improvement After XRT

In earlier series, Sheline et al. (1, 2, 28, 38) showed that patients with hemianopias were not likely to experience improvement following XRT. Transsphenoidal surgical resection showed improvements in the 75 to 90% range and often was performed to lead to prompt visual improvement (3, 39, 40). In a more recent analysis, Rush et al. (4) performed more detailed neuro-ophthalmologic evaluations before and after XRT. Seventy-eight percent of patients experienced visual improvement (4). In addition, the finding of optic atrophy was a significant marker for visual field and visual acuity outcome. Early visual improvement was seen in one-third of patients following XRT. Patients with a dense hemianopia were less likely to improve.

COMPLICATIONS OF XRT
Optic Neuropathy

Radiation injury to the optic nerves or chiasm can be a significant complication of pituitary tumor XRT. Tumors that compress the optic chiasm may reduce the radiation tolerance of that normal structure by ischemic mechanisms. Because improved tumor control rates have not been identified beyond 45 to 50 Gy, total doses beyond this level do not seem justified and may be associated with higher visual risks. Flickinger et al. (41, 42) evaluated the risk of optic neuropathy beyond 5 years in 100 patients with pituitary adenoma or craniopharyngioma. Most patients (and every patient with complications) were treated with dosage fractions of 1.8 or 2.0 Gy. There were no cases of optic neuropathy in the low-dose group with a median dose of 44 Gy (range, 38 to 45 Gy) as opposed to two patients in the high-dose group (60 to 70 Gy) for a risk of 13% at that dose level.

Either lower total doses and/or lower dosages per fraction (1.5 to 1.7 Gy per fraction) should be considered. Fortunately, radiation injury to other cranial nerves after pituitary XRT is rare.

Parenchymal Brain Injury

Using proper dose selection and a radiation delivery, there should be little or no risk for brain necrosis after pituitary irradiation (43). The dose threshold for brain necrosis is much higher than that for optic neuropathy. Although temporal lobe necrosis can be associated with high-dose fractionated XRT treated with parallel opposed lateral fields, this effect was seen primarily in prior years when lower-energy equipment was used.

Vascular Injury

Irradiation of the carotid arteries and other large vessels at the base of the brain places these vessels at risk for occlusion and stroke. The observed incidence of stroke in the University of Pittsburgh series compared with that based on age was two to three times higher at 10 and 20 years after XRT ($P = .08$) (41). Other investigators have reported strokes among relatively young patients after pituitary irradiation (44–46). The use of fractionated stereotactic irradiation may reduce the risk of radiation-related vascular problems if conformal planning reduces irradiation of the cavernous sinus and distal internal carotid artery as it branches into small vessels.

Pituitary Insufficiency

Hypopituitarism requiring hormone replacement eventually develops in many patients years after fractionated XRT to pituitary tumors. A wide range in the incidence of this finding is reported (37, 47–49). Littley et al. (47) studied 165 patients with pituitary tumors irradiated to dosages of 37.5 to 42.5 Gy in 15 to 16 fractions. Levels of GH, gonadotropin, corticotropin, and thyrotropin were present in 18, 21, 57, and 80% of patients, respectively, but these rates dropped to 0, 9, 23, and 58% 5 years after treatment. Radiation-induced hyperprolactinemia developed in 73 patients (44%), peaking at 2 years and then eventually declining to baseline.

Secondary Malignancy

A group of second tumors that developed in the radiation field years following pituitary radiation have been described. These include sarcomas, meningiomas, and glial tumors. A range of this finding between 0 and 3% was noted at 8- to 20-year evaluations (6, 13, 14, 29, 36).

STEREOTACTIC RADIOSURGERY USING THE GAMMA KNIFE

Stereotactic radiosurgery offers an alternative option for patients who do not require decompression of the optic apparatus or more rapid normalization of hormone hypersecretions than can be achieved with microsurgery (5, 50). For tumors extending into the cavernous sinus, radiosurgery provides an especially effective surgical strategy. Stereotactically focused charged particles have been used to irradiate pituitary tumors since the 1950s. This technique uses high-energy protons or helium ions generated by a cyclotron. In patients with acromegaly, Levy et al. (51) reported that the mean GH level in a cohort of 234 patients decreased by 70% within the first year and continued to decrease thereafter; normal levels were sustained during 10 years of follow-up (51). Kjellberg and Kliman (52) found that 60% of patients had a "normal" (defined as a GH level < 440 pmol/L [< 10 ng/mL]) GH level 24 months after treatment and that 80% of patients achieved normalization of GH level by 48 months after treatment. In patients with Cushing's disease, 95% of patients had normalization of either mean basal cortisol levels or the response to a dexamethasone suppression test. Fifteen percent of these patients relapsed, however, and required additional surgical procedures (adrenalectomy or sellar reexploration) (53). Kjellberg and Kliman (52) achieved normal cortisol status in approximately 65% of a cohort of 36 patients. Levy et al. (51) also reported that 60% of patients with prolactinomas eventually attained normal serum PRL levels. The incidence of pituitary insufficiency was lower in patients treated with charged particle radiotherapy than in patients who received fractionated photon radiotherapy (33% of patients required some form of hormone replacement). The incidence of new or worsened cranial nerve deficits unrelated to tumor growth in these series was 1 to 6% (53, 54). Most patients in these studies were treated before magnetic resonance imaging (MRI) and computed tomography became available to aid treatment planning.

Stereotactic hypophysectomy with the gamma unit was first reported by Backlund et al. (55) in eight patients with metastatic breast carcinoma. Examination of the pituitary gland in these patients at autopsy revealed a sharply demarcated area of necrosis at an area corresponding to a dose of 185 Gy. This information suggested that normal pituitary tissue has a relatively high tolerance to single high doses of irradiation.

During a 10-year interval, we performed radiosurgery

Table 31.1. *Distribution of Tumor Type for Stereotactic Radiosurgery (n = 88)*

Adrenocorticotropic hormone secreting	27 (31%)
Growth hormone secreting	22 (25%)
Nonsecreting	27 (31%)
Prolactinoma	10 (11%)
Mixed prolactin–growth hormone secreting	2 (2%)

on 88 patients with pituitary tumors (Table 31.1). Patient age varied from 9 to 88 years. Fifty-six patients were female and 32 were male. A prior surgical resection had been performed in 71 patients (81%), including a "gross total resection" in 11 patients. Fractionated external beam XRT had been delivered to 14 patients (16%), most within the 40- to 60-Gy range. Formal preoperative visual field testing in 38 patients showed normal fields in 27 patients (71%) and a visual field deficit in 11 patients (29%). Cavernous sinus involvement was present in 36 patients (41%).

Radiosurgery Technique

Radiosurgery was performed with a 201 source cobalt-60 Leksell Gamma Knife (Elekta Instruments, Atlanta, GA). First, the Leksell model G stereotactic frame was applied to the patient's head under local anesthesia. Following frame fixation, a stereotactic MRI scan was performed (or a computed tomographic scan in patients unsuitable for MRI). High-resolution coronal axial imaging was important for dose planning. Gammaplan software (Elekta Instruments) and high-resolution axial images were used to construct stereotactically accurate coronal and sagittal images. At present, we use volume acquisition imaging with 1-mm-thick slice intervals. Fat suppression imaging techniques have been used to improve tumor visualization when prior surgery had been performed. If an intrasellar tumor was identified with prior surgery or laboratory testing but not visualized on imaging, the entire sella served as the radiosurgical target. Images were transferred to a high-speed computer workstation via Ethernet for dose planning (Fig. 31.1). Combinations of 4-, 8-, 14-, or 18-mm-diameter beams were used to construct a dose plan conformal to the tumor margin (54). For the most part, smaller beam diameters were used for most patients. We used the 50% isodose line to target the tumor margin in most patients. Selected beam blocking was used to shift the peripheral isodose away from the optic apparatus, a technique more often employed in the model U Gamma Knife (Fig. 31.2) (56). We aimed to keep the dose to the optic apparatus less than or equal to 8 Gy (18). The dose also was reduced if the patient had received prior fractionated XRT. We aimed to deliver as high a dose as possible, the limiting feature being the optic apparatus (57). After radiosurgery, all patients were discharged from the hospital within 24 hours.

Follow-up imaging and endocrinologic studies are performed at 6-month intervals and then annually and biennially after radiosurgery (Fig. 31.3). Tumor dimensions are measured and entered into a database. Endocrine studies are maintained by the patient's endocrinologist. In patients with acromegaly, a normal fasting serum GH level was defined as less than 220 pmol/L (< 5 ng/mL). Somatomedin-C (IGF-1) levels were defined according to normal limits from various laboratories varying from 270 to 492 ng/mL. Patients with Cushing's disease were reported to have normal cortisol status if the fasting AM cortisol level was less than 690 nmol/L (< 25 μg/dL), the 24-hour urinary free cortisol level was less than 248 nmol (< 90 μg/dL), or the serum adrenocorticotropic hormone level was less than 18 pmol/L (< 82 pg/mL) (50).

Adrenocorticotropic Hormone-Producing Tumors

The effects of radiosurgery on hormone production in patients with Cushing's disease and Nelson's syndrome were evaluated (8). Results were evaluable in 16 of 22 patients at a mean of 20 months (range, 3 to 38 months). Eight patients (50%) had normalization of their adrenocorticotropic hormone/cortisol status at a mean latency interval of approximately 20 months. Two of these patients required ketoconazole to achieve normal cortisol levels. Two additional patients have had a significant improvement in their condition but have not yet achieved normalization. One of these patients was a 16-year-old male with Nelson's syndrome who has had a significant decrease in skin pigmentation and a 54% decrease in serum adrenocorticotropic hormone level 15 months after radiosurgery. The other patient was a 61-year-old female with Cushing's disease and a tumor in the right cavernous sinus who, 7 months after radiosurgery, lost 20 lb, had more energy, and had decreased requirements for blood pressure medication. Although we could not correlate radiation dose and hormone response, there seemed to be a trend toward a favorable response in patients whose tumors received higher maximum (46.5 Gy) and margin (24 Gy) doses (50).

Control of tumor growth was achieved in 15 (88%) of 17 patients who had follow-up imaging studies 5 to 39 months (mean, 20 months) after radiosurgery. Two patients with invasive tumors that had been refractory to previous microsurgery and XRT had progressive growth of their tumors with subsequent new cranial neuropathies.

Rahn et al. (7) reported 82 to 100% remission rates in patients with Cushing's disease who were treated based on pneumocisternogram and MRI, respectively. In the former group, patients received up to four separate procedures using doses of 70 to 100 Gy until remission was induced. There was a 20% incidence of pituitary insufficiency in this group. There has been no incidence of pituitary insufficiency in the group treated on the basis of MRIs, but follow-up in this group is shorter (2 to 4 years). In patients with tumors secreting these hormones, Rahn et al. (7) also reported a significant decrease in GH and PRL levels in

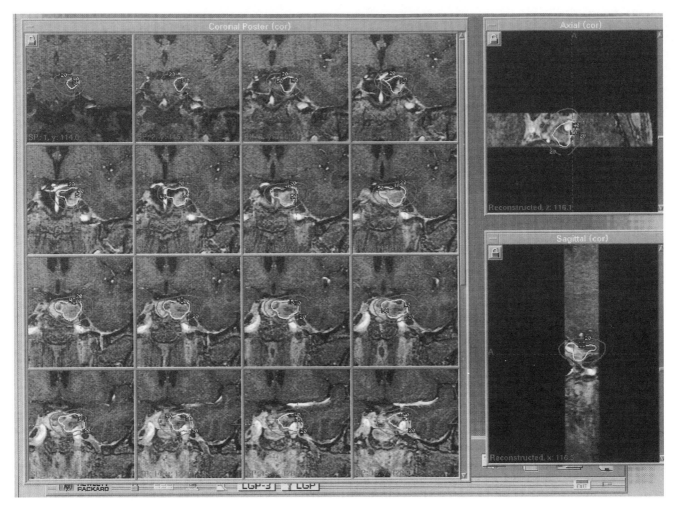

Figure 31.1. Dose planning for a pituitary tumor using the Gamma Knife. One-millimeter coronal images can be displayed simultaneously with axial and sagittal images. An irregular, conformal volume of irradiation is created using multiple isocenters.

21 and 5 patients, respectively. The incidence of pituitary insufficiency in patients with acromegaly was 13%.

Growth Hormone-Producing Tumors

The response of fasting serum GH levels to radiosurgery in patients with acromegaly was studied. Our results were evaluable in 12 of 16 patients at a mean of 32 months (range, 10 to 67 months). Levels of GH normalized in 8 patients (67%) at a mean of 32 months (50). Three of these patients required medication (bromocriptine or octreotide) to help achieve normalization. Five patients with normal GH levels reported a decrease in acromegalic features. Four patients had significant (> 50%) decreases in their GH levels. There were no apparent significant differences in the maximum and margin doses (within the range delivered) used in patients who attained normal levels.

The response of the serum IGF-1 level to radiosurgery was documented in 13 of 16 patients at a mean of 38 months (range, 10 to 83 months) after radiosurgery. Only 4 patients (30%) had normal IGF-1 levels. Two of these

patients reported a decrease in acromegalic features. The latency interval to normalization was 37.5 months in the 2 patients who were not taking medications. Two patients had normal levels but still required bromocriptine or octreotide therapy 10 to 17 months following radiosurgery. The 9 patients who continued to have elevated IGF-1 levels did not seem to have a significant response to radiosurgery in terms of this parameter. IGF-1 levels varied from 58 to 135% of their original values 15 to 83 months (mean, 37 months) after radiosurgery.

Control of tumor growth was achieved in 100% of the 14 patients who had follow-up imaging studies. These studies were obtained 10 to 83 months (mean, 38 months) after radiosurgery. Tumor volume decreased in 8 (57%) of these patients (50).

Prolactinoma

Stereotactic radiosurgery was evaluated in seven patients with prolactinomas. All seven patients had recurrent tumors following microsurgery and had failed or were intol-

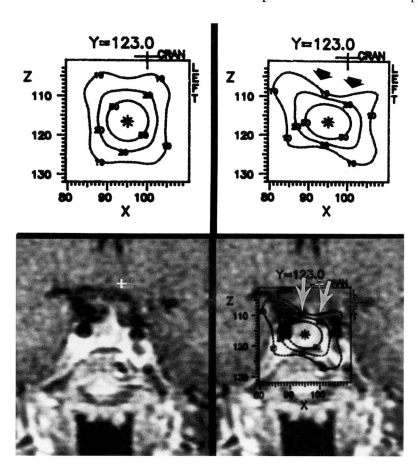

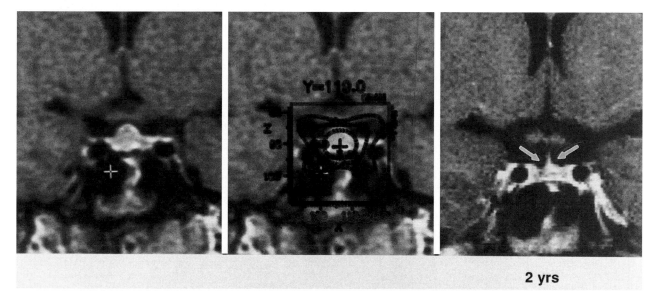

Figure 31.2. Selective beam blocking provides a modification in the isodose configuration. No beam blocking is shown for a small pituitary tumor (*left*). With blocking, the 10 and 20% isodose lines are moved away from the optic chiasm (*arrows*) to minimize irradiation of that structure (*right*). The tumor remains covered.

Figure 31.3. Serial coronal MRIs in a patient with Cushing's disease. Note the decrease in size of the pituitary tumor (*arrows*). The 2-year appearance remained unchanged 5 years after radiosurgery.

erant of medical therapy. Follow-up PRL levels were decreased in six patients. Follow-up imaging studies have been obtained in six of seven patients up to 3 years after radiosurgery. Tumor volume has decreased in four and remained stable in two. One patient has had disease progression refractory to further surgery and dopaminergic agents.

Nonsecreting Tumors

Follow-up imaging studies were acquired 3 to 72 months (mean, 28 months) after radiosurgery. The tumor control rate was 92%, with half of the patients showing tumor volume reduction (50). Other tumors of the sella and parasellar region include craniopharyngiomas, meningiomas, malignant skull base tumors (adenoid cystic carcinoma), and metastatic carcinoma. Tumor growth control rates above 90% have been documented for all these histologies. Again, the limiting feature for radiosurgery includes the proximity of the neoplasm to the optic nerve and chiasm.

New Neurologic Deficits

Five patients (6%) experienced new symptoms after radiosurgery. Three patients had symptoms related to tumor growth. Two complications occurred that may have been directly related to radiation. One patient with an aggressive nonsecreting tumor who had received prior XRT had decreased visual acuity and cognitive function 12 months after radiosurgery. An MRI scan showed an area of contrast enhancement in the hypothalamus. This patient had a seizure 4 months later and died. The second patient also had a nonsecreting tumor. This patient developed decreased visual acuity in the left eye and a right temporal visual field defect 7 months after radiosurgery despite a reduction in the size of the tumor.

One major difference between our results and the results in patients treated with fractionated radiation or charged particles is that none of our patients developed pituitary insufficiency. The absence of this complication in our series may be related to the generally sharp distinction on our stereotactic MRIs between tumor and normal gland. The absence of pituitary insufficiency may also be related to the sharp falloff of radiation that can be produced with the small-diameter beams available with the Gamma knife.

Secondary Malignancy

As discussed above, the development of a new, radiation-related neoplasm has been well characterized after large-volume fractionated XRT. To our knowledge, this finding has never been reported after stereotactic radiosurgery (for any indication). We believe that this is because of the extremely small volume of normal tissue irradiated and perhaps to a difference in the radiobiologic features of single-session radiation delivery. This potential advantage of radiosurgery should be considered as one factor in the decision to use different irradiation techniques for the management of young patients with pituitary tumors.

REFERENCES

1. Sheline GE, Goldberg MB, Feldman R. Pituitary irradiation for acromegaly. Radiology 1961;76:70–82.
2. Sheline GE, Tyrell JB. Pituitary adenomas. In: Phillips TC, Pistenma DA, eds. Radiation Oncology Annual. New York: Raven Press, 1983.
3. Cohen AR, Cooper PR, Kupersmith MJ, et al. Visual recovery after transsphenoidal removal of pituitary adenomas. Neurosurgery 1985;17:446–452.
4. Rush S, Kupersmith MJ, Leuch I, et al. Neuro-ophthalmologic assessment of vision before and after radiation therapy alone for pituitary macroadenomas. J Neurosurg 1990;72:594–599.
5. Pollock BE, Kondziolka D, Lunsford LD, et al. Stereotactic radiosurgery for pituitary adenomas: imaging, visual and endocrine results. Acta Neurochir (Suppl) 1994;62:5–10.
6. Tsang RW, Laperriere NJ, Simpson WJ, et al. Glioma arising after radiation therapy for pituitary adenoma: a report of four patients and estimation of risk. Cancer 1993;72(7):2227–2233.
7. Rahn T, Thoren M, Werner S. Stereotactic radiosurgery in pituitary adenomas. In: Faglia G, Beck-Peccoz P, Ambrosi B, et al., eds. Pituitary Adenomas: New Trends in Basic and Clinical Research. New York: Excerpta Medica, 1991:303–312.
8. Ganz JC, Backlund EO, Thorsen FA. The effects of gamma knife surgery of pituitary adenomas on tumor growth and endocrinopathies. Stereotact Funct Neurosurg 1993;61(suppl 1):30–37.
9. Degerblad M, Rahn T, Bergstrand G, et al. Long-term results of stereotactic radiosurgery to pituitary gland in Cushing's disease. Acta Endocrinol 1986;112:310–314.
10. Duma CM, Lunsford LD, Kondziolka D, et al. Stereotactic radiosurgery of cavernous sinus meningiomas as an addition or alternative to microsurgery. Neurosurgery 1993;32:699–705.
11. Kondziolka D, Lunsford LD, Flickinger JC. Current concepts in gamma knife radiosurgery. Neurosurg Q 1993;3:253–271.
12. Flickinger JC, Deutsch M, Lunsford LD. Repeat megavoltage irradiation of pituitary and suprasellar tumors. Int J Radiat Oncol Biol Phys 1989;17:117–175.
13. Flickinger JC, Nelson PB, Martinez AJ, et al. Radiotherapy of nonfunctional adenomas of the pituitary gland. Cancer 1989;63:2409–2413.
14. Brada M, Rajan B, Traish D, et al. The long-term efficacy of conservative surgery and radiotherapy in the control of pituitary adenomas. Clin Endocrinol 1993;38(6):571–578.
15. Ludecke DK, Lutz BS, Niedwovok G. The choice of treatment in incomplete adenomectomy in acromegaly: proton versus high voltage radiation. Acta Neurochir 1989;96:32–38.
16. Rush SC, Newall J. Pituitary adenoma: the efficacy of radiotherapy as the sole treatment. Int J Radiat Oncol Biol Phys 1989;17:165–169.
17. Barrow DL, Tindall GT, Kovacs K, et al. Clinical and pathologic effects of bromocriptine on prolactin-secreting and other pituitary tumors. J Neurosurg 1984;60:1–7.
18. Molitch ME, Celton RL, Blackwell RE. Bromocriptine as primary therapy for prolactin-secreting macroadenomas: results of a prospective multicenter study. J Clin Endocrinol Metabol 1985;60:698–705.
19. Mehta AE, Reyes FL, Faihnern C. Primary radiotherapy of prolactinomas. Am J Med 1989;83:59–68.
20. Rush S, Donahue B, Cooper P, et al. Prolactin reduction after combined modality therapy for prolactin macroadenomas. Neurosurgery 1991;28(4):502–505.
21. Trampe EA, Lundell G, Lax I, et al. External irradiation of growth hormone producing pituitary adenomas: prolactin as a marker of hypothalamic and pituitary effects. Int J Radiat Oncol Biol Phys 1991;20(4):655–660.
22. Tsagarakis S, Grossman A, Plowman PN, et al. Megavoltage pituitary irradiation in the management of prolactinomas: long-term follow-up. Clin Endocrinol 1991;34(5):399–406.
23. Tsang RW, Brierley J, Panzarella T, et al. Role of radiation therapy in clinical hormonally-active pituitary adenomas. Radiother Oncol 1996;41:45–53.
24. Caruso M, Shaw E, Davis D. Radiation treatment of growth hormone secreting pituitary adenomas. Int J Radiat Oncol Biol Phys 1993;21:121–122.
25. Werner S, af Trampe E, Palacios P, et al. Growth hormone producing pituitary adenomas with concomitant hypersecretion of prolactin are particularly sensitive to photon irradiation. Int J Radiat Oncol Biol Phys 1985 ;:1713–1720.
26. Eastman RC, Gorden P, Roth J. Conventional supervoltage irradiation is an effective treatment for acromegaly. J Clin Endocrinol Metab 1979;48:931–940.

27. Schoenthaler R, Albright NW, Wara WM, et al. Re-irradiation of pituitary adenoma. Int J Radiat Oncol Biol Phys 1992;24(2): 307–314.
28. Sheline GE, Wara WM. Radiation therapy of acromegaly and nonsecretory chromophobe adenomas of the pituitary. In: Seydel HG, ed. Tumors of the Central Nervous System. New York: John Wiley & Sons, 1975:119–131.
29. Fisher BJ, Gaspar LE, Noone B. Radiation therapy of pituitary adenoma: delayed sequelae. Radiology 1993;187(3):843–846.
30. Doban FC, Raventos A, Boucot N, et al. Roentgen therapy on Cushing syndrome without adrenocortical tumor. J Clin Endocrinol Metab 1957;17:8.
31. Edmonds MW, Simpson WJ, Meakeh JW. External irradiation of the hypophysis for Cushing's disease. Calif Med Assoc J 1972;107: 860.
32. Clarke SD, Woo SY, Buther EB, et al. Treatment of secretory pituitary adenoma with radiation therapy. Radiology 1993;188: 759–763.
33. Heuschele R, Lampe I. Pituitary irradiation for Cushing's syndrome. N Engl J Med 1967;285:243.
34. Grigsby PW, Simpson JR, Stokes S, et al. Results of surgery and irradiation or irradiation alone for pituitary adenomas. J Neurooncol 1988;6:129–134.
35. Estrada J, Boronat M, Mielgo M, et al. The long-term outcome of pituitary irradiation after unsuccessful transsphenoidal surgery in Cushing's disease. N Engl J Med 1997;336:172–177.
36. McCollough WM, Marcus RB Jr, Rhoton Al Jr, et al. Long-term follow-up of radiotherapy for pituitary adenoma: the absence of late recurrence after greater than or equal to 4500 cGy. Int J Radiat Oncol Biol Phys 1991;21(3):607–614.
37. Nelson PB, Goodman ML, Flickinger JC, et al. Endocrine function in patients with large pituitary tumors treated with operative decompression and radiation therapy. Neurosurgery 1989;24(3): 398–400.
38. Sheline GE. The role of conventional radiation therapy in the treatment of functional pituitary tumors. In: Linfoot JA, ed. Recent Advances in the Diagnosis and Treatment of Pituitary Tumors. New York: Raven Press, 1979:289–313.
39. Ciric I, Mikhael M, Stafford T, et al. Transsphenoidal neurosurgery of pituitary macroadenomas with long-term follow-up results. J Neurosurg 1983;59:395–401.
40. Laws ER Jr, Trautman JC, Hollenhorst RW Jr. Transsphenoidal decompression of the optic nerve and chiasm: visual results in 62 patients. J Neurosurg 1977;46:717–722.
41. Flickinger JC, Nelson PB, Taylor FH, et al. Incidence of cerebral infarction after radiotherapy for pituitary adenoma. Cancer 1989; 63:2404–2408.
42. Flickinger JC, Lunsford LD, Singer J, et al. Megavoltage external beam irradiation of craniopharyngiomas: analysis of tumor control and morbidity. Int J Radiat Oncol Biol Phys 1990;19:117–122.
43. Flickinger JC, Kalend A. Use of normalized total dose to represent the biological effect of fractionated radiotherapy. Radiother Oncol 1990;17:339–347.
44. Bowen J, Paulsen CA. Stroke after pituitary irradiation. Stroke 1992; 23(6):908–911.
45. Grattan-Smith PJ, Morris JG, Langlands AO. Delayed radiation necrosis of the central nervous system in patients irradiated for pituitary tumors. J Neurol Neurosurg Psychiatry 1992;55(10):949–955.
46. Sheline G, Wara W, Smith V. Therapeutic irradiation and brain injury. Int J Radiat Oncol Biol Phys 1980;6:1215–1228.
47. Littley MD, Shalet SM, Beardwell CG, et al. Hypopituitarism following external radiotherapy for pituitary tumors in adults. QJM 1989;70(262):145–160.
48. Tran LM, Blount L, Horton D, et al. Radiation therapy of pituitary tumors: results in 95 cases. Am J Clin Oncol 1991;14(1):25–29.
49. Wigg DR, Murray ML, Koschel K. Tolerance of the central nervous system to photon irradiation: endocrine complications. Acta Radiol Oncol 1982;21:49–60.
50. Witt T, Kondziolka D, Flickinger J, et al. Stereotactic radiosurgery for pituitary tumors. Radiosurgery 1996;1:55–65.
51. Levy RP, Fabrikand JI, Frankel KA, et al. Heavy-charged-particle radiosurgery of the pituitary gland: clinical results of 840 patients. Stereotact Funct Neurosurg 1991;57:22–35.
52. Kjellberg RN, Kliman B. Lifetime effectiveness: a system of therapy for pituitary adenomas, emphasizing Bragg peak proton hypophysectomy. In: Linfoort JA, ed. Recent Advances in the Diagnosis and Treatment of Pituitary Tumors. New York: Raven Press, 1979: 269–288.
53. Flickinger JC, Lunsford LD, Kondziolka D. Dose prescription and dose-volume effects in radiosurgery. Neurosurg Clin North Am 1992;3:51–59.
54. Flickinger JC, Lunsford LD, Wu A, et al. Treatment planning for gamma knife radiosurgery with multiple isocenters. Int J Radiat Oncol Biol Phys 1989;18:1495–1501.
55. Backlund EO, Rahn T, Sarby D, et al. Closed stereotaxic hypophysectomy by means of 60-cobalt gamma radiation. Acta Radiol Ther Phys Biol 1972;11:545–555.
56. Flickinger JC, Maitz A, Kalend A, et al. Treatment volume shaping with selective beam blocking using the Leksell gamma unit. Int J Radiat Oncol Biol Phys 1990;19:783–789.
57. Stephanian E, Lunsford LD, Coffey RJ, et al. Gamma knife surgery for sellar and suprasellar tumors. Neurosurg Clin North Am 1992; 3:207–218.

Note: Page numbers in italics refer to figures; page numbers followed by ''t'' indicate tables.

D